# Foundations of Kinesiology

## A Modern Integrated Approach

**Tinker D. Murray, Ph.D., FACSM**

Professor of Health and Human Performance and Honorary Professor of International Studies
Texas State University, San Marcos, Texas, USA

**James A. Eldridge, Ed.D.**

Professor and Chair of Kinesiology
University of Texas at the Permian Basin, Odessa, Texas, USA

**Harold W. Kohl III, Ph.D., FNAK, FACSM**

Professor of Epidemiology and Kinesiology

University of Texas Health Science Center at Houston and University of Texas at Austin, Austin, Texas, USA

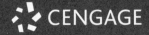
**CENGAGE**

Australia • Brazil • Mexico • Singapore • United Kingdom • United States

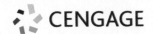

*Foundations of Kinesiology: A Modern Integrated Approach*

**Tinker D. Murray, James A. Eldridge, Harold W. Kohl III**

Product Director: Dawn Giovaniello

Product Manager: Krista Mastroianni

Content Developer: Jake Warde

Product Assistant: Marina Starkey

Marketing Manager: Ana Albinson

Content Project Manager: Carol Samet

Art Director: Michael Cook

Manufacturing Planner: Karen Hunt

Production Service: MPS Limited

Text and Photo Researcher: Lumina Datamatics

Text Designer: Ellen Pettengell

Cover Designer: Michael Cook

Cover Image: Main image, woman running: Michael Svoboda/iStockphoto; Therapist w/woman: Kali9/Getty; Fitness Ball: Kali9/Getty; Basketball Coach: Kidstock/Getty

Compositor: MPS Limited

For product information and technology assistance, contact us at **Cengage Customer & Sales Support, 1-800-354-9706.**

For permission to use material from this text or product, submit all requests online at **www.cengage.com/permissions.** Further permissions questions can be e-mailed to **permissionrequest@cengage.com.**

Library of Congress Control Number: 2017945212

ISBN: 978-1-337-39270-9

**Cengage**
20 Channel Center Street
Boston, MA 02210
USA

Cengage is a leading provider of customized learning solutions with employees residing in nearly 40 different countries and sales in more than 125 countries around the world. Find your local representative at **www.cengage.com.**

Cengage products are represented in Canada by Nelson Education, Ltd.

To learn more about Cengage platforms and services, visit **www.cengage.com.**

To register or access your online learning solution or purchase materials for your course, visit **www.cengagebrain.com.**

Printed in the United States of America
Print Number: 01     Print Year: 2017

## ABOUT THE COVER

The cover for the text reflects the fact that physical activity is the center of the kinesiology universe (see Chapter 1 for more) and is influenced by the multiple subdisciplines and foundations of the field. The four panels represent individuals and populations participating in varying types and intensities of physical activity (along a physical activity continuum) such as movement to increase and meet national physical activity guidelines, improve goal-oriented physical fitness levels, and/or, achieve peak performance. The cover also suggests that engaging in regular physical activity and exercise provides varying outcomes for individuals and populations such as rehabilitation, health, physical fitness, and peak performance across the lifespan based on one's functional abilities (mental/physical health).

The center panel shows a young woman with a running prosthetic limb designed for competitors trying to achieve peak performance. The panel to the upper left shows an older woman in a physical therapy setting engaging in resistance exercise through a range of motion, consistent with rehabilitation and improving joint mobility, increasing physical activity, and improving physical fitness. In the middle left panel, an older man is working with a personal trainer to increase his physical activity levels to meet national guidelines and to improve his physical fitness. In the bottom panel, a young girl is shown working with a coach to improve her sports skills, which can reinforce the odds of her participating in higher levels of physical activity for competition, fun, and health benefits.

The cover also symbolizes evolving and ever-changing kinesiology careers impacting individuals and populations across the lifespan (children, adolescents, adults, and older adults) and the integration of kinesiology into a variety of settings such as work, leisure, transportation, home, school sports, fitness facilities, and rehabilitation centers. The physical activity themes reinforce the need for kinesiology professionals to acquire, integrate, and apply knowledge, skills, and abilities about basic kinesiology subdisciplines such as biomechanics, motor learning, exercise physiology, public health, and sport/exercise psychology.

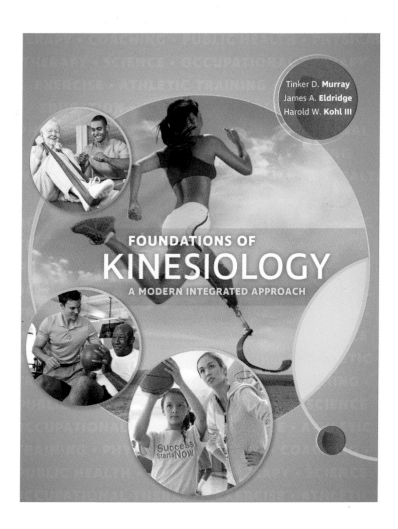

# Dedications

**Tinker Murray:** Special thanks to my loving wife Mary and her family for all their support during the development of this project. Also, thanks to my co-authors, relatives, all my friends, and professional colleagues who have help make this product possible.

**James Eldridge:** For my father and mother and all of the support they have given throughout life. Many thanks to all of those individuals who have mentored me to become the professional that I am today.

**Harold Kohl:** For my Father.

# Brief Contents

# Contents

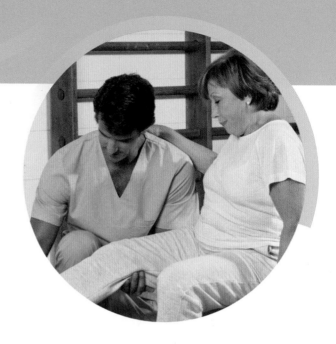

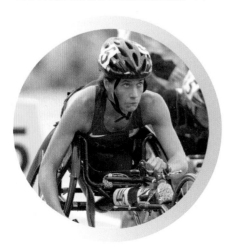

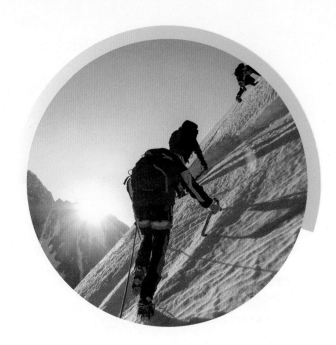

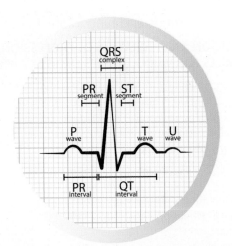

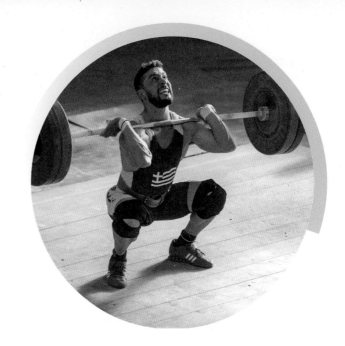

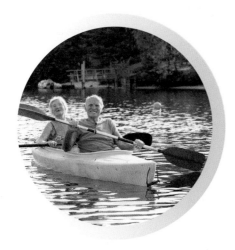

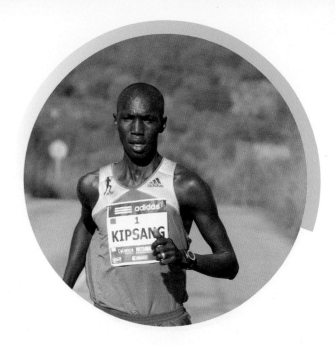

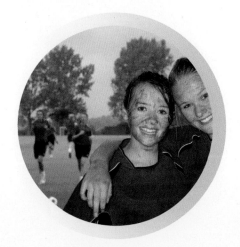

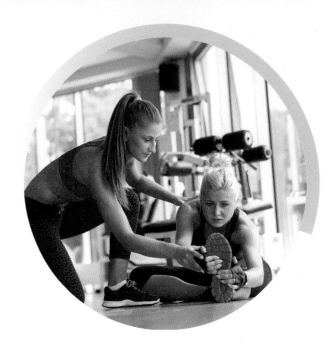

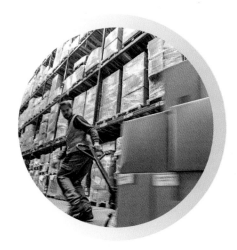

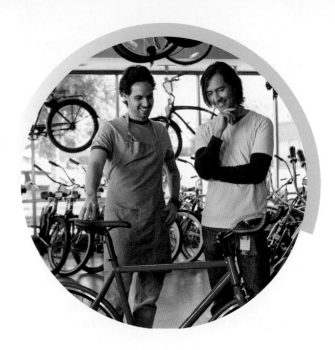

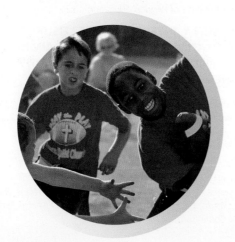

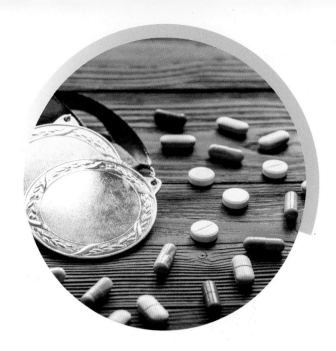

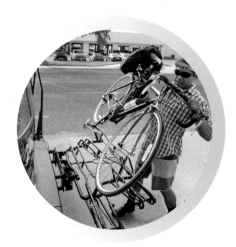

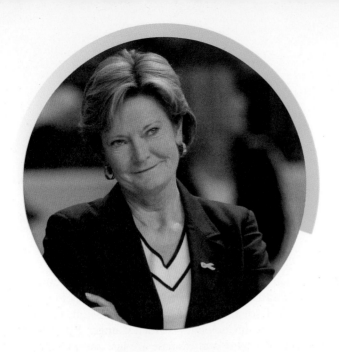

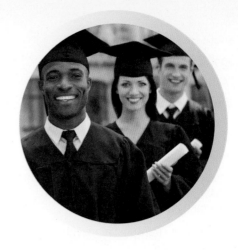

# Preface

## Introduction

Welcome to *Foundations of Kinesiology: A Modern Integrated Approach*. This text is meant to be used for an introductory or overview course and forms the basis for preparing undergraduates to incorporate evidence-based practice strategies in preparation for specific kinesiology professional careers such as those shown in the table.

### Possible Kinesiology Related Professional Careers

| | |
|---|---|
| Exercise physiologist | Physician assistant |
| Biomechanist | Medical doctor |
| Sports psychologist | Athletic trainer |
| Personal trainer | Physical therapist |
| Athletic coach | Wellness instructor |
| Public safety trainer | Physical education teacher |
| Chiropractor | Strength and conditioning specialist |
| Rehabilitation specialist | Occupational therapist |
| Physical activity public health practitioner | Other emerging career paths |

Integrating digital and traditional delivery methods, the text is designed to help students and instructors focus on physical activity as the center of the kinesiology universe (see Chapter 1 for details) and emphasize evolving and ever-changing kinesiology careers impacting individuals and populations across the lifespan (children, adolescents, adults, and older adults) and in a variety of settings such as work, leisure, transportation, home, schools, fitness facilities, and rehabilitation centers. The content is designed to help students develop skills and abilities about basic kinesiology subdisciplines such as biomechanics, motor learning, exercise physiology, and public health. Further, a critical and unique practical aspect of this text is the emphasis on required professional skills for developing an effective career path in kinesiology in areas such as design of physical activity training programs, promoting physical activity and public health, and managing energy balance and body composition.

## Kinesiology in Perspective

Although descriptions of human anatomy, including the muscles and how they move, can be traced back to the ancient Greek scientist Aristotle, the scientific study of kinesiology and its subdisciplines is much younger. Participation in physical activity and exercise are just naturally part of life if we are moving. Physical activity is any bodily movement that results in energy expenditure, while exercise is a specific type of physical activity that is planned, repetitive, and done for a specific purpose. As you can see, there are a broad range of applications to human movement, from an infant learning to walk and develop motor skills, to a stroke survivor learning to roll a wheel chair, to an elite athlete training for Olympic competition.

According to the American Kinesiology Association (AKA), kinesiology is an academic discipline, which involves the study of physical activity and its impact on health, society, and quality of life. It includes, but is not limited to, such areas of study as exercise science, sport management, athletic training and sports medicine, socio-cultural analyses of sports, sport and pre-professional training for physical therapy, occupational therapy, medicine, and other health-related fields.

Kinesiology has become one of the largest and fastest-growing undergraduate degree programs in universities in United States. According to the AKA, the number of undergraduate kinesiology majors grew 50% from 2003 to 2008, to more than 26,000 students, with multiple subdisciplines all focusing on movement. In a departure from traditional introductory texts for kinesiology, exercise science, human performance, and so forth, we have sought to effectively integrate, incorporate, and deliver evidence-based practice skills for students who must translate the information and apply it for potential career opportunities.

### A Modern Integrated Approach

Despite frequent calls by leaders in the field to integrate the subdisciplines of kinesiology, efforts to date have fallen short of this goal and the subdisciplines of kinesiology remained siloed. This new text focuses on a true integration of the field of kinesiology, with *physical activity* at the center, and on preparing undergraduates for careers in kinesiology promoted by the associations and groups such as the AKA, the National Physical Activity Plan Alliance (NPAPA), and the Physical Activity Guidelines for Americans. Our approach in this text is consistent with what many kinesiology scholars have advocated for the future of the field by supporting strong linkages to health and wellbeing of individuals and populations.*

With this textbook and associated digital resources, you will find an approach to presenting kinesiology concepts that is a modernized, integrated approach compared with more traditional "silo" methods of learning about the subdisciplines of kinesiology in an introductory course. For example, instead of a chapter fully dedicated to subdisciplines, this textbook integrates each subdiscipline into each chapter. Icons are used to highlight each subdiscipline thread for each area of instruction. Although each subdiscipline requires unique knowledge, unifying principles, such as a continuum of physical activity and place-based applications, provide common overlap for application in day-to-day practice. We believe strongly that promoting future career skills for kinesiology professionals that include the integration of the science and practice of physical activity (and exercise) with the numerous subdisciplines of the field will better prepare students for jobs in the field, now and in the future.

## Exercise for Fitness and Performance

Traditionally, exercise has been viewed as a way to train and improve physical fitness for a specific performance purpose such as preparing for a 10K race, a battery of fitness assessments, a 100-meter dash, or a weight lifting competition. Since the ancient times of the Greeks and Romans, athleticism and high levels of fitness have been associated with good health, vigor, and stamina. Even many of the early U.S. exercise practice guidelines (American Heart Association, American College of Sports Medicine) developed in the 1970s through the early 1990s were based primarily on performing endurance exercise to enhance performance, particularly aerobic capacity. The rationale for participating in regular exercise for improving fitness and peak performance, especially for individuals, by rapidly increasing intensity over time became a traditional approach that many came to understand, but could not necessarily achieve. In fact, physical activity and exercise goals that focus mainly on increasing levels of physical fitness and peak performance with a "more is better" philosophy often become additional barriers to people just struggling to find the time and the motivation to be physically active.

## Physical Activity for Health

Since the mid-1980s, science has advanced and expanded our under-

standing of kinesiology beyond training for performance to include physical activity for health. Strong scientific evidence has indicated that many children and adults are very inactive (or sedentary) and that even small amounts of physical activity and exercise can effect large positive changes in the health (cardiorespiratory, musculoskeletal, energy balance, mental health, and so on) of individuals and entire populations. The promotion of physical activity with or without exercise has become an effective tool in helping reduce chronic disease risk factors and prevalence, and has been helpful in chronic disease management. These advances have helped to solidify public health as a key subdiscipline of kinesiology.

We recommend that future kinesiology practitioners continue to study, understand, and promote traditional physical activity and exercise training strategies based on outcomes such as improved physical fitness and peak performance, especially for those who want to achieve higher order goals. Furthermore, kinesiology professionals should also learn about and promote additional physical activity and exercise goals for the achievement of positive individual and population-based health outcomes.

## Physical Activity Continuum

Because physical activity and exercise encompass varying types of outcomes such as health, physical fitness, peak performance across the life span as well as functional abilities (mental/physical health), it is important to understand that physical activity is not just a binary outcome, but can be conceptualized as a continuum. Movement can range from the smallest skeletal muscle contraction all the way to peak performance in athletic competition. Each type of movement is unique and, when applied with physiologic training principles of overload, specificity, and adaptation, can have a profound effect on the human body.

A core guiding principle in this text is the Physical Activity Continuum. The continuum begins at the sedentary level, which represents little to no movement. Proceeding left to right, minimal participation in physical activity, consistent with evidence-based guidelines, can result in positive health outcomes for children, adults, and older adults. Increases in physical fitness are based on achieving higher levels of physical activity and exercise for goals like lifting heavier weight, running a 10K, or improving agility. Finally, peak performance is consistent with achieving top athletic fitness or performance.

* All works cited are listed in the References section beginning on page 364.

### THE PHYSICAL ACTIVITY CONTINUUM

Sedentary

Health, Meeting the U.S. Physical Activity Guidlines (lowering your risk for chronic disease)

Increasing Physical Fitness (losing weight, running a 10K, or increasing your muscular strength and endurance)

Peak Performance

The Physical Activity Continuum icon is found throughout the text and was developed as a reminder that strategies and tactics discussed in the text should be used to promote physical activity and exercise concepts that can and should be applied at many different levels (based on participation goals, age, mental/physical health, and so on). In Chapter 4, the Physical Activity Continuum is introduced and highlighted regularly throughout the rest of the text as a reminder of how to integrate physical activity and exercise promotion into a variety of settings. The unifying physical activity principles of dose-response, overload, specificity, and adaptation as applied to the continuum are also introduced and reinforced throughout the text.

# How This Book Is Organized: Modules, Integration and the Practice of Kinesiology

The textbook consists of four modules containing 16 chapters with two lessons in each chapter. Lesson 1 provides core background information for the topics covered. Lesson 2 specifically challenges students and instructors to integrate the kinesiology subdisciplines into real life based on chapter topics specifically related to subdisciplines such as Exercise Physiology, Biomechanics, Sport/Exercise Psychology, Public health, and the Practice of Kinesiology.

The textbook has been developed such that the material can easily be delivered in a traditional classroom format, in a hybrid format, on-line, or through other popular content delivery pathways. The MindTap™ digital component provides engaging activities consistent with the goal of promoting future career skills for kinesiology professionals and the integration of the science and practice of physical activity (and exercise) with the subdisciplines of the field.

### Module 1: Chapters 1–3 Definitions, Careers, and Evidence-Based Practice

Module 1 provides an introduction to the various subdisciplines of kinesiology and how they are each related to physical activity and the use of evidence-based practices to help practitioners develop effective professional problem-solving skills. Students learn about the kinesiology universe and related academic preparation courses for various subdisciplines of kinesiology that are needed for professional training and future careers. Chapter 1 provides definitions and an overview of the textbook focus. Chapter 2 provides an in-depth look at kinesiology careers and professional development opportunities. In Chapter 3, students are introduced to concepts of evidence-based practices in kinesiology, and they are provided with several specific examples of the mechanics of evidence-based decision making.

### Module 2: Chapters 4–8 Common Deliverables for Kinesiology Majors

In Module 2, students learn about how kinesiology subdisciplines are integrated and the importance of being able to develop their physical activity programming skills to work with diverse populations seeking health, physical fitness, and peak performance goals. Students will also learn about common deliverables (such as aerobic fitness, muscular and skeletal strength, energy balance, body composition, and mental health) that provide knowledge, skills, and abilities (KSAs) in order to effectively promote physical activity and health, physical fitness, and peak performance goals across the lifespan. The Physical Activity Continuum and unifying physical activity principles of dose-response, overload, specificity, and adaptation are also introduced and applied in this module.

### Module 3: Chapters 9–13 Common Professional Settings and Occupational Challenges

The purpose of Module 3 is to provide opportunities to explore and interact about common and current professional and occupational settings that are dependent upon acquired kinesiology-related discipline KSAs. The module focuses on the integration of several of the sectors highlighted in the U.S. National Physical Activity Plan (www.physicalactivityplan.org)—business and industry; community recreation, fitness, and parks; education; faith-based settings; health care; mass media; public health; sport; and transportation, land use, and community design—to kinesiology and its subdisciplines. Module 3 links sectors presented to the common knowledge base of kinesiology (what every major should know) presented in Chapter 2:

- Physical activity in health, wellness, and quality of life
- Scientific foundations of physical activity
- Cultural, historical, and philosophical dimensions of physical activity
- The practice of physical activity

The specific chapters in Module 3 consist of topics addressing kinesiology in relationship to business and industry; home, leisure, and recreation; schools; sports; and, transportation.

### Module 4: Chapters 14–16 Professional Ethics, Leadership, and Continuing Education

This final module of the text is designed to provide opportunities to explore common and current professional standards regarding ethics, leadership, and continuing education skills for careers in kinesiology-related subdisciplines. It also reinforces the need to integrate the variety of academic disciplines undergraduate kinesiology majors experience so that they can master the knowledge base of kinesiology, translate that knowledge, and communicate it into intervention packages that help solve societal challenges. Themes in the module include integration of ethical decision making and the acquisition of leadership skills. Module 4 also provides general professional KSAs common to the subdisciplines of kinesiology. The final chapter in the module anchors the text with current professional practice recommendations on the unifying themes of kinesiology as supported by the American Kinesiology Association and the authors. Specifically, we support the importance of students understanding the following additional integrated concepts for preparing for their future career in kinesiology and promotion of the field as the whole:[2]

- The need to produce public goods or tangible products that contribute to solving societal problems. Examples of public goods in kinesiology are developing physical activity plans at the community level for specific populations or helping implement physical activity policies at the national, regional, or state levels. Examples of tangible kinesiology products are the development of wearable technology or programs like popup yoga classes conducted in park settings.

- The need to show that the kinesiology field and your role in the profession will continue to be valuable to society and that there are professional agendas that integrate kinesiology into national policy decisions and legislative actions such as public health–oriented goals.

- The need to focus on the future by being willing to change rapidly to meet emerging societal needs and able to evaluate the effectiveness of interventions, monitor them, and adjust them as needed.

By mastering the knowledge base of kinesiology, translating that knowledge, and communicating it by developing effective ways to enhance human movement, students can become better prepared to help solve societal challenges. The final thoughts section (Lesson 2) in Chapter 16 provides students with content on key lifetime learning concepts.

# Key Features of the Textbook and MindTap™

The textbook and the accompanying MindTap digital component together form a unique course solution for the introductory kinesiology course. Specific features found in the text are listed first followed by an introduction to the activities in MindTap. MindTap also includes a fully functional eBook edition of the printed text.

There are a number of key features that help students and instructors facilitate learning, interaction, and evaluation throughout an introductory kinesiology course. Specific key features include:

- **Student Learning Objectives (SLOs):** Listed at the beginning of each chapter, learning objectives require students to explain, justify, describe, integrate, provide examples, critically review, and develop materials related to the chapter material.

- **Case Studies:** This feature, used throughout the text, focuses on the Casey family as well as their extemded family and friends. The Caseys represent a busy but physically inactive family that you might find anywhere in U.S. society today. In most chapters, the case study is in two parts; part one in Lesson 1 describes a kinesiology related problem that requires the integration of the kinesiology subdisciplines to provide possible solutions. Part two in Lesson 2 provides possible solutions, based on the chapter material, for the case described.

- **Career Focus:** Each chapter has material related to various career opportunities based on obtaining a degree in kinesiology.

- **Call Out Boxes:** Chapters have additional information available for students and instructors about numerous topics mentioned in call out boxes.

- **Tables, Figures, Photographs:** The text is very visually oriented, with graphic features that enhance effective traditional or online learning.

- **Icons:** In addition to the Physical Activity Continuum icon described above, we have included special icons highlighting each subdiscipline of kinesiology discussed (Exercise Physiology, Biomechanics, Public Health, Motor Learning and Development, and Sport/Exercise Psychology). There is also an icon for The Practice of Kinesiology that includes history, philosophy, and sociology topics, plus practical integrated examples related to the subdisciplines of the field.

- **Chapter Summaries:** Each chapter has a brief but concise overview of topics and key points covered.

- **People Matter:** The "People Matter" feature in each chapter highlights various kinesiology professionals and how they practice kinesiology in their careers. The feature provides students with real life examples of how they can prepare for a variety of kinesiology careers by integrating the various topics and subdisciplines covered in the text.

- **Remember This:** The "Remember This" feature provides definitions for all terms explained throughout each chapter.

- **For More Information:** This key feature provides learners with numerous web links that allow learners to easily search for more information in each chapter.

- **Chapter References:** Each chapter includes sequentially numbered references to scientific works cited that provide evidence-based support for the concepts developed and presented in each chapter. The references provide students and instructors with additional opportunities to pursue more in depth learning about topics of special individual and/or class interest.

## MindTap for *Foundations of Kinesiology: A Modern Integrated Approach*

Beyond an eBook, homework solution, digital supplement, or premium website, MindTap is a digital learning platform that works alongside your campus learning management system (LMS) to deliver course curriculum across the range of electronic devices. The MindTap learning activities directly engage students with the content presented in the text.

▸ **Chapter Warm-Ups:** Each chapter includes a **Career Insights Video**, featuring both professionals and students discussing career-related topics. In addition, a short practice quiz helps students identify *what they already know* about the chapter topics.

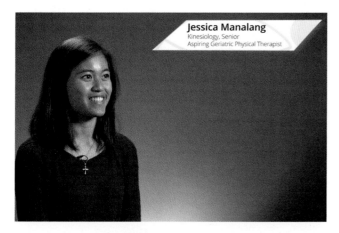

Jessica Manalang
Kinesiology, Senior
Aspiring Geriatric Physical Therapist

Kinesiology professionals share their experiences working in a wide variety of kinesiology-related careers.

▸ **Case Studies Activities:** In Chapter 1, the Caseys and their extended family are introduced. Throughout the text, the situations they face encourage students to develop their knowledge, skills, and abilities to devise solutions that promote physically active lifestyles despite the family's lifestyle, behavioral, and environmental challenges. Accompanying activities in MindTap offer student engagement with each of the cases presented in the text.

▸ **MindTap Engagement Boxes.** Throughout the text, students are encouraged to visit valuable websites related to the chapter content. For example, in Chapter 2, students are encouraged to visit the websites of organizations providing licensure and certification for a variety of careers. Related activities help students to evaluate and assimilate the content they have reviewed.

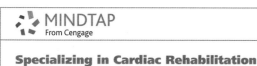

**Specializing in Cardiac Rehabilitation**

**Go to your MindTap course** to complete an activity that will help you understand more about becoming a cardiac rehabilitation specialist.

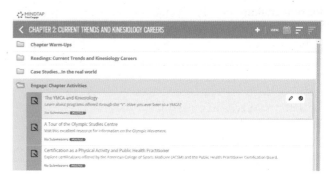

MindTap boxes in the text indicate an assignable follow-up activity is available in MindTap.

▸ **Take Action:** Students are presented with discrete career-oriented projects and targeted learning activities that help them develop the knowledge, skills, and abilities being presented in the text. Students can retain all the documents they create and use them to start developing career-oriented portfolios of their work.

# Acknowledgements

We wish to thank the many students and teachers who have inspired us to produce the first edition of *Foundations of Kinesiology: A Modern Integrated Approach*. First, we would like to thank all the reviewers of the textbook who provided their valuable insight, which improved our final work. It takes a great team to produce a textbook, and the members of the talented production team, listed on the copyright page, have made vital contributions to this product. Special thanks to our development editor Jake Warde, production manager Carol Samet, and marketing manager Ana Albinson. We would also like to thank Aileen Berg and Yolanda Cossio for helping initiate this project. Finally, a special thanks to Krista Mastroianni, our Health Product Team Manager at Cengage, and her dedicated team of highly talented people who have made this textbook a reality.

# Reviewers

Jeffrey Alexander
*Chandler-Gilbert Community College*

Diana Avans
*Vanguard University*

Jeffrey Beer
*Manchester University*

Evonne Bird
*Truman State University*

Amanda Bonikowske
*Carroll College*

Brian Brabham
*University of Mary Hardin-Baylor*

Stanley Brown
*Mississippi State University*

Ni Bueno
*Cerritos College (CA)*

Jacky Burke-Cherney
*Scottsdale Community College and Paradise Valley Community College*

Kay Daigle
*Southeast Oklahoma University*

Jordan Daniel
*Texas A & M University*

Judd Doryce
*University of North Dakota*

Alexandra Doussett
*California State University-San Bernardino*

Mike Fikes
*Wayland Baptist University*

Bob Filander
*Austin College (TX)*

Andrea Fradkin
*Bloomsburg University*

Christopher Kovacs
*Western Illinois University*

Cindy Kuhrasch
*University of Wisconsin*

Michele LeBlanc
*California Lutheran University*

Lisa Leininger
*California State University-Monterey Bay*

Sara Mahoney
*Bellarmine University*

Joe Marist
*Arizona State University*

Ileen Miller
*California State University-San Martin*

James R. Morrow, Jr.
*University of North Texas*

Gary Oden
*Sam Houston State University*

Rebecca Pena
*California State University-Northridge*

Karen Poole
*University of North Carolina-Greensboro*

Jesse Rhoads
*University of North Dakota*

Pamela Richards
*Central College (IA)*

Coty Richardson
*Northwest Christian University*

Russell Robinson
*Shippensburg University*

Greg Ryan
*University of Montana Western*

Paul Schempp
*University of Georgia*

Michael Schmidt
*University of Georgia*

Andrew Shim
*University of South Dakota*

Shannon Siegel
*University of San Francisco*

Duncan Simpson
*Barry University*

Kathleen Smyth
*College of Marin*

Dr. Kathleen Tritschler
*Guilford College*

Sarah Wall
*Eastern New Mexico University*

Kevin Weaver
*Western Kentucky University*

Valery Whereley
*Sacred Heart University*

Andrew Winterstein
*University of Wisconsin*

Gary L. Worrell
*University of New Brunswick-Saint John Campus*

Robyn York
*California State University-Fullerton*

Elizabeth Zicha
*Muskingum University*

# Author Bios and Career Linkages

In keeping with the strong career orientation of this text, we conclude this preface with brief biographies and statements on why we became kinesiology professionals. Note that at the end of every chapter, a section called "People Matter" features kinesiology professionals discussing their career choices in more detail as well.

### Tinker D. Murray, Ph.D., FACSM

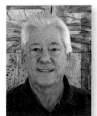

Dr. Tinker D. Murray is a professor of Health and Human Performance at Texas State University (formerly Southwest Texas State University [SWT]) in San Marcos, Texas. He earned a bachelor's of science degree in physical education and biology from the University of Texas in 1973. He earned his master's of education degree in physical education from Southwest Texas State University in 1976, and completed his Ph.D. in physical education and cardiac rehabilitation from Texas A&M University in 1984. He was also awarded a certificate in graduate studies in cardiac rehabilitation from Baylor College of Medicine in 1981.

Dr. Murray served as Director of Cardiac Rehabilitation at Brooke Army Medical Center from 1982 to 1984 where he was twice recognized for his exceptional performance. He has been at Southwest Texas and Texas State University since 1984 and served as the Director of Employee Wellness from 1984 to 1988, and Director of the Exercise Performance Laboratory from 1984 to 2000. He was a voluntary assistant cross country and track coach at Southwest Texas from 1985 to 1988 and helped win three Gulf Star Conference titles.

Dr. Murray is a Fellow of the American College of Sports Medicine (ACSM) and certified as an ACSM Program Director. He is a former two-time president of the Texas regional chapter of ACSM (1987 and 1994). He served on the national ACSM Board of Trustees from 1998 to 2001.

Dr. Murray has been a lecturer and examiner for the USA Track and Field Level II Coaching Certification Program (1988–2008). He also worked with the Professional Development Cooperative (PDC) in coordination with the Texas High School Coaches Association (THSCA) from 2003 to 2013 to promote continuing education experiences for coaches.

Dr. Murray served as the Vice Chair of the Governor's (Ann Richards) Commission for Physical Fitness in Texas from 1993 to 1994. He was named an Honorary Professor of International Studies at Texas State University in 2013.

Dr. Murray's research interests include school-based and clinical-based youth physical activity interventions for the prevention of obesity and diabetes and personal fitness, and training applications related to exercise physiology for youth, adults, and the elderly. Since 1984, he has worked with his colleagues to conduct and publish research and textbooks related to school physical education, public health, and clinical settings to promote physical activity in children, adolescents, and college students.

## Why I Became a Kinesiology Professional

I was an undecided major as an undergraduate at the University of Texas (UT) at Austin for my first semester. I was running as a freshman on the cross-country team at the time and our cross-country coach was, Jack T. Daniels, Ph.D., who was the first exercise physiologist I ever met. Years later *Runner's World Magazine* named Coach Daniels the world's best distance coach. As you can imagine, he had a major influence on me to learn about how to exercise for peak performance, while trying to stay healthy.

As I earned my bachelor's degree at UT, I was fortunate to have a who's who of professors who provided me with a quality undergraduate experience in Kinesiology (called Physical Education at the time). I then attended Southwest Texas State University for my master's degree and gained valuable practitioner skills as a graduate assistant teaching several physical activities that promoted the development of physical fitness. At the time, I also worked in a local family owned sporting goods store that provided me with valuable business skills.

By the time I was working on my doctorate at Texas A&M University, I was still interested in physical fitness and peak performance, but I had also developed an interest in preventing cardiovascular disease and the rehabilitation of cardiac patients. My post-doctoral internship at the Methodist Hospital and Baylor College of Medicine in in Houston, Texas, helped me develop clinical skills for helping prevent and manage chronic disease by integrating the various subdisciplines of kinesiology.

My academic training and acquisition of professional skills have served me well throughout my career. I am also very fortunate that I met professional colleagues like Dr. Eldridge and Dr. Kohl who share similar philosophies for student academic preparation and options for numerous careers in kinesiology as I do.

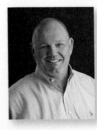

### James A. Eldridge, Ed.D.

Dr. James A. Eldridge is the chair and a professor of Kinesiology at the University of Texas of the Permian Basin (UTPB) in Odessa, Texas. He earned bachelor's of arts degrees in both physical education and biology from Texas Lutheran University in 1986. He earned his master of arts degree in physical education from Southwest Texas State University in 1989, and completed his Ed.D. in physical education and human performance from the University of Houston in 1996.

Dr. Eldridge served as a Biostatistician and Assistant Epidemiologist at M.D. Anderson cancer center from 1990 to 1995, where he worked on the largest funded NCI grant studying worksite behaviors and cancer risks. He then spent two years employed with Southwest Texas State University as the research associate for the Vice President of Student Affairs. He has worked at UTPB since 1997 and served as the Director of Exercise Physiology Labs from 1997 to 2010 and chairperson of the Kinesiology Department 2010 to present.

Dr. Eldridge is a member of the Texas chapter of the American College of Sports Medicine (TACSM) and served on the board of directors for the organization from 2005 to 2008. He also served as president of the organization in 2007.

Dr. Eldridge research interests include worksite injury reduction, rodeo injury occurrence, and school-based and clinical-based youth physical activity interventions for the prevention of obesity and diabetes and personal fitness. He has worked since 1989 with his colleagues to conduct and publish research and textbooks related to injury prevention and diagnosis, physical activity measurement, and health-related issues in medicine and nursing.

### Why I Became a Kinesiology Professional

I was a pre-engineering major as an undergraduate student at Texas Lutheran College for my first semester as a freshman; however, my study habits were less than stellar. I was lucky that Dr. Bill Squires saw potential in me and decided that he could use my help in his physiology lab working to collect data for grants he had acquired from NASA. I found out at that time that I really loved physiology and the ability to measure physiological parameters under adverse situations. Under his tutelage,

I presented a paper at TACSM in 1985 that gained the attention of several faculty members from other universities. Upon graduation in 1986, I was offered a graduate assistantship at Southwest Texas State University working with Dr. Tinker Murray.

Working with Tinker, I was able to hone my skills as a researcher and statistician by traveling across Texas collecting human performance data among high school and college students. I began presenting the data we collected at numerous state and national meetings. The ability to present and travel allowed me to meet future colleagues and set me up to receive a doctoral assistantship at the University of Houston working with Drs. Tony Jackson, Jim Morrow, and Jim Pivarnik. I was fortunate to have these well-recognized faculty as mentors. Each provided me with new perspectives on research and writing that has carried forward in my career.

In my first year of my doctoral work, a job opportunity with M.D. Anderson became available. The job included traveling across the nation collecting data in rural worksites and analyzing that data. I applied for the position and was hired. At the time, the NCI grant was the largest multi-site grant ever funded in behavioral science. As the biostatistician for the M.D. Anderson site portion of the grant, I was able to include questions within the questionnaire that would allow me to further my interests in physical activity in relation to worksite injury and cancer risk. While completing the NCI grant, I received funding from the Texas Tobacco Prevention grant to determine the relationship between print advertisements and youth smoking. Working on this grant brought me to the realization that technology enhances the capacity to collect data, intervene with large groups, and educate individuals through computer technology. At that time in 1994, application development was in its infancy. I was able to develop a computer-generated program that would help me collect data with a survey of de-emphasized print ads to determine how well youth could differentiate between tobacco ads compared to other ads. After completing the program, I had learned numerous new strategies for the use of technology and education, and have carried my love for creation of new learning strategies to the technological portion of this text.

I am very fortunate to have colleagues like Dr. Murray and Dr. Kohl who share the same excitement for student learning and the same drive to develop new learning technologies that will strengthen the academic preparation of kinesiology students.

### Harold W. Kohl III, Ph.D., FACSM, FNAK

Dr. Harold (Bill) Kohl is Professor of Epidemiology and Kinesiology at the University of Texas Health Science Center–Houston School of Public Health and the University of Texas, Austin. At the

University of Texas School of Public Health, he also serves as the Associate Regional Dean for Academic Affairs and International Health Affairs at the Austin Regional Campus. Prior to this appointment, he served as Lead Epidemiologist and Team Leader in the Physical Activity and Health Branch of the Division of Nutrition and Physical Activity at the Centers for Disease Control and Prevention in Atlanta.

He has worked since 1984 in the area of physical activity and health, including conducting research, developing and evaluating intervention programs for adults and children, and developing and advising on policy issues. He earned his doctorate in Epidemiology and Community Health Studies at the niversity of Texas Health Science Center - Houston School of Public Health, and a master of science in Public Health at the University of South Carolina.

Dr. Kohl's other areas of specialization are biostatistics and health promotion. His research interests include current focuses on physical activity, exercise, fitness, and health as well as and sports medicine surveillance systems for musculoskeletal injuries. In his recent efforts, he has concentrated on national and international physical activity surveillance and epidemiology issues, as well as program development and evaluation studies for the promotion of school-based physical activity for children and adolescents. He initiated Active Texas 2020, a state physical activity plan for Texas.

He has served as an elected trustee and is a Fellow of the American College of Sports Medicine and is a Fellow in the National Academy of Kinesiology. He is the founder and past president of the International Society for Physical Activity and Health. He has served in an editorial capacity for several scientific journals and is currently editor emeritus of the *Journal of Physical Activity and Health*. He served as Chair of an Institute of Medicine committee at the National Academies of Science on physical activity and physical education in school-based settings and is a past Chair of the Science Board of the President's Council on Physical Fitness, Sports, and Nutrition. He has published more than 200 papers, chapters, and monographs in the scientific literature and in 2012 co-authored the textbook *Foundations of Physical Activity and Public Health* with Dr. Tinker Murray.

## Why I Became a Kinesiology Professional

My path to becoming a kinesiology professional began with my interest and training in public health. I began with an interest in the physiology of acid/base chemistry compensation to environment challenges. My training in epidemiology, first under Dr. Carol Macera and later Dr. Milton Nichaman, opened my eyes to public health. Further inspired by Drs. Steven Blair and Ralph Paffenbarger, I came to see physical fitness and physical activity as not just a clinical issue for individuals, but a population and public health issue as well. I was able to combine my interest in physiology and my interest in public health into a new field: physical activity epidemiology.

My first job as an epidemiologist was at the Cooper Aerobics Center, where we were following thousands of patients of the Cooper Clinic in a prospective study to determine the role that precisely measured physical fitness plays in noncommunicable disease mortality. In those studies, led by Dr. Steven Blair, we were able to demonstrate that men and women who had higher levels of cardiorespiratory fitness, or who improved that fitness with physical activity, had a correspondingly lower risk of death due to all causes, cardiovascular disease, and some cancers. With these and studies from other groups at the time, the idea of physical activity and population health began to take its place in kinesiology.

Throughout my career I have been interested in the body's response to exercise and physical activity, how those responses can be quantified and studied as they may relate to noncommunicable disease outcomes, and how best to promote individual and population-level increases in physical activity, exercise, and physical fitness. This text provides a palette for us to create a teaching tool from our more than 90 collective years researching, teaching, and understanding the field of kinesiology.

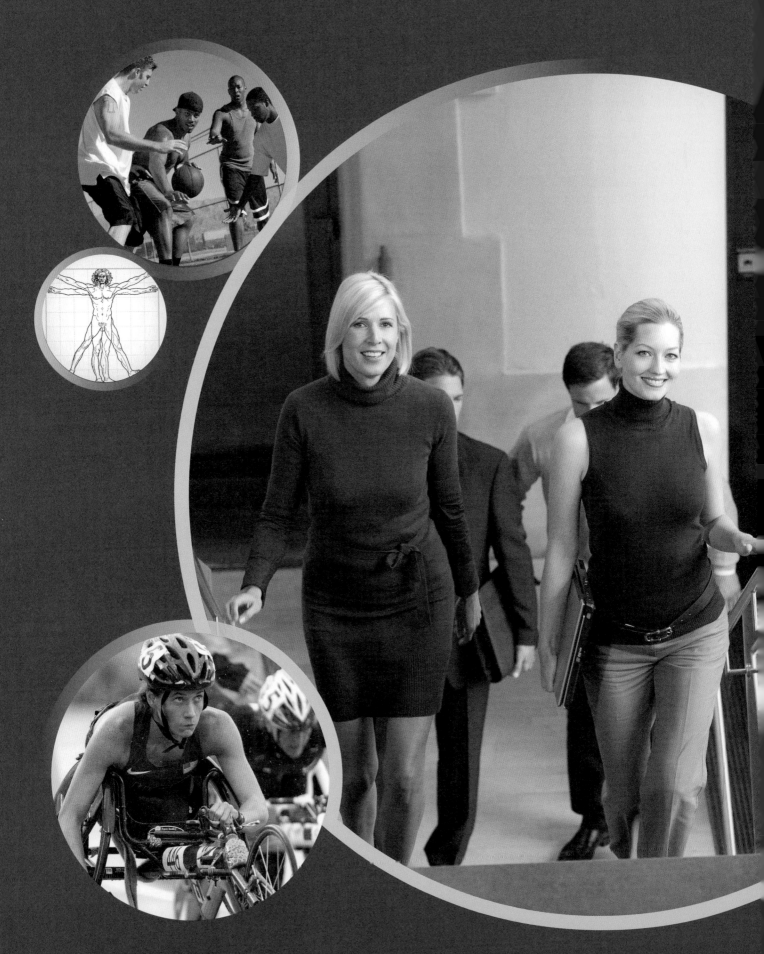

# Physical Activity and Society

*Why do you need this course?*

## Learning Objectives

*After completing this chapter, you will be able to:*

**Describe** the role and importance of physical activity within society.

**Describe** the role and importance of kinesiology as it relates to health, sports and occupational performance, and growth and development.

**Explain** the differences between physical activity, exercise, and physical fitness.

**Explain** briefly the field of kinesiology and the subdisciplines associated with it.

**Describe** the career options associated with kinesiology.

**Give** examples of professional training opportunities in the field of kinesiology.

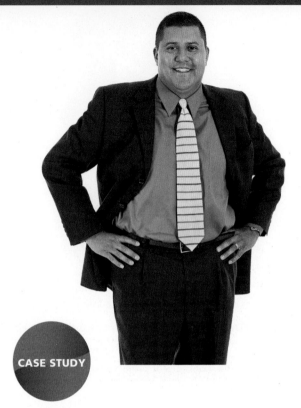

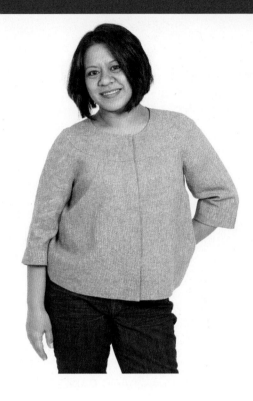

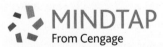

# In the real world . . .

Meet the Casey family. They represent a busy but physically inactive family that you might find anywhere in U.S. society today. We will follow the Caseys and their extended family and friends throughout the book. The situations they face will require you to use your knowledge, skills, and abilities to devise solutions that promote physically active lifestyles despite the family's lifestyle, behavioral, and environmental challenges.

The Casey family consists of William, Maria, Jerald, Cara, and Eugene. William is the 50-year-old dad and Maria is his 48-year-old wife and mother of the kids. Jerald is their 22-year-old son, Cara is their 14-year-old daughter, and Eugene is the 10-year-old youngest child of the family.

William is 6 feet tall and weighs 265 pounds. He is a former star high school football player who injured his right knee in his senior year and could not continue to play. He has been diagnosed with hypertension (controlled with prescription medication) and has suffered several recent bouts of chest pain that his cardiologist has identified as angina pectoris. He has been very sedentary for the past 15 years. He is an executive in a large business firm that requires a 1-hour commute daily and a 50+ -hour work week.

Maria is 5 feet, 4 inches tall, weighs 200 pounds, and is a stay-at-home mom, but paints and sells art on a part-time

## MINDTAP
From Cengage

Go to your MindTap course now to answer some questions and discover what you already know about physical activity and society.

## INTERACTIVE ACTIVITIES

**Research Focus**

Visit informative websites and complete an activity that will help you appreciate both past approaches to the study of human activity and exciting new directions.

**Career Focus**

Complete an activity that will help you understand the professional development process in many fields related to physical activity.

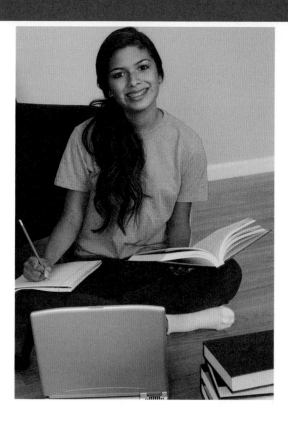

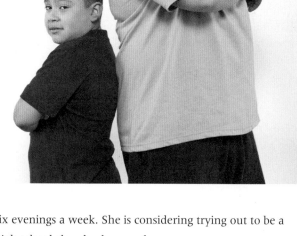

basis. She was very physically active until her later teen years and now struggles to be mobile regularly due to low back pain and physical challenges related to her type 2 diabetes (controlled with prescription medications), which was diagnosed four years ago.

Jerald, who is tall like his dad, started attending community college part time to study business after graduating from high school. He works full time as a server at a local restaurant to help pay for school. He was a youth athlete but stopped playing sports at age 13 years because he didn't like the way his baseball coach and teammates treated him, and it just was not fun anymore. He has been very physically inactive and gained 30 pounds in the last three years. He attends school in the late mornings and early afternoons, while working nights until midnight.

Cara is a healthy, academically successful eighth grader who loves to be physically active. She played basketball and baseball as a younger girl and now participates in club dance six evenings a week. She is considering trying out to be a high school cheerleader or a dancer.

Eugene is in the fifth grade, and he is struggling to make good grades in school. He finds school to be boring and would much rather text his friends and check his Twitter and Facebook accounts than study. He is a couch potato who only gets 45 minutes of moderate-intensity physical activity on one to two days per week. He is overweight, and William and Maria are worried that he will become an obese teen.

Now that you have met the Caseys, what kinesiology advice would you give each of the family members to increase/maintain their physical activity levels and mobility in the near future? As you move through the remainder of the course, use the In the Real World — Case Study feature to evaluate your ability to provide effective solutions for real-life kinesiology challenges that are related to health, physical activity, and performance.

# Introduction: Kinesiology, Movement, Physical Activity, and Exercise

**Kinesiology**, simply stated, is the scientific study of movement. The term has its origin in ancient Greek *kinesis* meaning "movement" and *logos* meaning "discourse." Although descriptions of human anatomy, including the muscles and how they move, can be traced back to the ancient Greek scientist Aristotle, the scientific study of kinesiology and its subdisciplines is much younger. Analysis of the human gait was advanced in the late nineteenth century by Christian Braune and Otto Fischer, who used the technological advancements of the early days of photography to evaluate the biomechanics of free walking and simple load-bearing movements. Our understanding of how muscles use oxygen was advanced in the early twentieth century by Nobel Laureate A. V. Hill. Clinical understanding of the effects of exercise training have recently been supplemented with the emergence of public health as a new subdiscipline in kinesiology. Taken together, these (and other) major advancements have helped to describe and define the field of kinesiology. Today it is a field that has a broad reach into many subdisciplines. These include, but are not limited to, biomechanics; motor learning and development; public health; human behavior; philosophy, history, and sociology; and exercise physiology.

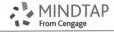

### History of Kinesiology

**Go to your MindTap course** now to visit informative websites and complete an activity that will help you appreciate both past approaches to the study of human activity and exciting new directions.

All human movement involves physical activity. Physical activity can thus be conceptualized as the center of kinesiology universe. Around this center are six academic subdisciplines, or areas of specialization, each of which focuses on some aspect of physical activity (Figure 1.1). These six areas of specialization—biomechanics; motor learning and development; public health; sport/exercise psychology/human behavior; philosophy, history, and sociology; and exercise physiology—provide the research and training core of kinesiology. Study in these subdisciplines helps to prepare students for careers in all things related to physical activity.

In addition to further studies in graduate education, studying kinesiology can prepare you for many different types of careers. Importantly, all such careers involve physical activity as their central focus. Seven are shown in Figure 1.1: Exercise science, athletic training, physical education, physical therapy/occupational therapy, public health practice, coaching, and sport management. Lesson 2 of this chapter covers each of the disciplines and career areas of kinesiology in detail.

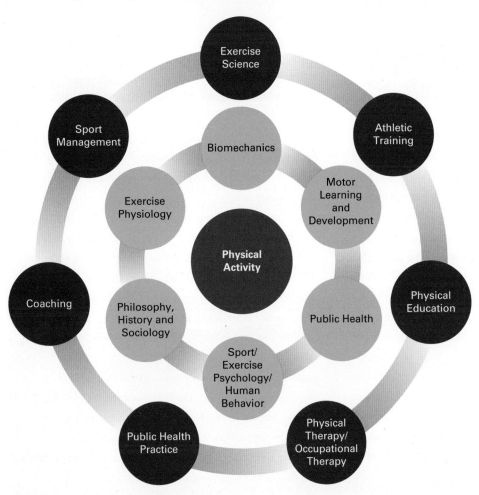

**Figure 1.1** | **An Integrated Vision of Careers and Fields of Study in Kinesiology.** Fields of study (green spheres) are united around physical activity as the center of kinesiology. Red spheres (outer ring) indicate some of the possible careers toward which various fields of study in kinesiology can lead.

# Physical Activity, Exercise, and Physical Fitness: What's the Difference?

These terms, although frequently used in kinesiology, can be confusing. Caspersen and Powell published generally accepted definitions.[1] **Physical activity** is any bodily movement that results in energy expenditure (burning of calories). Moving your arm up and down at your desk, skateboarding, lifting sacks of groceries out of the trunk of your car, and running a marathon are all different types of physical activity. **Exercise** is a specific type of physical activity that is planned, repetitive, and done for a specific purpose. Walking the dog for two miles every night, training for a soccer tryout, swimming laps, and working out at a gym are all examples of exercise. All athletes who train to improve components of their physical fitness exercise. Anyone who gets out of bed in the morning is doing some kind of physical activity.

The study of movement began with understanding how the muscles work to move the skeleton, proceeded to how the circulatory system provides fuel for movement and carries away metabolic by-products, and gradually expanded to include other systems in the body. This evolution in the science of studying human movement helped us to understand how to improve human performance in athletics and occupations and through rehabilitation. Today, kinesiology is widely viewed through three different lenses: health, sports and occupation, and growth and development.

# Kinesiology and Society

Although kinesiology has traditionally been considered a field where many subdisciplines come together, yet are separate in their study and application, a major purpose of this text is to demonstrate that kinesiology can be unifying. Physical activity is pervasive in society, and rather than thinking of kinesiology as a box with many parts, its linkages to society can make kinesiology larger than the sum of its parts.

### Kinesiology and Health

Only relatively recently in the history of kinesiology has health become a fundamental tenet. The emphasis on human performance made room for health in the early 1950s with the emergence of the hypothesis that exercise improves heart health and function. In 1953, Professor Jeremy Morris was one of the first to study this association by comparing deaths due to heart disease between bus drivers in London (who sat all day with limited movement) and the ticket takers (who moved all day collecting tickets from bus riders). Professor Morris

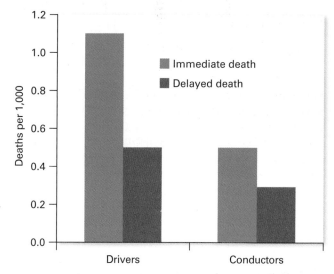

**Figure 1.2** | Mortality Study among Train Drivers and Conductors

*Source:* Adapted from J. N. Morris, A. Hagan, P. A. B Raffle, C. G. Roberts, and J. W. Parks, "Coronary Heart Disease and Physical Activity of Work," *The Lancet* 265 (1953): 1053–1057, 1111–1120.

showed very clearly that the ticket takers, because of their higher levels of physical activity, were much less likely to die from heart disease than their sedentary driver peers.[2] Evidence that movement was related to health began to emerge.

The main findings from this study are shown in Figure 1.2. The conductors, who were active all day taking tickets from passengers, had a significantly lower heart disease mortality experience than did the drivers who sat all day long during their shift. This was true for people who died immediately (within the first three days) of a heart attack as well as for those who survived the first three days but died up to three months after their heart attack (delayed). In each instance, conductors were at a significant heart health advantage. These findings were

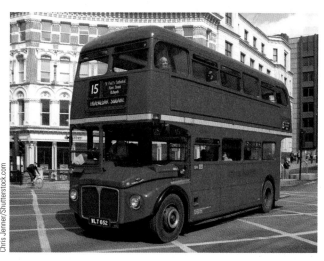

the first published data suggesting that physical activity could protect men against dying from a heart attack.

Since the early days of the London busmen studies, scientific literature around the world has grown exponentially with reports of the role that physical activity and exercise play in health. In fact, physical activity has been shown to play key roles in all five levels of disease prevention and rehabilitation, shown in Figure 1.3. The first level is **primordial prevention**, the most basic level of disease prevention. In primordial prevention, action is taken to prevent the precursors of a problem or disease state before they can begin to take harm. Preventing high blood pressure (which can damage the circulatory system), keeping blood sugar (glucose) in the normal range so that diabetes does not develop, or preventing a knee injury that could damage cartilage and result in osteoarthritis are three examples of primordial prevention. Physical activity and exercise have been shown to play substantive roles in primordial disease prevention. Primordial prevention can most frequently be used effectively in children and adolescents, as many chronic diseases have their beginnings in childhood.

The next level of disease prevention that physical activity can influence is **primary prevention**. Primary prevention involves efforts to prevent a condition or disease outcome from emerging by affecting its precursors. The key to primary prevention is that it takes place when no disease or condition has yet been diagnosed, but it is suspected that physiologic changes that can increase the risk of the disease or condition may be occurring. Physical activity acts to inhibit development or slow those changes before the clinical manifestations of the disease begin. Examples of how kinesiology is related to primary prevention of disease outcomes include lowering or normalizing of blood pressure and blood glucose levels with exercise, or muscular training for older adults to help prevent falls and the fractures that may result. Primary prevention is frequently focused on populations or groups of individuals rather than on individual people.

**Secondary prevention** involves a focus on individuals rather than populations and acts to prevent progression of a disease condition after it has been detected. Often referred to as "management," secondary prevention related to physical activity seeks to minimize the health impact of a disease by intervening as early as possible once a disease has been diagnosed. Physical activity in early-stage depression, physical activity for weight loss, and exercise for newly diagnosed type 2 diabetics are all examples of the role that kinesiology plays in secondary prevention.

**Tertiary prevention** involves improving or maintaining quality of life for people with diseases, their complications, and disabilities. Although physical activity may not affect progression of the diagnosed disease, the goal of tertiary prevention is to lessen the disease's impact on the individual. Physical activity for cancer survivors that is designed to improve their quality of life during and after treatments is an example of kinesiology in tertiary prevention.

**Rehabilitation** is the fifth area where kinesiology is related to health and disease outcomes. Although rehabilitation is often grouped with tertiary prevention in other fields, when viewed through a kinesiology lens, the goal of rehabilitation is restoration of health and physical function to the precondition or pre-disease state. In this case, physical activity is used as a primary method of helping a person overcome the health effects of a disease. Physical activity has proven to be a powerful part of rehabilitation. Cardiac rehabilitation after a heart attack and physical therapy after knee replacement surgery or after an occupation-related back injury are examples of applications of kinesiology in rehabilitation settings. Can you think of others?

The emergence of the health applications of kinesiology has been accelerated by a growing body of scientific literature on all aspects of health.

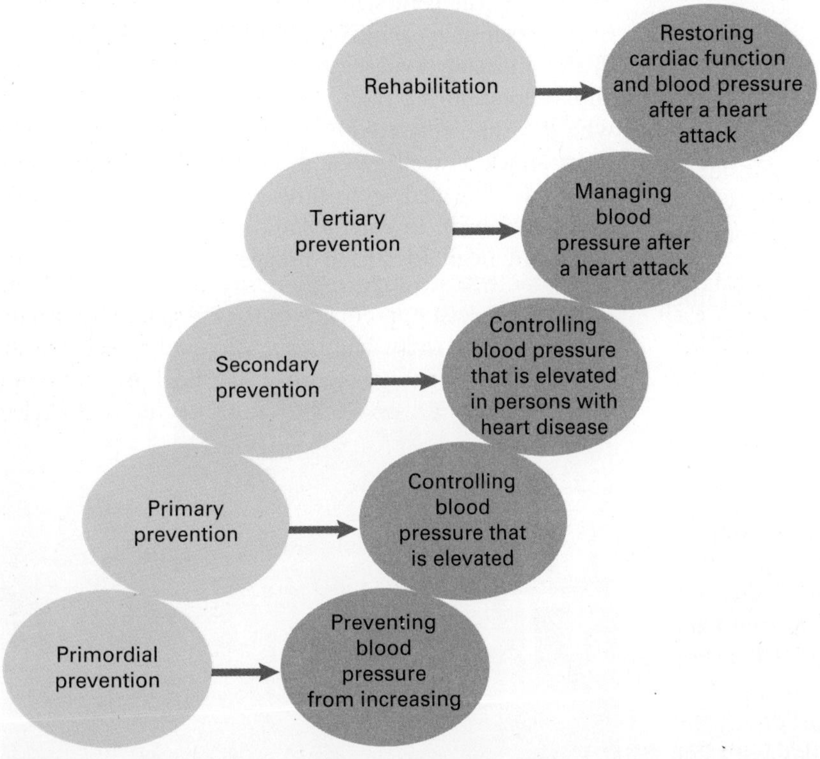

**Figure 1.3** | The Stages of Disease Prevention and How They Relate to the Problem of High Blood Pressure

Physical inactivity is associated an increased risk of a host of non-communicable diseases and conditions. In fact, in 2012 it was estimated that physical inactivity causes nearly as many deaths each year worldwide as tobacco use![3] Globally the problem of physical inactivity is so widespread (approximately 30% of all adults and approximately 80% of all adolescents are physically inactive) and has such serious implications for public health that it has been labeled a "pandemic."[4]

### What Is the Difference Between an Epidemic and a Pandemic?

An epidemic is the occurrence in a community or region of cases of an illness, specific health-related behavior, or other health-related events clearly in excess of normal expectancy. A pandemic is a much wider occurrence—an epidemic occurring worldwide, or over a very wide area, crossing international boundaries, and usually affecting a large number of people. Clearly the world has a problem with a pandemic of physical inactivity.

## Kinesiology: Sports and Occupational Performance

Training for sports performance has been a cornerstone of kinesiology for many years. Understanding the means and mechanisms through which athletes, elite and recreational, can improve their performance has provided the groundings for kinesiology. The idea of developing movement skills is central to kinesiology for sports performance. Although a sport is a physical activity, the activity is done for a purpose and practiced for mastery. There may be health benefits, but they are considered secondary to the performance benefits. Understanding the types of effective training, nutrition for optimal performance, and techniques to achieve optimal performance are all key areas of kinesiology for sports performance. These apply to the highest-performing athletes in the world as well as to children and adolescents and weekend warriors. Examples include mastery of a backhand stroke in tennis, techniques to conquer the high hurdles in track and field, or the speed and agility necessary to be a competitive wrestler. Can you think of more?

Similar to its place in sports performance is the role that kinesiology plays in occupational performance. Although jobs that require physical labor are rarer than they once were, we will always have a need for people working as firefighters, nurses, construction workers, and the like. To be successful in these jobs, people must move, sometimes substantially so. Firefighters need a fundamental level of fitness to be able to race into an emergency situation and perform rescues. Nurses need to move bedridden patients, push wheelchairs, and be prepared for a variety of other physical tasks. Even with mechanization, construction workers must lift, bend, stretch, and grasp items. Each requires movement to be successful, and kinesiology is a central part of understanding that movement.

## Kinesiology: Growth and Development

Human development is a process that occurs over a lifetime. The physical abilities that result from the development of gross and fine motor skills in early childhood often help determine the life course for many people. Acquisition of such skills requires movement and discovery and is a central theme in kinesiology. Development, however, does not stop in childhood; adults, too, begin with young adulthood and then eventually phase into old age. Each stage of life is associated with physical development or a lack thereof. Kinesiology is involved at each stage because each stage requires movement. Enhancing motor development in the young as well as overcoming motor impairment in the elderly all require a skill set central to kinesiology. Teaching a child to throw a ball and teaching a grandparent to walk again after suffering a stroke are remarkably similar pursuits from a kinesiology perspective.

Thus, kinesiology is really a topic central to society. Human movement affects all parts of our daily lives and is central to health, sport and occupational pursuits, and growth and development across the life span. Physical inactivity, on the other hand, is a true public health problem for the twenty-first century. The field of kinesiology is positioned impressively for the future and is changing dramatically.

## Introduction

In this text, the formal study of kinesiology refers to the curricula provided by a variety of community college and university-level departments such as physical education, exercise and sport science, human movement studies, health and human performance, and so on. The most common departmental division name in U.S. schools is "Kinesiology" as it applies to the major university association, the American Kinesiology Association (AKA), which "promotes and enhances kinesiology as a unified field of study and advances its many applications." The AKA advocates for kinesiology at national and international levels and supports its member departments by providing resource materials and leadership and educational opportunities for university administrators in kinesiology.

AKA is central to modernizing the field of kinesiology. Membership by a community college or university is not a prerequisite for using the recommendations that the AKA produces. For example, the Academy Papers contained in *Kinesiology Review*—such as "Back to the Future: Reflecting on the Past and Envisioning the Future for Kinesiology Research"—focus on where the field has been and where it is predicted to move in the future.[5] Key messages from the Academy Papers will be highlighted in chapters throughout the remainder of this text.

As covered in Lesson 1, kinesiology is the study of movement and how physical activity and physical fitness affect health, behavior, community, and quality of life. Although the field has its roots in physical education, it currently includes many subdisciplines. Each of these subdisciplines is associated, in one way or another, with the multitude of career opportunities available to the kinesiology graduate. Chapter 2 discusses the skill sets required for each subdiscipline and their usefulness within various careers. In this lesson, we will discuss the different subdisciplines of study the student will encounter while working toward a degree in kinesiology and link these subdisciplines to the numerous professional career choices available to the kinesiology graduate. Subdisciplines are classified into those that are primarily academic disciplines and those that are more traditionally practice-based, and they represent a type of "Kinesiology Universe," or "Knowledge Base for Kinesiology" as shown in Figure 1.4.

In Lesson 2 of future chapters, you will discover integrated kinesiology subdiscipline examples that can help you learn to apply and translate the science of kinesiology to practice. Since this is your first introduction to the field, we begin with an overview of the practice-based subdisciplines of kinesiology shown in Figure 1.4.

Lesson 2 in each chapter is about applying what you are learning to the real world. It is never too early to start considering how to use your college education to help build a career. Therefore, Lesson 2 in this chapter concludes with an overview of the many professional training options available once you have obtained an undergraduate degree in kinesiology.

The six subdisciplines highlighted in the green spheres in Figure 1.4 receive special focus in Lesson 2 for most chapters. When you see one of the six icons next to a heading, it is an indication that the coverage that follows provides specific information on how to apply knowledge from that subdiscipline into practice in kinesiology. Lesson 2 also ends with a special section called the "Practice of Kinesiology" to help you put the Lesson 2 information into practice (an icon introduces this section as well). Discussions related to the subdiscipline of philosophy, history, and sociology will appear as integrated examples (knowledge to practice) and will also be represented by the Practice of Kinesiology icon. The icons are shown below. You will see the same icons appearing in your MindTap course as well. It is a good idea, even at this early stage, to begin thinking about the practice of kinesiology in terms of integrating knowledge from the subdisciplines.

## Exercise Physiology

**Exercise physiology** is the study of the physiological/biological responses to physical activity and the effects of these responses on biological adaptations that occur with acute and chronic exercise. Topics within exercise physiology include energy metabolism, skeletal muscle function, cardiovascular function, disease pathology associated with physical inactivity, and physiological challenges among special populations. All of these topics will help to improve your understanding of the physiological mechanisms associated with acute and chronic physical activity.

In exercise physiology, topics you will study include the relationship of biology, chemistry, and math to physical activity and physical performance (Figure 1.5). In considering these topics, you will learn about energy transfer, energy expenditure, evaluation of the body's energy-generating capacities, the pulmonary system, the

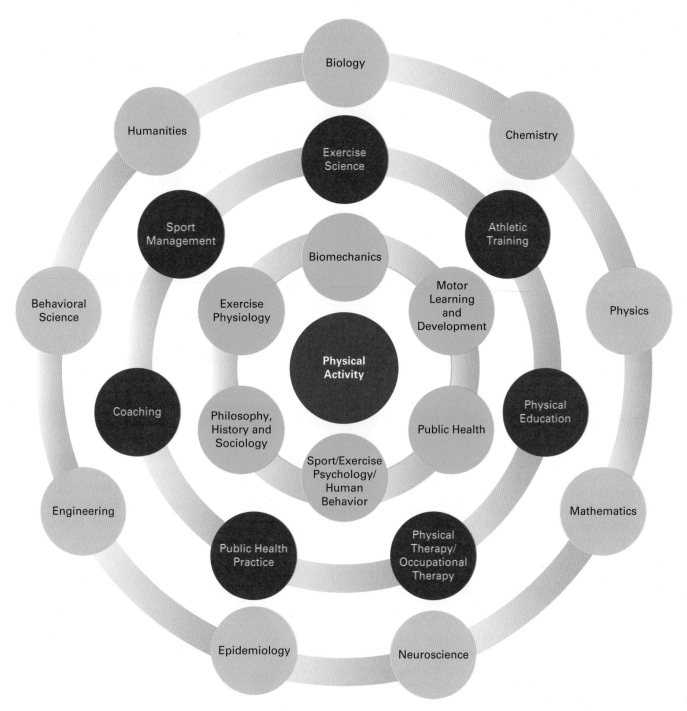

**Figure 1.4** | **Knowledge Base for Kinesiology.** In addition to the fields of study and potential careers, the kinesiology universe is highly influenced by multiple academic disciplines. The yellow spheres show the academic disciplines that inform the practice-based subdisciplines of kinesiology. Physical Activity is the center of the "Kinesiology Universe."

cardiovascular system, and the neuromuscular system. Beyond these topics, you will learn how to relate these basic principles to proper training methods for sports and exercise, how environmental factors affect the body and its performance capacities, and even how nutrition and ergogenic aids might enhance or hinder performance.

Nutrition, as it relates to improving human performance, is often included as a part of studies in exercise physiology, and we have addressed nutrition in relationship to energy expenditure, performance-enhancing strategies related to adverse events, and leadership challenges in Chapters 7, 12, and 14.

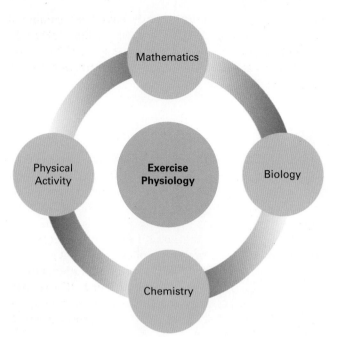

Figure 1.5 | Foundations of Knowledge for Exercise Physiology

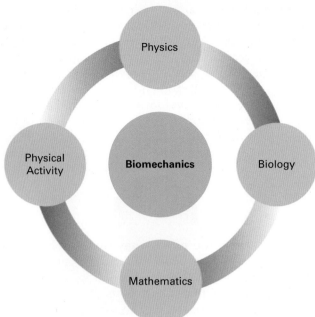

Figure 1.6 | Foundations of Knowledge for Biomechanics

# Biomechanics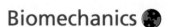

**Biomechanics** is the study of the relationship between physics and physical movement during sports and other physical activities. Biomechanists apply the laws of mechanics to the principles of movement during physical activity to better understand movement as it relates to performance and injury. Biomechanists study the actions of the muscles, joints, and skeleton during a specific movement to better understand the movement's effects on the associated skill or task. The study of biomechanics will help you understand and apply biomechanical principles to sports performance, sports mastery, injury rehabilitation, and injury prevention. In the subfield of biomechanics, you will study how the fields of biology, math, and physics relate to physical activity and physical performance (Figure 1.6). You will learn about torque, angular velocity, momentum, friction, and muscle joint and skeletal responses to external force.

# Motor Learning

**Motor learning** is the study of the relationship between neuroscience and biology as it applies to physical movement during sports and physical activity, and methods to produce permanent changes that will enhance these movements. Motor learning specialists study movement. They apply the factors associated with neural encoding and central nervous system processing to explain or improve both simple and complex movements needed to complete a movement task. Motor learning specialists can help improve physical activity and physical performance through their understanding of how practice and training

can affect the learning of specific movements and how to make changes in the practice steps to improve performance. The study of motor learning will help you understand how the neural and muscular systems produce a movement and how practicing these movements will affect and improve changes in the movement. In motor learning, you will study how biology, neuroscience, and physics relate to the development of and generation of both simple and complex movements (see Figure 1.7).

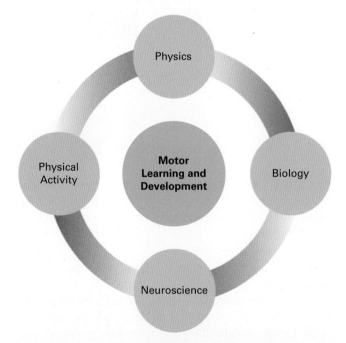

Figure 1.7 | Foundations of Knowledge for Motor Learning and Control

These studies will help you understand how to improve movements through practice of a task to enhance physical activity and physical performance. You will learn about neural signaling, motor recruitment, proprioception, timing, signal organization, and feedback as they apply to learning both sport and activity movements.

In this text, we have developed the motor learning and development icon to refer to examples of the integration of motor learning, motor control, motor development, and motor behavior with kinesiology. Please see Chapter 2 for more details and explanations.

## Sport/Exercise Psychology

**Sport and exercise psychology** is the study of psychology in relation to sports performance and physical activity. Sport psychology focuses on the psychological or mental factors that affect sports performance; exercise psychology focuses on the psychological factors that affect exercise and physical activity. Sport psychologists specialize in identifying cognitive and behavioral factors that may enhance sports performance (winning and losing) or act as a barrier to sports performance, as well as studying the effect of physical performance on psychological performance related to stress, anxiety, and well-being. Exercise psychologists (sometimes called behavioral scientists) specialize in identifying psychological factors that may enhance or act as a barrier to physical activity participation or exercise adherence (Figure 1.8). Sport psychology and exercise psychology are usually grouped together in the field

of psychology and more recently have been combined within the field of human behavior in kinesiology. In Chapter 2 you will learn more about sport and exercise psychology as it relates to the study of human behavior and its applications.

## Public Health

**Public health** is the science and practice of protecting, promoting, and improving the health of populations and communities. When we think of public health, notable achievements such as vaccinations against disease, quarantine rules for controlling disease outbreaks, reductions in deaths due to motor vehicle accidents, fluoridation of public water supplies to improve dental health, and food safety and restaurant inspections to reduce food-borne illnesses come to mind. Kinesiology and public health come together when we must promote policies and environments that support physical activity (see Figure 1.9).

Public health science is characterized not just by the accumulation of new knowledge, but also by the application of that knowledge to improve health. Public health research must be translatable to action for disease prevention, health promotion, or both. There are five key topical areas in public health—epidemiology, environmental health, health promotion/education, health administration/policy, and biostatistics—with many more specializations, including physical activity and public health (see Chapter 2 for more).

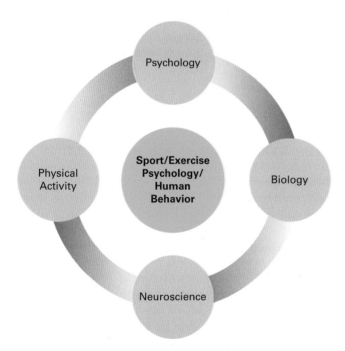

**Figure 1.8** | Foundations of Knowledge for Sports and Exercise Psychology/Human Behavior

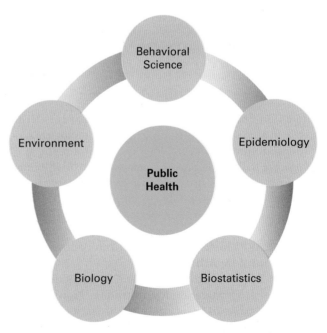

**Figure 1.9** | Foundations of Knowledge for Public Health

## Epidemiology and Disease Control

**Epidemiology** is the basic science of public health. The word *epidemiology* has Greek origins: *epidemia* ("on people") and *-ology* ("to study"). Although it may be defined in several ways, a modern-day definition of epidemiology is "the study of distributions and determinants of disease and disability in populations."[6] Notable in this definition, as pointed out in the preceding discussion, is the word *populations*. Epidemiologists are most interested in a defined population and how a disease or disability affects that population. What causes the disease to spread? How can it be prevented? How many people are affected? What types of people or other organisms might be affected more than others? Who is at risk? How many could be affected in the future? These are all questions that epidemiologists are trained to answer.

Epidemiology is a quantitative scientific discipline that relies heavily on statistics and study design. During the twentieth century, the patterns of health and disease transitioned from communicable to primarily noncommunicable diseases. Epidemiologic methods have evolved to apply not only to infectious disease outbreak investigations but also to longer-term chronic disease investigations. For example, much of what we know about risk factors for heart disease (e.g., poor lipid and lipoprotein profile, high blood pressure, cigarette smoking, physical inactivity) came from early and ongoing epidemiological studies of (mostly) men with and without these characteristics. Researchers used epidemiological methods to compare study participants with and without these characteristics and then calculated the associated risk of the occurrence of a disease. These techniques have evolved as the need to address more complicated analytical questions has increased.

## Environmental Health

The environment can be defined as "all that is external to the host organism" including physical, biological, and cultural influences.[7] Our physical environment (i.e., where we live, work, and play) has a powerful influence on our health. The air we breathe, the water we drink, the food we eat, the safety of our work environment, radiation exposure, and the ways we control these environmental influences can promote or hinder public health. Thus, a large part of public health addresses **environmental health**.

Major advances have been made in public health as a result of environmental health studies. Prohibition of lead-based paint to reduce the risk of learning disabilities in children, fluoridation of water supplies to reduce dental caries in communities, air quality regulations for automobile manufacturers and industrial polluters to promote cleaner air and water, and food safety standards to reduce the risk of food-borne diseases are all examples of public health initiatives that came about because of environmental health studies. Can you think of others?

---

### Environmental Influences

Clearly, people should be aware of the environmental influences on health and the importance of physical activity and exercise.

"Physical activity has been engineered out of people's lives through urban planning and transportation investments that favor travel by automobile, labor-saving devices at home and in the work place, and a proliferation of electronic entertainment options. Built environments are worthy of special attention because they can affect virtually all residents of a community for many decades..."

—Quote from J. F. Sallis et al.[8]

---

Systematic approaches to studying the environmental influences on health, quantifying these influences, and prioritizing resources and approaches to eliminate the health hazards have been advanced only recently. Our understanding of the role of the environment in promoting or inhibiting physical activity has advanced rapidly since the mid-1990s. We can now identify barriers and correlates in the physical, social, and cultural environments that influence physical activity participation. This has been, and will continue to be, a major growth area in the field of physical activity and public health.

## Health Promotion and Health Education

Why do some people exercise consistently, avoid tobacco, eat well, use alcohol responsibly, avoid illicit drugs, see their doctors regularly, and do other things necessary for health maintenance, whereas others do not? How can we best teach basic health concepts for lasting effectiveness? How can population-level health behaviors be changed to maximize life expectancy and quality of life? These are examples of key questions those in the health promotion and health education sectors of public health routinely address. Although the environment and our genetic makeup contribute substantially to our health status, the way we deal with health threats through our behavior has become a major focus of public health.

Much of the basis for health promotion and health education comes from the concept of social justice, which is central to public health. Social justice in public health refers to the assumption (some call it an imperative) that the health burdens and benefits in a population should be distributed equitably. We have known for centuries that poverty is a predictor of disease, disability, and poor quality of life. Health promotion and health education strategies in public health aim to devise solutions to reduce health disparities such as those between low- and high-income groups.

## Health Administration and Policy

Health administration and policy is the fourth pillar of public health and focuses on the delivery of public health services. This area of expertise addresses important skills such as budgeting, policy development and analysis, planning and prioritization, and communication. In keeping with the theme that public health is action oriented, health administration and policy skills support the appropriate implementation of programs that, theoretically, are derived from research evidence. A good example is the application of study results in addressing the HIV/AIDS epidemic. Research has shown that needle exchange programs likely reduce hypodermic needle sharing, and thus the risk of transmission of HIV/AIDS, among intravenous drug users.[9] Health administration and policy experts can use such research data to plan community-based projects that promote needle exchange programs.

In the field of physical activity and public health, experts continue to discover the effects of policies and program administration. Policies that provide places to be physically active show promising results for the promotion of physical activity. Such polices include physical education requirements in schools, transportation policies that emphasize active travel for physical activity, and worksite policies that create incentives for employees to be physically active. Expertise in health administration and policy is critical for the implementation and evaluation of such efforts.

## Biostatistics

Public health relies on both qualitative and quantitative methods to move from knowledge to action. **Biostatistics** provides the basis for the quantitative branch. Is the difference in efficacy between two interventions to promote breast cancer screening in a community due to the effect of the intervention, or simply to chance? What is the predicted number of cases of influenza in the upcoming year? Based in mathematical theory, biostatistics allows for the practical and rational analysis of data, the interpretation of study results, and the translation of those results into action. Biostatisticians and epidemiologists work closely to advance the science of public health.

Kinesiology students interested in public health may pursue any of a variety of possible career options. Working in state, local, and federal health departments to reduce the burden of chronic diseases due to physical inactivity has broad appeal. Project managers for programs that promote physical activity in defined groups of people are in demand, and expertise in kinesiology is needed to design and deliver such programs. Advanced study in public health or in health education is also useful.

# Philosophy, History, and Sociology

The final subdiscipline in kinesiology has its foundation in humanities and social/behavioral sciences. Sport philosophy embodies the values of human movement including ethics, the importance of human movement to societies (developing and developed), and the intersection of sport, art, and physical culture. Sport history involves an assessment of the historical contexts, forces, and people that have helped to define sport and human movement. Studying the evolution of the Olympic movement and its role in shaping societies is an example application of sport history. Finally, sport sociology addresses the role that sports and human movement play in cultural and social development. Sport sociology is a subdiscipline and straddles a line between kinesiology and sociology. Questions around access to sports and racial/ethnic disparities in sports participation are examples of topics in sport sociology.

Academic preparation for a career in philosophy, history, or sociology most likely will require skills in one of these subdisciplines. Graduate education for further specialization at the master's and doctoral levels could follow (see Figure 1.10).

While philosophy, history, and sociology represent an important subdiscipline of kinesiology and should always be included in the practice of kinesiology, an in-depth discussion is beyond the scope of this text. Thus, when discussions of philosophy, history, and sociology appear in the text, they will be highlighted with the Practice of Kinesiology icon. Please see Chapter 2 for more about philosophy, history, and sociology.

An example of how the concepts from philosophy, history, or sociology can be integrated in kinesiology has been proposed by Gill.[10] She recommends that to sustain the profession (i.e., meet the needs of the present without compromising the ability of future generations to meet their needs), kinesiology professionals need to use historical, philosophical, and sociological approaches to integrate kinesiology as (1) an academic discipline, (2) a professional discipline, and (3) a discipline that promotes inclusion and social justice.

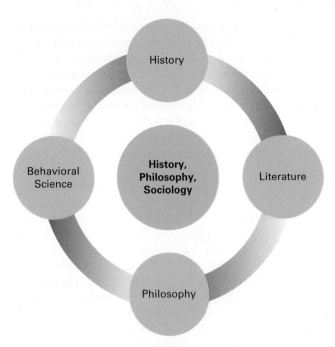

**Figure 1.10** | Foundations of Knowledge for Philosophy, History, and Sociology

From a socio-cultural perspective, you should learn how to seek higher levels of evidence-based research from the academic discipline to help guide your professional decision making; participate in problem-solving activities through public service or "service learning activities;" and learn to promote physical activity for all, regardless of gender, race/ethnicity, and disabilities. An appreciation and basic understanding of philosophy, history, and sociology in relationship to kinesiology can help you avoid re-inventing the wheel or using outdated/ineffective intervention strategies to promote physical activity to clients and populations.

## Professional Training

Hopefully, it is clear that kinesiology involves a diversity of subdisciplines and multiple opportunities for preparation for professional careers. In this section, we present many of the common professional training options that are available once you have obtained your undergraduate degree in kinesiology. We will limit our discussion here to the following professional training areas (i.e., degree specialties; there are others, and new opportunities are continuing to emerge): exercise science, athletic training, physical education teaching, physical therapy/occupational therapy, physical activity and public health practice, coaching, and sport management.

In addition to an undergraduate degree in kinesiology, you will most likely need to consider obtaining **professional certification** (documentation that you possess the essential knowledge, skills, and abilities—KSAs—to perform a specific job) through a professional association or organization. For instance, you might be certified as a personal trainer, an exercise specialist, or a strength and conditioning coach. Professional certification is sometimes optional for a career field based on typical job descriptions (like coaching certification is in some states), but often certification is required (or becomes required over time). Professional certification is often voluntary or optional for a career field based on typical job descriptions (like coaching certification is in some states), but often certification is required (or becomes required over time). For many career fields, maintenance of professional certification is tied to continuing education requirements like those found in other professions such as medicine, law, and business.

Professional certification is big business and very profitable for the various certifying entities. It is important to pursue academically rigorous and broadly recognized and accepted certifications that can help your career. On the other hand, those that lack academic rigor and are awarded in exchange for little more than a fee are not respected by many kinesiology professionals. Look for the numerous web links to KSAs for various professional certifications throughout the remainder of the textbook (see Chapter 2 to explore your options for professional certification opportunities). For degrees and careers such as physical education teaching, athletic training, and physical therapy you will also need to obtain professional **licensure** (granting of a license to practice) and registration prior to working in your career field.

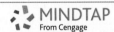

### Professional Development in Fields Related to Physical Activity

**Go to your MindTap course** now to visit informative websites and complete activities related to career options and appropriate certification/licensure in the following fields:

▸ Exercise Science
▸ Athletic Training
▸ Physical Education Training
▸ Physical Therapy/Occupational Therapy
▸ Public Health
▸ Coaching
▸ Sport Management

## Exercise Science

Professional training in exercise science is usually designed to prepare individuals for careers in nonpedagogical professions that include basic undergraduate requirements with an emphasis in the kinesiology content areas of anatomy, physiology, biomechanics, nutrition, fitness, and exercise prescription. Students who pursue exercise science training should also acquire specific professional certifications that then can lead to careers in personal training, cardiac rehabilitation, or preparation for graduate studies.

## Athletic Training

Professional education in athletic training is based on guidelines developed by the National Athletic Trainers' Association (NATA) and can lead to careers in sports (at all levels), hospitals, business/industry, the military, the performing arts, and public safety. Basic training includes the normal core undergraduate course work with extensive study directed toward immediate emergency care, prevention of injury, rehabilitation, and other clinical skills. Students who pursue athletic training should also acquire specific professional state and/or national certifications and licensure.

## Physical Education Teaching (Pedagogy)

Professional training in physical education teaching usually focuses on academic and practice experiences for pre-kindergarten (pre-K) through high school level students. Teachers of physical education can train to work in specialty areas such as adapted physical education and outdoor education. In most kinesiology programs, teacher education programs in physical education are supervised by pedagogy professionals (specialists in the art and science of teaching) who can provide students with a general knowledge base about kinesiology along with application skills appropriate for specific school populations (pre-K, elementary, middle school, or high school). Current, up-to-date physical education teaching programs include experiences with the Centers for Disease Control and Prevention (CDC) Whole School, Whole Community, Whole Child (WSCC) model and with health-related physical education (HRPE, also referred to as health-optimizing physical education or HOPE).[11] Students who pursue professional training in physical education teaching will need to acquire a state license and certification for the state in which they apply for work.

## Physical Therapy/Occupational Therapy Training

Many universities have undergraduate kinesiology degree plans for pre-physical therapy (PT) and/or pre-occupational therapy (OT) preparation, which require acceptance into and completion of advanced degrees (master's or doctoral levels) in allied health-related programs. Physical therapists work in rehabilitation to help patients reduce pain and improve or restore mobility and will find job opportunities in a variety of settings such as hospitals, home care, schools, business and industry, fitness centers, and research facilities. Occupational therapists help patients across the aging lifespan who have disabilities, are recovering from injury, and/or have cognitive and physical limitations master their everyday occupational tasks. Pre-PT and pre-OT programs are designed to give students the prerequisites they will need to work as licensed and registered physical or occupational therapists. Students who pursue physical or occupational therapy training should also acquire specific professional state and/or national certification and licensure. Adaptive physical education/activity, therapeutic recreation, and chiropractic practice all rely on kinesiology professional training subdisciplines that have linkages to many physical therapy and occupational therapy skill sets.

## Physical Activity and Public Health Practice

Public health deals with populations rather than individuals. Physical activity and public health practitioner training is a new and emerging field of training that combines the disciplines of kinesiology and public health. In the United States, the National Physical Activity Society (NPAS) has developed a set of core competencies that include many KSAs that are related to the basics of kinesiology (exercise physiology, biomechanics, behavioral science, and exercise testing and prescription). Students interested in physical activity and public health practice training will need to apply the kinesiology skills that they have acquired from working with individual interventions (to increase physical activity, fitness, etc.) to populations or communities representative of public health targets. Specific curricula related to physical activity and public health practitioner training have emerged and have been recognized by the National Academy of Kinesiology (NAK)/American Kinesiology Association (AKA) as a new professional focus area for those pursuing degrees in kinesiology.

## Coaching

Professional training in coaching can prepare you to coach individuals and teams associated with schools, clubs, and/or agencies. Basic training includes the normal core undergraduate course work with additional coursework in safety (First Aid, CPR, AED), basic athletic training, sports skills, competitive strategies, and communication/leadership. Usually coaches need a minimum of an undergraduate degree in kinesiology-related training to gain an entry-level position in coaching and a master's degree (in a related discipline

## People Matter Blake Thedinga, Physical Therapist*

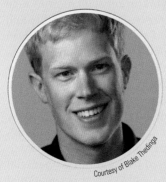

Courtesy of Blake Thedinga

**Q: Why and how did you get into the field of kinesiology?**

**A:** *My fascination, some say obsession, with kinesiology and its subdisciplines began at a young age. I was always enamored with how body movement patterns and physical abilities were so different between people, yet everyone found their way to play sports and other physical activities. This inspired me to pursue an occupation where I was able to help people restore their function, which is incredibly fulfilling.*

**Q: What was the major influence on you to work in the field?**

**A:** *During my undergraduate education, I dislocated my shoulder and was left with significant pain and loss of function. Physical therapy changed my life and completely restored my shoulder function and mobility. I changed my minor in kinesiology to a major so that I could more easily pursue a career in physical therapy.*

**Q: What do you do to keep your knowledge base current to be the most effective in your work?**

**A:** *Each state requires a minimum number of credit hours towards courses approved by your state. Fortunately, the physical therapy world is evolving and there are endless courses to expand your knowledge. Typically your employer will provide you with a continuing education allocation for these courses. In this day and age, social media/blogs are also an excellent source of information to review courses and collaborate with like-minded physical therapists.*

**Q: How do you stay physically active yourself and promote good health to others directly around you?**

**A:** *Staying physically active has always played a prominent role in my life. I enjoy hiking, skiing, and a variety of other sports. For me this is imperative, as I believe people will not adhere to your education and instruction if you don't "walk the talk." Every client I see, regardless of their diagnosis, is an opportunity for me to help them promote their own health and wellness through physical activity.*

**Q: How have you had to integrate the subdisciplines of kinesiology in your professional practice?**

**A:** *Since I have the pleasure of working with people of all ages and capacities, I utilize most subdisciplines of kinesiology on a daily basis. Everyone can benefit from a biomechanical analysis to improve recruitment of certain musculature and efficiency of movements to decrease pain and enhance function. It is also fun to integrate motor development strategies with adults, such as rolling with the upper and lower extremities, to improve trunk mobility and stability.*

*Dr. Thedinga earned his Doctorate in Physical Therapy from Des Moines University in 2011. He practices with Discovery Physical Therapy near Seattle, Washington. He specializes in sports physical therapy, foot/ankle rehabilitation, running analysis, and movement retraining.

area) to coach at the higher education level. It is helpful for students interested in coaching training to identify a "coach mentor" that they can shadow and interact with to gain the appropriate coaching application experiences required for success (see Chapter 2 for more on mentoring experiences).

## Sport Management

Professional training in sport management is usually designed to prepare individuals for careers related to organized sports (across a spectrum from youth to professional levels including nonprofit, corporate, and for-profit/club levels) and fitness. Basic training includes the normal core undergraduate course work with additional emphasis on the business and management of sports and on communication and leadership, along with 480 hours of internship, which provides future job opportunities (see Chapter 2 for more on internships). Students who pursue sport management training should also acquire specific professional certifications that can enhance their career opportunities.

---

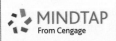
**MINDTAP** From Cengage

Now that you have completed this chapter, go to your MindTap course to complete all assigned activities. Check out the additional resources developed to help you apply the material in this chapter to your course and career goals.

---

# Chapter Summary

- Kinesiology, simply stated, is the scientific study of movement.
- Six areas of specialization provide the research and training core of kinesiology: biomechanics; motor learning and development; public health; human behavior; philosophy, history, and sociology; and exercise physiology.
- The five levels of disease prevention and rehabilitation are primordial prevention, primary prevention, secondary prevention, tertiary prevention, and rehabilitation.
- The study of kinesiology is important to understanding and optimizing a variety of societal outcomes like health, occupational performance, growth and development, sports performance, and other human movement experiences.
- The primary subdisciplines of kinesiology discussed in Lesson 2 include exercise physiology, biomechanics, motor learning, sport and exercise psychology, public health, and philosophy/history/sociology.
- Public health and kinesiology overlap relative to five topical areas: epidemiology, environmental health, health promotion and health education, health administration and policy, and biostatistics.
- Professional training areas in kinesiology include, but are not limited to, exercise science, sport management, athletic training, physical therapy/occupational therapy, physical education training, coaching, and physical activity and public health practice.

# Remember This

| | | | |
|---|---|---|---|
| biomechanics | exercise physiology | primary prevention | secondary prevention |
| biostatistics | kinesiology | primordial prevention | sport and exercise |
| environmental health | licensure | professional certification | psychology |
| epidemiology | motor learning | public health | tertiary prevention |
| exercise | physical activity | rehabilitation | |

# For More Information

Access these websites for further study of topics covered in the chapter:

- Search for further information about topics like epidemiology, physical activity, and exercise at the Centers for Disease Control and Prevention (CDC) website: www.cdc.gov.
- Search for information about the American Kinesiology Association (AKA) at www.americankinesiology.org.
- Search for information about physical activity and the International Society of Physical Activity and Health at www.ispah.org.

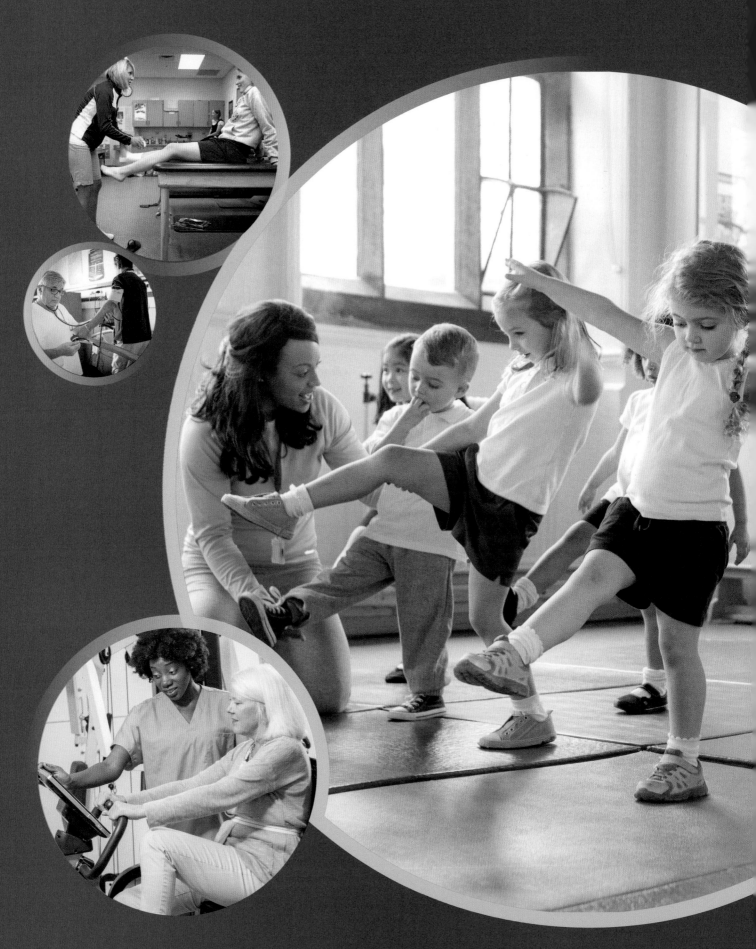

# Current Trends and Kinesiology Careers

*Have you thought about the first professional kinesiology job or potential career that you will pursue after graduation?*

**LESSON 1** INTEGRATION OF PROFESSIONAL SKILLS FOR VARIOUS KINESIOLOGY CAREERS

**LESSON 2** CAREER PLANNING IN KINESIOLOGY

## Learning Objectives

*After completing this chapter, you will be able to:*

**Describe** and explain the common knowledge, skills, and abilities (KSAs) acquired with an undergraduate kinesiology degree.

**Explain** in detail how physical activity is related to health, wellness, and quality of life.

**Explain** why it is important to integrate your academic training in kinesiology with its subdisciplines to optimize evidence-based learning and your problem-solving skills.

**Optimize** your problem-solving skills through evidence-based learning.

**Integrate** academic knowledge of kinesiology with the professional practical fields within it.

**Plan** your preparation for professional training in detail.

**Discuss** twenty-first century skills for professional career success and the importance of using readily available career service tools.

**Use** reliable investigation techniques to expand your successful career-planning skills.

# INTEGRATION OF PROFESSIONAL SKILLS FOR VARIOUS KINESIOLOGY CAREERS

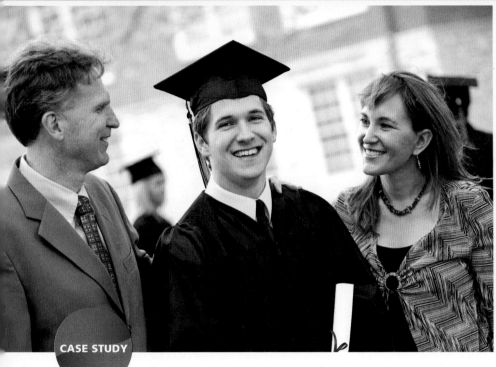
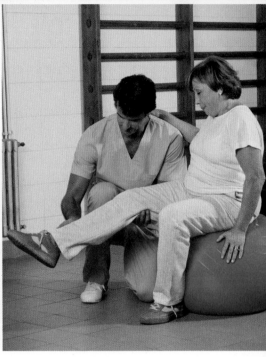

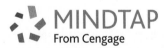

## In the real world . . .

Martijn is a close friend of the Casey family that you met in Chapter 1. Martijn is attending a state university with a large kinesiology department (more than 800 undergraduates). Now in his junior year, he has decided to major in pre-physical therapy (PT) because, as a former high school quarterback, he would like to specialize in treatment of sports injuries when he completes his academic and professional preparation. Martijn's father, Gijs, has a Ph.D. in kinesiology (health/fitness promotion) and works in health promotion for a nonprofit organization. Gijs hopes his son will pursue more clinical training and acquire a recognized professional certification such as occupational therapy, athletic training, or physical therapy. He knows that good job opportunities are becoming very competitive, and possessing numerous career skills will provide multiple options for professional employment. Martijn's mother, Kay,

## MINDTAP
### From Cengage

Go to your MindTap course now to answer some questions and discover what you already know about current trends and careers in kinesiology.

## INTERACTIVE ACTIVITIES

### Research Focus

Does your state have a physical activity plan? Go to you MindTap course to complete an activity that allows you to view the physical activity plan for your state or, if your state does not have a plan, the National Physical Activity Plan.

### Career Focus

What grades and skills do you need to meet your career goals? Go to your MindTap course to complete an activity based on what professional organizations such as the American Kinesiology Association and the National Association for Sport & Physical Education (now SHAPE) recommend for general requirements for success.

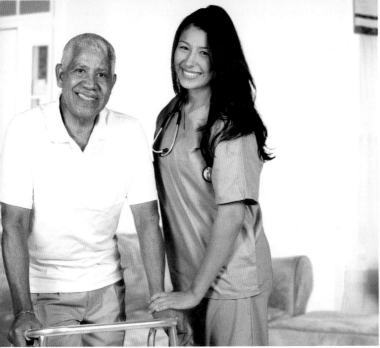

## Introduction: Common Basic KSAs in Kinesiology

At the 2009 American Kinesiology Association (AKA) meeting, a group of kinesiology higher education leaders representing 33 institutions proposed the development of a new core of essential educational elements that all undergraduates of kinesiology should commonly share (from www.americankinesiology.org). Speakers at the meeting defined the **knowledge base of kinesiology** as one that "integrates information gained through experiencing physical activity, through professional application, and through multidimensional scholarly approaches to the study of physical activity—biological, medical, and health-related aspects, psychological and social-humanistic." Or, as H. A. Lawson simply described it, "What should every undergraduate kinesiology major know or be able to do?"[1]

The proposed AKA 2009 common core or knowledge base of kinesiology included the following:

- Physical activity in health, wellness, and quality of life
- Scientific foundations of physical activity
- Cultural, historical, and philosophical dimensions of physical activity
- The practice of physical activity

For example, regarding the role of physical activity in promoting health and wellness across the lifespan, the kinesiology student would be expected to exhibit the following KSAs:[2]

1. Students will be able *to describe* the role of physical activity in promoting health and wellness across the lifespan.
2. Students will be able *to explain* the role of physical activity in promoting health and wellness across the lifespan.
3. Students will be able *to develop* physical activity programs that promote health and wellness across the lifespan.
4. Students should be able *to assess* the effectiveness of physical activity programs that promote health and wellness across the lifespan.

The primary curricular strategy in this text is integration of the variety of academic disciplines you will experience as an undergraduate kinesiology major so that you can master the knowledge base of kinesiology, translate that knowledge, and communicate it into intervention packages that help solve societal challenges related to kinesiology (examples of interventions include physical activity, weight loss, and sports performance programs). Another important integrating factor for kinesiology majors is the ability to use effective measures to determine intervention outcomes and to evaluate the intervention or program.

who operates her own business out of their home, hopes Martijn acquires some business skills to complement his kinesiology training.

Put yourself in Martijn's shoes: What unique academic preparation challenges do you think he is already facing if he is to be successful in reaching his career dream and addressing his parents' concerns? What professional challenges are common for pre-PT majors, and why should he consider a professional back-up plan? We'll follow up with Martijn later in the chapter, after you have had a chance to learn more about the integration of professional skills required for various kinesiology careers and more specifics about professional training preparation.

For example, in the classic 1985 research review paper of the "efficiency of human movement," the authors noted that quantifying efficient movement (work done with respect to energy expended) seems simple, and this efficiency can be easily evaluated using observational techniques.[3] Although explaining the concept of movement efficiency appears to be easy, it really requires an integrated, multidisciplinary investigation of the variety of factors (psychological–psychomotor, physiological, biomechanical, biochemical factors, and others) that affect the efficiency and metabolic cost of running at various speeds. For example, when only a unidimensional explanatory approach, such as assessing a runner's biomechanics, is used to quantify and define efficiency of movement, the variance in efficiency between individuals is large and can be difficult to identify. In fact, when coaches, physiologists, and biomechanists are asked to review films of endurance athletes to determine visually who is the most efficient runner, the rankings by simple observation do not correlate well with actual measures of oxygen uptake, which are now used as the criterion for the newer term for efficiency, **economy** (oxygen cost at given speed or workload).

The integration of subdisciplines of kinesiology is shown in Figure 2.1, which illustrates how individual efficiency or running economy is influenced by psychomotor factors (motivated, tired, or over-trained), physiological factors (trained or untrained, maximal heart rate, stroke volume),

biomechanical factors (gait movements, muscle and joint geometry), biochemical factors (lactate threshold, glycogen depleted, number of muscle fibers recruited at a given speed), and other factors (training level, gender, experience, age). By understanding and obtaining measures of the factors in the figure, you can gain a better understanding of the economy of running and predict performance more accurately.

In this chapter, you will learn about the knowledge base of kinesiology and why you need to integrate the knowledge of subdisciplines of kinesiology into your academic training to optimize evidence-based learning and your problem-solving skills. You will also learn about concepts that you can use in your preparation for careers in kinesiology now and for your future.

## Physical Activity in Health, Wellness, and Quality of Life

As you learned in Chapter 1, physical inactivity is the fourth leading cause of death worldwide. Youth, adults, and older adults throughout the world are not active enough to achieve optimal health. Physical activity promotion is based on health behavior, health education, and public health programming efforts that extend well beyond the prevention of overweight and obesity. Increased mortality is not the only result of inactivity. Disability prevention is also one of the other key areas (like cardiovascular health, energy balance, musculoskeletal health, and mental health) where physical activity seems to make important health contributions. For example, studies using physical activity interventions to prevent falls among older adults provide strong evidence that the integration of kinesiology concepts is required to successfully promote physical activity in health, wellness, and quality of life across the lifespan.

The 2008 Physical Activity Guidelines for Americans Advisory Committee Report (PAGAC) reviews the scientific evidence that lower levels of functional health are related to low levels of musculoskeletal health (low muscle mass and low muscle function). **Functional health** (also called Health-Related Quality of Life) has been defined by Raven and colleagues as the ability to maintain health and wellness by reducing or controlling your health problems and maintaining your physical independence through **functional abilities** (such as physical movement for transportation, walking, and preventing avoidable falls), activities of daily living (ADL; such as dressing and self-feeding), and instrumental activities of daily living (IADL; such as housework and shopping for groceries).[4]

**Figure 2.1** | Kinesiology Subdiscipline Performance Factors Related to Individual Runners That Impact Running

*Source:* Adapted from P. R. Cavanagh and R. Kram, "The Efficiency of Human Movement: A Statement of the Problem," *Medicine and Science in Sports and Exercise* 17 (1985): 304–308.

The close relationship between physical activity and the lower risk for functional/mobility limitations based on nine research studies is shown in Figure 2.2. As one gets more physically active (versus remaining inactive–level 1) at moderate (level 1) to higher levels (4 and 5) for extended periods of time (like 150 minutes per week), their risk of functional limitations or decreased mobility is reduced. Most falls among older adults are associated with declines in muscular strength, reaction time, and balance that can all be counteracted at least to some degree with appropriate physical activity interventions that reduce fall risk. A basic understanding of the kinesiology subdisciplines of exercise physiology, biomechanics, behavioral sciences, and public health as well as others is necessary to determine how to help people, particularly older adults, avoid a sedentary lifestyle, develop and maintain functional health, and cope with and adapt mentally and physically to mobility challenges, medical management issues, and rehabilitation situations.

## Scientific Foundations of Physical Activity

Many university undergraduate kinesiology departments place a major emphasis on academic preparation in science-based courses such as exercise physiology, biomechanics, motor learning/motor development, sports medicine, psychology of physical activity or sport, and others that often require prerequisites from other science-related fields (biology, chemistry, etc.) as part of a common curricular theme. However, these course offerings are usually delivered without integration with each other (stuck in silos) with the hope that you as a student will use the scientific concepts from these courses independently to solve real-life professional challenges such as:

▸ How do you increase teens' physical activity during school physical education classes?

▸ How do you optimize the physical rehabilitation experience of a patient after hip replacement so she can return to full mobility?

▸ How do you coach and manage an elite club soccer team for success?

▸ How do you develop an adult kettle bell conditioning class for weight management?

The evolution of the scientific foundations in kinesiology has been rapid, but many undergraduates have not been able to acquire evidence-based practice skills to apply to their careers. As a result, some have suggested that the field, particularly surrounding professionals who guide and prescribe exercise for individuals and populations, has become rife with "misinformation and bogus facts."[5] Although you should embrace and master the scientific foundations of kinesiology in your own academic undergraduate preparation, it is also wise for you to focus on how to apply the science you are learning—that is, how to translate that information into your own problem-solving skill sets for in-school and out-of-school challenges.

## Cultural, Historical, and Philosophical Dimensions of Physical Activity

Are you regularly physically active? Why or why not? Are you aware of the history of kinesiology? Do you know why it is the primary discipline shaping your future career, or how the curricula you are studying have been shaped by cultural, historical, and philosophical changes over time? What is your personal philosophy about why the concepts of kinesiology are important to society as a whole? The answers to all of these questions—which address the present social relevance of kinesiology—require not only your personal reflection, but also a working knowledge and application of cultural, historical, and philosophical concepts.

Cultural, historical, and philosophical factors all have shaped the subdisciplines of kinesiology and continue to enhance their evolution as fields of study. By understanding the influence of these factors on kinesiology, you will be better at predicting and developing successful strategies for future programming related to the discipline, and better at avoiding strategies from the past that did not work and likely will not now. Whether or not you have enjoyed the study of these topics in the past,

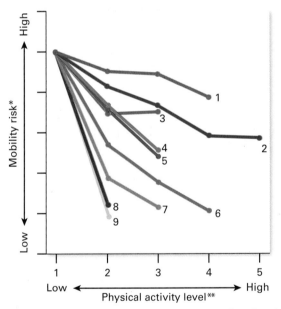

*High mobility risk is associated with lower functional health and an increased risk for falls.
**Based on results of nine large studies.

**Figure 2.2** | Relationship between Higher Physical Activity Levels and the Risk of Functional Limitations or Decreased Mobility

*Note:* The largest improvements occur when one moves from being inactive to moderate levels of physical activity.

*Source:* Adapted from "Physical Activity Guidelines Advisory Committee Report, 2008" (Washington, DC: U.S. Department of Health and Human Services, 2008), G6–7.

it is important for you now to learn to draw upon cultural, historical, and philosophical knowledge to answer simple questions that are commonly posed in everyday kinesiology decision-making situations, such as developing a business model approach to health and fitness. For instance, in strategic organizational planning sessions in a business setting, colleagues often develop mission/vision statements based on questions like: Where are we in terms of performance? Are we meeting our customers' expectations? Where have we been and what have we been doing? Where are we going now, and how are we going to get there?

Since the 1800s, the YMCA (now known as the Y) has been an example of a classic business model of health/fitness that integrates the cultural, historical, and philosophical aspects of kinesiology. Currently the Y's areas of focus include promoting youth development, healthy living, and social responsibility.

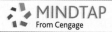

### The Y and Kinesiology

**Go to your MindTap course** now to learn more about the cultural, historical, and philosophical aspects of and the diverse activities offered through the Y. Have you ever been to a Y facility?

The importance of having an appreciation for the culture, history, and philosophy of kinesiology and the ability to integrate these dimensions becomes evident when, for example, you consider the Olympic movement and its global impact on sports. Do the Olympic Games affect physical activity behaviors of the people who watch these events? The leadership and promoters of numerous Olympic Games (past and present) have pronounced that the games as national and international events often stimulate more physical activity and sports participation worldwide, and yet there is no scientific evidence to support such statements.[6] Indeed, one might argue that the games promote sedentary behavior for spectators, which is just the opposite of common promotion messages we see in the media concerning many other sporting events.

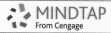

### Tour the Olympic Study Center

**Go to your MindTap course** now to learn more about the Olympic Movement and resources available at the Olympic Resources Centre.

## The Practice of Physical Activity

If you are a kinesiology major or minor, it makes sense that you should be part of the culture by being physically active yourself. As with any academic discipline, professionals are always judged at least to some degree by behaviors—such as being physically active or sedentary—they display to other professionals and others. Just as it seems logical for a health care professional to refrain from smoking cigarettes or using tobacco, it makes sense that you, as a kinesiology professional, should be a role model of sorts for others who are inactive and "lead from the front" by engaging in physical activity. Being physically active during your kinesiology training can take many forms, such as participating in a physical activity skills course, participating in your own regular exercise routine, playing on a collegiate team or in a club sport, participating in campus recreation activities, or working in a professional physical activity–related practicum or internship. You do not necessarily need to be an elite athlete or someone who can demonstrate all levels of accomplishment, but you should recognize that your professional credibility may suffer if you yourself do not practice and exhibit positive physical activity behaviors.

However you choose to practice physical activity as a kinesiology student, it should become part of your professional credentials. Although your participation in specific physical activities most likely will change over your professional career and lifespan (see Chapter 1), by remaining in the culture you can more effectively integrate your personal experience with the science and art of kinesiology to help others solve their physical activity challenges.

# Academic Kinesiology Course and Professional Preparation

By now you should be very familiar with the requirements, including the coursework, you must complete at your academic institution to obtain your undergraduate degree in a kinesiology-related field. Figure 2.3 is an integration model showing how many of the kinesiology subdiscipline courses you will encounter are related to achieving goals such as functional health, goal-oriented physical fitness outcomes, and peak performance. The model shows how functional health should be a common goal that you encourage individuals and populations you work with to achieve. By integrating and applying your KSAs from the various kinesiology subdisciplines, you can also help a diversity of populations achieve their high-order goals such as physical fitness and peak performance. The proposed model shown in Figure 2.3 also links professional training for jobs and careers that promote physical activity concepts supported by the U.S. National Physical Activity Plan (NPAP) (see page 36 for NPAP MindTap activity later in this chapter).

*Why should all kinesiology majors and minors take an interest in history, philosophy, and culture?*

We discussed the link between sociology of sports and kinesiology in the previous section. But how do history and philosophy link to kinesiology? A current example of historical linkages can be found in the American College of Sports Medicine (ACSM) initiative Exercise Is Medicine (EIM), which is a program designed to help physicians emphasize regular physical activity and exercise for their patients. Although this program initiative integrates exercise across several disciplines, it is not a new social message as the concept was first promoted by the Greek physicians Hippocrates and Galen as the "original laws of health."[7]

Philosophy in kinesiology involves the study of the mind and body and how they are related to factors such as the laws of nature, truth, individual goals/beliefs, and social experiences. Various areas of interest in the philosophy of kinesiology include ethics, moral decisions in sport, and studies of values related to play, games, and physical activity, to name a few. Philosophy within kinesiology addresses important questions related to the social values of sports and physical activity, the ethical implications of performance doping, and how sports mimic art (and vice versa).

Six traditional philosophies—existentialism, pragmatism, idealism, realism, naturalism, and humanism—have been applied to kinesiology and continue to influence thought in this area. Within the context of kinesiology, existentialism is the study of the individual (as opposed to society) as the center for sport philosophy. Pragmatism refers to attempts to explain the meaning of physical activities in our personal lives. Idealism is based on the premise that the reality of movement depends on what is contained within the individual's mind rather than what is outside of it. Realism suggests that there are facts (truths) that are independent of what we may believe or even of the available evidence. Naturalism refers to a belief that the laws of nature (rather than spiritual laws) govern fundamental decisions about physical activity and sports participation. Finally, humanism is a series of ideas that view movement and human development as holistic, and propose that the mind, body, and spirit cannot be divided related to physical activity. Although each of these principles, as well as others, help drive thought in the philosophy of kinesiology (philokinesiology), an in-depth discussion of them is beyond the scope of this text. A basic understanding of philosophy will help you to develop your own personal philosophy about effective physical activity promotion. See the table, which highlights standards of a physically educated person based upon expert opinions and the philosophy of the Society of Health and Physical Educators (SHAPE America).[8]

## SHAPE America Definition of a Physically Educated Person

SHAPE America's National Standards define what a student should know and be able to do as result of a quality physical education program. States and local school districts across the country use the National Standards to develop or revise existing standards, frameworks, and curricula.

A physically educated person:

| | |
|---|---|
| **Standard 1:** | The physically literate individual demonstrates competency in a variety of motor skills and movement patterns. |
| **Standard 2:** | The physically literate individual applies knowledge of concepts, principles, strategies, and tactics related to movement and performance. |
| **Standard 3:** | The physically literate individual demonstrates the knowledge and skills to achieve and maintain a health-enhancing level of physical activity and fitness. |
| **Standard 4:** | The physically literate individual exhibits responsible personal and social behavior that respects self and others. |
| **Standard 5:** | The physically literate individual recognizes the value of physical activity for health, enjoyment, challenge, self-expression, and/or social interaction. |

*Source:* SHAPE America, Society of Health and Physical Educators, "National Standards for K-12 Physical Education," www.shapeamerica.org/standards/pe. Copyright 2013, SHAPE America – Society of Health and Physical Educators, 1900 Association Drive, Reston, VA 20191, www.shapeamerica.org. All rights reserved. Used with permission.

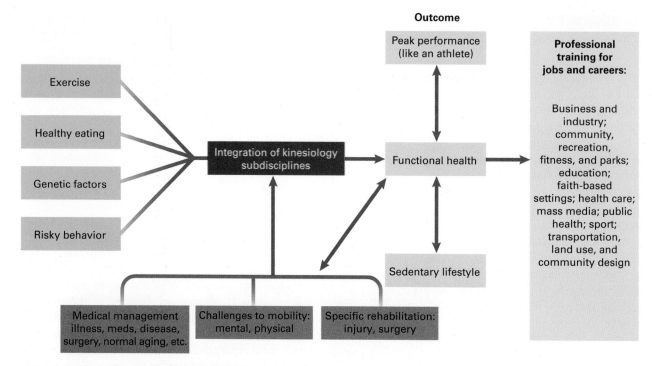

**Figure 2.3 | Factors That Influence the Promotion of Physical Activity and Health, Physical Fitness, and Peak Performance for Kinesiology Professionals.** The arrows indicate the integration of multiple factors that should be considered by kinesiologists to help individuals and populations achieve health, physical fitness, and peak performance goals based on their professional training experiences.

By effectively evaluating the lifestyle behaviors and health status of individuals and populations, you can and should promote functional health through any of the kinesiology-related careers for which you are academically prepared. The following subsections of the text are adapted from the American Academy of Kinesiology and highlight various subdiscipline courses that you will likely encounter during your academic preparation and the KSAs from each course required to succeed in your career goals.

An earlier section mentioned the introductory courses in other disciplines that prepare you for your courses in kinesiology. These courses include but are not limited to biology, math, physics, and psychology. In the following section you will first learn why it is important to integrate previous coursework with the courses you are taking in kinesiology and how to do so, using real-life, specific examples. You will also learn, through examples, about integrated problem solving in relationship to professional preparation.

### Exercise Physiology

Exercise physiology is a common core course for all major and minors in kinesiology. Exercise physiology has its foundations in biology and how the body's various systems respond to exercise training and detraining. As described in the previous chapter, exercise physiology will help you describe the biological factors that affect exercise and sports performance. The general applications of

exercise physiology include: (1) human performance; (2) physical activity and fitness; (3) growth, development, and aging; and (4) prevention and rehabilitation from disease.[9] Figure 2.4 illustrates how you might use the concepts that you will learn about in your exercise physiology course, including:

- Epidemiology, physical activity, exercise, and health
- Basic training principles for exercise
- Neuromuscular responses and adaptations to exercise
- Basics of exercise metabolism
- Fuel use during exercise
- Hormonal regulation of metabolism during exercise
- Exercise, obesity, metabolic syndrome, and diabetes
- The cardiovascular system and exercise
- Cardiovascular adaptations to an exercise program
- The respiratory system and exercise
- Measurement of common physiological responses to exercise
- Basics of nutrition and exercise
- Nutritional strategies and ergogenic aids to enhance exercise
- Body composition and weight management
- Adaptations to environmental extremes: heat, cold, altitude, and air pollution

## Biomechanics

Biomechanics is a diverse field of study that primarily focuses on the mechanical aspects of human movement. These aspects include concepts such as acceleration, velocity, force, mass, torque, and angular velocity. As described previously, biomechanics has its roots in the application of physics to human movement. The study of biomechanics includes numerous areas of interest related to kinesiology including muscle mechanics and modeling, human factors, ergonomics, sports techniques, and others. Hamill (2007) reviewed the guidelines recommended for undergraduate biomechanics in 2003 by the Biomechanics Academy of the National Association for Sport and Physical Education (NASPE) and suggested that students should recognize and achieve the following goals: (1) apply biomechanics competencies to human movement and (2) apply anatomical bases to human movement.[10]

Figure 2.5 illustrates how you might think about using the concepts from your biomechanics course to understand and evaluate movement, coordination, movement disorders associated with injury, muscle imbalances, aging effects on movement, and congenital conditions.

## Motor Learning, Motor Control, and Motor Development or Motor Behavior

Motor learning and **motor control** are sciences that generally focus on learning and the process of skill acquisition associated with human movement. How do children learn skills related to baseball or soccer? Why do some do better than others? Can a patient who has

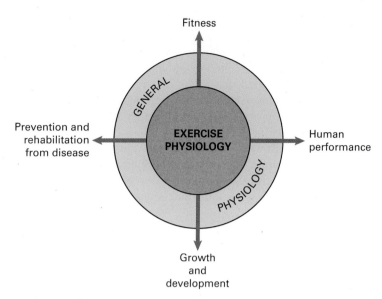

**Figure 2.4** | Exercise Physiology, a Subdiscipline of General Physiology. Prerequisites to an exercise physiology course should be a basic understanding of anatomy and systems physiology. The general applications of exercise physiology for the undergraduate kinesiology major consist of (1) human performance, (2) fitness, (3) growth and development, and (4) prevention and rehabilitation from disease.

*Source:* Adapted from J. Ivy, "Exercise Physiology: A Brief History and Recommendations Regarding Content Requirements for the Kinesiology Major," *Quest* 59 (2007): 39.

had a massive stroke learn to move or walk again? As compared with motor learning, motor control is more focused on how the neuromuscular system activates and coordinates movement patterns and stability with respect to behaviors and environmental factors (such as smooth versus rough surfaces). **Motor development** is generally the study of changes in motor behavior over

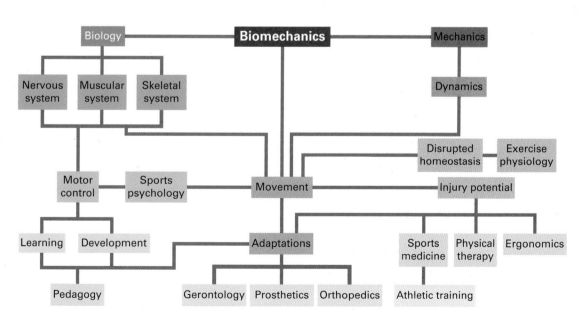

**Figure 2.5** | Integration of Biomechanics and Movement-Related Disciplines

time or the lifespan. In most undergraduate kinesiology programs, students will take core courses such as motor learning and/or motor development with concepts from motor control integrated into one or both courses. Ulrich and Reeve have argued that at the undergraduate level it may be more effective to study motor learning, motor control, and motor development together as facets of **motor behavior**.[11]

Figure 2.6 illustrates some of the concepts you will learn in your motor behavior coursework and how you might apply the KSAs you acquire to problem-solving motor skill challenges for individuals and populations across the lifespan.

## Public Health

Public health encompasses many disciplines in an effort to promote and protect health and prevent disease and disability in defined populations and communities.[12] How can physical inactivity be treated as a public health problem in the same way that cigarette smoking is? Are there effective public policy changes (such as creating safe, accessible places to be physically active) that a city government can enact? As you learned in Chapter 1, physical activity in public health has emerged as a new subdiscipline of kinesiology that provides opportunities to become certified as a physical activity and public health practitioner by the National Society of Physical Activity Practitioners in Public Health (NSPAPPH) and the American College of Sports Medicine.

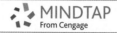

### Certification Process

**Go to your MindTap course** to complete an activity that will help you understand the process for certification as a physical activity and public health practitioner.

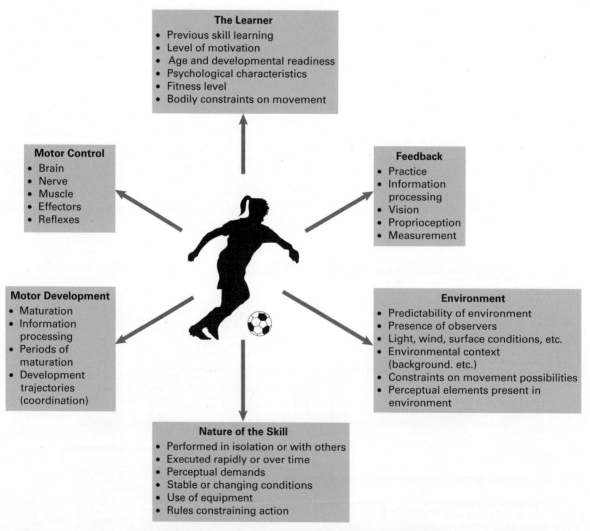

**Figure 2.6** | Integration of Motor Learning with Motor Control, Motor Development, Motor Behavior Factors, and Physical Activity

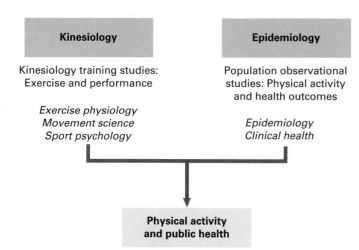

Figure 2.7 | The Merger of Kinesiology and Epidemiology to Create Physical Activity and Public Health

*Source:* Based on H. W. Kohl and T. D. Murray, *Foundations of Physical Activity and Public Health* (Champaign, IL: Human Kinetics, 2012).

Physical activity and public health has emerged as a global field of academic study that includes overlapping fields of study from epidemiology and kinesiology as shown in Figure 2.7. Figure 2.8 shows that the epidemiology and exercise science fields have emerged since 1900 to include population studies (how physical activity can improve health, physical fitness, and peak performance), behavioral science, and environment and policy concerns. For example, public health and physical activity has been used to reorient traditional school physical education courses toward health-related physical education (HRPE) that provides opportunities for students to be active, have fun, learn movement and behavioral skills, and promote current and future physical activity and fitness.[13]

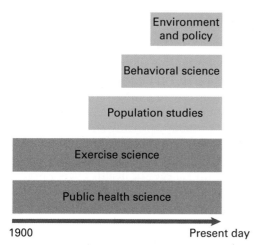

Figure 2.8 | Physical Activity and Public Health—The Emergence of a Subdiscipline

*Source:* Based on H. W. Kohl and T. D. Murray, *Foundations of Physical Activity and Public Health* (Champaign, IL: Human Kinetics, 2012).

## Human Behavior

In this text, we include **human behavior** as a study area that incorporates the traditional kinesiology study areas of sport/exercise psychology (review Figures 1.1 and 1.8) as well as behavior change for physical activity promotion. Study of human behavior in kinesiology is also linked to numerous aspects of mental health and physical activity (see Chapter 8 for more).

Human behavior in kinesiology historically is grounded in basic psychology and applies psychological principles to sports and exercise. How can athletes (professional golfers, for example) mentally train to become better competitors? What behavioral techniques can be used to help people begin and maintain a personal physical activity program? Academic preparation with an emphasis on the basic KSAs related to human behavior involves integrating and applying topics such as those listed in Table 2.1. McCullagh and Wilson have recommended that undergraduates in kinesiology understand both how psychological variables impact physical activity participation and how physical activity participation can impact psychological variables.[14]

## Philosophy, History, and Sociology

Academic preparation for a career in kinesiology most likely will require acquisition of knowledge in one of these areas should you decide to go on for a graduate degree. You would follow up by taking specialized

Table 2.1 | Key Topics in Human Behavior for Kinesiology

| |
| --- |
| 1. History of sport and exercise psychology |
| 2. Personality and sport |
| 3. Motivation |
| 4. Arousal, anxiety, and stress |
| 5. Group behavior |
| 6. Feedback and behavioral principles and applications |
| 7. Performance modification |
| 8. Self |
| 9. Injuries, overtraining, and burnout |
| 10. Addictive and unhealthy behaviors |
| 11. Social variables |
| 12. Individual variables |
| 13. Children in sports and coaching behaviors |

*Source:* Modified from P. McCullough and G. Wilson, "Psychology of Physical Activity: What Should Students Know?" *Quest* 59 (2007): 49.

kinesiology graduate courses related to philosophy, history, or sociology at the master's and/or doctoral levels. Review Chapter 1, pages 15–16 to re-examine the recommendations of Gill related to philosophy, history, and sociology applications to kinesiology.[15]

## Exercise Science

A key tenet of this text is the importance of integrating multiple subdisciplines into kinesiology. Exercise science is frequently referred to as an integration of multiple kinesiology subdisciplines, particularly for a professional application or career. As you learned in Chapter 1, effective professional training in exercise sciences requires you to integrate core information from areas such as exercise physiology, biomechanics, human behavior, motor behavior, and clinical interventions. For example, a cardiac rehabilitation specialist might have a patient who wants to participate in a phase 2 program (outpatient hospital-based) including clinical exercise electrocardiogram (ECG) monitoring, but hopes to safely transition to a phase 3 out-patient (non–hospital-based) program in which he can swim in his own backyard pool. To optimize his rehabilitation success, the specialist should consider the following questions regarding the safety and potential effectiveness of a plan for the patient:

▸ How well does the patient swim?

▸ Is he an economical (lower physiological energy cost) swimmer biomechanically (does he use smooth or thrashing strokes)?

▸ Is the patient self-motivated enough to begin and then maintain a home swimming program (human behavior and motor behavior)?

▸ Is he likely to be compliant in taking his medications, recognizing side effects with exercise, and consistently staying within his exercise limitations (clinical interventions)?

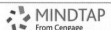 **MINDTAP** From Cengage

**Specializing in Cardiac Rehabilitation**

**Go to your MindTap course** to complete an activity that will help you understand more about becoming a cardiac rehabilitation specialist.

## Sport Management

The most common job requirements for sport management professionals are event development, promotion, and implementation. How can city recreation leagues be optimized to maximize physical activity participation?

How can mass events such as 5K fun runs for children be managed safely and for maximal participation? For example, a program manager at a large city nonprofit sports organization might be placed in charge of administrating and coordinating a large (20,000 participants) marathon run (26.2 miles). In order to have a safe and successful fund-raising event, the manager will need to draw from her or his undergraduate course preparation and service learning/internship experiences to resolve issues such as:

▸ How many medical support staff do I need for safety? What kinds of medical issues should be expected and what types of medical specialists do we need (cardiologists, orthopedics specialists, general practitioners, volunteers)?

▸ How do I decide when to close the course (incidence of injuries increases dramatically after 5 to 6 hours due to fatigue—physiological and biomechanical factors)?

▸ What is the most effective way to communicate to participants and volunteers throughout the course (communication and leadership skills)?

▸ How much money should participants be charged to enter the run based on the economics of providing a quality event and also generating sufficient revenue for the organization (business skills)?

To learn more about sport management issues in administrating and coordinating a large running event, use your favorite Internet search engine to search for the phrase "how to organize your own race for runners." In Chapter 12 of this text, you will learn much more about kinesiology, sport, and sport management, as well as specific career opportunities in these areas.

## Athletic Training

How can athletes be managed to maximize their participation and keep the risk of injury to a minimum? What are evidence-based strategies for athletic rehabilitation that allow an athlete to return to competition as quickly as possible after an injury? The majority of accredited athletic training programs currently are found in kinesiology departments, although there is a recent move promoted by the National Athletic Trainers' Association (NATA) to align more with colleges of health-related professions.[16] Some current undergraduate level subject matter areas associated with kinesiology academic preparation are shown in Table 2.2.

A listing of the primary practice settings for athletic trainers is shown in Table 2.3. As you can see, career field opportunities are quite diverse. Please see the NATA website for current updates about job options for athletic trainers (www.nata.org).

**Table 2.2** | Common Athletic Training Core Requirement Subject Matter Areas

| FOUNDATIONAL COURSES |
| --- |
| ▶ Human physiology |
| ▶ Human anatomy |
| ▶ Exercise physiology |
| ▶ Kinesiology/biomechanics |
| ▶ Nutrition |
| ▶ Therapeutic modalities |
| ▶ Acute care of injury and illness |
| ▶ Statistics and research design |
| ▶ Strength training and reconditioning |

| PROFESSIONAL COURSE CONTENT AREAS |
| --- |
| ▶ Risk management and injury/illness prevention |
| ▶ Pathology of injury/illness |
| ▶ Assessment of injury/illness |
| ▶ General medical conditions and disabilities |
| ▶ Therapeutic exercise; rehabilitative techniques |
| ▶ Health care administration |
| ▶ Weight management and body composition |
| ▶ Psychosocial intervention and referral |
| ▶ Medical ethics and legal issues |
| ▶ Pharmacology |
| ▶ Professional development and responsibilities |

*Note:* See www.nataec.org for more information.

*Source:* From D. H. Perrin, "Athletic Training: From Physical Education to Allied Health," *Quest* 59 (2007): Table 6, 118.

**Table 2.3** | Primary Practice Settings for Athletic Trainers

| |
| --- |
| High school: 15.76% |
| College/university: 19.53% |
| Professional sports: 10.52% |
| Sports medicine clinics: 18.29% |
| Clinical/industrial: 4.27% |
| Hospital: 3.45% |
| Other: 28.18% (Public safety, military, occupational health, etc.) |

*Note:* See www.nata.org for more information.

*Source:* From D. H. Perrin, "Athletic Training: From Physical Education to Allied Health," *Quest* 59 (2007): Table 7, 118.

Athletic trainers constantly are required to integrate their kinesiology course work preparation into clinical practice. Table 2.4 provides an example of this application of knowledge in practice, listing the numerous factors that are associated with anterior cruciate ligament (ACL) injury and noting how they are integrated with kinesiology.

## Physical Therapy/Occupational Therapy

Professional training or careers in physical therapy (PT) or occupational therapy (OT) will require an integration of kinesiology course work and clinical volunteer/nonvolunteer work to problem-solve as part of your day-to-day practice. What is the most optimal way for a patient who has had an artificial knee implanted to rehabilitate after the surgery? What complications might be expected? An example of the application of academic and clinical skills that is common to PT and OT professionals alike is conducting functional capacity testing of employees at worksites. Functional capacity testing can include evaluation of the cognitive and physical abilities of employees.

In many business and industry settings such as oil and gas refineries, overnight freight delivery services, public safety organizations such as police and fire departments, and hospitals, employees often have to perform physical tasks like lifting, carrying, climbing, opening valves, firefighting, and product loading. These types of work tasks require that employees be regularly evaluated for physiological factors (such as muscular strength and muscular

**Table 2.4** | Examples of Athletic Training/Kinesiology Linkages Using the Anterior Cruciate Ligament (ACL) Injury Model

| ACL ISSUE | KINESIOLOGY PROGRAM, COURSE, OR LABORATORY |
| --- | --- |
| Access of girls to organized youth sport | Philosophy/history of physical activity |
| Impact of Title IX on ACL injuries | Sociology of physical activity |
| Limb alignment issues | Biomechanics of physical activity |
| Laxity/neuromuscular response | Biomechanics and motor development |
| Sex hormones, laxity, and injury risk | Physiology of physical activity |
| Surgery and restoration of function | Motor behavior and pedagogy |
| Rehabilitation compliance | Sport and exercise psychology |

*Source:* From D. H. Perrin, "Athletic Training: From Physical Education to Allied Health," *Quest* 59 (2007): Table 9, 120.

endurance) and biomechanical factors (such as balance and mobility) as well as psychological factors (such as work satisfaction or concentration during monotonous work) that are related to levels of job performance and quality management. Functional capacity testing can help worksite leadership answer questions such as:

1. Can an employee physically perform a job task safely without assistance?

2. What jobs can an employee do safely and effectively post-employment?

3. How effective is functional capacity testing at predicting future job injuries?

4. What testing strategies are effective for optimizing injured employees' return to work?

Physical therapists and occupational therapists are constantly challenged to integrate effective tests selected based upon valid and reliable measures, potential legal disputes, and economic screening procedures.

---

### Kinesiology in Practice: Measurement Issues in Kinesiology

Andrew S. Jackson, PED, and colleagues were some of the first investigators to use employment strength assessment in the oil and gas industry to determine the strength requirements of many job tasks. Dr. Jackson is an expert in measurement issues related to kinesiology and has conducted several studies to answer questions such as:

1. What are the critical physically demanding tasks of a specific job?

2. What strength tests actually measure job-specific strength (validity—whether a test measures what it should accurately)?

3. How reliable (consistent) are strength tests used to predict performance at the worksite?

4. Can a battery of strength tests be developed with reasonable cut scores that evaluate safe and effective job performance?

Dr. Jackson identified isometric (static) strength testing as an effective way to predict performance for a variety of specific job tasks such as valve cracking (opening and closing a tightly-closed valve—a challenge for refinery workers). In numerous technical reports, he reported that he could accurately predict the ability to crack valves, as well as perform other job tasks, successfully at worksites by using the sum of three static tests: grip, arm lift, and back lift on an electronic load cell.

As you can tell from the static strength-testing example described, the discipline of kinesiology requires that you learn to apply measurement techniques regularly to solve real-life problems.

---

### Physical Standards for Public Safety Employees

A very real-world application of kinesiology involves public safety employees (police and other law enforcement personnel, firefighters, etc.). How much fitness is necessary for public safety employees to do their job effectively? How much upper body strength does a firefighter need to be able to carry an adult victim to safety in an emergency? How fast must a police officer be able to run to capture a suspect? These are critical occupational kinesiology questions that arise every day. For more on physical standards for public safety employees, see your local public safety physical testing standards for firefighters and police.

## Teaching Physical Education/Pedagogy

Students interested in working as physical education (PE) teachers will need to integrate a variety of **pedagogy** (art and science of teaching) strategies to help their pupils achieve the goals of health-optimizing PE (HOPE) (see Chapter 1). For example, if you teach PE to sixth and seventh graders, you most likely will be required to assess the fitness levels of your students and collect data yearly as part of state accountability measures for effective teaching. Many school districts throughout the United States have used assessments such as the FITNESSGRAM®, which has been adopted by the President's Council on Fitness, Sports and Nutrition (see www.fitness.gov for more information), to determine the physical fitness levels of their students. FITNESSGRAM is based on a variety of assessments, such as mile run or PACER, body mass index (BMI), curl-ups, trunk lift, push-ups, and the back-saver sit and reach in the predetermined healthy or at-risk zones, evaluated on criterion-related levels of health. You may also find that you will have to develop lesson plans and integrate and implement effective strategies to achieve 50% of class time with students engaged in vigorous or moderate-intensity physical activity, with an emphasis on increasing physical activity and fitness performance outcomes.

---

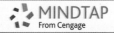
MINDTAP
From Cengage

**FITNESSGRAM®**

**Go to your MindTap course** to complete an activity that will help you understand the basics of this comprehensive educational, reporting, and promotional tool used to assess physical fitness and physical activity levels for children.

---

## Coaching

Professional preparation for successful coaching careers based on kinesiology focuses not only on integration of kinesiology subdisciplines that help optimize performance such as physiology, biomechanics, motor behavior, and human behavior, but also on safety and public health outcomes. So, how does a coach integrate various aspects of kinesiology into coaching? The following scenario is just one example.

Imagine a football coach has an athlete who experiences helmet-to-helmet contact with another player while tackling an opponent in a game, and then comes to the sideline in a bit of a "fog" or "zoned out" state but does not lose consciousness. What should the coach do? If you are a veteran coach or a former athlete who has experienced this situation, you know that this is a difficult question because concussion management has become a moving target in recent years. In the past, a coach would acknowledge the athlete had his "bell rung" and then send him back into the game, maybe even on the next play. However, the science of head injury or trauma has evolved greatly, and a coach would be considered negligent for such actions today. So now what does a competent coach do?

Perhaps a first step would be for the coach to be familiar with laws in his or her state concerning concussion care and be certified in basic first aid, cardiopulmonary resuscitation (CPR), and automated electrical defibrillators (AED). If the coach has attended a recent coaching clinic, he or she will likely be aware of the latest scientific evidence regarding concussions based on the American College of Sports Medicine [ACSM] Team Physician Consensus Statement, 2012, produced in collaboration with six major professional sports medicine organizations.[17] If so, the coach should know to suspect that the athlete has a head injury and refer the athlete to a health care provider who is available at the game (team physician, certified athletic trainer, etc.). The coach should recognize that when concussion is suspected there is no same-day return to play for the athlete.

---

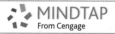

**Concussions**

**Go to your MindTap course** to complete an activity that provides coaches with the latest updated policies for preventing and managing concussion injuries in sport.

---

You may be asking yourself, "Why does a coach need to know about a team physician consensus statement? I'm not a physician. Why should I need to know anything about this problem? I'll just refer the athlete properly and I'll have met my obligation. I only care about when the athlete can return to play." Yes, those comments would be partly correct, but today coaches at all levels are expected to be part of a management team that works with physicians, athletic trainers, and other health care personnel to maintain the health and safety of their athletes. In fact, if today's coach has not learned to integrate kinesiology into coaching, he or she will be lost with regard to proper concussion management and perhaps become negligent after the fact. For example, the following scientific and clinical factors are involved in the current climate of effective concussion management (ACSM):

- Biomechanics of the contact
- Epidemiology
- Preseason planning and assessment
- Same-day evaluation and treatment
- Post-day evaluation and treatment
- Diagnostic testing
- Return to play (RTP)
- Complications of concussion
- Prevention
- Legislative actions

Therefore, if a coach thinks his athlete will have no problems with RTP, he is mistaken and will be disappointed because he lacks understanding of at least the scientific basics of current best practices related to concussions.

## Physical Activity and Public Health Practice

As you learned in Chapter 1, an emerging field that combines kinesiology and public health involves training physical activity and public health practitioners. If you are interested in preparing for careers related to this emerging area, you will have numerous opportunities to integrate your academic and practical skills as they relate to developing and implementing community and population interventions. If you are asked to develop and implement a physical activity plan for your local community as part of your job, you will need to seek out existing plans/guidelines that can help you be successful, such as a state plan like Active Texas 2020.[18]

Active Texas 2020 is one of a few state plans that have been developed thus far.[19] It reflects the U.S. National Physical Activity Plan and is designed to help meet more state and local needs for translation and mobilization of physical activity plans for local communities. Active Texas 2020 provides key strategies that can help physical activity and public health practitioners develop and implement physical activity interventions to improve the health of individuals and populations at the community level. Active Texas 2020 encourages the incorporation of the following eight guiding principles that require the integration and mastery of concepts from kinesiology and public health:

1. Physical activity improves health. This requires a strong understanding of the 2008 Physical Activity Guidelines for Americans and the 2008 Physical Activity Guidelines Advisory Committee Report.

2. Public health approaches to increasing physical activity are needed to improve the health of populations. One source that helps provide insight about this principle is "The Community Guide,"[20] which provides information about effective physical activity intervention strategies.

3. Make the healthier choice. Physical activity/public health practitioners need to consider effective strategies that help increase physical activity by creating more options and removing more barriers for communities and populations.

4. All health is local. You will need to understand how to recruit local leaders to implement national and state policies that promote physical activity considering factors such as safety, access, and local health care benefits.

5. Health is everyone's business. This requires an understanding of how physical activity can improve individual/population health and well-being and have positive effects on business productivity, health insurance costs, and a community's growth and quality of life.

6. Prioritize leadership, collaboration, and partnerships. To be effective you will need to help build relationships that bring community leaders together in partnerships that contribute to a shared vision of physical activity interventions in the community.

7. Work from the evidence base. Instead of "reinventing the wheel" by developing and implementing physical activity interventions that are either unproven or have failed in the past, practitioners should seek out and use/modify evidenced-based programs that work such as those described by "The Community Guide."

8. Evaluate the effectiveness. All physical activity and public health practitioners should learn to effectively measure and document how well their program interventions work and adopt strategies to make them more effective for the future.

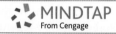

### National Physical Activity Plan

**Go to your MindTap course** to complete an activity that allows you to view the U.S. National Physical Activity plan with attention to the following sectors: business and industry; recreation, fitness and parks; education; faith-based settings; healthcare; mass media; public health; sports; transportation, land use, and community design.

## Special Populations

Finally, one area that has been often overlooked or minimized within kinesiology is working with special populations or those with special needs. Historically, kinesiology majors usually defined special populations as those individuals who are physically or intellectually challenged. In the past, kinesiology majors would only come in contact with the intellectually challenged in pedagogical practices within school systems. More recently, the topic of special populations has expanded beyond the historical context and now can be considered a subdiscipline within kinesiology pedagogy, exercise science, and public health. An emerging definition of **special populations** includes those individuals who have either acute or chronic conditions that limit or require modifications to standard physical activity practices.[21] Subpopulations within special populations include children, the elderly, pregnant women, the physically disabled, those with chronic diseases, and the intellectually challenged. Each of these groups has special needs or limitations that could hamper their ability to be physically active, and yet we know that physical activity improves health and increases the lifespan. So it is the kinesiology practitioner's goal to develop modified activities that can improve the health of the individual while recognizing his or her limitations.

### Exercise for Everybody

Want to learn more about physical activity and special populations? **Go to your MindTap course** and read excerpts from "Exercise Is for Everybody," a series of articles from the American College of Sports Medicine.

# CAREER PLANNING IN KINESIOLOGY

*In Lesson 2, you will learn about examples of how physical activity promotion concepts in schools are integrated with the subdisciplines of kinesiology.*

- Exercise Physiology
- Biomechanics

- Sport/Exercise Psychology/Human Behavior
- Public Health
- Motor Learning and Motor Development

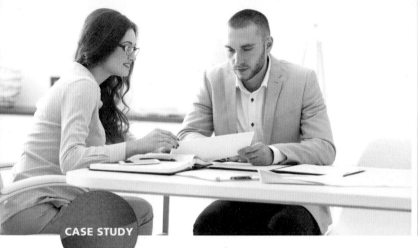

CASE STUDY

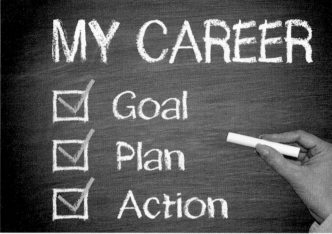

## In the real world . . .

Let's revisit Martijn and his goals: to earn an undergraduate degree in pre–physical therapy preparation in kinesiology, to secure his acceptance into and success in physical therapy school, and to eventually practice as a licensed and registered physical therapist. Read on about his career preparation challenges and take some time to apply what you learn from Martijn's experiences to your own academic professional preparation. Practice the career planning tips from the continued Real World feature that follows.

### Academic and Professional Plan One

When we last visited Martijn, he was a junior taking course work (such as exercise physiology, biomechanics, and motor learning) in kinesiology as prerequisites for his pre-PT degree. While Martijn was a good student (cumulative grade point average [GPA] of 2.95 with a 3.2 GPA in science-based courses), his grades were below the national GPA average that is required for acceptance to PT schools. He faced a lot of competition within his own department (which is common nationally) because more than 500 other students were also classified as pre-PT majors. Additionally, even though his university had an entry-level professional program leading to the doctor of physical

therapy (DPT) degree, which is designed for students who have a bachelor's degree and who are seeking a professional degree in physical therapy, this program only admitted 40 students per academic year. Even when looking statewide, there were only 12 institutions that offered DPT opportunities (average entering class size of 40). Thus, there were only 480 total spaces available yearly for those applying from pre-PT programs.

Martijn knew that other pre-PT skills are considered when evaluating candidates for admission to DPT programs, such as:

- Leadership roles as an undergraduate and/or graduate student
- Experience in various kinesiology laboratories
- Teaching assistant experiences
- PT volunteer activities in clinics and in the community
- Recommendations from professors, mentors, and employers

He felt very good about his own ancillary pre-PT skills, especially his volunteer experiences. Martijn had really enjoyed volunteering at a progressive local PT clinic where he learned about traditional PT treatments and therapies but also about other programs like workers' compensation testing, post-offer employment testing, drug testing, and functional health maintenance programs, which are becoming common revenue-generating programs for PTs nationally.

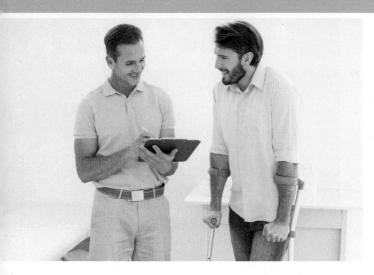

Have you ever thought about your career goals in the context of your own kinesiology GPA and external professional preparation such internships, practicums, work experiences, and service learning events? What careers do you think you will be qualified for with your degree, and what specific skills (besides a good GPA) do you think you will need to get hired? Perform a web search on two to three of the career fields from the AKA and NASPE websites and evaluate yourself by comparing what others recommend as general requirements for success to your own current credentials.

---

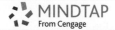
**MINDTAP**
From Cengage

**Matching Careers, Organizations and Degrees**

**Go to your MindTap course** to visit the American Kinesiology Association career center. Complete activities related to organizations that support various careers in kinesiology and degrees required.

---

## Reality Checks

Although Martijn had anticipated a lot of competition to get into PT school, he had not prepared himself for the real possibility of not getting accepted into PT school, and he had not developed a backup plan (or two) for an alternative career based on his kinesiology degree and the integration of the various subdisciplines. Despite his anxiety about his chances of getting accepted to DPT school, he applied to five schools and got an invitation for an interview at a program 30 miles away from where his parents lived. He felt fortunate to get an interview, but because he was so busy with his current schoolwork and lacked practical experience with interviewing, he just relied on his pre-PT buddies for advice about interviewing and the general PT admission process. Although his PT school interview was over a month away, Martijn decided to take his chances in the interview process without any additional preparation. One day prior to his PT school interview, he learned that there were 160 students interviewing for 40 spots, and it made him very anxious.

The night before the interview, Martijn didn't get much sleep and kept waking up wondering what questions he might be asked. How, realistically, could he compete against other candidates who had better grades and GRE scores? On the day of the interview Martijn arrived 15 minutes early. He noticed that, though he was nicely dressed (business causal), the other interview candidates he saw all looked more professionally dressed (traditional business). Martijn's interview lasted 30 minutes. Afterward, he felt like he had connected well with the interviewer. However, he thought he could have answered the general questions about his professional goals, strengths, and limitations much better if he had anticipated some of these questions ahead of time and practiced his answers, and also relaxed a bit more during the whole process. He found out a month later that he did not get into PT school and scored in the lowest third of all applicants interviewed. Although he was not too surprised by the results of the whole process, he felt a bit empty; though he was going to graduate with a degree in kinesiology, he did not know what job or career opportunities to pursue now that his dream of practicing physical therapy was not going to come true any time soon, if ever.

Although Martijn's DPT admission process turned out negatively for him, he knew he had learned a lot about aspects of this process he had not thought or been adequately educated about during his academic training preparation. For instance, he learned from other applicants that completing the DPT program would be costly (at least $75,000) and he would have had additional student loans to pay if he had been accepted. Although his parents had covered much of the costs of his undergraduate program, he still had $15,000 to pay back and would have had to rely primarily on loans for the DPT program. He also had not given much thought to potentially better alternative options such as pursuing an associate's degree in PT from a community college (PT assistant) first. An associate's degree would allow Martijn to begin work and thus finance his future educational opportunities. Have you thought realistically about the costs and benefits related to your pursuit of your own college education? It is always important to examine all your options for acquiring and repaying loans/grants as well as part-time and full-time employment opportunities to offset your current and future (post-graduation) financial obligations.

What would you have done differently than Martijn if you had been in his shoes during the PT application process? What sources of information would have better prepared Martijn for the process and its multiple potential outcomes?

## Postscript and Professional Plan Two

So what happened to Martijn after graduation? Well, things turned out just fine, but it took him a while to develop and implement a back-up career plan. The week after graduation he traveled to Sydney, Australia (a graduation gift from his parents) to spend a couple of weeks seeing the city and getting in some surf time. As he climbed the Sydney Harbor Bridge, Martijn envisioned how his future career planning was a lot like his bridge-climbing experience: it depended on several small initial steps, would take time, and would require the support of his fellow climbing teammates. When he returned home he took his parents' advice and visited an old friend of the family—a college professor/mentor—who suggested that Martijn pursue a master's degree in health administration and focus on future employment opportunities in health care management related to physical therapy. Martijn was ultimately successful and completed his master's of health administration (in two years) with a thesis on a PT-related topic. Upon graduation, he was employed immediately at a health promotion company as a junior executive. He has been with the company now for two years and is happy there.

| 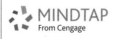 | Go to your MindTap course to complete the Case Study activity for this chapter.<br>Additional engagement activities related to this Case Study include Becoming a Physical Therapist and Finding Your Mentor. |
|---|---|

# What About You and Your Career?

Okay...what about you? What are your career plans? What plan do you have now and for the future to be successful with your kinesiology degree? Do you have a backup plan or two (unlike Martijn)? What professional KSAs do you currently have, and which ones do you need to develop for success? Where should you start? Perhaps one way to begin is to develop a vision about what you want to do. You should also strive to acquire twenty-first century learning skills, explore various accessible resources, become and remain coachable, develop and maintain a positive attitude, and become a life-long learner.

If you have visited some of the websites highlighted in this text or recommended by your instructor thus far, you probably already have an initial vision of what you want to do professionally. What twenty-first century learning skills do you need to be aware of and acquire to be competitive and happy as a kinesiology professional?

A framework of twenty-first century learning skills is illustrated in Figure 2.9.

By exploring a variety of accessible resources, you should be able to devise an initial career plan and acquire the skills to tweak the plan over time, become and remain coachable, develop and maintain a positive attitude, and become a lifelong learner. We suggest that you initiate (but not necessarily limit) your kinesiology career planning by accessing your own academic institution's career services website and then exploring multiple specific sites for professional success.

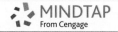

**Planning Your Career**

**Go to your MindTap course** to learn more about practical career-building tips usually available on your own college's website.

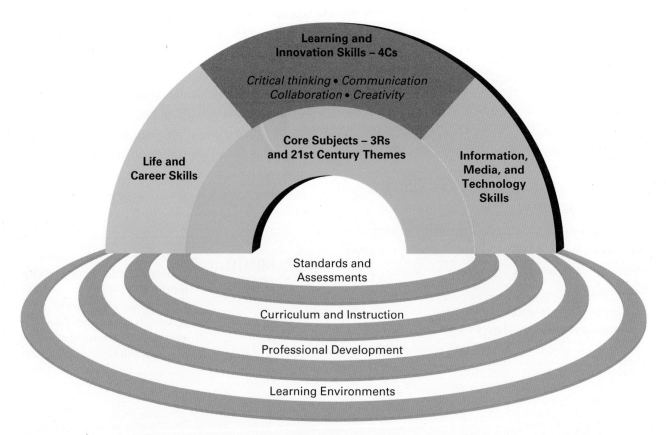

**Figure 2.9** | A Framework of 21st Century Learning Skills

*Source:* From J. Bellance and R. Brandt, *Century Skills: Rethinking How Students Learn* (Bloomington, IN: Solution Tree Press, 2010).

# People Matter Jack W. Berryman, Professor of Bioethics and Humanities*

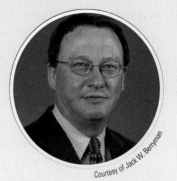

Courtesy of Jack W. Berryman

**Q: Why and how did you get into the field of kinesiology?**

**A:** *I wanted to be a high school baseball coach and physical education teacher, so I pursued an undergraduate degree in physical and health education at the same college my high school coach attended. During my senior year, after realizing that graduate credits were needed for permanent teacher certification in my state, I applied and was accepted into a master's degree program featuring exercise science and sports studies. Here, my interest shifted from coaching to studying the historical and sociological significance of sports in society.*

**Q: What was the major influence on you to work in the field?**

**A:** *My interest in the field came from a love of physical activity and sports. Several faculty members at the colleges I attended further influenced my career. The sports studies faculty at the University of Massachusetts, Amherst, were leaders in their respective fields: Guy Lewis (history), Harold Vander-Zwaag (philosophy), John Loy (sociology), and Ellen Gerber (history). My Ph.D. work was directed by Marvin Eyler at the University of Maryland, and he was a pivotal figure in my career.*

**Q: What are your current research interests, and how do you translate your research results to practitioners?**

**A:** *My research interests currently and over the past 40 years have been the historical study of sports, physical education, exercise science, and sports medicine. I have published my research in the literature of these fields to be readily available for practitioners. I have taught several different history classes for kinesiology majors and contributed chapters and summaries of historical trends to anthologies devoted to sports history, sports medicine, public health, and exercise science. My work*

*has been used in government publications pertaining to physical activity and public health. My expertise has also been solicited by medical and health writers to provide context and perspective for the reading public. As historian for the American College of Sports Medicine, my work is regularly disseminated to the membership.*

**Q: How do you stay physically active yourself and promote good health to others directly around you?**

**A:** *I have been a physically active person all of my life and greatly enjoy and appreciate the role that strength, endurance, and overall fitness play in my daily life. Before retirement, I exercised every lunch hour at the student gym on campus and did a combination of lifting and cardio. Now, at almost 70 years of age, I walk regularly, fish, canoe, and maintain two properties, which includes mowing, trimming, chopping wood, and general yardwork on more than seven acres. I try to promote good health to others by my example and with lectures and consultations explaining the centrality of physical activity in the medical regimens of ancient physicians like Hippocrates and Galen.*

**Q: How have you had to integrate the subdisciplines of kinesiology in your professional practice?**

**A:** *My teaching and research career has been guided and informed by my early studies that focused on the historical, sociological, psychological, and philosophical aspects of physical activity and sports. In addition, my research on the history of exercise science and sports medicine has been more meaningful and contextual because of the classes I took in exercise physiology and biomechanics.*

*Jack W. Berryman is Professor Emeritus in the Department of Bioethics and Humanities at the University of Washington. He is also an Adjunct Professor Emeritus, Department of Orthopaedics and Sports Medicine at the University of Washington School of Medicine.

In Chapter 1, we suggested that students review the Occupational Handbook of the Bureau of Labor Statistics (www.bls.gov/ooh/), which provides detailed information including descriptions, salaries, future forecasts for employment, and so on for a variety of career opportunities.

What resources does your school provide to help you develop your career plans? You should take the time to check out the websites referred to in this lesson and search for other Internet resources that will help you develop your initial career plan and future alternatives for backup. Learn from Martijn and others you know how to clarify and evaluate your kinesiology career goals.

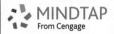 **MINDTAP** From Cengage | Now that you have completed this chapter, go to your MindTap course to complete all assigned activities. Check out the additional resources developed to help you apply the material in this chapter to your course and career goals.

## Chapter Summary

▸ The knowledge base of kinesiology "integrates information gained through experiencing physical activity, through professional application, and through multidimensional scholarly approaches to the study of physical activity—biological, medical, and health-related aspects, psychological and social-humanistic."

▸ The common core or knowledge base of kinesiology includes physical activity in health, wellness, and quality of life; scientific foundations of physical activity; cultural, historical, and philosophical dimensions of physical activity; and the practice of physical activity.

▸ Examples of integrating kinesiology concepts for solving societal issues include fall prevention and the promotion of functional health in the elderly.

▸ It is important to learn to integrate your KSAs from the subdisciplines of kinesiology including, but not limited to, exercise physiology, biomechanics, motor learning, motor control, motor development, human behaviors, philosophy, history, sociology, pedagogy, and measurement.

▸ It is important to recognize that physical activity and exercise are for everyone, and the field of kinesiology is expanding in reference to career opportunities to serve traditionally underserved populations.

▸ Your own career planning should include accessing and maximizing the use of your academic institution's career services website.

▸ One future vision for career success in kinesiology might include becoming and remaining coachable, developing and maintaining a positive attitude, and becoming a lifelong learner.

## Remember This

economy
functional abilities
functional health
human behavior

knowledge base of kinesiology
motor behavior
motor control
motor development

pedagogy
special populations

## For More Information

- Find updates and quick links to these and other epidemiology and exercise physiology-related sites in MindTap.

- Search for information about the American Kinesiology Association (AKA) and the knowledge base of kinesiology at www.americankinesiology.org.

- Search for information about kinesiology-related careers at the Society of Health and Physical Educators (SHAPE) America at www.shapeamerica.org.

- Search for information about kinesiology-related careers and certifications from the American College of Sports Medicine (ACSM) at www.acsm.org.

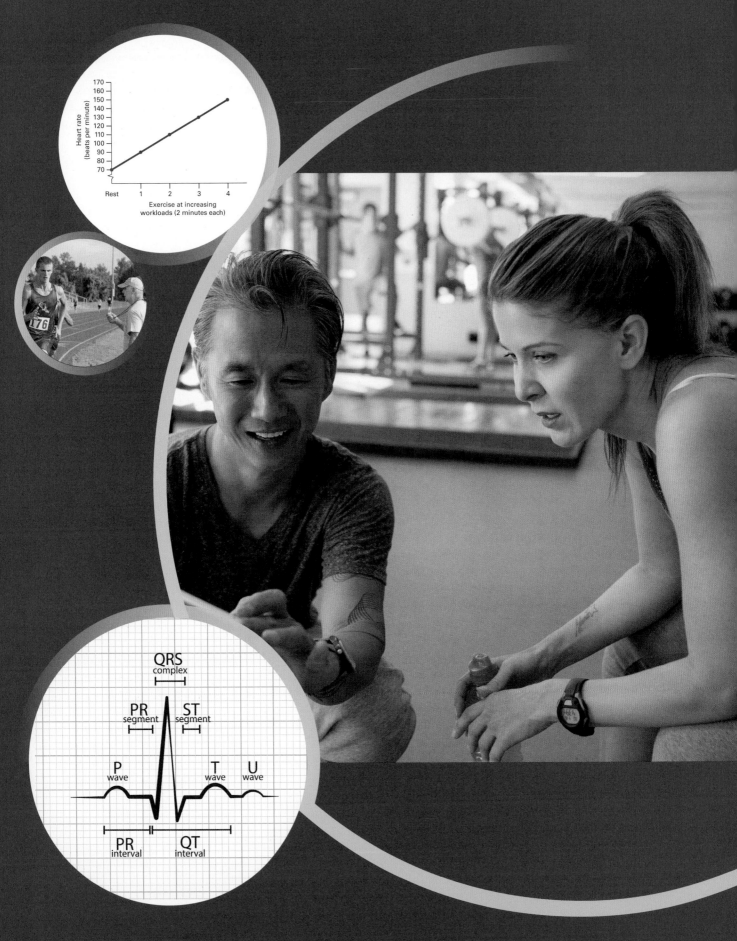

# Evidence-Based Practice in Kinesiology

*Have relatives or friends ever asked you for advice about the best ways to participate in physical activity and exercise to maximize health and fitness? How might you improve your knowledge, skills, and abilities to better answer kinesiology-related questions? Where would you find scientific evidence that you could rely on as recent, up-to-date, and accurate?*

**LESSON 1** DEFINITIONS, THE SCIENTIFIC METHOD, AND THE MECHANICS OF EVIDENCE-BASED PRACTICE

**LESSON 2** EXAMPLES OF EVIDENCE-BASED PRACTICES IN KINESIOLOGY

## Learning Objectives

*After completing this chapter, you will be able to:*

**Describe** the steps involved in effective evidence-based practice.

**Differentiate** between the levels of available evidence.

**Segregate** the available evidence within the quality of evidence pyramid.

**Describe** the pros and cons of evidence-based practice.

**Explain** how to incorporate evidence-based practice into your future professional careers.

**Give** examples of evidence-based practices in kinesiology.

**Explain** the examples of evidence-based practices in kinesiology.

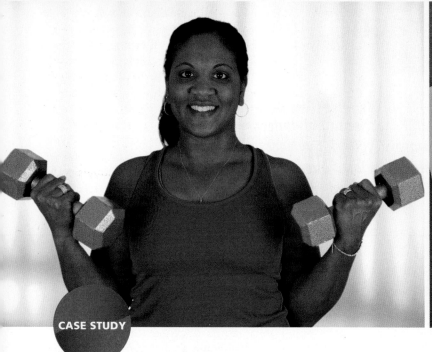

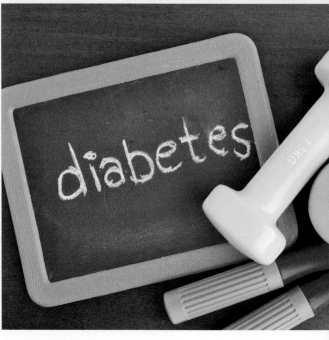

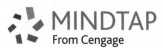

## In the real world . . .

Maria Casey was at a local spring festival selling some of her art pieces when she overheard a conversation that caught her attention. A young lady named Ava, a personal trainer who had recently graduated with an undergraduate kinesiology degree, was chatting with one of Maria's customers about the benefits of resistance training for health and improved performance. Maria was interested in trying to do some resistance training herself. Her type 2 diabetes limited her mobility, and she thought resistance training might help make her stronger and improve her metabolism so she could better control her blood sugar. However, Maria was unsure about what resistance exercises she should do, or how to do them. As she listened to Ava's conversation, she learned about some general resistance training concepts but could not help wondering what the advice she was hearing was based upon. Was Ava an expert? Would these techniques work for her and her diabetes? Ava kept using the term "evidence-based practice" when she referred to

---

## MINDTAP
From Cengage

Go to your MindTap course now to answer some questions and discover what you already know about evidenced-based practice in kinesiology.

## INTERACTIVE ACTIVITIES

### Research Focus

Go to your MindTap course to view a tutorial on evidence-based practice.

### Career Focus

When you fail to take evidence into account, personal biases can steer you in the wrong direction. Go to your MindTap course to participate in a survey about some common fitness practices and the amount of evidence to support that the fitness practice has real benefits.

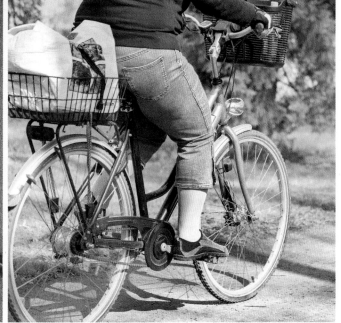

## Introduction: Evidence-Based Practice in Kinesiology and Related Definitions

All academic fields such as kinesiology rely on science to generate knowledge so the field can advance. The evolution of knowledge in kinesiology has occurred so rapidly since the middle of the twentieth century that traditional degree programs in kinesiology, exercise science, human performance, and the like have sometimes lagged in teaching the most up-to-date science. Nonetheless, knowledge of current research findings is particularly important to kinesiology students who must later translate and apply the information that they have learned in class into real-world settings. Many kinesiology majors go on to work with individuals and groups to help them be more physically active, fitter, and healthier. However, some experts have suggested that the field of kinesiology has become rife with "misinformation and bogus facts," particularly among practitioner professionals, such as physical therapists, personal trainers, and exercise physiologists, who guide and prescribe exercise for individuals and populations.[1] Others have reported that a theory-to-practice gap exists in kinesiology and that in order for this field to gain more respect as an academic discipline, its students and practitioners must acquire and apply scientific research results in their everyday practices.[2]

**Evidence-based practice (EBP)** refers to a model in which clinical decisions are based on the best research knowledge or evidence available.[3] Evidence-based practice in kinesiology is essentially decision-making for action that is based on, or informed by, the best available science. Actions in this case can include our own physical activity behaviors (What is the ideal training program for completing a 10K race?) or the behaviors of others (What kind of rehabilitation schedule will help strengthen a knee after a meniscus repair surgery?).

resistance exercise, yet Maria had no idea of what she meant. Put yourself in Maria's shoes. How should Ava explain evidence-base practices related to kinesiology to Maria? How can resistance exercise help in the management of type 2 diabetes? What types and frequency of resistance exercises would be best for Maria? What evidence do you have, or can you find, to support or refute Maria's ideas about the benefits of exercise? We will follow up with Maria in Lesson 2 of this chapter after you have learned more about evidence-based practices in kinesiology and how to gather and interpret trustworthy data.

### Science and Truth

As Ariel Ruiz i Altaba (a molecular biologist at the University of Geneva) has stated:

> Science is based on the idea that there is truth, whether or not we have access to it. What we know depends on systems of knowledge, and we may never be able to get to specific truths, but the idea is that there is a reality: there is a way, humans evolved or cancers grow, for instance. And science is a way to get to that.

Evidence-based practice in kinesiology is a concept that is consistent with the knowledge base of kinesiology that you learned about in Chapter 2 (see pages 23–24). It is important to learn to implement evidence-based practices to help in critical thinking, problem solving, and effective, informed decision making during your undergraduate training and future professional activities. Although evidence-based practice does not guarantee that you will never make errors, it does allow you to perform better than you could by guessing with limited information and to avoid perpetuating misinformation.

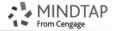

**Evidence-Based Practice**

**Go to your MindTap course** to view a tutorial on evidence-based practice.

## Isolated Facts versus Evidence

It has been said that everyone is entitled to their own opinion but not to their own facts. Have you ever been in a discussion about an issue and found yourself using facts that you have learned in one of your classes or read on the Internet to defend your position? For example, what would you say if someone told you that children and adolescents are less physically fit than they were 60 years ago? Would you agree or disagree? How would you support your point of view: with random facts, or with a solid body of scientific evidence? Where would you go to find the information? What is the difference between an accumulation of random facts and a body of evidence?

In this case, the answer to the question "Are children and adolescents less physically fit than they were 60 years ago?" is probably "Yes," though there is less scientific evidence than we would like to see to support the statement. The concept that youth are less physically fit than in the past is consistent with commonly held assumptions—often based on observations of adults, intuition, and bias—that are promoted to the general public but supported with only limited scientific data.

For the purposes of this text, we define **isolated facts** as ideas and concepts that tend to generalize simple solutions to complex problems. We encounter isolated facts from science each day in the media and on the Internet: "a study shows that eating red meat causes cancer"; "a new study concluded that reducing the time you spend sitting each day can lower blood pressure"; "stretching before exercise will reduce the risk of musculoskeletal injuries." Additionally, these "isolated facts" will sometimes contradict each other. For example, the results of a newly published study showing that vigorous intensity exercise lowers blood pressure among people with hypertension may be contradicted by another that shows no such effect. Unfortunately, these isolated facts—taken alone and out of context—are frequently mistaken for the truth and acted upon accordingly. Reasons for such errors are varied—the new study could be flawed, it could have been conducted in a different population, it could have measured some variables inadequately, etc. Without an understanding of context and an overall view of *all* the facts, even the best scientific findings are isolated facts, and isolated facts may or may not equate to the truth.

In contrast to isolated facts, **body of evidence** refers to an accumulation of all the facts in a particular area. A body of evidence is built through scientific inquiry and includes a systematic evaluation process that occurs over time, usually many years. The body of evidence may yield relatively simple solutions to a problem but much more often uses a multiple-systems approach to develop effective solutions. Remember that the facts you can acquire by reading or hearing about one research journal study do not prove or disprove anything. Most scientists would argue that scientific research never really proves or disproves popular beliefs or established truths. Rather, the results of one study add to the body of evidence on a particular topic. We only rethink and restudy topics and questions when we have shifts in paradigms (models) that support or refute previous documentation and our beliefs. Unfortunately, in our media-rich society, we are all likely to regularly experience confusion about what we should recognize as truth with regards to kinesiology as well as to daily local, national, and global news reports.

Evidence-based practice has emerged as a way to optimize clinical practice not only in medicine but also in other health-related disciplines such as nursing, physical therapy, and athletic training. The most informed practices related to exercise and physical activity are those that rely on the body of evidence, the "big picture," rather than on random facts. It has been difficult to integrate evidence-based practices into kinesiology for several reasons, including the lack of applied research that resolves the ever-changing professional questions that arise, as well as the lack of interdisciplinary and integrated research summaries. Questions related to kinesiology, such as "What are the benefits of the new legal dietary supplement 'Y,' which some have claimed improves physiological, biomechanical, and psychological performance?" are difficult to answer. How would you answer such a question if information about the supplement and its influence on human performance were limited? Would you believe the manufacturer's claims without any independent testing or evidence of effectiveness? What about any side effects? Even if a well-designed study on the effects of the supplement on human performance were to be conducted, it might not be safe or ethical to administer the dosages recommended by the manufacturer to the subjects. Once research results are available, trying to integrate the findings of a study or studies to evaluate three separate performance areas (physiological, bio-mechanical, and psychological) poses even more difficulties. A strong evidence-based approach is essential for kinesiology but difficult to establish unless you learn to use the scientific method and critical thinking to effectively problem solve every-day professional challenges.

## The Scientific Method

You may have learned about the scientific method as early as your third or fourth grade science studies. The **scientific method**, which is a sys-tematic process for testing hypotheses, provides the basis for evidence-based practice in kinesiology and the steps or mechanics of applying this method help optimize the process. Scientists conduct re-search in an ordered way using the scientific method. By reviewing and applying the basics of the scientific method, you can become a better and more effective kinesiology professional as well as a more analytical problem solver. You have proba-bly used the scientific method without realizing it to problem solve and provide friends or relatives with quality feedback that helped improve their performance or understanding of kinesiology con-cepts through critical thinking. For example, what if a collegiate male long jumper who consistently jumped 26 feet told you that in recent practices he could jump only 24 feet? You would probably want to observe him. Most likely you would make a video of several jumps to observe his takeoff speed, steps, technique, and landing. If he jumped poorly, and you noticed that he took off a foot be-hind the takeoff board and had a slow approach, you could help him correct those factors and regain his 26-foot form. In making this analysis, you have applied the scientific method.

The traditional structure of the scientific method is shown in Figure 3.1. Although this traditional model is consistent with the method most of us would expect laboratory scientists such as chemists, molecular biolo-gists, and geneticists to follow, we should also consider a simpler model that is closely linked to the application of evidence-based practice to modern-day kinesiology inter-ventions and programming. A simplified model of the sci-entific method, which you should begin to apply as you problem solve both in and outside of your kinesiology classes, is shown in Table 3.1.

You do not have to be a research scientist to use the scientific method. You can use it in the locker room, on the playing field, in the clinic, or in the classroom just by thinking more critically and seeking out resources that can help you make better decisions. You can prac-tice the steps of the scientific method in many situa-tions, and the tips that follow can help you apply them

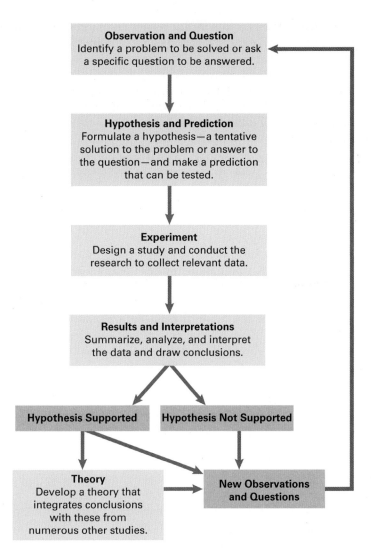

**Figure 3.1** | **The Scientific Method.** The figure represents a traditional structure of the scientific method that you probably first learned about in high school.

**Table 3.1** | The Steps of the Simple Scientific Method Model

1. Make sure you have a good kinesiology-related question to resolve—one that can be answered—and a hypothesis that can be tested to answer the question.

2. Observe or test the situation related to the question, if possible.

3. Describe what you observe.

4. Explain your observation(s) and description(s).

5. Predict future outcomes related to the question more pre-cisely than you would by guessing.

effectively. In each of the remaining chapters in the text, you will find examples of how kinesiology profession-als have used the scientific method to address questions important to their work. Through the collection and translation of scientific evidence related to physical activity, new knowledge is acquired and the entire field of kinesiology advances.

## Steps Toward Evidence-Based Practices

### Step 1: Developing the Question

The first step is to think about the way a question is asked. For example, consider the question, "What is the best replacement fluid to drink during exercise to avoid serious dehydration?" The first answer that comes to mind might be "water." And, although water is an excellent replacement fluid in sporting activities at moderate intensity that last 30 minutes or less, for events that last several hours (like a cycling race) or those that have elimination rounds (like an all-day soccer competition) there are probably better choices. For example, many exercise physiologists would recommend that an athlete drink a nutrient replacement drink because these beverages contain a variety of substances like protein, carbohydrates (sugar), and electrolytes such as sodium and magnesium that are associated with enhanced performance. These components are also needed to help athletes restore what they have lost (by expending calories and sweating) during longer periods of exercise and within hotter climates.

So, to get a good answer to commonly asked exercise science questions, you will probably have to ask more specific questions relevant to effective planning for particular clients or a certain population. For example, Amonette and colleagues have suggested that, in order to develop an effective exercise program, a kinesiology professional would want to ask questions such as the following to narrow in on specific evidence needed for successful implementation:[4]

1. What are the desired outcomes after training (e.g., improved strength, balance, cardiovascular fitness)?
2. Are there underlying clinical issues (e.g., heart disease, compromised circulation, or high blood pressure)?
3. What is the training experience/physical activity background of the target (client or population)?
4. What is the age of the target group?
5. What adherence issues are apparent?

### Step 2: Searching and Gathering Evidence

Once you have a good question or set of questions, the next step is deciding how to gather the best scientific evidence to help you develop an evidence-based approach to answering the question. It is here that the scientific method should help guide decisions about the strength of evidence. Three primary sources of evidence can assist in the search for the best professional practices: your

research knowledge, your academic preparation, and your professional experience.[5] The interpretation of scientific evidence is critical to your ability to minimize any personal bias in your professional decision making and programming.

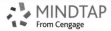 MINDTAP
From Cengage

**Personal Bias**

Bias can be defined as a systematic prejudice in favor of or against a thing, person, or group. In kinesiology, personal bias can manifest itself in many ways; favoring one kind of exercise over another, avoiding recommending some rehabilitation protocol, or eating one type of food prior to exercise are three of many possible examples. When you fail to take evidence into account, personal biases can steer you in the wrong direction. Can you think of other examples? Understanding and using evidence-based practice skills can help the kinesiology student avoid personal bias and understand the field much better!

**Go to your MindTap course** to participate in a survey about some common fitness practices and the amount of evidence to support that the fitness practice has real benefits.

**Research Knowledge.** There are three general levels of scientific research evidence that you can use to make more informed decisions through the scientific method:

1. The body of evidence built by scientific results from many published, peer-reviewed research reports
2. The best scientific evidence available based on a limited number of reports in the published literature
3. Expert or "want to be" expert opinion

**A Note about Wikipedia**

Although Wikipedia or other general definitional websites have many documented scientific facts, many of them are reported to be scientifically questionable. For example, Wikipedia is a good beginning reference source, but we suggest you seek deeper understanding of topics by evaluating multiple levels of evidence. See the text for more information on how to do this.

The best evidence to answer a question is found at level one, the body of evidence. The next-best evidence would come from level two, but it may not be possible to access recent research reports, particularly if only a few studies have been conducted in an area. When using evidence from level three, expert opinion, it is important to look carefully at the expert whose opinion you are using, especially if you rely on opinions expressed on television or in popular publications. The "experts" may really want to sell certain products and may have little regard for scientific evidence.

Even if your only goal in taking this course and reading this book is to be a kinesiology practitioner, you should understand that all scientific disciplines require you to read and understand the research, which provides the basis of knowledge in that discipline. In the case of kinesiology, professionals such as physical educators, athletic coaches, exercise leaders, personal trainers, and physical therapists all practice in occupations based on scientific discovery in the medical sciences.

Peer review is important in building a body of scientific evidence. With peer review, results of studies are reviewed by other experts in the field prior to their release and publication. The better studies pass through peer review and are published, while those of lower quality frequently do not. Many information sources you will find on the Internet are not peer-reviewed, making them less credible; they should thus be interpreted carefully. Reading and referring to peer-reviewed research published in scientific journals, along with research presentations from open forums such as scientific meetings, is considered critical to promoting the scientific method in kinesiology. Peer-reviewed journals have editorial boards and expert reviewers from the field that help professionals edit and interpret their research findings with the ultimate goal of achieving agreement on scientific issues. The peer-review process helps ensure that more questions are raised about scientific issues, and this enables kinesiologists to accept or refute hypotheses over time.

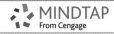

**MINDTAP**
From Cengage

**What Is Science?**

**Go to your MindTap course** to read a brief article entitled "What Is Science?" (P. B. Raven and W. G. Squires, *Medicine and Science in Sports and Exercise* 21, no. 4 (1989): 351–352).

### Step 3: Evaluating the Evidence

To expand your research knowledge base and to evaluate the evidence you gather, it is important for you to have a basic understanding of how to (1) identify kinesiology-related misinformation; (2) read, analyze, and interpret news stories from various media sources related to kinesiology; (3) read and analyze a kinesiology research article at a basic level; and (4) recognize a study's basic research design and its relationship to the quality of evidence the study contributes to the knowledge base. Common sources of misinformation related to the field of kinesiology are shown in Table 3.2. These misinformation sources are often associated with fantastic and unrealistic promises that are not based on scientific inquiry and are typically driven by self-proclaimed "experts" seeking easy and large profits. The common thread in all these sources is that they are not peer-reviewed. A good rule of thumb is: when in doubt, seek the best peer-reviewed information available.

When you read or hear about kinesiology-related stories from various media sources such as magazines, television, or the Internet, it is important to use critical thinking skills to form your own educated opinion about the topic. The following tips can help you avoid being fooled by sensational media accounts that catch your attention but can mislead you professionally:[6]

> For scientific research studies, determine whether the study has been (or will be) published in a peer-reviewed

**Table 3.2** | Common Sources of Misinformation in Kinesiology

**Advertorials:** lengthy advertisements in newspapers, magazines, or on Internet sites that read like feature articles but are written to tout the virtues of products and may or may not be accurate.

**Anecdotal Evidence:** information based on interesting and entertaining, but not scientific, personal accounts of events.

**Conflict of Interest:** situation in which a kinesiology professional or paraprofessional promotes devices or products for personal gain without disclosing that they have a personal interest in the success of the device or product.

**Fraud or Quackery:** the promotion, for financial gain, of devices or products claimed to improve health, well-being, or appearance without proof of safety or effectiveness. (The word *quackery* comes from the term *quacksalver*, meaning a person who quacks loudly about a miracle product [lotion or salve].)

**Infomercials:** feature-length television commercials that follow the format of regular programs but are intended to convince viewers to buy products and not to educate or entertain them. The statements made may or may not be accurate.

**Urban Legends:** stories, usually false, that may travel throughout the world via social media, gaining strength of conviction solely on the basis of repetition.

*Source:* Modified from F. S. Sizer and E. Whitney, *Nutrition, Concepts and Controversies*, 14th ed. (Cengage Learning, 2016), 24.

journal such as the *Journal of Physical Activity and Health*, because if it is unpublished or not peer-reviewed you have no way of knowing if the study has been scrutinized. Be careful, though, because sometimes even a peer-reviewed study can have inaccuracies.

‣ The news report should describe the methods used in the study—though few reports include this information. For example, it matters if the number of subjects studied is only 8 as compared to 8,000 and whether researchers actually measured physiological, biomechanical, or behavioral variables instead of relying solely on self-reported data.

‣ The news report should define the study participants (e.g., cells, animals, or humans) and include their ages.

‣ Valid news reports compare new findings with results of previous research. News writers who do not have specific expertise in a kinesiology-related field may superficially assume nothing else has been reported about the topic of interest.

---

### What Are Review Articles?

Review articles provide a broad perspective about a single topic and appear in most kinesiology-related research journals. Review articles describe the findings of numerous studies and usually discuss the major trends reflective of the research topic.

---

‣ Finally, does the news report make sense to you? Is it a single study that suggests a remarkable discovery or a study that adds significantly to a body of evidence?

Reading research articles related to kinesiology should become part of your daily or weekly routine as an aspiring professional. Practicing and improving your research reading skills can help you make better professional kinesiology decisions. It will be helpful for you to develop an approach to reading research papers for better understanding by asking three general questions: (1) What was the research question, and what existing knowledge in this area led researchers to pose it? (2) What are the gaps in the research literature (e.g., "a, b, and c are known, but more evidence is needed about x, y, or z")? (3) Did the researchers use the scientific method to answer their research question?

When you read a kinesiology research article, you will typically see the following sections: abstract, introduction, methods, results, discussion, conclusions, and references. Table 3.3 contains descriptions of the sections in a typical kinesiology-related research article for you to learn to understand when you read them.

Finally, to expand your research knowledge it is important to learn about research design terminology and the major types of research studies, which are featured in Tables 3.4 and 3.5. Your basic understanding of research terminology and research methods will enable you to understand the kinesiology pyramids (see Figure 3.2) and examples for evidence-based practices and decision making discussed in Lesson 2.

The pyramids of evidence in kinesiology that summarize evidence-hierarchies from observational, experimental and secondary studies are illustrated in Figure 3.2. Evaluating the strength of scientific evidence involves many factors, including the types of studies that make up the evidence. In general, studies higher in each hierarchy shown are considered more methodologically rigorous with respect to determining cause and effect. With observational studies, the researchers do not control what "exposure" study participants have. Experimental studies involve some kind of manipulation of study

---

**Table 3.3** | Descriptions of the Sections in a Typical Kinesiology-Related Research Article and Evidence-Based Questions to Consider

**Abstract:** provides a brief overview of the article, its purposes, and its conclusions. It helps you decide whether to read the article in more detail.

**Introduction:** explains why the study is important and provides a review and evaluation of relevant previous literature. Look for the "purpose of the study" statement and research question(s).

**Methods:** explains who the study participants were and what measures and procedures were conducted. The Methods section should provide all the information needed to conduct the study again, simply by repeating the methods used. Read with a close, critical eye to determine if researchers gathered evidence systematically.

**Results:** describes the findings of the study and usually includes tables and figures. Only the facts should be presented in the Results section.

**Discussion:** interpretation and evaluation of the study results as compared to other findings in the literature. Important to determine if the results seem logical and whether the researchers may have bias.

**Conclusions:** summarizes the answer to the research question(s) and the strengths and limitations of the study, which you should consider carefully. It is also important to identify and evaluate any constructive suggestions for future research provided by the researchers.

**References:** list of important and relevant studies that can help you understand the research question(s) and topic better.

**Table 3.4** | Common Research Design Terms

**Variable:** any factor that can be measured, controlled, or changed in a scientific study.

**Dependent Variable:** the main outcome of interest. It can be observed or the result of experimental manipulation.

**Independent Variable:** the main "exposure" variable that is observed or controlled (treatment).

**Statistical Significance:** the probability (e.g., $p<0.05$) that the results of a study would occur by chance and not due to an actual effect or association.

**Experimental Group:** participants in an experiment who receive the treatment (process or intervention) under investigation.

**Control Group:** a group of individuals who are similar in all possible respects to the experimental group but do not receive the treatment. Results in the experimental group are compared to those in the control group.

**Blind Experiment:** an experiment in which the subjects do not know whether they are members of the experimental group or the control group. In a double-blind experiment, neither the subjects nor the researchers know to which group the members belong until the end of the experiment.

**Placebo:** a sham "treatment" with no therapeutic effect, such as a harmless sugar pill, often used in scientific studies. Placebos are frequently used for control group participants in experimental studies.

**Instruments:** tools used to collect and quantify the data, such as skinfold calipers, heart rate monitors, metabolic carts, and questionnaires.

**Measurement:** the process of quantifying the physical qualities of objects and individuals such as age, weight, height, density, and so on. If a variable is important in a scientific study, it should be measured with as much precision as possible; this often results in a numerical value.

**Evaluation:** the process of using measures to develop evidence-based practices about policies, performances, processes, and so on.

**Randomization:** a statistical process (like flipping a coin) wherein subjects in an experiment have an equal opportunity to be assigned to various experimental (or control) groups.

**Causality:** the degree to which an event (cause) results in an outcome. In kinesiology and other areas of science, causality refers to the strength of the evidence that one condition causes another. This is opposed to correlation, in which two conditions or variables may be related (move in the same or opposite direction) but one does not necessarily cause the other.

**Validity:** the ability of an instrument to measure what it is supposed to measure. For example, does your performance (time) on the one-mile run test actually reflect your cardiorespiratory fitness level? Validity cannot exist without reliability.

**Reliability:** the ability of an instrument to yield consistent results when used repeatedly to measure the same thing. For example, if you use a skinfold caliper to estimate the percentage of body fat for an individual one day and measure the same person again the next, how closely do the two measures agree?

**Quantitative Analysis:** a process that uses numerical values to explain the outcomes of a research project as they pertain to the hypothesis or research question.

**Qualitative Analysis:** a process that uses words and phrases (such as interviews or personal stories) to explain the outcomes of a research project as they pertain to the hypothesis or research question.

**Quality Assurance:** a process that allows researchers and practitioners to develop outcomes measures that provide evidence about health-related quality and effectiveness.

**Surveillance:** a process that provides quantitative information about a health-related issue and its determinants in a defined population. Surveillance includes measures of incidence, morbidity (disease state of an individual or the incidence of illness in a population), survival, and mortality (death). It can also include measures related to genetics, environmental and behavioral risk factors, screening, and action related to quality of care outcomes. Examples of physical activity and exercise surveillance systems are the Behavioral Risk Factor Surveillance System (BRFSS) and the Youth Risk Behavior Surveillance System (YRBSS, see www.cdc.gov for more).

participants. Secondary studies rely on data that are previously collected or studies that have been previously published.

### Step 4: Incorporating the Evidence into Practice

Your individual academic preparation will include exposure to research findings in kinesiology, primarily through the required textbooks selected by instructors. You should consider the suggestions in this section to help you to effectively locate valid and reliable information about kinesiology, and then incorporate it into your professional practice. Although many professors strive to use textbook material based on current scientific research, the material is often already outdated to at least

**Table 3.5** | Types of Studies with Descriptors

**In Vitro (test tube) Research:** studies (such as those in experimental biology) in which parts (such as tissue) from an organism can be isolated (e.g., in a test tube) and evaluated.

**In Vivo Research:** studies using the whole living organism.

**Animal Research:** study of animals (usually rats and mice) that can provide further understanding of health-related issues (like disease management) in humans.

**Ideas, Editorials, Opinions:** published reports that provide research analyses about topics primarily based on individual or group opinions.

**Case Series and Case Studies:** studies of individuals. Clinically, researchers can observe treatments and their apparent effects.

**Cross-Sectional Studies:** studies that quantify the association between a hypothesized exposure and outcome at a single point in time.

**Case Control Studies:** studies in which participants with and without an outcome are compared to determine differences in exposure.

**Cohort Studies:** studies that follow similar individuals who are initially outcome-free over time to determine the health effects of an existing trait or behavior.

**Randomized Controlled Trials:** human research studies that are tightly controlled (often double blind) and are used to compare the health outcomes of a control group(s) to those of an experimental group.

**Systematic Reviews:** research studies that use controlled statistical techniques to review a large body of scientific evidence about a topic and then provide conclusions and recommendations for effective practices.

**Meta-Analysis:** a form of systematic review that uses quantitative statistical analyses to provide insight about consistent results from a variety of similar studies.

**Primary Research:** studies that are experimental (such as those comparing randomized control group outcomes to those of a treatment group) or observational (control and treatment groups are not randomized).

**Secondary Research:** review studies of the scientific body of evidence relevant to a kinesiology-related topic.

some degree (one year or so) by the time it is published. In addition, lectures and class activities are often based upon the individual instructor's own personal bias, which may include teaching the way they were taught, with little new or current research integrated into the course.

The philosophy of the authors of this text includes encouraging all those in academia (professors, students, and professional staff) to effectively use all electronic media linked to the Internet to expand their personal and professional opportunities. Obviously the meaning of "effective use" varies greatly among students, faculty, and staff, and we all know some of the downsides to inappropriate use (e.g., embarrassing e-mail or text messages, excessive spam, and exposure

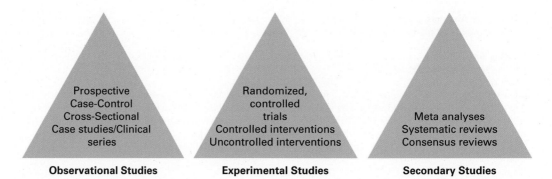

**Figure 3.2** | The Pyramids of Scientific Evidence for Kinesiology. Evidence-Based Hierarchies: Evaluating the strength of scientific evidence involves many factors, including the types of studies that make up the evidence. In general, studies higher in each hierarchy are considered more methodologically rigorous with respect to determining cause and effect. With observational studies, the researchers do not control what "exposure" study participants have. Experimental studies involve some kind of manipulation of study participants. Secondary studies rely on data that were previously collected or studies that have been previously published.

to electronic viruses and spying). The following tips are provided to help you and others use the Internet more effectively for kinesiology research and general information gathering.

1. Seek out credible sources of kinesiology-related information such as professional organizations like the International Society of Physical Activity and Health (www.ispah.org), government agencies like the Centers for Disease Control and Prevention (www.cdc.gov), library sites like the U.S. National Library of Medicine's PubMed (www.ncbi.nlm.nih.gov/pubmed), or commercial sites like Exercise Prescription (www.exrx.net).

   Also, determine if the sites you are using are providing trustworthy information by reviewing and judging them based on the following questions: Who has developed and maintains the site? Is the sponsoring organization for-profit or nonprofit? Is the information that is provided properly referenced? Is the site updated regularly?

2. When you use Internet search engines, remember that the links you will view vary from source to source, and your first few hits, while term specific, may lack real substance relative to what research information you are seeking. If you do not find specific research information about a question by conducting one general Internet search, don't assume that no research has been conducted on the topic. Most likely another Internet search or two will be needed to verify that little or no information is available about the topic.

3. For best results on Internet research sites it is wise to go beyond the first few pages of the site and get very familiar with the linkages and resources available in more detail so that you can take full advantage of the site's features.

### Step 5: Routinely Re-Evaluating the Evidence

Your cumulative professional experience, in combination with a strong research base and solid academic preparation, are all important to optimizing evidence-based practice skills. Your academic mentors and fellow students will expose you to kinesiology concepts and methods that are valid and effective, and if you become a professional life-long learner your occupational experiences will provide you with the "art" of application of the "science" of effective decision making. On the other hand, if you do not continually strive to stay current with emerging kinesiology research findings, and rely only on your professional experiences, you will risk becoming less objective and more biased in your decision-making processes. This, in turn, can leave you less professionally effective.

*In Lesson 2, you will learn about examples of evidence-based practice related to the six various subdisciplines of kinesiology that were highlighted in* *Chapter 1 and the common core or base of knowledge from Chapter 2.*

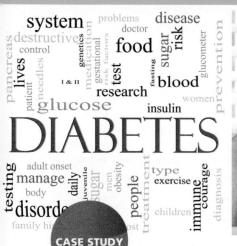

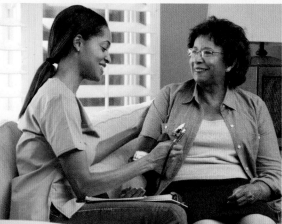

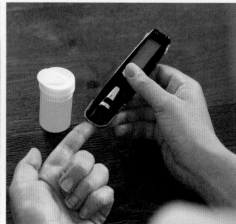

**CASE STUDY**

## In the real world . . .

As you will recall from the beginning of this chapter, Maria Casey overheard a conversation regarding evidence-based practice for resistance training, and it sparked her interest because she was thinking about starting a resistance training program to help in the management of her type 2 diabetes. Now that you know about evidence-based practice in kinesiology, where would you start to help Maria understand the concept and develop a resistance training program that can effectively help manage her type 2 diabetes?

## Introduction

In Lesson 1, you learned about the importance of using evidence-based practices in kinesiology. Some kinesiology professionals would argue that evidence-based practice minimizes the importance of practitioner experience and eliminates the "art" or creativity in kinesiology problem solving and programming. The reality, however, is that the most effective kinesiology professionals are those who integrate the science base with their experience into a toolbox with a variety of tools. Current and future kinesiology professionals should depend upon research and evidence-based practice to guide their planning and programming, while adapting implementation strategies in creative ways to meet the needs

of various target populations. Societally there currently is much more emphasis on data-driven decision making than in the past, and evidence-based practice has become a significant driving force of many other professions including law, medicine, nursing, physical therapy, orthopedics, and athletic training. The art of application in kinesiology is important but should coexist with a strong dependence on evidence-based practices, which can help to minimize misinformation, the perpetuation of bogus facts, and the theory-to-practice gap that is the emerging norm. As you move through your career, you should strive to incorporate evidence-based practices into your daily decision making and encourage your colleagues to do likewise (see Table 3.6).

## Example of an Evidence-Based Practice Plan

### Step 1: Question

How do you help Maria understand the concept of evidence-based practice? How can you help her to develop an exercise program including resistance training that can effectively help manage her type 2 diabetes?

### Step 2: Searching and Gathering Evidence

Websites such as those for the American Diabetes Association (ADA, www.diabetes.org), the American College of Sports Medicine (ACSM, www.acsm.org), and the

**Table 3.6** | Steps to Evidence-Based Practice in Kinesiology

| |
|---|
| 1. Develop the question |
| 2. Search and gather evidence |
| 3. Evaluate the evidence |
| 4. Incorporate the evidence into practice |
| 5. Routinely re-evaluate the evidence |

National Strength and Conditioning Association (NSCA, www.nsca-lift.org) are all reputable places to start gathering basic information to answer Maria's questions. At the ADA site there is plenty of general information about the differences between type 1 and type 2 diabetes as well as specific research information about how to manage type 2 diabetes with lifestyle adjustments including moderate weight loss/weight maintenance and participating in regular physical activity. One article archived under the diabetes research icon is a combined ADA and ACSM position statement (evidence-based research practices paper) published in *Diabetes Care* in 2010 that provides exercise recommendations for effective diabetes management.[7]

Table 3.7 contains evidence grading categories from the ACSM (quality levels from highest [A] to lowest [D]) and clinical practice recommendations from the ADA (quality levels from highest [A] to lowest [D]). Seek out level A evidence when it is available; however, much of the guiding evidence in kinesiology is based upon categories B, C, and D. Category D evidence can be very suspect depending on the credentials of the experts. The information in Table 3.7 provides an important link between the analyses of statistics from the literature and their clinical implications. Similar concepts are often applied in investigating such questions as "Is an athlete fit enough to return to play after injury?" or "Is it safe for a patient can go back to full-time work after a heart attack?"

### Step 3: Evaluating the Evidence

Colberg and colleagues summarized the following physical activity participation recommendations to help persons with type 2 diabetes to more effectively manage their condition:[8]

▸ Persons with type 2 diabetes should undertake at least 150 minutes per week of vigorous or moderate-intensity physical activity (such as walking or cycling) spread out over at least three days during the week, with no more than two consecutive days between bouts of aerobic activity.

▸ In addition to aerobic training, persons with type 2 diabetes should undertake resistance training (such as weight lifting or elastic bands exercises) at least two to three days per week.

▸ Supervised and combined aerobic and resistance training may confer additional health benefits, although milder forms of physical activity (such as yoga) have shown mixed results. Persons with type 2 diabetes are encouraged to increase their total unstructured physical activity. Flexibility training may be included, but should not be undertaken in place of other recommended types of physical activity.

### Step 4: Incorporating the Evidence into Practice

To help Maria incorporate the evidence provided by Step 3 into her lifestyle, you will need to learn how to develop physical activity and *exercise* programming that achieves the recommended goals, but also use clinical skills to prevent possible complications. For example, you could use a variety of evidence-based resources you are already aware of (2008 Physical Activity Guidelines for Americans, and organizations such as the International Society for Physical Activity and Health and the American College of Medicine) to help Maria develop a regular physical activity and exercise plan to meet the 2010 ACSM/ADA recommendations. You should use practical considerations such as those in Table 3.8 to aid in

**Table 3.7** | Evidence Categories for ACSM and Evidence-Grading System for Clinical Practice Recommendations for ADA

| I. ACSM EVIDENCE CATEGORIES | | |
|---|---|---|
| EVIDENCE CATEGORY | SOURCE OF EVIDENCE | DEFINITION |
| A | Randomized, controlled trials (overwhelming data) | Provides a consistent pattern of findings with substantial studies |
| B | Randomized, controlled trials (limited data) | Few randomized trials exist, which are small in size, and results are inconsistent |
| C | Nonrandomized trials, observational studies | Outcomes are from uncontrolled, nonrandomized, and/or observational studies |
| D | Panel consensus judgment | Panel's expert opinion when the evidence is insufficient to place in categories A-C |

| II. ADA EVIDENCE-GRADING SYSTEM FOR CLINICAL PRACTICE RECOMMENDATIONS | |
|---|---|
| LEVEL OF EVIDENCE | DESCRIPTION |
| A | Clear evidence from well-conducted, generalizable, randomized, controlled trials that are adequately powered, including the following:<br>▶ Evidence from a well-conducted multicenter trial<br>▶ Evidence from a meta-analysis that incorporated quality ratings in the analysis<br>Compelling nonexprimental evidence, i.e., the "all-or-none" rule developed by the Centre for Evidence-Based Medicine at Oxford<br>Supportive evidence from well-conducted, randomized, controlled trials that are adequately powered, including the following:<br>▶ Evidence from a well-conducted trial at one or more institutions<br>▶ Evidence from a meta-analysis that incorporated quality ratings in the analysis |
| B | Supportive evidence from well-conducted cohort studies, including the following:<br>▶ Evidence from a well-conducted prospective cohort study or registry<br>▶ Evidence from a well-conducted meta-analysis of cohort studies<br>Supportive evidence from a well-conducted case-control study |
| C | Supportive evidence from poorly controlled or uncontrolled studies, including the following:<br>▶ Evidence from randomized clinical trials with one or more major or three or more minor methodological flaws that could invalidate the results<br>▶ Evidence from observational studies with high potential for bias (such as case series with comparison to historical controls)<br>▶ Evidence from case series or case reports<br>Conflicting evidence with the weight of evidence supporting the recommendation |
| D | Expert consensus or clinical experience |

S. R. Colberg et al., "Exercise and Type 2 Diabetes: The American College of Sports Medicine and American Diabetes Association, Joint Statement," *Diabetes Care* 33, no. 12 (2010): e149.

**Table 3.8** | Prevention of Hypoglycemia or Hyperglycemia during Exercise

| BEFORE EXERCISE |
| --- |

1. Estimate intensity, duration, and the energy expenditure of exercise.

2. Eat a meal 1–3 hours before exercise.

3. Administer insulin in accordance with anticipated requirements.
   a. Administer insulin .1 hour before exercise so that the peak insulin action does not coincide with the exercise period.
   b. Decrease the does of insulin to compensate for increased insulin action during exercise.

4. Assess metabolic control.
   a. If blood glucose is 5 mmol/L (90 mg/dl), extra calories before exercise will likely be required.
   b. If blood glucose is 5–15 mmol/L (90–270 mg/dl), extra calories may not be required.
   c. If blood glucose is 15 mmol/L (270 mg/dl), delay exercise and measure urine ketones.
      i. If urine ketones are negative, exercise can be performed, and extra calories are not required.
      ii. If urine ketones are positive, take insulin and delay exercise until ketones are negative.

5. Do not use an exercising extremity as an injection site.

| DURING EXERCISE |
| --- |

1. Monitor blood glucose during long sessions.

2. Always replace fluid losses adequately.

3. If required, use supplemental carbohydrate feedings (30–40 g for adults, 15–25 g for children) every 30 minutes during extended periods of exercise.

| AFTER EXERCISE |
| --- |

1. Monitor blood glucose, including overnight, if amount of exercise is not habitual.

2. Adjust insulin therapy to decrease immediate and delayed insulin action (intensive therapy regimens provide increased flexibility in adjusting insulin).

3. If required, increase calorie intake for 12–24 hours after activity, depending on the intensity and duration of exercise and risk for hypoglycemia.

*Source:* From P. Raven, D. Wasserman, W. Squires, and T. Murray, *Exercise Physiology* (Boston: Cengage Learning, 2013), 199.

the prevention of hypoglycemia (low blood sugar) or hyperglycemia (high blood sugar) during exercise.

### Step 5: Re-Evaluating the Evidence

Finally, you can explain to Maria that in order to stay up-to-date with current recommendations for exercise in the management of type 2 diabetes like those provided by the ACSM/ADA, she should watch for regular updates on joint position or consensus statements. These usually appear every 5 or so years and are published by professional organizations or governmental agencies.

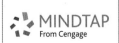 **MINDTAP** From Cengage

Go to your MindTap course to complete the Case Study activity for this chapter.

## Physical Activity in Health, Wellness, and Quality of Life

In Chapter 2, prevention of falls was used as an example of evidence-based practice, which integrated physical activity in health, wellness, and quality of life through the acquisition and maintenance of functional health. In this section, we provide some examples of other evidence-based practices for the kinesiology subdisciplines of human behavior and exercise physiology/coaching, using the same five-step process.

### Human Behavior

#### Step 1: Question

Imagine you are a personal trainer and your business, which serves young, fit athletes, is booming. One day, a 55-year-old man with a family history of heart disease contacts you to help him to begin and maintain an exercise program. You accept him as a client but don't really have any personal experience working with middle-aged clients who are unfit. Where do you begin, and how do you build a program that will help your client safely meet his goals?

#### Step 2: Searching and Gathering Evidence

Because you don't have experience working with this type of client, it is critical to understand the science base on behavior change for physical activity promotion. Critical information would include what the behavioral science literature tells us about strategies that work and the types of behavioral theories that seek to explain this kind of human behavior. You would also want to review the physiologic adaptations (cardiovascular, musculoskeletal, metabolic) that might be expected when moving your client from sedentary to active, including how long it may take for these changes to appear. Finally, you would be interested in learning more about exercise safety and the cardiac risks associated with physical activity because he has a family history of heart disease. Fortunately, you can search the National Library of Medicine's PubMed database of peer-reviewed scientific publications for current and past scientific literature on these questions.

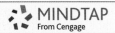

**The PubMed Database**

**Go to your MindTap course** now to take a tour of the National Library of Medicine's PubMed database.

#### Step 3: Evaluating the Evidence

To help your client meet his goals, a plan must be developed and implemented according to the best available

scientific evidence. Relevant questions that an interview of the client combined with the scientific evidence can help you answer include:

- What is your client's history with exercise and physical activity?
- What are his current barriers? Why isn't he physically active now?
- Who can he rely on to help support him?
- Where is he likely to experience setbacks in his program?
- Are there any types of physical activity he enjoys more than others?
- Does he have any biomechanical or other musculoskeletal limitations?
- What training dose (exercise frequency, intensity, duration) should you begin with and how can that be changed to accommodate training effects as he becomes more active?
- What strategies might work to help him maintain the behavior change once it begins?
- What risk factors should you work to minimize?

#### Step 4: Incorporating the Evidence into Practice

Based on the first two steps, an initial training plan for your client could include walking at a moderate intensity on three or four days for the first two weeks along with some modest resistance training exercises (wall push-ups, for example). If he has a support system—his family, for instance—engaging their help (such as scheduling walks with your client) could be a useful strategy. Also, helping him recognize potential barriers (e.g., work or travel schedule encroaching on his exercise time) and strategies to overcome those barriers would be critical. As he becomes more active, his body's systems will adapt and the dose of physical activity can be increased toward a minimum goal of 150 minutes per week of moderate-intensity physical activity or 75 minutes per week of vigorous-intensity physical activity. As he transitions to maintenance of his behavior change, identifying rewards, prompts, and cues to help him continue to be physically active is critical.

#### Step 5: Re-Evaluating the Evidence

Because science is dynamic, evidence is continually emerging. Staying abreast of changes in this area is critical for maximally effective evidence-based practice.

## Scientific Foundations of Physical Activity

In this section, we will provide you with evidence-based practice examples using the five-step process for the kinesiology subdisciplines of exercise physiology, public health, biomechanics, and motor learning.

## Exercise Physiology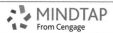

### Step 1: Question

Suppose you are working with Mary, a 17-year-old high-school female miler from a small town who has a 5:20 personal best time. How would you, as her coach, design a successful training program for her final track season? In order to proceed, you might first need to understand that her 5:20 time would make her very competitive at the state championship level throughout the United States. One of your goals as a coach would be to design sport-specific activities that would help her improve her time in the mile and perhaps even win the state championship.

### Step 2: Searching and Gathering Evidence

In searching for resources with which to coach Mary, you would want to focus on gaining an understanding of the components of successful training that predict success for the mile run, such as those promoted by groups like USA Track & Field (www.usatf.org) and expert distance running coaches like Jack T. Daniels, Ph.D. (named world's best distance coach of the century by *Runner's World* magazine, 2005). Dr. Daniels is an author, coaching consultant, and an active coaching education advocate.[9]

---

**MINDTAP**
From Cengage

**Additional Web Resources**

**Go to your MindTap course** for direct links to all websites referenced in this chapter including:

- www.usatf.org. The USA Track & Field website for insight about track and field events and best times nationally.

- www.coacheseducation.com. The Coaches Education website assists coaches at all levels by sharing information, both theoretical and practical, among coaches and other sports science professionals.

---

### Step 3: Evaluating the Evidence

The research and practical coaching evidence would suggest that to prepare Mary properly for the one-mile track season, you would need to, at a minimum, develop workouts to challenge the following physiological, biomechanical, and psychological factors that are predictive of mile run success:

- Maximal oxygen uptake ($VO_2$ max, or maximal oxygen uptake, a common measure of maximal cardiorespiratory endurance)

- Long, slow distance runs (pace for three to five miles)
- Lactate threshold runs (pace at lactate threshold)
- Running economy pace (oxygen uptake at given submaximal pace)
- General upper body resistance conditioning (exercises, sets, and repetitions)
- Mental conditioning, injury prevention, and recovery strategies

### Step 4: Incorporating the Evidence into Practice

A basic plan for Mary might include the following initial goals for meeting the challenges from evaluation of the evidence (there are certainly other possible coaching solutions to achieve success as well):

- Maximal oxygen uptake ($VO_2$ max): Intervals improve this factor. Interval pace in this case works well for improvements by working at 90% of $VO_2$ max. This can be predicted by running two miles all out for time ($VO_2$ max = $0.2 \times$ speed in meters/min).

- Long, slow distance runs (pace for three to five miles): Can run these at 60 to 70% of $VO_2$ max speed.

- Lactate threshold runs (pace at lactate threshold): Initial speed of 70% of $VO_2$ max speed.

- Running economy pace: Repetition runs like $5 \times 1$ min at 2–3 seconds faster than $VO_2$ max speed with a 1-min slow jog rest between bouts.

- General upper body conditioning that might include pushups, pull-ups, bicep curls, and upright rowing exercises all at initial three sets of 10 repetitions.

- Help Mary develop strategies to incorporate mental imagery (practice) during racing, an eating and hydration recovery plan, sleeping/rest tips, and injury prevention tactics.

The training recommendations of Mary's plan would then need to be coordinated by you, as her coach, into a sequential (periodization) weekly program for the spring track season.

### Step 5: Re-Evaluating the Evidence

Did the plan work? Was Mary competitive? Did her mile time decrease? As a coach, you should sit down with Mary after the spring track season, re-evaluate the effectiveness of your coaching plan, and accumulate additional evidence to modify your plan as needed to help Mary move toward her goals.

## Public Health

### Step 1: Question

Obesity is defined by various public health and medical groups as having a body mass index (BMI; weight for height) $> 30.0$ kg/m². For years, public health leaders have claimed that a high BMI increases the risk of many kinds of diseases, including heart disease and diabetes. Imagine that, for a class project, you have been asked to do Internet search on "overweight athletes" and found that a high percentage of professional athletes (50% or greater) are considered overweight or obese based on BMI calculations. Can an athlete be at risk for disease even if she or he is physically active and otherwise healthy with a BMI $> 30.0$ kg/m²? The topic of overweight or obese athletes has been a popular media message without much real scientific evidence available to determine the accuracy of the information. To determine if information from the Internet is accurate, you need to know the definition of BMI and that it provides a ratio of weight to height, and requires a true understanding of how to evaluate it (see Steps 2 and 3 in the next sections).

### Step 2: Searching and Gathering Evidence

According to Raven and colleagues, and the Centers for Disease Control and Prevention, body mass index (BMI) is equal to one's weight in kilograms (kg) divided by one's height in meters squared (m²). BMI can be classified as shown in Table 3.9. A BMI between 18.5 and 24.9 kg/m² is considered normal or healthy, whereas a BMI of between 25 and 29.9 places an adult in the overweight category, and a BMI greater than 30 is consistent with obesity.

### Step 3: Evaluating the Evidence

BMI is a better indicator of obesity than weight alone and can be used to predict percentage of body fat. However, BMI is subject to a large measurement error. Moreover, a person's body mass is made up of water, lean (nonfat) tissue, and fat, whereas BMI accounts for only the total weight of these components together. Thus, BMI does not consider the amount of lean tissue a person has. Athletes with a large proportion of muscle

#### Table 3.9 | Weight Classifications Using Body Mass Index (BMI)

| BODY MASS INDEX (kg/m²) | CLASSIFICATION |
| --- | --- |
| <18.5 | Underweight |
| 18.5–24.9 | Healthy weight |
| 25.0–29.9 | Overweight |
| 30 | Obese |

*Source:* From P. Raven, D. Wasserman, W. Squires, and T. Murray, *Exercise Physiology* (Boston: Cengage Learning, 2013), 436.

(lean tissue) or other muscular adults can easily be misclassified as being overweight or obese. Lean tissue is thought not to increase the risk of poor health. You should consider using additional body composition assessment methods to effectively evaluate athletic adult populations.

### Step 4: Incorporating the Evidence into Practice

So, was the Internet right about 50% of athletes being overweight? Well, maybe, if you define *overweight* based solely on BMI criteria. In fact, most professional athletes have lots of lean muscle mass and are therefore misclassified by their BMIs as being overweight or obese. Perhaps another way to approach the issue would be to compare professional athletes' BMI measures and weight-to-hip ratios (WHR; WHR $\geq 0.95$ in males or WHR $\geq 0.85$ in females is considered high). An athlete with a high BMI and a high WHR is more likely be overweight or obese than one with a high BMI and a normal WHR. An athlete's weight status could be further evaluated with more precise body composition methods (such as dual-energy x-ray absorptiometry, DXA) when necessary based upon the athlete's health risks and playing performances.

### Step 5: Re-Evaluating the Evidence

As noted in Step 1, based on literature reviews and the opinions of the authors of this text, the topic of overweight or obese athletes has not been effectively studied. It is apparent that the majority of professional athletes are not overweight or obese, as, if they were, they most likely would be unable to perform at an optimal level necessary for their profession. The topic of overweight or obese athletes would probably be more relevant for young athletes who are trying out for the first time for sports participation and are deconditioned, or for athletes who have stopped competing and have become deconditioned.

## Biomechanics

### Step 1: Question

Suppose the school board for the district where you are the athletic director is reviewing contracts for cleats for the soccer athletes in the district. They have asked you to review the contracts and make recommendations on which are the best shoes for the players. As you look at the technical descriptions of shoes, you see that two companies have reported data for traction coefficients and offer cleat designs for different surfaces (field turf, artificial turf, and natural grass). You remember from a recent state coaching clinic that shoe traction and surface-specific cleat designs can increase the likelihood of noncontact lower limb injuries in athletes. Although you are not a trained biomechanist, you do have a degree in kinesiology, and you have had practice reviewing biomechanical research and recognize that doing so can help you make an informed recommendation to the school board.

### Step 2: Searching and Gathering Evidence

You begin your online search by retrieving articles from the National Library of Medicine using the search term "shoe traction." Immediately you are inundated with over 300 articles. Because all the soccer fields in the district are grass, you decide to refine your search by adding "grass" to the previous search terms. Your search has now retrieved a manageable number of articles (< 150). As you review articles with titles that seem specific to your topic, you find that many of the articles discuss cleat design, cleat material, and load as the dominating factors that affect traction on grass. Furthermore, you find no consistent means of measuring load among the articles; although a few discuss torque on the lower limb, even these describe torque of different areas of the leg (ankle, tibia, and knee). You have found a recent article that suggests that shoes with the traditional round cleat design compared to an aggressive mixed cleat design (bladed cleats on the outer edge with round central cleats) produce higher levels of peak torque on the lower limb under all loading conditions.[10] Although this is a promising article, it by no means represents a body of evidence for decision-making.

### Step 3: Evaluating the Evidence

There is no consensus or preponderance of evidence regarding which shoe designs are best for soccer players within the currently available research because shoe development is continually evolving and changing based upon manufacturers' designs and marketing needs; the number of independent scientific studies evaluating shoe performance has lagged the evolution in shoe manufacturing. Furthermore, you have found that measurement techniques and instrumentation used to determine the best shoe design vary significantly between the studies.

### Step 4: Incorporating the Evidence into Practice

While there is no apparent consensus among researchers regarding the best shoe type for the soccer player, you still have a decision to make; you can either recommend to the school board that they purchase the rounded traditional cleats similar to those that have been historically used by most teams, or you can gamble on the single article that states that the aggressive mixed cleat design had lower peak torque on the lower limb under all loading conditions. What do you do?

### Step 5: Re-Evaluating the Evidence

Suppose you have now made the decision and advised the school board accordingly. No matter what choice you made, it is clear from the current literature that claims by shoe manufacturers are not necessarily supported by independent research. Even if you choose to maintain the status quo and order the traditional cleats for your soccer players, you now know that evidence emerging through independent research may someday be able to determine the best cleat design to minimize lower limb injuries. If you choose to try the new aggressive cleat design, which was supported by the single research study as reducing peak torque on the lower limb, you will need to follow the rate of injuries over the next few seasons and compare those injury rates to historical injury rates to determine whether lower limb injuries were minimized. No matter what decision you made, you should depend upon evidence-based practices to guide your future decision-making.

## Motor Learning

### Step 1: Question

Imagine that you are a physical therapist who wants to find ways to reduce the time between rehabilitation and return-to-play for women athletes who have undergone anterior cruciate ligament (ACL) repair surgery. At a recent state meeting, you overheard a colleague discussing a new technique called cross-education training as a means to minimize muscle atrophy during the postsurgical weeks of phases 1 (1 to 14 days post operation) and 2 (often two weeks to six weeks post operation) of rehabilitation. You wonder if you can incorporate this type of training in your practice and if it will have an impact on the rehabilitation to return-to-play time interval. To determine whether cross-education training would be useful in your practice, you need to know what cross-education training is and what the current literature says about its efficacy and use.

### Step 2: Searching and Gathering Evidence

Your first order of business in learning about cross-education of muscles is to visit the National Library of Medicine's PubMed site to search for articles than can help you understand the technique. To limit your search, you decide to search for articles that have the term "cross-education" in the title. Your search returns about 20 articles that have cross-education in the title, and of those 20, only 5 are pertinent to muscle strength or rehabilitation. Then, according to one article, cross-education strength refers to the strength increases that occur when unilateral limb resistance training improves muscle strength of the contralateral (opposite) limb.[11] By reading this article, you discover two new terms to search for further information: *unilateral* and *contralateral resistance training*. You also notice that although the authors found an increase in strength measures in the contralateral limb, there was no increase in muscle mass. This finding does not support what you heard about cross-education reducing muscle atrophy, since muscle atrophy results in the loss of muscle mass. You decide to search further to see if you can find more recent articles on cross-education to help you better understand how this type of training works.

### Step 3: Evaluating the Evidence

Upon completion of your literature search, you determine that cross-education affects the neural (nervous system) components associated with strength and not the physiological or morphological (appearance) characteristics of the muscle. Although morphologic and physiologic adaptations do not appear to occur, you have found that cross-education training seems to, at a minimum, maintain strength in the contralateral limb, and may improve strength on the average of 7.6% in the contralateral limb.[12] Furthermore, recent studies suggest that cross-education resistance training during rehabilitation may improve the recovery and rehabilitation time of post-operative immobilized limbs.

### Step 4: Incorporating the Evidence into Practice

Your review of the research literature about cross-education resistance training reveals that there is a preponderance of evidence suggesting resistance training of the unilateral limb improves contralateral strength. Although there is still no consensus on whether the cross-education adaptations occur at the motor unit (muscle) level or within the spinal cord circuitry (nervous system), the current literature does support the use of resistance training exercises of the unilateral limb in the rehabilitation process. Because none of the studies suggested that there are deleterious effects associated with cross-education training, you decide to add unilateral limb resistant training techniques to the first four weeks of the rehabilitation process for post-operative ACL repair patients.

### Step 5: Re-Evaluating the Evidence

Once you have implemented the cross-education resistance training program in your physical therapy practice, you will need to conduct two ongoing evaluation activities. The first evaluation activity is collection of data to confirm that the cross-education training program is indeed improving the time for return-to-play. You will need to compare previous records of patients, including these athletes' time for full rehabilitation and strength values, with data for the new patients who undergo the cross-education resistance training program you have implemented. The second continuing evaluation activity will be to review new articles on cross-education training as they are published. This means that you should save your search terms in the journal databases that were used to find the previously reviewed articles. You can then go to the online database monthly or bimonthly and run the search to see if any new evidence was added to the knowledge base. By doing these two activities, you can remain up to date with the newest evidence from others as well as collecting data on your own specific practices.

# Cultural, Historical, and Philosophical Dimensions of Physical Activity

In this section, we provide an example of integration of evidence-based practice using the five-step process for the kinesiology subdisciplines of history, philosophy, and sociology.

## An Integrated Problem

### Step 1: Question

At the beginning of this chapter, we used the example of the common perception that children are less fit today than they were 60 years ago. Assume that you have been asked to serve on a federal task force to determine how previous governmental policies may have impacted the decline in adolescent physical fitness and to make recommendations for new policies to counteract the decline. From reading the chapter, you may have discovered that some questions such as this are multi-faceted and complex in nature. To answer the questions of whether and why children's physical activity and physical fitness have declined in the past 60 years, you must fully understand the historical, cultural, and philosophical paradigm shifts that have occurred during that 60-year time frame.

### Step 2: Searching and Gathering Evidence

In starting your search for information, you come across a recent journal article: a systematic review of previous research in physical activity and youth fitness over 50 years.[13] Although this is a great starting place, you decide to delve deeper into the research to find original research studies as well. You review the references from this article as well as those in other articles that express a similar premise for other nations and cultures.

### Step 3: Evaluating the Evidence

As you review numerous articles, you find common trends associated with physical activity and physical fitness among the U.S. articles and articles from other nations. These trends include changes over time in the population's socioeconomic status, the evolution of technology, the transition from a rural/agricultural lifestyle to urban settings, dietary intake changes, and changes in opportunities to participate in school-based physical education. Research from emerging countries suggests that upward movement into higher socioeconomic status classifications tends to be related to an increase in BMI and a decline in fitness levels. You also learned that factors such as genetics and growth and development can significantly influence fitness scores in children. In addition, changing state and federal policies over time were shown to impact how physically active and fit children and adolescents are.

### Step 4: Incorporating the Evidence into Practice

In your review of the literature you find that physical education, at least in the United States, evolved between the late 1940s and early 1950s, when physical education was driven by fitness to meet the demands of military readiness, and the 1980s and 1990s, when the focus became achieving higher levels of physical fitness and athletic performance. Since the late 1990s, there has been a growing movement toward promoting health-related physical education for health, fun, and leisure. However, in most states, physical education requirements have been systematically eliminated in schools. After reviewing the historical, cultural, and philosophical information related to physical activity and fitness levels of children, your task force might be motivated to recommend standards that require all school-age children to participate in 60 minutes of daily school physical education as an intervention to increase physical activity and fitness levels of children in the United States.

### Step 5: Re-Evaluating the Evidence

In a perfect world, if the task force's recommendations were accepted and converted to policies without changes, this school physical education requirement might be implemented throughout the country. However, despite a new universal federal policy, the real question becomes: Does the policy have an impact by reversing the trends or claims of declining physical activity levels and physical fitness among youth? The only way to answer this question would be to conduct future studies to compare fitness levels of students prior to the inception of the policy with those of children who are impacted by the policy.

# The Practice of Kinesiology

In this section, we provide an example of evidence-based practice using the five-step process for the kinesiology subdisciplines of athletic training and physical therapy.

### Step 1: Question

Return-to-play following a sports concussion has become a challenging clinical problem for coaches, athletic trainers, and physical therapists, as you learned in Chapter 2. In the practice of kinesiology, you must use evidence-based practices to optimize return to functional health as well as to competition, or else you will compromise the healing/recovery process and most likely complicate the rehabilitation process economically and psychologically for patients. What basic considerations (steps/stages) must an athletic trainer or a physical therapist account for to optimize return-to-play following a concussion?

### Step 2: Searching and Gathering Evidence

The topic of sports concussions has generated a tremendous amount of media and professional interest. Many kinesiology professionals consider it a "moving target" for effective management because the body of knowledge about concussions is rapidly changing. For example, a summer 2016 Internet search using the phrase "concussion management 2016" provided over 4,000,000 hits. As you learned in Lesson 1 of this chapter, deciding what represents quality evidence-based practice is difficult, but often one can look for the best and latest evidence from professional organizations such as the National Athletic Trainer's Association (NATA), the American Physical Therapy Association (APTA), the American College of Sports Medicine (ACSM), the National Collegiate Athletic Association (NCAA), and the American Academy of Neurology (AAN).

The AAN recently published a research review paper that provides evidence-based recommendations to answer the following questions:[14]

1. What factors increase or decrease the risk of a sports concussion?

2a. For athletes who have sustained a concussion, what diagnostic tools are useful for identifying those with a concussion?

2b. For athletes suspected of having a concussion, what diagnostic tools are useful for identifying those with a concussion?

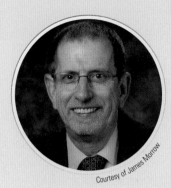
3. For athletes with concussion, what clinical factors are useful in identifying those at increased risk for severe or prolonged early post-concussion impairments, neurologic catastrophe, recurrent concussions, or chronic neurobehavioral impairment?

4. For athletes with concussion, what interventions enhance the recovery process, reduce the risk of recurrent concussion, and diminish long-term problems?

## Step 3: Evaluating the Evidence

As an athletic trainer or physical therapist, you will need to be aware of the basic stages and strategies of general rehabilitation. These include the acute or healing stage, recovery/remodeling stage, return-to-function stage, and return-to-play stage. Each one of the general stages of rehabilitation coincide with clinical applications and a progressive process such as passive care (acute or healing stage), the active assistive stage (recovery and tissue remodeling), active stage (return-to-function), and the rehabilitation stage (return-to-play).

## Step 4: Incorporating the Evidence into Practice

Based on the available evidence, the authors of the AAN review paper made the following determination about effective recovery interventions for sports concussions: "Data are insufficient to show that any intervention enhances recovery or diminishes long-term sequelae postconcussion." However, the AAN 2013 review does recommend that practitioners such as athletic trainers

*of physical activity throughout life. It is indeed nearly impossible to read the lay or professional literature without seeing data supporting the important role that living a physically active lifestyle has on personal health outcomes, as well as the influence on the general population. As such, my hope is that my work, and that of my colleagues, is relevant and influential to the point that people will adopt and maintain physically active lifestyles. This results in sharing one's professional research with other scientists so that they can critique and further the work, and also sharing research in a way that can be read, used, adopted, and influence the lives of people across the globe.*

**Q: How do you stay physically active yourself and promote good health to others directly around you?**

**A:** *I have retired now but both my wife and I attempt to remain physically active throughout the week. We are members of the local fitness club and exercise there regularly. Additionally, I enjoy golfing and do so several times a month. We enjoy walking and generally attempt to engage in movement through means that result in our not always taking the modern mechanized way of getting to and from places and generally moving about. In general, it is our attempt to meet the national physical activity guidelines that have been developed since 2008. We visit with our family and friends about these recommendations and encourage them to engage in health lifestyles.*

**Q: How have you had to integrate the subdisciplines of kinesiology in your professional practice?**

**A:** *None of the so-called kinesiology subdisciplines really stands alone well. Certainly, there are scientists who specialize their work and focus their research on specific topics. Nevertheless, physical activity and movement crosses all of these areas (e.g., physiology, psychology, biomechanics, sociology, media, measurement, statistics, etc.). Regardless of the nature of any specific research study, or field of interest in kinesiology, one can interpret the results of research and imagine how that specific piece of work might influence other kinesiology areas.*

*James Morrow, Regents Professor Emeritus of Kinesiology at the University of North Texas, was named the 2011–2012 Alliance Scholar by the American Alliance for Health, Physical Education, Recreation and Dance for his research on the measurement and assessment of physical activity in children, youth, and adults. He received the National Academy of Kinesiology's Hetherington Award in 2016. His research on physical activity has been published widely as well as presented in Europe and Asia.

or physical therapists participating in a concussion management team, which would include coaches, licensed health care providers (LHCP), parents, and others, consider the following:[15]

1. Provide pre-participation counseling about concussions and screen for those at higher risk (based on factors such as age, sex, sport played, level of sports participation, and equipment used).

2. For those with a suspected concussion, use effective valid and reliable checklists and screening tools to track progress.

3. Have those with a suspected or documented concussion undergo neuro-imaging.

4. Return-to-play should be managed and signed off on by an LHCP and should include special considerations for the age of the athlete, possible gradual return to physical activities, and recovery time for cognitive restructuring.

5. Lastly, for those with chronic concussion challenges, retirement-from-play counseling should be provided.

### Step 5: Re-Evaluating the Evidence

The practice of kinesiology requires practitioners to constantly keep up with the scientific research literature regarding topics such as sports concussions to provide the best evidence-based practices and most up-to-date care for their patients. Science is continually advancing in kinesiology, and new evidence must be considered for greatest effectiveness.

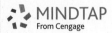
## Chapter Summary

▸ Evidence-based practice (EBP) refers to a model in which clinical decisions are based on the best research knowledge or evidence available. Evidence-based practice is essentially practice-based decision-making that is based on, or informed by, the best available science.

▸ The most informed decisions in exercise and physical activity kinesiology practice are those that rely on the body of evidence, the "big picture," rather than on isolated facts. It has been difficult to integrate evidence-based practices into kinesiology for several reasons, including the lack of applied research to explain every changing and emerging professional question that arises, as well as the lack of interdisciplinary and integrated research summaries.

▸ The major steps for integrating the scientific method into evidence-based practice are (1) developing the question, (2) searching and gathering evidence, (3) evaluating the evidence, (4) incorporating the evidence into practice, and (5) routinely re-evaluating the evidence.

▸ There are numerous sources of misinformation in kinesiology, including advertorials, anecdotal evidence, fraud, conflicts of interest, infomercials, and urban legends.

▸ Research journal articles in kinesiology include the following sections: abstract, introduction, methods, results, discussion, conclusions, and references.

▸ A basic understanding of research terminology and research methods is required to understand the pyramids of evidence in kinesiology practices.

▸ The pyramids of evidence in kinesiology provide examples of the levels of evidence and how various types of research studies contribute to the body of knowledge about various kinesiology topics. All types of research including basic (test tube) research, case studies, clinical studies, and systematic reviews contribute to the body of knowledge of kinesiology.

## Remember This

| | | | |
|---|---|---|---|
| abstract | control group | independent variable | randomized controlled |
| advertorials | cross-sectional studies | infomercials | trials |
| anecdotal evidence | dependent variable | instruments | references |
| animal research | discussion | isolated facts | reliability |
| blind experiment | evaluation | measurement | results |
| body of evidence | evidence-based practice | meta-analysis | scientific method |
| case control studies | (EBP) | methods | secondary research |
| case series and case | experimental group | placebo | statistical significance |
| studies | fraud or quackery | primary research | surveillance |
| causality | ideas, editorials, opinions | qualitative analysis | systematic reviews |
| cohort studies | in vitro (test tube) | quality assurance | urban legends |
| conclusions | research | quantitative analysis | validity |
| conflict of interest | in vivo research | randomization | variable |

# For More Information

Access these websites for further study of topics covered in the chapter:

- Find updates and quick links to these and other evidence-based practice related sites in your MindTap course.

- Search for further information about topics like evidence-based practice as related to kinesiology at the National Registry of Evidence-Based Programs and Practices (NREPP) website at www.nrepp.samhsa.gov.

- Search for information and for the evidence-based practice tutorial at the Health Sciences Library at the University of Minnesota: http://hsl.lib.umn.edu.

- Learn about resources for evidence-based practices from this online article: J. A. Jacobs et al., "Tools for Implementing an Evidence-Based Approach in Public Health Practice," *Preventing Chronic Disease* 9 (2012): 110324, doi: http://dx.doi.org/10.5888/pcd9.110324.

- Search for research about evidence-based practice at the National Center for Biotechnology Information: www.ncbi.nlm.nih.gov.

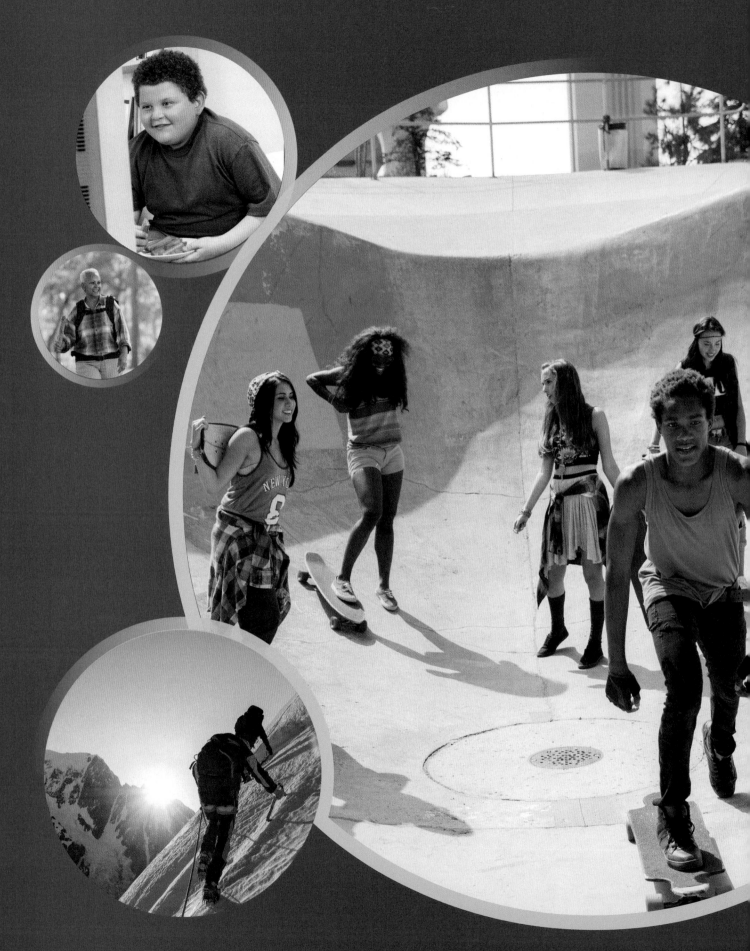

# The Physical Activity Continuum: Applications to Kinesiology

4

*What is the physical activity continuum? How can it be applied to career choices in kinesiology?*

**LESSON 1** PHYSICAL ACTIVITY AND EXERCISE OVER THE LIFESPAN

**LESSON 2** EXAMPLES OF APPLYING TRAINING FUNDAMENTALS IN KINESIOLOGY SUBDISCIPLINES

## Learning Objectives

*After completing this chapter, you will be able to:*

**Describe** the physical activity continuum.

**Distinguish** between traditional and emerging concepts regarding the importance of physical activity and exercise across the lifespan.

**Understand** traditional kinesiology-based individual exercise training models and peak performance goals.

**Understand** emerging concepts of physical activity and exercise for the improved health of populations.

**Distinguish** between the traditional individual exercise prescription model and the emerging population physical activity planning model.

**Describe** the Human Capital Model.

**Describe** the overall benefits of physical activity and exercise for health and human performance.

**Explain** the position of physical activity and exercise in relation to the SLOTH model.

**Define** the unifying characteristics of overload, specificity, and adaptations.

**Explain** how the unifying characteristics of overload, specificity, and adaptations apply across the continuum of movement.

**Give** examples of integration of stress (overload), specificity, and adaptations with achievement of peak performance and health-related outcomes.

**Describe** a simple systems approach for planning physical activity and exercise interventions.

**Give** examples of applying training fundamentals in kinesiology subdisciplines.

**Explain** the examples of application of training fundamentals in kinesiology subdisciplines.

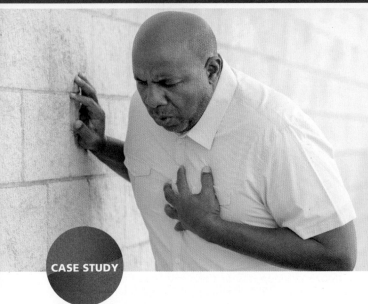

**CASE STUDY**

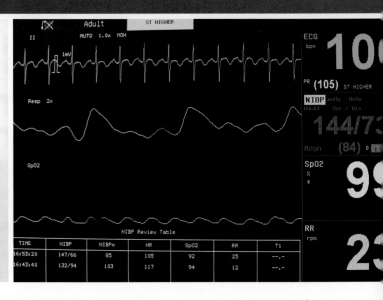

# In the real world . . .

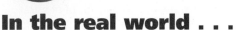

Harry Casey—a.k.a. Grandpa—is the father of William Casey. He is 72 years old and lives several hundred miles away from the family. Harry is a large man: he is 6 feet 2 inches tall and weighs 295 pounds. He smoked two packs of cigarettes daily for 20 years and quit at age 50. He has had hypertension (high blood pressure) for 10 years and high cholesterol for five years. His blood glucose is also high and consistent with pre-diabetes. He is physically inactive, but works part time (20 hours a week) as a salesperson in a lumberyard to supplement his Social Security earnings.

The Caseys just received news that Grandpa suffered a myocardial infarction (heart attack) two days ago. Of course, everyone in the Casey family was worried when they first heard the news, but they all felt much better when, four hours after the event, Harry's physician called to tell them that he was stable and would survive. Because William's mother had

passed away three years previously and Harry lived alone, William and his wife Maria traveled to Omaha as soon as possible to be with Harry. When William and Maria arrived at the hospital, they were concerned about how serious Harry's condition was and about what his future health outcomes might be. Fortunately, the medical center had a high-quality cardiac rehabilitation program, and Harry's cardiologist ordered Phase I cardiac rehabilitation, an inpatient program involving early assessment of the ability of post–heart attack patients to be physically active and successfully perform activities of daily living. Late on Harry's second day in the hospital, William and Maria met the cardiac rehabilitation coordinator, Helen. Helen has an undergraduate and a master's degree in kinesiology, and she is a certified clinical exercise specialist.

The Caseys were relieved to learn from Helen about the core components of cardiac rehabilitation and how Harry could benefit by participating. They also learned that Harry was eligible for Phase II cardiac rehabilitation at the hospital

---

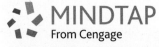

Go to your MindTap course now to answer some questions and discover what you already know about the physical activity continuum and its applications to kinesiology.

## INTERACTIVE ACTIVITIES

### Research Focus

Go to your MindTap course to read an article and answer questions about the global pandemic of physical inactivity and global action for public health.

### Career Focus

Go to your MindTap course to learn about physical activity infographics and various physical activity reports from the United States and globally.

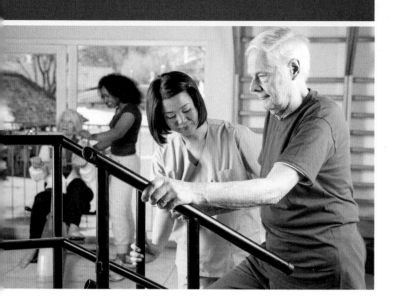

## Introduction: Kinesiology—Emerging Concepts and Influences Related to Physical Activity

As you learned in Chapter 2, physical activity is at the center of the kinesiology universe. Physical activity is any bodily movement that results in energy expenditure (burning of calories).[1] Moving your arm up and down at your desk, skateboarding, lifting sacks of groceries out of the trunk of your car, and running a marathon are all types of physical activity. Exercise is a specific type, or subset, of physical activity that is planned, repetitive, and performed specifically to attain a physical fitness goal such as improved cardiorespiratory fitness. Walking the dog for 2 miles (3.2 km) every night, training for a soccer tryout, swimming laps, and working out at a gym are all examples of purposeful physical activity that can be labeled as exercise. All athletes who train to optimize components of their physical fitness exercise. Anyone who gets out of bed in the morning is engaged in physical activity.

post discharge (Phase II cardiac rehabilitation often begins a few days after discharge and continues for about 6 to 12 weeks). William, Maria, and Harry had many questions for Helen and the cardiologist. What kinds of questions do you think you'd have if you or a loved one suffered a heart attack? What do you think the core components of cardiac rehabilitation are? When should someone who has had a heart attack begin to exercise? Does cardiac rehabilitation work? Can someone safely return to work after a heart attack? What are some of the principles necessary to help Harry move from being totally sedentary to physically active again in his job and at home? We will follow up with Harry Casey's story later in Lesson 2 of this chapter, after you have had a chance to learn more about the physical activity continuum.

As you might imagine, physical activity encompasses a broad range of movement that can be placed along a continuum from sedentary behavior (sleeping and sitting) to the intense exercise needed to train for marathon competition. Particular physical activities can be placed along this continuum based on their difficulty (intensity), the frequency (e.g., times per week) with which they are performed, and the duration of an individual physical activity bout. The product of these three attributes yields the **volume of physical activity** (proportional to the total calories burned; see Chapter 7 for more details about caloric expenditure).

$$V \text{ (volume)} = F \text{ (frequency)} \times I \text{ (intensity)} \times D \text{ (duration)}$$

For example, based on the above equation, if a 165-pound adult walked at 3 mph for 150 minutes per week, that person would expend 620 calories:

$$620 \text{ Total Calories} = 5 \text{ times per week} \\ \times 4.13 \text{ calories per minute} \\ \times 30 \text{ minutes}$$

Each of these three characteristics can be changed (moved up or down along the continuum), which results in a change in the total volume of physical activity. The health and fitness benefits of physical activity and exercise are dose related, and the adaptations/benefits are dependent upon overload of total volume and its components as well as the specificity of physical activity. The volume of physical activity can and should be adjusted for individuals and populations across the lifespan as you will learn in later chapters.

In addition to volume, there are multiple domains in one's life where the continuum of physical activity can be manifested. The **SLOTH model** (SLOTH stands for sleep, leisure-time, occupation, transportation, and home-based activities) has been used by public health researchers to describe the domains of physical activity. Within each domain, physical activity can be performed for very different purposes—to train for a marathon within the leisure-time domain, or to walk to school within the transportation domain, for example. Later in this chapter, we will discuss the SLOTH model and three key unifying characteristics of kinesiology (overload, specificity, and adaptations/benefits). In the kinesiology field, these concepts have traditionally been emphasized in lessons about increasing physical fitness and achieving peak athletic performance. With the understanding that the physical activity continuum offers health benefits at all levels, kinesiology professionals are in a unique position to make full use of the continuum for improving health and performance across the entire life and ability spans.

In Chapter 4, you will learn about applying physical activity and exercise concepts across a continuum (from sedentary status to peak performance) in relation to all age groups and functional statuses. You will also learn about the wide variety of benefits of physical activity in terms of **capital** (resources related to health and well-being). Physical activity can positively affect many forms of capital including physical capital, emotional capital, individual capital, social capital, intellectual capital, and financial capital.

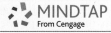

**The Global Pandemic of Physical Inactivity**

**Go to your MindTap course** to read an article and answer questions about the global pandemic of physical inactivity and global action for public health.

## The Physical Activity Continuum

The importance of physical activity and exercise can be visualized and conceptualized in numerous ways by kinesiology professionals. It is critical, however, to understand physical activity as a continuum (a gradual progression or transition among physical activity levels).[2] The **physical activity continuum** can be visualized as a possible progression (and regression) of movement of individuals or populations from sedentary behaviors (physical inactivity) toward functional health (see Chapter 2), then goal-specific physical fitness outcomes (such as weight loss, improved cardiorespiratory fitness, and others), and ultimately, if desired, toward peak performance (see Figure 4.1). As illustrated in Figure 4.1, increasing levels of physical activity (versus remaining

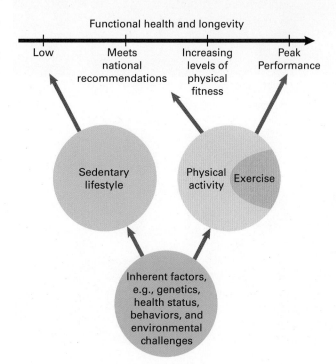

**Figure 4.1** | A Model of the Influences That Affect Increasing Physical Activity Levels along a Continuum

or becoming sedentary) are dependent upon several factors. For, example inherent factors like genetics and health status, personal or population behaviors, and environmental challenges significantly influence the engagement in physical activity. In the next several sections of Chapter 4, two additional figures (Figure 4.8 and 4.10) are used to illustrate additional important exercise principles with the goal of translating theories into practice that conceptualize other aspects of the continuum of physical activity. Once you have learned the additional continuum concepts, you will be encouraged to use Figure 4.10 to represent a simple model of the physical activity continuum that you should use in your kinesiology practices, and we will refer to it throughout most of the remaining chapters in the text.

Why are some people physically active while others are not? What causes people to move up and down the physical activity continuum or to remain in one spot for many years like elite marathon runners do? Do these causes (or predictors) differ by age? This is a field of aggressive research in kinesiology. Many different reasons have been hypothesized, yet few can be clearly demonstrated. When a definite cause or predictor of physical activity is determined, the question of whether it is appropriate across the human life span must still be answered. For example, do the same predictors in 20- to 30-year-olds apply for people older than 70 years? An example of an ecological model of some of the determinants of physical activity being studied is shown in

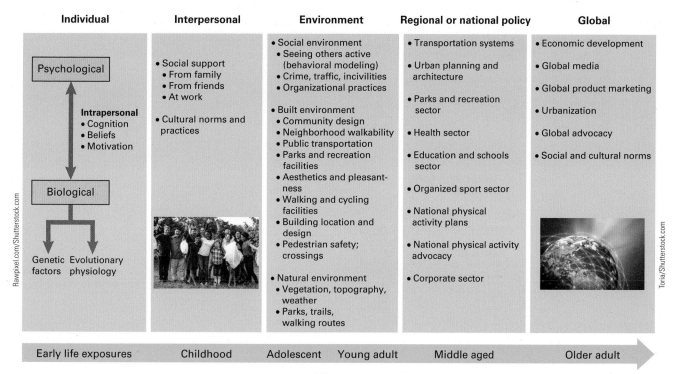

| Individual | Interpersonal | Environment | Regional or national policy | Global |
|---|---|---|---|---|
| Psychological ⇅ Intrapersonal • Cognition • Beliefs • Motivation ⇅ Biological → Genetic factors Evolutionary physiology | • Social support • From family • From friends • At work • Cultural norms and practices | • Social environment • Seeing others active (behavioral modeling) • Crime, traffic, incivilities • Organizational practices • Built environment • Community design • Neighborhood walkability • Public transportation • Parks and recreation facilities • Aesthetics and pleasantness • Walking and cycling facilities • Building location and design • Pedestrian safety; crossings • Natural environment • Vegetation, topography, weather • Parks, trails, walking routes | • Transportation systems • Urban planning and architecture • Parks and recreation sector • Health sector • Education and schools sector • Organized sport sector • National physical activity plans • National physical activity advocacy • Corporate sector | • Economic development • Global media • Global product marketing • Urbanization • Global advocacy • Social and cultural norms |

Early life exposures   Childhood   Adolescent   Young adult   Middle aged   Older adult →

Lifecourse

**Figure 4.2** | A Detailed Model of Factors That Affect the Adoption of Physically Active Lifestyle Throughout Life

*Source:* Adapted from A. E. Bauman et al., "Correlates of Physical Activity: Why Are Some People Physically Active and Others Not?," *The Lancet* (2012), 258–271.

Figure 4.2. Importantly, these causes range from characteristics that are unique to an individual (such as cognition and belief systems) to the most global influences (such as the level of economic development in a country or societal norms). Can you think of some specific examples of what "causes" people to be physically active at these various levels?

Some of the most convincing evidence regarding the vast reach of physical inactivity's impacts on health and society is illustrated in Figures 4.3 through 4.5. Each of these figures, developed and published in *Designed to Move: A Physical Activity Action Agenda*, illustrates the vast consequences, not just to individuals but to society as well, of physical inactivity.[3] The *Designed to Move* materials target primarily children and adolescents with physical activity and exercise suggestions and interventions, but the negative implications of being physically inactive also apply to those in early adulthood, middle age, and older adulthood.

The compounding economic costs and the increasing economic drains on society that are associated with physical inactivity from childhood through adolescence and then adulthood are shown in Figure 4.3. For example, an inactive child who grows up into an inactive adult may have much greater lifetime health care costs than an active child who continues to be physically active throughout her life. Figure 4.3 illustrates

the challenging cycle of physical inactivity that regularly confronts kinesiology practitioners trying to promote increased physical activity for improved health/fitness, peak athletic performance, disease prevention and management, or rehabilitation.

The interrelationships among levels of the physical activity continuum (low to high), keys to positive growth and development outcomes, and observed and documented benefits (such as improved brain function, cardiovascular function, musculoskeletal function, and motor movement skills) are shown in Figure 4.4. Better growth and development outcomes among young children who are physically active can be hypothesized to make it easier to be physically active in early adolescence. This positive experience can then yield more physical activity that continues to reinforce the behavior through life. As the old saying goes: success breeds success. Strong research evidence indicates that inactive children are much more likely than active children to grow up to be inactive adults. The pathways in Figure 4.4 clearly suggest that early positive physical activity experiences for children can affect their behavior over a lifetime.

Finally, the potential compounding economic and social benefits for individuals who are physically active throughout life—and for the society they belong to—are illustrated in Figure 4.5. Emerging evidence suggests

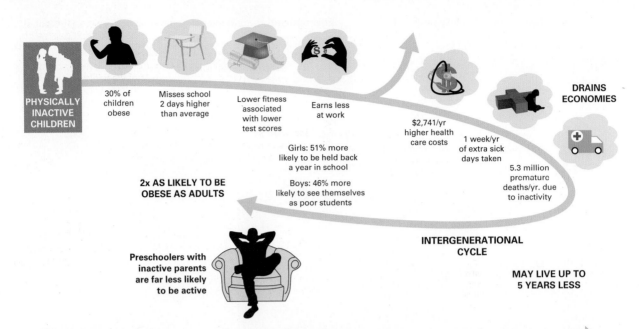

The above illustration is based upon select studies from a range of countries. The graphic shows how physical inactivity across the lifespan is associated with negative health, educational, and economic consequences. See reference source for more details.

**Figure 4.3** | Various Factors That Affect the Increased Economic Costs of a Lifestyle of Physical Inactivity

*Source:* Adapted from Nike, Inc., "Designed to Move: A Physical Activity Action Agenda," 2012, 7.

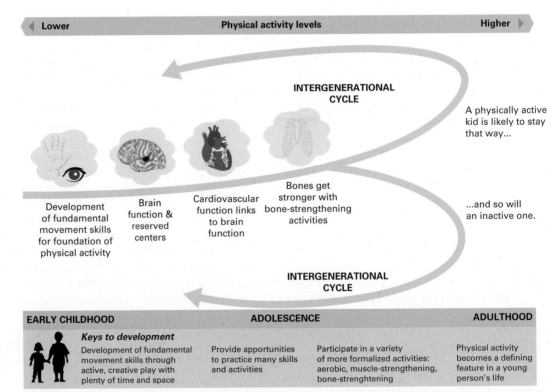

The above illustration is based upon select studies from a range of countries. The graphic shows how participation in regular physical activity and exercise across the lifespan is associated with positive physiological and developmental outcomes. See reference source for more details.

**Figure 4.4** | Impact of Physical Active and Physically Inactive Lifestyles on Growth and Development, Motor Skills, and Future Quality of Life

*Source:* Adapted from Nike, Inc., "Designed to Move: A Physical Activity Action Agenda," 2012, 13.

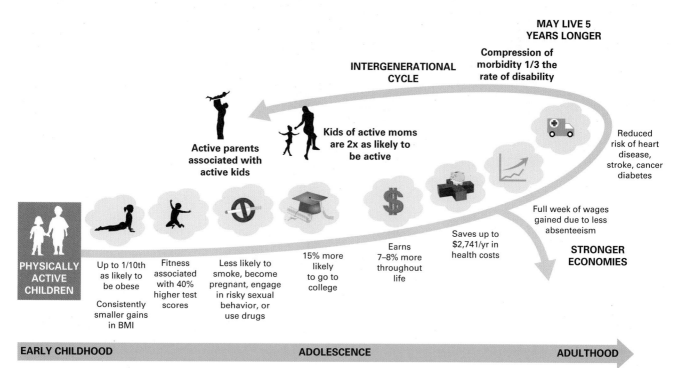

MAY LIVE 5
YEARS LONGER

INTERGENERATIONAL
CYCLE

Compression of
morbidity 1/3 the
rate of disability

Kids of active moms
are 2x as likely to
be active

Active parents
associated with
active kids

Reduced
risk of heart
disease,
stroke, cancer
diabetes

Full week of wages
gained due to less
absenteeism

STRONGER
ECONOMIES

PHYSICALLY
ACTIVE
CHILDREN

Up to 1/10th
as likely to
be obese

Consistently
smaller gains
in BMI

Fitness
associated
with 40%
higher test
scores

Less likely to
smoke, become
pregnant, engage
in risky sexual
behavior, or
use drugs

15% more
likely
to go to
college

Earns
7–8% more
throughout
life

Saves up to
$2,741/yr in
health costs

EARLY CHILDHOOD          ADOLESCENCE          ADULTHOOD

The above illustration is based upon select studies from a range of countries. The graphic shows how participation in regular physical activity and exercise across the lifespan is associated with positive health, educational, and economic outcomes. See reference source for more details.

Figure 4.5 | The Benefits of a Physically Active Lifestyle Throughout Life

*Source:* Adapted from Nike, Inc., "Designed to Move: A Physical Activity Action Agenda," 2012, 14.

that physically active children tend to perform better academically than inactive children.[4] Imagine the effects on a generation's health and economic productivity if all children were active and reached their full academic potential! These topics are rarely discussed in traditional kinesiology courses, but because physical activity is central to the kinesiology universe, they become incredibly important, as they extend beyond any one individual to society in general.

## Traditional Individual Exercise Prescription and Emerging Population Physical Activity Planning

As noted in Chapter 2, the Greek physicians Hippocrates (460–370 BC) and Galen (AD 129–210) were the first to promote the health benefits of physical activity and exercise.[5] In early writings, concepts such as "humoral theory," which was composed of "naturals" (physiology), "non-naturals" (hygiene), and "contra-naturals" (pathology of disease) were discussed. The non-naturals included six items related to hygiene (or what today we might call wellness): air, food and drink, motion and rest, sleep and wake, exertions and retentions, and passions of the mind. Both Hippocrates and Galen believed that the six non-naturals were influenced and regulated by (1) quantity, quality, time, and order (excess leads to imbalance and disease); (2) temperature and humidity; and

(3) disease states. How do you think some of the modern concepts of kinesiology that you have learned would relate to what Hippocrates and Galen described as the non-naturals?

The traditional kinesiology professional model of the past 30 years encouraged practitioners to focus almost exclusively on exercise training regimens that promoted the development of high levels of physical fitness and peak performance, rather than on the maintenance of or improvements in health achieved through physical activity along the continuum. In the 1970s, even kinesiology practitioners in pedagogy or sports management were less focused on health programming outcomes for their clients than measures related to optimizing performance. A sample of the traditional exercise training model that focused on individual exercise prescription targeting maximum performance as the key outcome is shown in Figure 4.6. What is missing from this model? The answer, of course, is the health effects of physical activity. Modern kinesiology professionals must embrace both the health and performance aspects of physical activity across the physical activity continuum.

The 1990s saw an expansion of the traditional performance-based approach to kinesiology to include research on the health aspects of physical activity. The publication of the Physical Activity Guidelines Advisory Committee Report, 2008[6] and the 2008 Physical

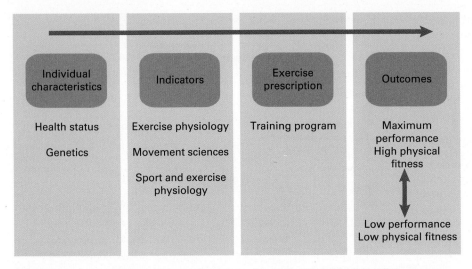

**Figure 4.6** | A Traditional Kinesiology-Based Exercise Training Model Focused on Increasing Peak or Maximum Performance

*Source:* H. W. Kohl and T. D. Murray, *Foundations of Physical Activity and Public Health* (Champaign, IL: Human Kinetics, 2012), 19.

Activity Guidelines for Americans[7] provided the first examples of an integration of the traditional kinesiology exercise training model concepts with population physical activity planning strategies from public health. The U.S. Physical Activity Guidelines represent a paradigm shift for kinesiology practitioners such that we now need to not only consider the initial (baseline) health levels of our clients but also strive to maintain or improve their health through their physical activity and exercise experiences. Even kinesiology practitioners who are interested solely in maximizing human performance should consider how to manage new health challenges related to accountability outcomes for their clients and their loved ones, in addition to meeting leadership goals. Health challenges that influence prevention of, rehabilitation from, and return to play after injury or illness might include, but are not necessarily limited to, musculoskeletal injuries, concussions, *Staphylococcus* infections, and asthma.

A graphical example of how the **dose** (amount or volume of physical activity or exercise including frequency, intensity, and duration) of physical activity and exercise can affect (often maintain or improve) health outcomes is shown in Figure 4.7. Although not all beneficial health outcomes are illustrated, this figure is intended to show health effects across the physical activity continuum. The dose of physical activity or exercise associated with each of the health outcomes illustrated in Figure 4.7 (such as osteoporosis, stroke, coronary artery disease) varies. Differences in patterns of health risks for varying diseases and problems with higher volumes of physical activity are shown in Figure 4.7. An additional consideration is that individual differences exist between people in how they respond to regular physical activity or exercise.

Lastly, in many cases, too much physical activity can be associated with negative side effects (injury). For example, if a person engages in too much weight bearing physical activity they increase their risk for musculoskeletal injury (see the musculoskeletal injury curve in Figure 4.7).

In Chapter 2, a new model for the integration of kinesiology subdisciplines and a continuum along which individuals move from physical inactivity (sedentary behavior)

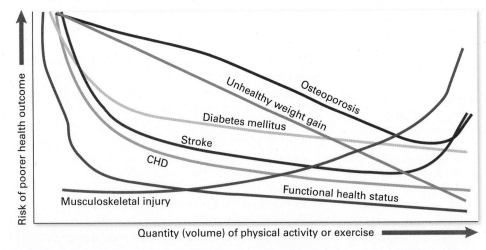

**Figure 4.7** | Physical Activity and Exercise Dose Response Curves That Influence Health Outcomes: The association between increasing physical activity and risk of adverse chronic disease health outcomes is shown. In general, risk of chronic disease drops dramatically with a relatively small amount of physical activity. The risk continues to drop along the continuum. The risk of musculoskeletal injuries, however, increases along the continuum.

*Source:* Adapted from H. W. Kohl and T. D. Murray, Foundations of Physical Activity and Public Health (Champaign, IL: Human Kinetics, 2012).

to functional health, then to physical fitness (based on higher order personal goals), and optionally toward peak performance (see Figure 2.3) was introduced. In this figure, the kinesiology subdisciplines and professional training are based upon the 2008 Physical Activity Guidelines for Americans and the National Physical Activity Plan.[7,8] Figure 4.8 (further modified from Figure 2.3) represents a comprehensive physical activity continuum and kinesiology model that helps kinesiology practitioners use various volumes and training principles to achieve desired physical activity levels for traditional individual exercise prescriptions as well as for population-based physical activity plans. The arrows linking each step (from low to high physical activity) in Figure 4.8 represent the application of the unifying training principles to improve conditioning over time, concepts you will learn more about later in this chapter.

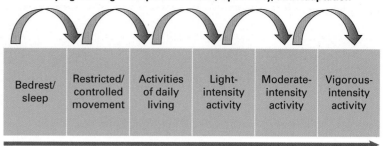

**Unifying Training Principles: Overload, Specificity, and Adaptation**

| Bedrest/ sleep | Restricted/ controlled movement | Activities of daily living | Light- intensity activity | Moderate- intensity activity | Vigorous- intensity activity |

Low      Physical activity/exercise levels      High

**Figure 4.8** | Overload, Specificity, and Adaptation: Training Principles That Affect Conditioning across a Physical Activity Continuum. The arrows linking each step (from low to high physical activity) represent the application of the unifying training principles to improve conditioning over time along a physical activity continuum.

## 2008 Physical Activity Guidelines for Americans

A key question that often faces kinesiology practitioners is: "How much physical activity or exercise is enough?" In light of the Chapter 3 discussion on evidence-based practice, you would probably need to clarify the previous question by asking a second one—"What is the desired outcome?"—in order to answer it appropriately. The answer to the question "How much exercise is enough?" will vary greatly depending upon, for example, whether the client is seeking to achieve good health, peak cardiovascular athletic performance, or a combination of both in relationship to the physical activity continuum. Numerous commercial exercise programs advertise that you can "get a total body workout" and reach peak performance in 5 to 10 minutes per day, 3 to 5 days per week, if you buy and use their product or service. However, the results among individuals following a given regime typically vary dramatically (this is often pointed out in advertising disclaimers), and these varying results often do not meet the desired goals of the participant. For example, one person might lose weight and gain cardiovascular endurance, while another person does not due to potential differences in dosages related to the concepts of overload and specificity. Therefore, the answer to the original question, "How much physical activity or exercise is enough?" is probably easier to answer relative to improving or maintaining health based on the current scientific evidence than for other common goals (such as weight loss) or outcomes (such as running a 10K in under 60 minutes) that you may encounter.

The 2008 Physical Activity Guidelines for Americans provide detailed information regarding what is known and not known about the health benefits of physical activity and exercise.[9] Scientific evidence indicates that participation in regular physical activity and exercise is associated with positive health outcomes, and the U.S. guideline papers contain major findings related to the following categories:

- All-cause mortality
- Cardiorespiratory health
- Metabolic health
- Energy balance
- Musculoskeletal health
- Functional health
- Cancer
- Mental health
- Children and youth
- Adverse events

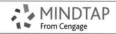

### MINDTAP
From Cengage

**2008 Physical Activity Guidelines for Americans**

**Go to your MindTap course** to read more about the latest U.S. physical activity guidelines.

Tables 4.1, 4.2, and 4.3 contain the current recommendations for physical activity and exercise from the U.S. Department of Health and Human Services. Tables 4.1, 4.2, and 4.3 contain key guidelines for children

**Table 4.1** | Key Guidelines for Children (Less Than 6 Years) and Adolescents

> ▸ Children and adolescents should do 60 minutes (1 hour) or more of physical activity daily.
>
> - *Aerobic:* Most of the 60 or more minutes a day should be either moderate- or vigorous-intensity aerobic physical activity, and should include vigorous-intensity physical activity at least 3 days a week.
> - *Muscle-strengthening:* As part of their 60 or more minutes of daily physical activity, children and adolescents should include muscle-strengthening physical activity on at least 3 days of the week.
> - *Bone-strengthening:* As part of their 60 or more minutes of daily physical activity, children and adolescents should include bone-strengthening physical activity on at least 3 days of the week.
>
> ▸ It is important to encourage young people to participate in physical activities that are appropriate for their age, that are enjoyable, and that offer variety.

*Source: 2008 Physical Activity Guidelines for Americans* (Washington, DC: U.S. Department of Health and Human Services, 2008), 16.

**Table 4.2** | Key Guidelines for Adults

> ▸ All adults should avoid inactivity. Some physical activity is better than none, and adults who participate in any amount of physical activity gain some health benefits.
>
> ▸ For substantial health benefits, adults should do at least 150 minutes (2 hours and 30 minutes) a week of moderate-intensity, or 75 minutes (1 hour and 15 minutes) a week of vigorous-intensity aerobic physical activity, or an equivalent combination of moderate- and vigorous-intensity aerobic activity. Aerobic activity should be performed in episodes of at least 10 minutes, and preferably, it should be spread throughout the week.
>
> ▸ For additional and more extensive health benefits, adults should increase their aerobic physical activity to 300 minutes (5 hours) a week of moderate-intensity, or 150 minutes a week of vigorous-intensity aerobic physical activity, or an equivalent combination of moderate- and vigorous-intensity activity. Additional health benefits are gained by engaging in physical activity beyond this amount.
>
> ▸ Adults should also do muscle-strengthening activities that are moderate or high intensity and involve all major muscle groups on 2 or more days a week, as these activities provide additional health benefits.

*Source: 2008 Physical Activity Guidelines for Americans* (Washington, DC: U.S. Department of Health and Human Services, 2008), 22.

(> 6 years) and adolescents, adults (> 21 years), and older adults (> 65 years), respectively. The U.S. physical activity and exercise recommendations apply across the lifespan except for those younger than 6 years of age, because a scientific consensus for recommending specific dosages of physical activity and exercise for the health of young children has not yet been reached.

**Table 4.3** | Guidelines for Older Adults (same as for adults plus the following)

> ▸ When older adults cannot do 150 minutes of moderate-intensity aerobic activity a week because of chronic conditions, they should be as physically active as their abilities and conditions allow.
>
> ▸ Older adults should do exercises that maintain or improve balance if they are at risk of falling.
>
> ▸ Older adults should determine their level of effort for physical activity relative to their level of fitness.
>
> ▸ Older adults with chronic conditions should understand whether and how their conditions affect their ability to do regular physical activity safely.

*Source: 2008 Physical Activity Guidelines for Americans* (Washington, DC: U.S. Department of Health and Human Services, 2008), 30.

# The Human Capital Model and the Domains of Physical Activity and Exercise

In 2012, Bailey and colleagues reported that a diverse group of sports scientists, medical researchers, psychologists, and other experts brought together by Nike, Inc. had developed a conceptual model of physical activity called the **Human Capital Model (HCM)**.[10] The model, illustrated in Figure 4.9, demonstrates how participation in and socialization through physical activity contribute holistically to the development of positive individual and population attributes; these attributes, in turn, can yield successful societal investments such as well-being, economic worth, academic achievement, and so on. Clearly, physical activity is not just about how to improve on a personal best in a 10K run or winning a tennis championship. Like kinesiology, physical activity can be viewed as an important center of our societal achievement.

The HCM includes the following six domains that impact health and social challenges: (1) physical capital, (2) emotional capital, (3) individual capital, (4) social capital, (5) intellectual capital, and (6) financial capital.

1. **Physical capital:** Includes the direct benefits of participating regularly in physical activity and exercise and the prevention/treatment effects of physical activity on disease processes; physical activity/exercise participation may also reduce risky behaviors.

2. **Emotional capital:** Includes the mental health and psychological benefits of regular participation in physical activity and exercise. Physical activity and exercise can also reduce the risks of excessive stress, depression, and anxiety.

3. **Individual capital:** Includes the positive character developmental factors associated with regular participation in physical activity and exercise.

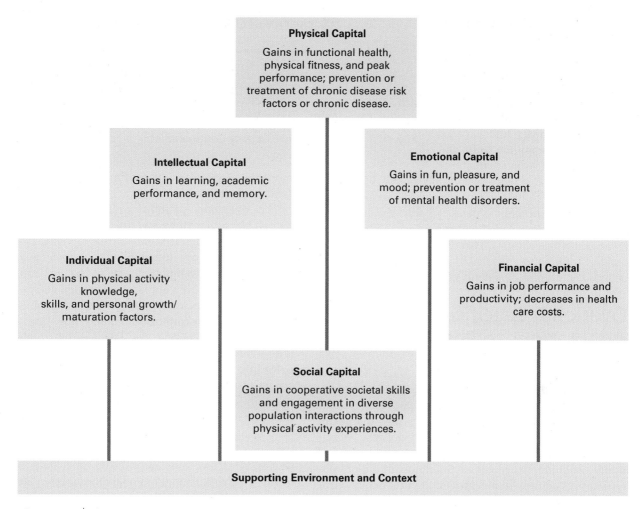

**Physical Capital**

Gains in functional health, physical fitness, and peak performance; prevention or treatment of chronic disease risk factors or chronic disease.

**Intellectual Capital**

Gains in learning, academic performance, and memory.

**Emotional Capital**

Gains in fun, pleasure, and mood; prevention or treatment of mental health disorders.

**Individual Capital**

Gains in physical activity knowledge, skills, and personal growth/maturation factors.

**Financial Capital**

Gains in job performance and productivity; decreases in health care costs.

**Social Capital**

Gains in cooperative societal skills and engagement in diverse population interactions through physical activity experiences.

**Supporting Environment and Context**

**Figure 4.9** | The Human Capital Model: Benefits of Participating in Regular Physical Activity

*Source:* R. Bailey, C. Hillman, S. Arent, and A. Petitpas, "Physical Activity as an Investment in Personal and Social Change: The Human Capital Model," *Journal of Physical Activity and Health* 9 (2012): 1053–1055.

4. **Social capital:** Includes the effects related to interactions with people and groups during regular participation in physical activity and exercise experiences.

5. **Intellectual capital:** Includes the cognitive developmental, academic, and educational gains associated with regular participation in physical activity and exercise.

6. **Financial capital:** Includes job success and productivity and lower health care costs associated with regular participation in physical activity and exercise.

The HCM, which is based on scientific evidence, illustrates why kinesiology majors must integrate their professional skills through undergraduate academic training to achieve successful client and population-based outcomes. The HCM provides a vision of how you might use your kinesiology common core or knowledge base to understand the underlying factors linking the practice of kinesiology to well-being and success. (See Chapter 2 sections on physical activity in health, wellness, and quality of life; scientific foundations of physical activity; cultural,

historical, and philosophical dimensions of physical activity; and the practice of physical activity.)

As Bailey and colleagues suggest, "Ultimately, the Human Capital Model is a call to consider investments in physical activity as powerful catalysts for personal and social change."[11]

## Details of the SLOTH Model

The SLOTH model has been described as a time-budget model incorporating key economic factors that may influence individuals' choices about their use of time and physical activity.[12] The SLOTH model highlights how physical activity (and inactivity such as sleep) is integrated into every person's day. It illustrates how we as practitioners can and should encourage participation in regular physical activity for better sleep experiences, for leisure (recreation and entertainment), occupationally (working or studying), for transportation (active commuting), and at home (domestic activities, e.g., mowing, gardening).

The SLOTH model can be useful to a kinesiology practitioner, particularly during development and implementation of interventions and recommendations to increase physical activity. For example, many opportunities for encouraging physical activity and exercise are dependent upon the **built environment** (constructed structures affecting physical activity opportunities). The built environment might include open spaces/parks, urban design/land use, transportation systems, schools, and buildings/workplaces. By understanding the barriers and facilitators associated with the built environment, kinesiology practitioners can be better prepared to promote positive physical activity and exercise experiences.

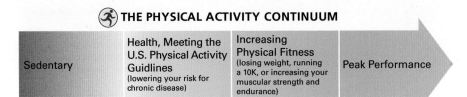

**Figure 4.10** | The Physical Activity Continuum

## Overload, Specificity, and Adaptations to Physical Activity and Exercise

The center of the kinesiology universe is physical activity. The effects of physical activity on human body systems result in the physiologic changes from which the health and performance benefits of physical activity arise. Oftentimes, kinesiology professionals use the terms *training* and *conditioning* interchangeably as descriptors of the physiologic results gained from a specific physical activity program. The authors of this text, on the other hand, define training as a *process* that encompasses specific groups of exercises based on physiologic "training principles" and conditioning as the *physiologic outcomes* or *long-term effects* of training. **Training** is a consistent or chronic progression of exercise sessions designed to improve physiologic function for better health or sports performance. **Conditioning** includes the persistent physiological changes or adjustments resulting from training or training adaptation.

Notice the cause and effect relationship that is established when we define training and conditioning in this manner. Training is the cause and conditioning is the effect. Thus, training results in achieving and maintaining conditioning, and both universally relate to moving people and populations along the physical activity continuum. For example, effective training and conditioning messaging and programming developed by kinesiology practitioners are essential to producing increased physical activity and exercise in models like that shown in Figure 4.8 or, in a simple form, in Figure 4.10. The physical activity continuum presented in Figure 4.10 is also represented by this simple icon that you will see frequently through the remainder of this text. 🏃

**Training principles** are fundamental guidelines that form the basis for training the body's systems with physical activity. Three unifying training principles that apply across the physical activity continuum are overload, specificity, and adaptation.

The **overload principle** refers to increasing the dose of physical activity and exercise to stress the body's physiologic systems beyond normal homeostasis (rest) in order to improve function (e.g., metabolic, muscle, biomechanical, psychological, and so on). For example, if you want to improve your fitness level and decrease your 10K run time, increasing your speed during training runs will overload your cardiovascular and muscular systems. This overload will then translate to improvements in fitness compared with where you began. The **specificity principle** refers to the fact that training adaptations are very specific to the imposed demands on the body. *Specificity* refers to the adaptations that occur within specific tissues of the body, which vary based on the level (low to high) of training demand. For example, weight training of the upper body (physical activity) will result in a specificity because only those upper-body muscles being trained will undergo adaptations (gain strength/endurance). Finally, the **adaptation principle** refers to how the body reacts over time to overload and specificity related to physical activity—for instance, one might be progressing (making improvements), at a plateau, in a maintenance mode, or actually losing (or reversing) the positive conditioning changes associated with training anywhere along the physical activity continuum.

The unifying training principles—overload, specificity, and adaptation—are illustrated in Figures 4.11 through

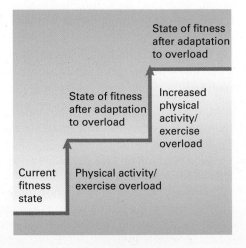

**Figure 4.11** | The Overload Principle

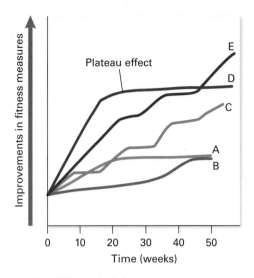

Figure 4.12 | Specificity and the Trainability Principle

A–E = Different individuals

4.13. The general aspects of the overload principle are illustrated in Figure 4.11. Figure 4.12 illustrates how some specific adaptations over 50 weeks of physical activity training (trainability) are affected by the rate of change and maximal potential of various individuals (labeled A–E in the figure). Notice the plateau in training effect for individual D. A general model of training and conditioning adaptations related to meeting and exceeding the adult 2008 Physical Activity Guidelines for Americans is shown in Figure 4.13; as you can see, it includes an initial stage, an improvement stage, and a maintenance stage for

conditioning and improvements in functional health and fitness.

Other training principles related to progression, plateau, maintenance, and reversibility describe the conditioning effects of specific adaptations to training. *Progression* refers to improvements or decreases in performance based upon regular participation in physical activity or exercise. With each increase (or decrease) in activity, physiologic systems in the body progress to higher (or lower) fitness levels. Decreases in performance are associated with becoming or remaining sedentary for long periods of time (weeks to months). The *plateau principle effect* refers to reaching a stage where there are no improvements or declines in performance with changes in physical activity. The *maintenance principle* refers to reaching a physical activity or fitness goal and then performing enough physical activity to remain at the desired level. The *reversibility principle* refers to the loss of physical activity benefits that occurs when a previously active person becomes physically inactive and remains so for long periods of time. Studies of the effects on human physiology of the absence of physical activity during space flight and bed rest are good examples of reversibility.

## Examples of the Integration of Overload, Specificity, and Adaptations with Health-Related Outcomes and Peak Performance

A classic theory known as **general adaptation syndrome (GAS)** proposes that stress (psychological, physiological, or environmental) causes numerous physiological reactions beyond rest or **homeostasis**.[13] The

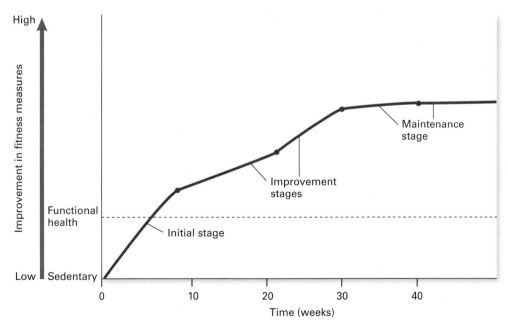

Functional health = *2008 Physical Activity Guidelines for Americans* (Adults; at least 150 minutes per week)

Figure 4.13 | General Model of Training and Conditioning Adaptations Related to Meeting and Exceeding the Adult 2008 Physical Activity Guidelines for Americans

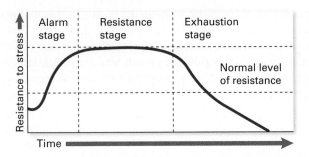

**Figure 4.14** | An Example of Selye's General Adaptation Syndrome

physiological response to a stressor begins the process of adaptation. Figure 4.14 graphically represents the physiological reaction to any stress as described by Selye, the researcher who first described GAS. As adaptations occur, the reaction to the stressor is minimized. Selye further described and explained this adaptation process as having three stages: alarm reaction, resistance, and exhaustion.

The first stage of GAS is the alarm reaction stage. This is the immediate or acute response to a perceived stressor. Stage 1 deals with the flight-or-fight response associated with the sympathetic nervous system (the part of the human nervous system that maintains body functions such as heart rate, digestion, and perspiration without our conscious awareness). During physical activity and exercise, this response to the stressor is regulated through release of hormones into the blood by nerve cells simply in anticipation of beginning the activity. This anticipatory stress is an acute response that immediately occurs with the first bout of exercise. The end product of these events is a physiological response to the perceived stress such as an increase in heart rate.

In relationship to the physical activity continuum, if one remains sedentary or, even worse, is challenged by two to three weeks of prolonged bed rest, the body will adapt in negative ways physiologically, psychologically, and biomechanically, which is called **detraining**. Bed rest is an extreme example of detraining, but 20 days of complete bed rest in 20-year-olds has been shown to cause a greater deterioration in cardiorespiratory capacity than 30 years of aging.[14]

It is important to recognize that the benefits of physical activity may be lost at different rates depending upon an individual's characteristics. For example, if an individual detrains by reducing aerobic (cardiovascular) workouts for four weeks, you may notice that his cardiovascular fitness level drops significantly, while his strength may not decrease by the same degree. You should also realize that individuals do not lose significant fitness benefits in a day or two, or even three. Therefore, it is not harmful—and, in fact, always a good idea—to have clients take off a day or two on occasion, especially if they are unusually tired, sick, or have significant conflicts of schedule.

The second stage of GAS, resistance, refers to the chronic effects of stress. When physical activity or exercise is the stress stimulus, the end product of this stage is true physiological adaptation. The resistance stage can be described as a sensitization to the stressor whereby physiological adaptations bring the body back into homeostasis, thus alleviating the impact of the stressor. In the resistance stage, the chain of events that occurs during the first stage is reduced due to changes or adaptations in physiology.

The relationship between GAS and physical activity and exercise can be observed even with a very simple day-to-day activity. What happens if you decide to begin walking up and down six flights of stairs instead of taking the elevator every day at your workplace or your apartment building? As you look at the stairs on the first day and decide to begin to take the first steps toward better fitness, the perception of stress (the anticipatory response) causes a neural trigger that stimulates an immediate physiological response to increase your heart rate and respiration rate and illustrates Stage 1 of GAS. As you repeat this process each day, the perception or anticipation dissipates due to desensitization of the challenge. In other words, after a week of taking the steps, you become accustomed to the sight of the staircase and realize that it is not a barrier for you.

In Stage 2, as you take the steps each day, the stressor for this activity is the increase in work required to move your body up the incline of the stairs. We can define *work* with the simple mathematical equation: work = force × distance. In the case of taking the stairs, work = body weight (the force) × the product of the vertical and horizontal incline (distance). As you repeatedly complete this activity over the course of several weeks, adaptations in one or more of the physiological systems (such as your thigh muscles, your pulmonary system, or your heart) will occur to resist the effects of the stressor. One additional physiological adaptation that might occur after weeks of taking the steps is the loss of body fat. That loss of body fat changes (decreases) your weight, which in turn decreases the amount of work required to move your body up the steps. As Selye observed, prolonged stress ultimately forces physiological accommodations (adaptations) to maintain a relative homeostasis in the presence of continued stress.

Remember that previously we described physical activity and exercise as the stressor; however, we should be more specific and name the exercise load—or, to use a more appropriate term, the exercise volume—as the true stressor. With this in mind, we can then assume from our stairs example that once you have adapted to the exercise volume (distance traveled up the stairs), you again reach physiological homeostasis. Once you have reached physiological homeostasis, no further adaptations will occur and the current exercise volume is no longer a stressor.

If you maintain the same exercise volume for the rest of your life, theoretically you will remain in the same state of fitness once the full adaptation process is complete. In other words, unless you increase the exercise volume (overload), you will remain in a maintenance state. So, to further improve your fitness levels, whether health related or sports specific, you will overload yourself and move along the physical activity continuum.

The third stage of GAS is exhaustion. The exhaustion stage is attained when stress persists with enough intensity (overload) that the individual reaches a point beyond which adaptations are no longer possible and physiological, biomechanical, and psychological function suffer. In other words, if stress of physical activity or exercise persists long enough or with a great enough intensity, the individual begins to experience a decline in performance (**over-training**). This means that kinesiology practitioners must be aware that individuals may react to physical activity and exercise volume in the form of overload in a negative fashion such that they cause a detriment to training and ultimately performance. Although over-training is typically a characteristic of the upper end of the physical activity continuum, it can happen at any stage along the continuum.

One extreme example of excessive exercise volume and over-training involves peak performance training. A young man who was training for the Toronto Marathon had a personal goal to complete the marathon in less than three hours (7:02 per mile pace for 26.2 miles). While the young man had been a good cross-country runner (3 miles) in high school, he had no experience running a marathon. When asked about his training volume, he stated that he was training himself and running about 200 miles per week (an extremely high volume even for elite competitive marathoners who train closer to 100 miles per week). His actual training method during most days of the week was to rise at 2:00 a.m. and go for a 10-mile run, followed by breakfast and a rest period of reading or watching TV. At 9:00 a.m. he went out for a 5-mile run, followed by a snack, and then he attended classes at the university. At 4:00 p.m. on some days, he would complete 10 more miles, followed by dinner and some reading. On Saturday or Sunday, he would run 20 to 30 miles continuously. As you have probably figured out, the "stress" he experienced far exceeded his ability to adapt within just a couple of weeks. The negative physiological and psychological symptoms he developed in response to the stress were sleeplessness, lethargy, some pulmonary problems, and an aversion to running—an activity that had once been fun. The young man was burned out on running, was over-trained and exhausted, and was not even able to show up to run the marathon.

The two examples provided above illustrate how GAS can positively or negatively influence physical and mental performance related to movement. Elements of Selye's stress model should be integrated with the unifying physical activity and exercise training principles (overload, specificity, and adaptation) by kinesiology practitioners to help people and populations reach realistic physical activity and exercise goals, while avoiding both detraining and over-training.

# A Systems Approach for Planning Physical Activity and Exercise Interventions for Kinesiology Practitioners

According to Kohl and colleagues, we are currently experiencing a global pandemic of physical inactivity; moreover, future economic and social transitions appear likely to increase the prevalence of physical inactivity even more for many years to come.[15] However, physical activity continues to be undervalued despite strong evidence that it is important for good health and contributes positively, economically and socially, to all societies.[16] Previous attempts to increase physical activity levels have focused on individuals rather than populations (similar to the traditional training models used in kinesiology). A key recommendation is that future physical activity intervention strategies should consider additional factors besides biology (e.g., genetics and disease risk), behavior (e.g., lifestyle actions), and environment (e.g., low versus high socioeconomic status) with regards to changes in the prevalence of inactivity. Kohl and colleagues suggest using a systems approach to understanding the complex elements that influence physical activity comprehensively. Figure 4.15 illustrates traditional public health and physical activity interventions focusing on behavioral and environmental approaches (A) as compared to a more comprehensive systems approach (B).[17]

For kinesiology professionals, the global challenge of physical inactivity is an opportunity to refocus on the real value of physical activity and exercise within our field. This new focus should include a systems approach to understanding the complex pathway to adopting physical activity and exercise, beyond simple descriptions of individual pieces of the puzzle such as specific health behaviors and environmental factors. A **systems approach** (Figure 4.15) allows kinesiology practitioners to study contributing factors including (1) barriers to physical activity, (2) enablers that promote physical activity adoption, (3) accelerants that speed up adoption of physical activity, (4) competing actions affecting adoption of physical activity, (5) effects of the built environment on physical activity, (6) the impact of physical activity adoption in schools, the workplace, sports and recreation, and transportation, and (7) and other influences. Some of the contributing factors in systems approach

**(A) Behavioral and Environmental Approaches**

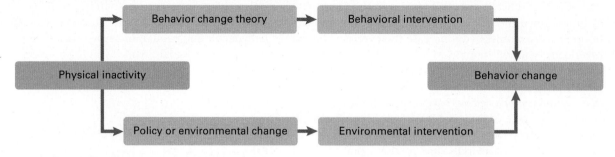

**(B) Systems Approaches**

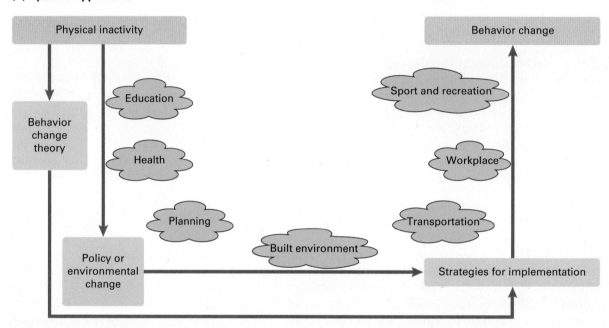

**Figure 4.15** | Behavioral and Environmental Approaches versus Systems Approaches to Physical Activity Behavior Change. Systems approaches to population change in physical activity. In addition to behavior and environmental changes, various places and sectors where people live must be engaged.

*Source:* Adapted from H. W. Kohl III et al., "The Pandemic of Physical Activity: Global Action for Public Health," *The Lancet* 380 (2012): 295–305.

analyses for physical activity are included as resources for the Designed to Move program. These can be used by practitioners to promote physical activity while recognizing potential behavioral and environmental barriers to successful adoption.

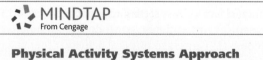

**Physical Activity Systems Approach**

**Go to your MindTap course** to learn about physical activity infographics and various physical activity reports from the United States and globally at Designed to Move.

By all means, kinesiology professionals should continue to embrace and practice the effective traditional physical activity and exercise strategies for human performance (focused more on individual change) of the past 30 years. However, it is also essential that kinesiology practitioners embrace the full physical activity continuum and the health benefits of physical activity. Not everyone will be an elite athlete; nonetheless, everyone deserves the health benefits associated with physical activity. It is important that you learn and apply new models and systems approaches (including the physical activity continuum, 2008 Physical Activity Guidelines for Americans, SLOTH model, Kohl and colleagues' model, and Designed to Move: Physical Activity Systems Maps) to promote changes in populations served by future kinesiology practitioners.

# EXAMPLES OF APPLYING TRAINING FUNDAMENTALS IN KINESIOLOGY SUBDISCIPLINES

*In Lesson 1, we emphasized the importance of understanding the physical activity continuum and models that can help kinesiology practitioners understand how to better optimize the adoption of physically active lifestyles such as SLOTH and the HCM. In Lesson 2, you will learn about examples of applying the subdisciplines of kinesiology to problem solving across the physical activity continuum.*

- Public Health
- Exercise Physiology
- Motor Learning
- Sport/Exercise Psychology
- Biomechanics
- The Practice of Kinesiology

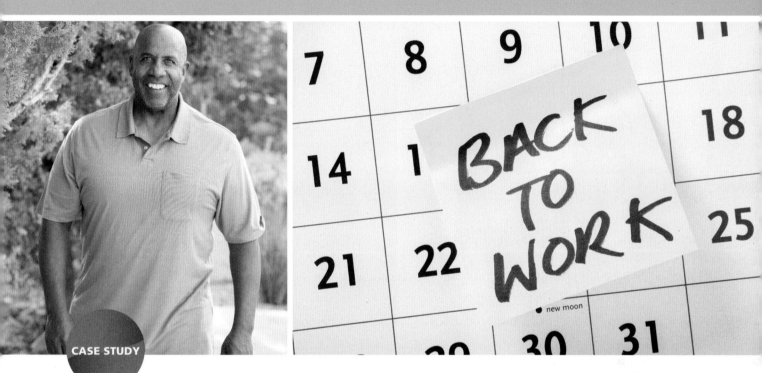

CASE STUDY

## In the real world . . .

Recall from the beginning of this chapter that Harry Casey suffered a myocardial infarction (MI). William and Marie visited with the cardiac rehabilitation coordinator, Helen, and learned about the core components of cardiac rehabilitation secondary/prevention programs. Helen told the Caseys that the medical center used evidence-based practices and integrated multi-factorial plans for their cardiac rehabilitation programming based on the American Heart Association (AHA) and American Association of Cardiovascular and Pulmonary Rehabilitation (AACVPR) guidelines.[18] The medical center's cardiac rehabilitation model included a Phase I component, or in-patient program (including items like medical history, physical examinations, risk factor management, physical therapy range-of-motion exercises, a nutritional consult, a psychosocial consult as needed, and weight management counseling) prior to discharge. Harry was diagnosed with a right-sided, mild, and uncomplicated MI, so his hospital stay lasted four days. He was given a medically supervised symptom-limited submaximal graded exercise test (with a 5-MET maximal workload) with electrographic monitoring (ECG) on day four. (1 MET equals the energy expended at rest, so 5 METs refers to 5 times resting energy expenditure.) Harry was discharged by his cardiologist and Helen with a documented plan including short-term goals (promote healing of heart damage and train to obtain functional health) and long-term goals (return to part-time work status). He started the Phase II cardiac rehabilitation program (outpatient phase lasting 12 weeks and covered by Harry's supplemental insurance).

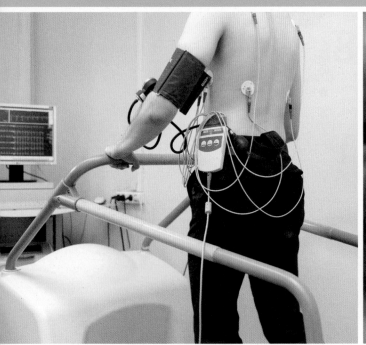

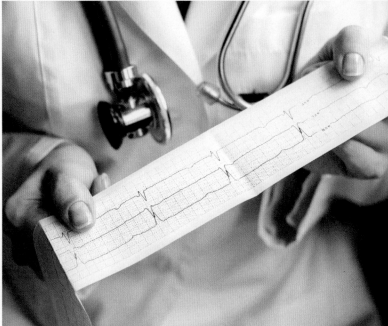

The Phase I case scenario described above provides you with a typical example of the diversity of skills and clinical knowledge that a kinesiology practitioner like Helen must acquire and integrate into her or his daily practice. A working knowledge of models like those you learned about in this chapter—such as the Human Capital Model and the systems approach to physical activity—helps professionals like Helen to enhance patient compliance and program outcome success.

For Harry's Phase II programming, Helen designed an individual plan based upon population-based evidence (in this case, the population consists of post–heart attack patients). Harry's rehabilitation plan included evaluation, interventions, and expected outcomes for the following areas: blood pressure management, lipid management, diabetes management, tobacco cessation, psychological management,

physical activity counseling, and exercise training. Helen provided Harry with specific physical activity and exercise training recommendations based on the 2007 AHA/AACVPR recommendations. The specific recommendations are shown in Appendix I.

In conclusion, comprehensive and detailed planning is part of most kinesiology professionals' daily duties. Gaining practical experiences with integrating system-based approaches to physical activity and exercise training for the future is essential to the effective practice of kinesiology.

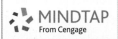 **MINDTAP** From Cengage | Go to your MindTap course to complete the Case Study activity for this chapter.

## Public Health and Exercise Physiology ⚕ 〽

The physical activity continuum is very much a part of the public health subdiscipline of kinesiology. Public health guidelines for physical activity for youth indicate that each child and adolescent should get 60 minutes of moderate-intensity or vigorous-intensity physical activity each day of the week. In the past, we have depended on physical education classes in schools to provide daily physical activity for children and adolescents. With changes in the school day and increasing emphasis on standardized testing, physical education has frequently been cut and modified such that in many school districts it is no longer reliable as a means for children to be sufficiently active.

The Institute of Medicine (IOM) has coined the term *Whole of School* for their recommended approach to physical activity.[19] With the Whole of School approach, physical activity opportunities before, during, and after school are maximized to help children and adolescents achieve the recommended 60 minutes per day of physical activity, using all the time spent in school. For example, active transport to school (biking, walking, skateboarding) can contribute a certain amount of activity. Active lessons and recess breaks, physical education, intramural and extramural sports, after-school programs, and active transport back home from school can all be leveraged as opportunities for physical activity. Schools are in a good position to succeed with this approach and thus affect a large swath of the population because (1) most children are in schools and (2) schools already have many of the resources needed for these programs in place. If physical activity was a health (and education) priority for all schools, as is called for in the report, many children would be moved along the physical activity continuum and health and other important benefits would follow. (Review Chapter 1 and see Chapter 11 for further details about the Whole of School approach.)

## An Integrated Kinesiology Scenario Related to the Physical Activity Continuum

This section provides an integrated example regarding movement and the physical activity continuum and including areas of study related to motor behavior, sport/exercise psychology, and biomechanics.

### Motor Learning

To understand the physical activity continuum fully, you must recognize that motor behavior—defined as the study of movement acquisition—is the foundation of any exercise skill or physical activity. As you learned in Chapter 2, motor behavior encompasses the areas of motor development (the development of movement skill), motor learning (the acquisition and improvement of movement skills through practice), and motor control (the neural control and fine tuning of movement skills). Motor behavior determines whether movement occurs and, if so, how that movement is implemented. To put motor behavior into context within the physical activity continuum, you need only to understand that without movement, there is no physical activity, and without physical activity there is no continuum. Any physical activity skill, whether it is running, jumping, throwing, etc., involves motor behavior because movement of the body is required.

Progressing from the sedentary area of the physical activity continuum to the physically active area requires body movement (motor behavior) with a subsequent increase in energy expenditure due to the movement. So, whether you are a parent, teacher, coach, or exercise instructor, at some time in your career, you will use information from the motor behavior subdiscipline to teach a movement skill to an individual, and hopefully that skill will move the individual further along the physical activity continuum. You should strive to teach movement skills effectively, or unwanted consequences that can limit the individual's movement along the physical activity continuum may occur due to lack of skill development.

One example of how the lack of motor skill development can impact lifetime physical activity relates to the skill of running and the inherent pacing necessary to properly run a given distance. Think back to all of the physical education classes you had as a child. Most students in elementary school and many students in middle and high school are asked to complete a physical fitness test each year. That fitness test usually includes an aerobic component (running) such as the 1.5-mile run (timed), 12-minute run (number of laps completed), or shuttle run (timed) that is required of all students. If you ever participated in one of these, do you remember ever being taught *how* to practice/prepare for the fitness test? For most students, the teacher probably looked at a daily lesson plan and declared it was fitness test day, probably without allowing students to prepare for the evaluation. Elementary students who have not been taught proper running techniques (such as pacing and related growth and development factors) typically start the test moving as fast as they can in an inefficient running style (usually at a sprint on the balls of their feet with short strides). Within a few minutes, they become tired and have to walk or cannot complete the test, thereby performing poorly on the aerobic portion of test.

In the above scenario, the question is, who failed? Was it the student who did not have the proper running technique and pacing strategy, or the teacher who did not teach that student the proper running technique and pacing? And because the student failed, it might be harder to move him or her from the sedentary to active portion of the physical activity continuum because no one enjoys failure or poor performance.

## Sport/Exercise Psychology

To demonstrate how sport/exercise psychology relates to the physical activity continuum and how this subdiscipline of kinesiology is linked to the motor behavior subdiscipline, we will differentiate between sport psychology and exercise psychology to introduce two new tools and examples that can affect and influence the physical activity continuum. As discussed in the motor behavior example, teaching proper movement skills to students is paramount to achieving desirable outcomes. One tool the sport psychologist can use to improve and fine-tune those skills is called mental imagery. Mental imagery is a technique in which the student imagines what the perfect movement looks like in her or his mind and then mentally practices that movement. As they mentally practice the movement, students can compare the perfect movement to their own performance. By using mental imagery, they can determine areas of improvement in their own movement activities and correct any faulty movements, thereby "fine-tuning" and improving their skill in the activity. As the student improves in the activity, his or her feeling of "self" increases, which can motivate the individual to move on to more physically demanding activities; this, in turn, moves the individual along the physical activity continuum.

For the exercise psychologist, a tool that is most helpful in moving a person along the physical activity continuum is the stages of motivational readiness (stages of change) model.[20] The stages of change model describes the mental readiness of a person to move from inaction to action. The model includes five main categories that characterize a person's desire to move from inaction to action: precontemplation, contemplation, preparation, action, and maintenance (see Chapter 7 for more about the model). The precontemplation category describes a person who does not yet embrace change because of perceived barriers or previous failure. The contemplation category describes the person who is willing to think about changing when previously perceived barriers are lessened or removed. The action stage describes the person's willingness to move to action and participate in the activity. Finally, the maintenance stage is the stage in which the person continues to participate in the activity, improving her or his performance. Have you noticed how the stages of change relate to the physical activity continuum? The precontemplation and contemplation stages describe the sedentary individual whereas the action and maintenance stages describe the physically active person. The exercise psychologist understands these stages and intervenes to move the individual from precontemplation to maintenance. For physical activity, this translates to moving the person from physical inactivity to physical activity and then to improved performance through maintenance of the physical activity task, thereby moving the person along the physical activity continuum. In our real world example, Harry may need assistance in overcoming his reasons for staying in the precontemplation or contemplation stages and moving along to action and maintenance to get the most out of his cardiac rehabilitation programming.

## Biomechanics

The field of biomechanics relates to the physical activity continuum through both healthy and disease states associated with the aging process. In the healthy individual, the knowledge of muscle mechanics can help improve physical activity efficiency, whereas in the person in the disease state it may help maintain the current stage of the physical activity continuum. As individuals age, certain diseases such as arthritis and joint deterioration—conditions that create pain and discomfort upon movement—may cause a slow regression to more sedentary behaviors, moving the individual from a physically active lifestyle back toward a sedentary lifestyle.

Other, more deleterious diseases that can occur suddenly such as strokes or the onset of Parkinson's disease can have an immediate impact on the person's stage along the physical activity continuum. The physical therapist or rehabilitation specialist often must combine a knowledge of motor behavior with a knowledge of biomechanics to help rehabilitate a person and return him or her to a more active lifestyle. In the case of Parkinson's disease, where no cure is available, the rehabilitation specialist likely will attempt to improve the quality of life of the afflicted individual and to slow the progression of the disease.

Parkinson's disease is a degenerative disease that affects the motor pathways of the brain. The motor symptoms include tremors, slowed movement, stiffness in the limbs, and loss of core stability. You can likely imagine how changes in these functions would reduce the person's physical activity level. The rehabilitation specialist uses her or his knowledge of biomechanics and motor behavior to improve the client's gait speed (walking speed), flexibility, and strength. With improvement in these areas, the person can enjoy a better quality of life.

Specifically, rehabilitation specialists work to maintain the biomechanical properties of the individual such as muscle flexibility and joint range of motion. For example, the kinesiologist working with Harry should initially ensure fundamental joint motion in his knees, hips, and ankles as a prerequisite to moving him into more challenging rehabilitation settings. By working with these biomechanical properties, the specialist can facilitate some improvement in mobility and physical function, which will maintain and sometimes improve the individual's physical activity ability. This intervention can at the

## People Matter  Amanda Peterson, Clinical Exercise Physiologist*

**Q:** Why and how did you get into the field of kinesiology?

**A:** *I grew up playing sports and was always on the move. I originally thought I wanted to go into education and coaching. It wasn't until my junior year in my undergraduate work that I realized I was more interested in the field of kinesiology and exercise physiology. After completing an internship at the Cooper Fitness Center in Dallas, Texas, I knew I was where I needed to be professionally.*

**Q:** What was the major influence on you to work in the field?

**A:** *A few of my undergraduate professors played a role in my interest to learn about cardiovascular physiology and how the body responds to activity. Dr. Carl Foster became more of a major influence after I was accepted to UW-La Crosse, where I attended graduate school and obtained a Masters in Clinical Exercise Physiology. Now, as a young professional in my career, my colleague Mark Vitcenda keeps me inspired that there is always something new to learn within the field of exercise physiology and cardiac rehab.*

**Q:** What are your current research interests, and how do you translate your research results to practitioners?

**A:** *I am currently not actively involved in any research; however, I have always been interested in the psychological aspect of health and chronic disease. I feel that we, as clinicians, play a major role in our patients'* day-to-day moods, as well as their outlook on life as they can be dealing with serious health conditions.

**Q:** How do you stay physically active yourself and promote good health to others directly around you?

**A:** *In order to practice what I preach, I stay physically active by swimming, walking, and riding my bike. I also enjoy lifting weights and competed in my first powerlifting meet recently. I love the outdoors and enjoy outdoor activities as well, such as camping, canoeing, hiking, and skiing. I tend to silently lead by example, and always try to be encouraging to others of not only the physical benefits of exercise, but the psychological ones as well.*

**Q:** How have you had to integrate the subdisciplines of kinesiology in your professional practice?

**A:** *I spent the first two years of my post-MS career working in a cardiac rehabilitation center in Dallas, TX, that was part of what might be called a work hardening center. It became obvious that muscle strength and endurance, as well as lifting mechanics, were co-equal with aerobic capacity in terms of achieving the rehabilitation goal of patients being able to return to the lives they want to live.*

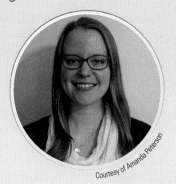
Courtesy of Amanda Peterson

*Amanda Peterson is a Clinical Exercise Physiologist in Cardiopulmonary Rehabilitation at UW Hospitals and Clinics in Madison, WI. She is a member of the American Association of Cardiovascular and Pulmonary Rehabilitation (AACVPR). Her interests also include research and progressive thinking within the field.

least help maintain the individual's current stage along the physical activity continuum, and in some cases improve their physical activity status. At a minimum, the understanding and proper use of biomechanics can maintain the quality of life of the individual and slow the regression toward a sedentary lifestyle.

### The Practice of Kinesiology—Return to Work

The physical activity continuum is strongly related to a person's ability to return to work after a life-changing event like Harry Casey's heart attack, which was described in the case study. An individual can, in a worst-case situation, remain physically inactive and psychologically stressed or, in the best case, regain the previous level of functional health by being physically active, while managing his or her disease and future health status.

As you may remember from Lesson 1, Harry was employed part time as a salesman in a lumberyard prior to his heart attack. If he wants to return to work, how would a kinesiology practitioner like Helen help him? Patients like Harry often want or need to return to work for financial reasons and/or for the socialization and self-esteem benefits associated with working and being a productive citizen, which improve quality of life. The following scenario presents one approach to addressing the challenge of returning to work after a heart attack.

Although medical variables (heart attack severity and the resulting damage to the heart muscle) are often used as strong predictors of a patient's ability to return to work, they may not affect return to work as much as psychological factors. Mood disturbances such as depression are a major factor that limit a patient's ability to return to work. Therefore, an evaluation of Harry's beliefs and self-efficacy designed to determine if he is psychologically ready to return to work after Phase II rehabilitation (about two months post–heart attack) would be helpful for Harry as well as for his employer and primary care physician. It is important to encourage cardiac patients who wish to return to work to do so within two to three months post cardiac event, or the probability of successful return to work becomes much less likely.[21]

A common approach in cardiac rehabilitation for return to work is to conduct an energy cost and psychological work assessment of the actual job requirements. In Harry's case, most of his sales duties would only require 2 to 3 times resting energy expenditure (2–3 METs). Since Harry successfully completed his Phase II cardiac rehabilitation programming with Helen, he should be good to go once he has a return-to-work plan. A return-to-work plan might include the following:

▸ Phase back gradually into duties (e.g., 5–10 hours the first couple of weeks)

▸ Avoid heavy lifting or lifting items that require breath holding (contraindicated because they increase heart rate and blood pressure)

▸ Include additional rest periods as needed when fatigue occurs

▸ Rehabilitation specialist to obtain feedback about performance from Harry and employer

In Harry's case it may be important to observe him actually working because, as the majority of his work duties will be categorized as light on the physical activity continuum, he may become overconfident about his physical abilities and try to do too much too soon. In his return-to-work plan it would be wise to encourage him to ask for help from colleagues when he needs to lift a heavier item on the sales rack, or to slow the rate at which he lifts and stacks stock items, for example.

Harry should be encouraged to return to work and continue the physical activities that he participated in during Phase II of cardiac rehabilitation. As he regains his functional health and previous position on the physical activity continuum, he will be more likely to achieve and maintain his physical independence and a higher quality of life.

---

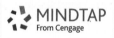 Now that you have completed this chapter, go to your MindTap course to complete all assigned activities. Check out the additional resources developed to help you apply the material in this chapter to your course and career goals.

---

## Chapter Summary

▸ Physical activity is any bodily movement that results in increased energy expenditure. Exercise is a subset of physical activity that is performed specifically for the purpose of increasing physical fitness. The two concepts are related but not synonymous.

▸ Physical activity encompasses a continuum of behaviors—from sedentary behavior (sleeping and sitting) to the intense exercise needed to train for marathon competition. Activities are placed along the continuum based on their difficulty (intensity), the frequency (e.g., times per week) with which they are performed, and the duration of an individual physical activity bout.

▸ The ecological model describes determinants of physical activity and includes characteristics that span from those that are unique to an individual (such as cognition and belief systems) to the most global influences (such as a country's economic development or global societal norms).

▸ The traditional kinesiology professional model encouraged practitioners to focus almost exclusively on exercise training regimens that promoted the development of high levels of physical fitness and peak performance, rather than on the maintenance of or improvements in health achieved through physical activity. Modern kinesiology professionals must embrace both the health and performance aspects of physical activity across the physical activity continuum.

▸ The Human Capital Model includes six domains that impact health and social challenges: (1) physical capital, (2) emotional capital, (3) individual capital, (4) social capital, (5) intellectual capital, and (6) financial capital.

▸ The SLOTH (sleep, leisure-time, occupation, transportation, and home-based activities) model has been described as a time-budget model incorporating key economic factors that may influence individuals' choices about their use of time and physical activity.

▸ Training principles are fundamental guidelines that form the basis for training the body's systems with physical activity. Three unifying training principles that apply across the physical activity continuum are overload, specificity, and adaptation.

- For kinesiology professionals, the global challenge of physical inactivity is an opportunity to refocus on the real value of physical activity and exercise within our field. This new focus should include a systems approach to understanding the complex pathway to adopting physical activity and exercise, beyond simple descriptions of individual pieces of the puzzle such as specific health behaviors and environmental factors.

## Remember This

| | | | |
|---|---|---|---|
| adaptation principle | financial capital | intellectual capital | social capital |
| built environment | general adaptation syndrome (GAS) | over-training | specificity principle |
| capital | overload principle | systems approach |
| conditioning | homeostasis | physical activity continuum | training |
| detraining | Human Capital Model (HCM) | | training principles |
| dose | | physical capital | volume of physical activity |
| emotional capital | individual capital | SLOTH model | |

## For More Information

Access these websites for further study of topics covered in the chapter:

- Find updates and quick links to these and other evidence-based practice-related sites in your MindTap course.
- Search for further information about topics such as the global physical activity pandemic at *The Lancet* journal website: www.thelancet.com/series/physical-activity.
- Search for more information about the Human Capital Model at the website for *Designed to Move: A Physical Activity Action Agenda*, http://designedtomove.org.

- Search for information and resources for strategies to promote physical activity and exercise in the United States at the U.S. Physical Activity Guidelines webpage (http://health.gov/paguidelines) and the U.S. Physical Activity Plan webpage (http://physicalactivityplan.org).
- Search for research about the built environment and its effects on physical activity and exercise at the Global Physical Activity Network, www.globalpanet.com.

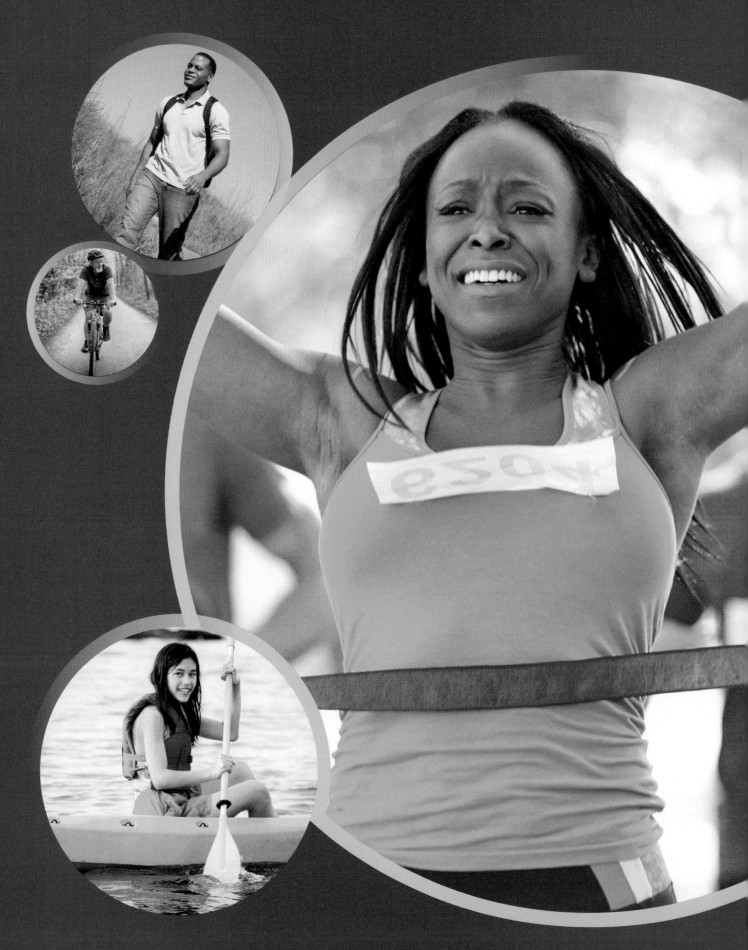

# The Physical Activity Continuum: Integration of Principles of Aerobic Physical Activity

*What are aerobic physical activity principles? How do these principles align along the physical activity continuum?*

**LESSON 1** INTEGRATION OF AEROBIC PRINCIPLES INTO KINESIOLOGY

**LESSON 2** EXAMPLES OF APPLYING AEROBIC PRINCIPLES IN KINESIOLOGY SUBDISCIPLINES

## Learning Objectives

*After completing this chapter, you will be able to:*

**Define** the term aerobic physical activity.

**Explain** how aerobic physical activity relates to health and human performance.

**Justify** the importance of understanding the relationship between aerobic physical activity principles and the various subdisciplines of kinesiology.

**Describe** the specific health benefits of participating in aerobic activities across the physical activity continuum.

**Explain** how the health benefits acquired through participation in aerobic activities influence the prevention and management of chronic diseases and affect longevity.

**Explain** common physiological, behavioral, and biomechanical responses to aerobic physical activity.

**Give** examples of common central and peripheral responses to aerobic activity.

**Give** examples to show how overload, specificity, and adaptation are related to participation in aerobic activities.

**Describe** various methods and measures by which aerobic activities and aerobic fitness can be evaluated and monitored.

**Give** examples of application of aerobic principles in kinesiology subdisciplines.

**Explain** the examples of application of aerobic principles in kinesiology subdisciplines.

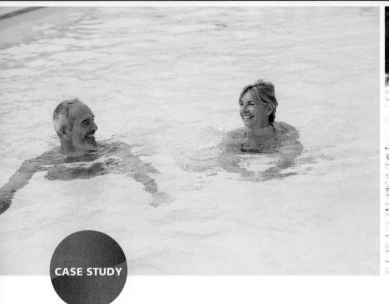

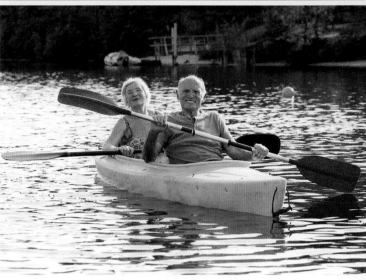

**CASE STUDY**

# In the real world . . .

Jerald Casey traveled to San Diego to visit one of his old high school buddies, James, during the summer. While visiting, he ran into some friends of his parents, Dan and Beth, at a marina where he and James had rented a kayak for fun one afternoon. Jerald told James that as he was growing up he was always amazed to see how physically active Dan and Beth were compared to most other adults he knew, including his own parents, who had become sedentary by middle age.

Dan is a 62-year-old college professor and Beth is a 50-year-old third grade elementary school teacher. Dan and Beth like to walk and jog regularly, but they also like to cycle, hike, and kayak together. As Jerald visited with Dan and Beth, he learned that they had only been kayaking three times, but they had just purchased a tandem kayak and they were looking forward to participating in a five-mile kayak charity fundraiser event in six weeks. Jerald and James had kayaked half a dozen times together but were not very confident that they had the skills or conditioning to do five miles themselves. So, they asked Dan to explain to them how he and Beth were planning to train to complete the five-mile course comfortably, without having to overexert themselves.

What do you think Dan and Beth included in their plan? Do you know the difference between aerobic and anaerobic activities? Is kayaking mainly an aerobic or anaerobic activity? How could Dan and Beth use the principles of overload, specificity, and adaptation in their preparation plan? What are some of the basic skills associated with efficient kayaking? Would biomechanical and motor behavior factors influence Dan and Beth's preparation and performance on race

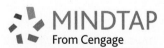

**From Cengage**

Go to your MindTap course now to answer some questions and discover what you already know about applying the integration of principles of aerobic physical activity.

## INTERACTIVE ACTIVITIES

**Research Focus**

Go to your MindTap course to read an article and answer questions about the Compendium of Physical Activities, a document developed by researchers to describe intensity of a variety of common physical activities.

**Career Focus**

Go to your MindTap course to read more information about aerobic benefits for individuals and populations across the physical activity continuum. Resources from several resources are reviewed.

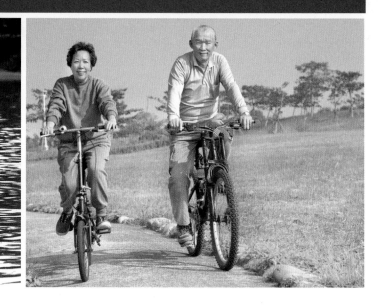

## Introduction: Aerobic Physical Activity and Kinesiology

Physical activities can generally be classified as anaerobic (nonoxidative), aerobic (oxidative), or combined anaerobic and aerobic (interval training). The term *oxidative* means "combining with oxygen." You probably have already heard terms like *aerobic* and *anaerobic* applied to physical activities or exercise that you have performed. **Aerobic** activities depend on good heart/lung (cardiorespiratory) function and heavily on metabolic reactions in muscle cells that require large amounts of oxygen (hence the word "aerobic") and that allow an individual to reach **steady state**. Steady state (homeostasis during exercise) during aerobic activities means that you are working at a level at which your heart and lungs can deliver adequate oxygen through the blood stream to meet the demands for oxygen by the working muscles.

Aerobic activities include walking, jogging, swimming, cycling, rowing, cross-country skiing, and activities such as raking leaves as well as other longer-term, vigorous or moderate-intensity physical activities. In addition to good cardiorespiratory function, some aerobic activities require a minimal amount of sport-specific skills, while others require higher levels of sport-specific skills. For example, walking, hiking, or jogging do not require high levels of skill. On the other hand, more specialized activities such as swimming, cycling, skiing, and rowing require your neuromuscular system to function at higher levels (balance, coordination, timing, etc.). The popularization of the concept of "aerobics" by Kenneth H. Cooper, MD in 1968[1] helped lead to the founding of the Cooper Institute in Dallas, TX, which has become one of the world's primary integrated research centers investigating aerobic fitness, health, and well-being (see example in Lesson 2 of this chapter spotlighting the Cooper Institute). The work at the Cooper Institute was preceded by the work of exercise physiologists at facilities in the United States like the Harvard Fatigue Laboratory (1927–1946), and facilities like the Karolinska Institute Medical School in Stockholm (featuring Per-Olof Astrand; 1946–1987) and the August Krogh Institute – University of Copenhagen (1970–Present), which you can learn more about through independent Internet searches. The foundational work at the Cooper Institute has also been reinforced and expanded in the 1996 U.S. Surgeon General's Report on Physical Activity and Health,[2] and the U.S. Department of Health and Human Services Physical Activity Guidelines Advisory Committee Report.[3]

As you will learn later in this chapter, aerobic activities are associated with numerous health benefits, and higher levels of aerobic fitness are associated with increased longevity and quality of life. Improvements in aerobic fitness include significant changes in one's ability to pump

day? Is six weeks enough time to prepare for a five-mile kayak race? We will follow up with Dan and Beth's story later in Lesson 2 of the chapter, after you have had a chance to learn more about the integration of aerobic principles into the physical activity continuum.

Dan told Jerald that Beth and he were already physically active and used to training, therefore Dan feels that they can easily prepare for the five-mile kayak within six weeks just by practicing in their new kayak at least two to three times per week. Beth and Dan hope to complete the five-mile San Diego Bay course in about an hour. However, just to verify his assumptions Dan conducted a computer search using the search phrase, "training to complete a 5-mile kayak race." He was a bit surprised to find several resources through his search, including a couple of six-week kayak training plans. Dan reviewed several websites and developed a list of training tips and considerations to share with Beth so that they could establish their own individual training plan.

oxygenated blood to the tissues (especially muscle cells) and to extract or use oxygen in the tissues to produce large amounts of energy. Regular participation in aerobic activities increases one's maximum capacity for using oxygen at higher intensities (**maximal oxygen uptake or VO$_2$ max**) and to work at higher percentages of one's VO$_2$ max for longer periods of time. You will learn more about VO$_2$ max later in the chapter. **Aerobic capacity** (also known as aerobic fitness) is a broad measure of a human's ability to work for several minutes and is an indicator of how well the body is able to deliver oxygen and fuel to, and clear metabolic products from, working muscles.

**Anaerobic** activities depend heavily on metabolic reactions (or bioenergetics) in muscle cells that do not require high levels of oxygen to provide chemical energy for movement. Unlike aerobic activities, anaerobic activities do not allow individuals to reach a true steady state in which the body's demand for oxygen equals the ability to supply oxygen at a given workload. Examples of anaerobic activities include sprints, many specific sports drills, weight lifting, and weight training, as well as other short-term, high-intensity (or explosive) muscle power activities, such as shot put, discus, or hammer throw. Oxygen is needed to perform anaerobic activities, just not in the quantity demanded by aerobic activities. We will further discuss anaerobic activities, particularly those that strengthen the musculoskeletal system, in Chapter 6.

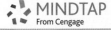

## MINDTAP
From Cengage

### What Is the Cooper Institute?

Many of the scientific foundations for our knowledge of the health benefits of cardiovascular fitness and exercise have come from the Cooper Institute. Founded in 1970 by the "Father of Aerobics," Kenneth H. Cooper, MD, the Cooper Institute, and particularly Dr. Steven Blair, has advanced our understanding of how and why people who are fit and active are healthier than those who are not fit and physically active. By following thousands of people for many years, scientists at the Cooper Institute were able to identify low physical fitness as a key factor that influences risk of early mortality as well as heart disease and other chronic diseases. Moreover, studies from the institute have demonstrated that people who improve their fitness can lower their risk of early mortality. **Go to your MindTap course** to learn more about the Cooper Institute and aerobic fitness.

Although the aerobic/anaerobic classification is helpful, many physical activities performed in real life are both anaerobic and aerobic in nature. Examples of such activities include tennis, stairclimbing, racquetball, soccer, rugby, field hockey, and lacrosse. All of these activities

include components of a program of **intervals** (or interval training) and require moderate-to-high levels of sport-specific skills as well as adequate cardiovascular fitness.

Interval activities require participation in a high-intensity (more anaerobic than aerobic) bout of activity followed by participation in a lower-intensity (more aerobic than anaerobic) bout of activity, or vice versa. Interval activities may allow individuals to achieve a greater total volume of physical activity and exercise than they would if they worked at only a single lower intensity continuously (review Chapter 4, p. 73). Interval-type training has been used by athletes for almost 100 years to systematically improve their aerobic capacity and other aerobic abilities. Optimizing an interval-type training program for high levels of performance requires developing an appropriate work-recovery interval—for example, 30 seconds of vigorous-intensity activity (largely anaerobic) followed by 90 seconds of light- to moderate-intensity activity (largely aerobic) before the next vigorous bout of activity during training, as well as allowing an appropriate amount of recovery between training sessions to enable aerobic training adaptations to occur. In the last five years, high-intensity interval training has been shown to improve a wide variety of physiological functions (aerobic and anaerobic) quickly and thus specific training programs with these benefits are said to provide "a lot of gain for a little pain."

The concept of interval training provides the basis for many popular commercial fitness training programs developed for consumers (Figure 5.1). These programs, although popular, may also be detrimental because they may not allow enough recovery time between intervals for individuals of low and average fitness levels to continue participating, and/or they may increase the risk of orthopedic injury for participants as you learned in Chapter 4 (see Figure 4.7). Nonetheless, even low-fit individuals can engage in interval activities, such as repeatedly alternating one minute of brisk walking with

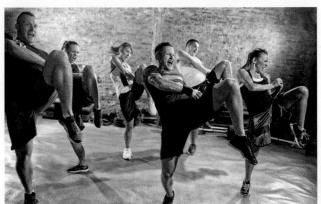

**Figure 5.1** | Individuals Participating in Group Interval Training

one minute of slow walking, to achieve higher intensities of exertion while achieving a greater total volume of work to improve their health and fitness levels.

In this chapter, you will learn more about how to apply and integrate aerobic principles across the physical activity continuum (review Chapter 4). Regular participation in aerobic activities affects physiologic, biomechanic, psychologic, motor behavior, and other factors of interest to practitioners of the subdisciplines of kinesiology. Likewise, physiologic, biomechanic, psychologic, and other influences affect performance of aerobic physical activities. Specifically, this chapter is designed to help all kinesiology students to understand (1) the relationships among participation in aerobic physical activities, health, and well-being; (2) the scientific basics of participating in aerobic activities and how to monitor and evaluate them; (3) some of the cultural, historical, and philosophical factors associated with participation in aerobic activities; and (4) why it is important to participate in aerobic activities throughout life.

## Aerobic Activity: Basic Terms, Training Concepts, and the Physical Activity Continuum

Energy expenditure can be quantified using units called kilocalories, often referred to simply as calories. Any time you move your body—from getting out of bed in the morning, to walking to the bus stop, to playing basketball, to walking down the hallway—you are being physically active and using calories. Along the continuum of aerobic physical activity, four key issues are relevant to caloric expenditure during physical activity or exercise: frequency, intensity, duration, and total volume. **Frequency** refers to the number of occasions (or bouts) of physical activity that occur within a unit of time. Sessions per day or per week, sessions per month, or active weeks per year are all examples of measures of frequency of physical activity. Obviously frequency must include some unit of time referent.

**Intensity** is the second physical activity parameter of interest. A bit more complicated than frequency, intensity refers to the amount of work that a single session of physical activity or exercise requires. The typically used unit of measure for exercise intensity is the **metabolic equivalent of task (MET)**. A MET is defined as the ratio of the energy cost (in kilocalories) of a certain physical activity to the energy cost of rest.

$$1 \text{ MET} = 1 \text{ kcal/kg (body weight)} \times \text{hour}^{-1}$$

Although METs are commonly used to estimate the intensity of energy expenditure, other measures such as percentage of maximal heart rate (%MHR) can be used, and it is important to realize that all estimates of energy expenditure have some error of accurately

predicting energy expenditure (acceptable errors are about 10% compared with laboratory measures such as $VO_2$ max, which is discussed later in the chapter). Because heavier people require more energy to perform the same physical activity than do lighter people (think of a defensive lineman and a wide receiver from the same football team doing the same 100-meter dash), use of the MET is a way to standardize intensity for purposes of comparison (i.e., take the body weight factor out of the way). The intensity of physical activities is usually measured as a multiple of 1 MET (rest). A brisk walk is approximately 3 METs (3× rest); a slow jog, 6 METs (6× rest); and an intense game of soccer, as much as 12 to 15 METs at certain points. Often, studies will group many different intensities of physical activity into a few broad categories. Light-intensity activities are those physical activities that require anywhere from 1.2 to 2.9 METs. Moderate-intensity physical activities require anywhere from 3.0 to 5.9 METs. Vigorous-intensity physical activities require 6 or more METs of energy expenditure. Intensity is the most difficult parameter of physical activity and exercise to measure accurately.

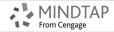

**MINDTAP**
From Cengage

**The Intensity of Common Physical Activities**

**Go to your MindTap course** to complete an activity related to the Compendium of Physical Activities. The Compendium of Physical Activities was developed by researchers to describe the MET intensity of a variety of common physical activities.

The third physical activity parameter of interest is **duration**. Duration refers to the length in time of a specific physical activity or exercise event. Swimming for 60 minutes is an example of physical activity duration. In many cases assessing duration of physical activity is not straightforward, however. For example, a standard soccer game is composed of two halves of 45 minutes each. Based only on this information, one might assume that all the players participating in a soccer game are physically active for 90 minutes, but in fact, this may not be the case. At any point during the game, many of the players not currently in the game are sitting or standing on the sideline using far less energy than those who are playing. Moreover, the goal keeper has a very different physical activity profile than the rest of the team. As a result of these factors, each player in a soccer game has a unique profile of physical activity duration. Contrast this with a long-distance runner who runs a half-marathon in 90 minutes.

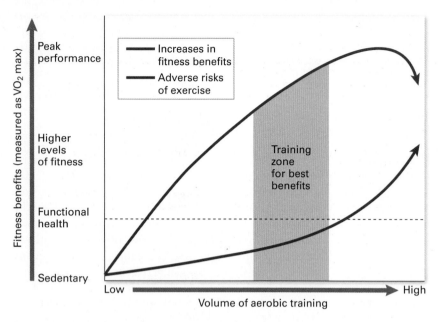

Functional health = *2008 Physical Activity Guidelines for Americans*
(Adults; 150 minutes per week)

**Figure 5.2** | Achieving the Conditioning Benefits of Aerobic Training.
The figure illustrates a training zone for achieving better aerobic benefits, but as explained in the text, benefits improve along the physical activity continuum based upon the volume of training.

Different manipulations of physical activity and exercise frequency, intensity, and duration have different training effects on aerobic capacity. Elite athletes and their coaches will customize a training program that may increase speed or stamina differentially. On the other hand, in discussions of physical activity for promotion of health rather than athletic performance, total volume is the physical activity parameter of most interest. As you learned in Chapter 4, total volume (an estimate of caloric expenditure) is the product of the three previous individual parameters: frequency, intensity, and duration.

$$\text{Volume (kcal)} = \text{Frequency} \times \text{Intensity} \times \text{Duration}$$

As shown in the preceding equation, changes in frequency, intensity, or duration of physical activity will directly affect the total volume or energy expenditure of an individual. For example, if two women walk together around a local park for the same amount of time (duration) and at the same intensity three days each week (frequency), they should have nearly the same total volume of physical activity. If one of the women adds another walk around the park on a different day of the week (increasing the frequency but not the intensity or duration of the exercise bout), her total volume will increase proportionately.

An example of how intensity, duration, and frequency of aerobic training (volume of training) might

be optimized (sometimes called the training zone) to move a person from being sedentary to obtaining basic functional health and beyond (physical activity continuum) is illustrated in Figure 5.2. As the volume of training increases, so do the risks of overtraining (see Chapter 4) or adverse effects of exercise such as orthopedic injuries, cardiovascular risks, and lowered immune responses. Figure 5.2 indicates a zone of optimal improvement and benefits by participating in physical activities (training zone); however, benefits can be gained at all training volumes as compared to being physically inactive. In fact, the Physical Activity Guidelines Advisory Committee Report of 2008 supports the concept that some physical activity is better than none, and too much leads to problems such as increased risks for orthopedic injuries, upper respiratory infections, and depressed immune function.[4,5] Aerobic fitness outcomes will vary based on the design of an aerobic physical activity or exercise program.

Figure 5.2 further illustrates the concept of the physical activity continuum and the unifying training principle of overload, specificity, and adaptation introduced in Chapter 4. When individuals engage in a specific aerobic physical activity, they increase their $VO_2$ max and aerobic capacity based upon their personal goals, genetic potential, and the volume of their participation over time.

Traditionally it has been recommended that someone who is sedentary should consult a physician or health care provider prior to beginning a physical activity or exercise program. However, there is no evidence that people who visit a physician or other health care provider prior to starting such a program are any safer than individuals who do not.[6] In fact, the message can create a significant barrier to people who may use it as another excuse not to exercise. If practitioners are still concerned about the basic health screening of individuals, they can use the American College of Sports Medicine recommended risk stratification tool, the Physical Activity Readiness Questionnaire or PAR-Q. The PAR-Q contains seven health screening questions, and if an individual answers "yes" to any questions, they should consult a physician or health care provider before participating in further exercise programming (see Figure 5.3).

# PAR-Q & YOU

**(A Questionnaire for People Aged 15 to 69)**

Regular physical activity is fun and healthy, and increasingly more people are starting to become more active every day. Being more active is very safe for most people. However, some people should check with their doctor before they start becoming much more physically active.

If you are planning to become much more physically active than you are now, start by answering the seven questions in the box below. If you are between the ages of 15 and 69, the PAR-Q will tell you if you should check with your doctor before you start. If you are over 69 years of age, and you are not used to being very active, check with your doctor.

Common sense is your best guide when you answer these questions. Please read the questions carefully and answer each one honestly:  check YES or NO.

| YES | NO | |
|---|---|---|
| ☐ | ☐ | 1. Has your doctor ever said that you have a heart condition <u>and</u> that you should only do physical activity recommended by a doctor? |
| ☐ | ☐ | 2. Do you feel pain in your chest when you do physical activity? |
| ☐ | ☐ | 3. In the past month, have you had chest pain when you were not doing physical activity? |
| ☐ | ☐ | 4. Do you lose your balance because of dizziness or do you ever lose consciousness? |
| ☐ | ☐ | 5. Do you have a bone or joint problem (for example, back, knee or hip) that could be made worse by a change in your physical activity? |
| ☐ | ☐ | 6. Is your doctor currently prescribing drugs (for example, water pills) for your blood pressure or heart condition? |
| ☐ | ☐ | 7. Do you know of <u>any other reason</u> why you should not do physical activity? |

**If you answered**

## YES to one or more questions

Talk with your doctor by phone or in person BEFORE you start becoming much more physically active or BEFORE you have a fitness appraisal. Tell your doctor about the PAR-Q and which questions you answered YES.

- You may be able to do any activity you want — as long as you start slowly and build up gradually. Or, you may need to restrict your activities to those which are safe for you. Talk with your doctor about the kinds of activities you wish to participate in and follow his/her advice.

- Find out which community programs are safe and helpful for you.

## NO to all questions

If you answered NO honestly to <u>all</u> PAR-Q questions, you can be reasonably sure that you can:

- start becoming much more physically active – begin slowly and build up gradually.  This is the safest and easiest way to go.

- take part in a fitness appraisal – this is an excellent way to determine your basic fitness so that you can plan the best way for you to live actively. It is also highly recommended that you have your blood pressure evaluated.  If your reading is over 144/94, talk with your doctor before you start becoming much more physically active.

**DELAY BECOMING MUCH MORE ACTIVE:**
- if you are not feeling well because of a temporary illness such as a cold or a fever – wait until you feel better; or
- if you are or may be pregnant – talk to your doctor before you start becoming more active.

**PLEASE NOTE:** If your health changes so that you then answer YES to any of the above questions, tell your fitness or health professional. Ask whether you should change your physical activity plan.

<u>Informed Use of the PAR-Q</u>: The Canadian Society for Exercise Physiology, Health Canada, and their agents assume no liability for persons who undertake physical activity, and if in doubt after completing this questionnaire, consult your doctor prior to physical activity.

**No changes permitted. You are encouraged to photocopy the PAR-Q but only if you use the entire form.**

NOTE: If the PAR-Q is being given to a person before he or she participates in a physical activity program or a fitness appraisal, this section may be used for legal or administrative purposes.

"I have read, understood and completed this questionnaire. Any questions I had were answered to my full satisfaction."

NAME _____

SIGNATURE _____ DATE _____

SIGNATURE OF PARENT _____ WITNESS _____
or GUARDIAN (for participants under the age of majority)

Note:  This physical activity clearance is valid for a maximum of 12 months from the date it is completed and becomes invalid if your condition changes so that you would answer YES to any of the seven questions.

**Figure 5.3** | Physical Activity Readiness Questionnaire (PAR-Q) & You. The PAR-Q is a basic health screening tool that is helpful to kinesiology professionals to identify individuals or populations at higher risk for physical activity and exercise.

*Source:* From the Canadian Society for Exercise Physiology, 2002, available at www.csep.ca/CMFiles/publications/parq/par-q.pdf.

For those people who already have underlying health issues such as hypertension (high blood pressure), cardiac problems, or musculoskeletal limitations and who plan to participate in high intensity physical activities, appropriate pre-program health screening should occur prior to participation. Healthy and/or low risk (no chronic health problem like heart disease, diabetes, or musculoskeletal injures) individuals who want to start a walking program at light to moderate intensity would not need a prior consultation with a physician or health care professional.[7]

## Health, Longevity, and Quality of Life Benefits of Aerobic Activities

Today, there is little doubt that regular physical activity maintains health and can improve myriad health conditions. This is true for young children and the oldest adults. More than 50 years of scientific research has helped us understand the strong relationship between physical activity and the prevention or delaying of coronary artery disease, stroke, hypertension, and poor blood lipid profiles.

---

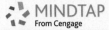

**What Is a Lipid Profile?**

Lipids are fats and fat-like substances found in the body. They are either produced in the body or are the metabolic products of the food you eat. High levels of "bad" blood lipids like low-density lipoproteins (LDL) or very-low-density lipoproteins (VLDL) can increase your risk of heart disease. High levels of "good" blood lipids like high-density lipoproteins (HDL) can lower that risk.

**Go to your MindTap course** to read and complete an activity about lipid profiles.

---

**Table 5.1** | Summary of Health Benefits of Participating in Aerobic Physical Activity or Exercise

| |
|---|
| Reduced all-cause mortality (all causes of death) (30% reduction) |
| Reduced risk of developing type 2 diabetes* and metabolic syndrome** (30%–40% reduction) |
| Maintenance of weight loss and prevention of weight regain |
| Improved bone (lower risk of osteoporosis), joint, and muscle health |
| Reduced risk of loss of mobility (30% reduction) |
| Reduced risk of colon cancer (30% reduction) and breast cancer (20% reduction) |
| Reduced depression, distress/negative well-being (20% reduction), and dementia (30% reduction) |

\* Type 2 diabetes is associated with abnormal glucose (blood sugar) levels and obesity.

\*\* Metabolic syndrome is a condition that often leads to type 2 diabetes and is associated with a cluster of risk factors including hypertension, abnormal blood lipids (fats), abnormal glucose and/or insulin levels, and obesity/increased waist girth.

---

Regular participation in aerobic physical activity and exercise improves cardiorespiratory fitness and lowers the risk for cardiovascular diseases and stroke by 20% to 35%. The benefits of physical activity and exercise on cardiorespiratory health apply effectively for men and women and for individuals of all ages, and there is no evidence for race/ethnic differences when adjusted for volume of activity.[8]

How much is enough? That is, how much physical activity is necessary to improve health? For adults, the broad public health recommendation based on scientific evidence is that at least 150 minutes per week of moderate-intensity aerobic physical activity, 75 minutes of vigorous-intensity aerobic physical activity, or an equivalent combination of both intensities is the minimum amount necessary for health promotion and disease prevention. This is roughly equivalent to a brisk 30-minute walk on five or more days each week. (A MindTap activity introduced later in this lesson will help you learn more about moderate and vigorous intensity levels.) A summary of the health benefits of regular physical activity in adults is shown in Table 5.1.

The amount of physical activity recommended for children and adolescents (ages 5–18 years) is somewhat different than that recommended for adults. For youth, the guideline is to engage in 60 minutes of moderate-intensity physical activity every day. They should also engage in three or more days of muscle-strengthening and bone-strengthening activities (see Table 5.5

for examples). Why the difference? In recent years, it has become clear that children and adolescents are not just "little adults" and need physical activity and exercise that are tailored to their specific needs. Because of growth and development needs, physical and cognitive maturation, and other differences, children clearly need more physical activity each day than adults. Moreover, recent scientific studies are beginning to show that, in addition to enjoying health benefits, children who are more active do better in school than children who are less active.[9]

In the United States, the average life expectancy at birth is approximately 80 years for women and 75 years for men. However, a lifetime of sedentary behavior can accelerate a loss of functional health long before death and often results in a reduction of quality of life. Regular participation in physical activity and exercise has been shown to not only improve health, but also predict increased longevity with better quality of life. This phenomenon is sometimes referred to as the "compression of morbidity," as shown in Figure 5.4.

Two scenarios are shown in Figure 5.4. First, the physically inactive situation (left line) where health (broadly defined) declines slowly with age until death. In this scenario, only about 50% of maximal health is achieved about mid-life. Second, the physically active situation, where health is maintained for much longer throughout life until a fairly short (compressed) time period until death. In the second scenario, a 50%

decline in health isn't reached until relatively late in life.

Scientific evidence provided by leading researchers such as Ralph Paffenbarger and Jeremy Morris, along with Steven N. Blair (University of South Carolina), Harold W. Kohl (University of Texas), William Haskell (Stanford University), Arthur Leon (University of Minnesota), and others suggests that fit, physically active persons have a lower risk of dying prematurely than physically inactive or unfit persons. More recently, Jackson and colleagues reported that individuals who remain physically active, maintain their weight, and abstain from smoking as they age maintain their functional fitness levels—in this case, cardiorespiratory or aerobic fitness—longer than those who do not.[10] Figure 5.5 illustrates how normal declines in cardiorespiratory fitness with age and the age at which

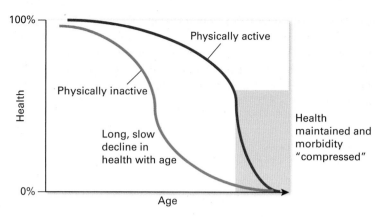

**Figure 5.4** | Example of the Compression of Morbidity: Comparing a Sedentary Lifestyle to a Physically Active One

functional health is lost vary with regards to the individual's sex, physical activity index (PAI; 0-low to 3-high), and BMI.

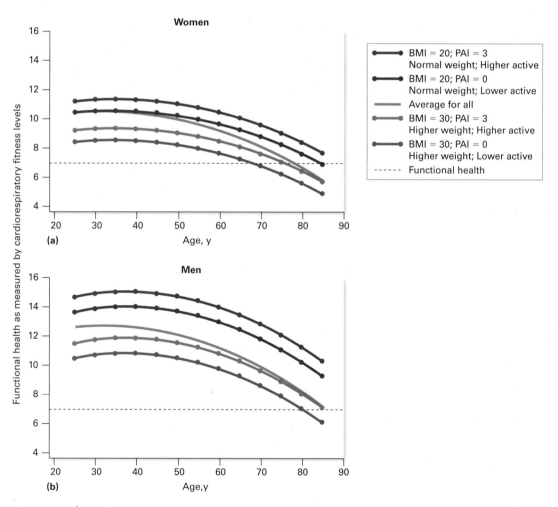

**Figure 5.5** | Cardiorespiratory Fitness Levels in Relationship to Aging and Changes in Weight and Physical Activity Levels over Time. Notice that for both men and women, those with higher BMI and lower physical activity levels are predicted to lose functional health (dotted line) sooner than those who are leaner and more physically active.

Indeed, the research findings reported by these investigators and the many kinesiologists who continued their work were instrumental in persuading the surgeon general of the United States to classify physical inactivity as an independent risk factor for cardiovascular disease.[11] This means that the effects of physical inactivity contribute over and above the effects of previously established risk factors such as high blood pressure, poor lipid profile, and cigarette smoking.

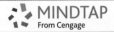

### The Framingham Heart Study

This long-term study, begun in 1948, followed thousands of men over many years to discover the causes of heart disease. Much of our understanding of the risk factors for heart disease came from the Framingham Heart Study. **Go to your MindTap course** to learn more about the Framingham Heart Study.

## Peak Performance and Aerobic Activity

Intensive aerobic training and interval training over many years are associated with dramatic changes in performance for those who are genetically gifted to adapt to the training stimuli and those who can resist or recover rapidly from musculoskeletal injuries associated with the overload. U.S distance runner Meb Keflezighi (born 1975; height = 5 feet 5 inches; weight = 126 pounds) is an excellent example of an individual who has achieved superior levels of performance with aerobic training and intervals. Meb ran a 5:20 mile in junior high and became a high school champion and a four-time NCAA champion at UCLA. Meb has enjoyed a long, distinguished running career, earning a silver medal in the 2004 Athens, Greece, Olympic Games Marathon and fourth place in the 2012 London, England, Olympic Games Marathon (following a win in the U.S. Olympic trials). In 2014, at the age of 37, he won the Houston Aramco Half Marathon in 62 minutes. In 2014, Meb won the Boston Marathon and established himself as an American hero by winning the race after the fatal bombing incident of 2013.

Meb often trains by running 100 miles or more for several weeks prior to major races. Based on his personal best marathon speed (2:09:08 in 2012 or approximately 4:55 per mile pace), we could estimate that he would need to accumulate 600 to 720 minutes of running per week—considerably more than the 150 minutes per week recommended for functional health.

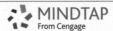

### Aerobic Benefits for Individuals and Populations

**Go to your MindTap course** to learn more about how to optimize the aerobic benefits for individuals and populations across the physical activity continuum. The following resources are reviewed:

▸ Physical Activity Guidelines Advisory Committee Report 2008

▸ The American College of Sports Medicine (ACSM) Position Stand, *Quantity and Quality of Exercise for Developing and Maintaining Cardiorespiratory, Musculoskeletal, and Neuromotor Fitness in Apparently Health Adults: Guidance for Prescribing Exercise*

▸ The American College of Sports Medicine (ACSM) website information on professional competencies related to aerobic physical activity principles

## Basic Physiological Responses and Benefits of Participation in Aerobic Physical Activities

The physiologic effects of (and adaptation to) participation in aerobic physical activities will be covered in detail in your undergraduate exercise physiology course. However, there are several basic responses that all kinesiology practitioners should be familiar with and be able to readily explain. The following section provides you an overview of how participating regularly in aerobic physical activities can improve health, physical fitness, and peak performance.

One of the most important concepts to understand regarding the basics of participation in aerobic activities and improving aerobic capacity for improved health is the relationship among maximal oxygen uptake, heart rate, and stroke volume. The relationship is represented by the **FICK equation**:

$$\text{Maximal Oxygen Uptake (VO}_2\text{ max)}$$
$$= (\text{Maximal Heart Rate} \times \text{Stroke}$$
$$\text{Volume}) \times \text{Arterial-Venous Oxygen}$$
$$\text{Difference}$$

This can be rewritten as: $\text{VO}_2$ max
$$= \text{Cardiac Output} \times \text{A-VO}_2 \text{ diff}$$

**Maximal Heart Rate (MHR)** = your maximal heart rate (HR) in beats per minute or approximately 220 − your age; **Stroke Volume (SV)** = the amount of blood pumped per beat of your heart in milliliters/minute;

**Table 5.2** | Central and Peripheral Adaptations to Long-Term Aerobic Conditioning

| CENTRAL CHANGES | PERIPHERAL CHANGES |
|---|---|
| Increased $VO_2$ max (on average 5%–20%). Greater improvements are associated with lower initial values and factors like genetics, age, sex (males on average have a 1 MET higher value than females), volume of training, and body composition. | Increased size and number of mitochondria and metabolic enzymes. Positive changes in gene regulation related to cellular aerobic metabolism and reduced inflammation due to oxidative stress improving the immune system. |
| Increased SV and cardiac output. The primary muscles of respiration (diaphragm and intercostals) adapt and allow for greater breathing rates and volumes to be maintained over time. | Increased number of capillaries for blood supply and improved A-$VO_2$ diff. Improved ability of the peripheral nerves (sympathetic and para-sympathetic) to regulate blood flow to the organs during exercise. |
| Decreased resting HR and lower blood pressure (BP) and HR at lower or submaximal workloads; i.e., **economy** (oxygen cost for a given workload—speed/grade). | Increased storage and ability to use energy (glycogen—stored glucose and triglycerides—fats). |
| Improved recovery HR and return to homeostasis. | Increased ability to regulate blood lipids (fats like cholesterol and triglycerides) and blood glucose. |

**Cardiac Output** = HR × SV, or the amount of blood pumped per minute in liters/minute; **Arterial-Venous Oxygen Difference (A-$VO_2$ diff)** = the amount of oxygen the tissues (like muscles) can extract or use from arterial blood and return to venous blood.

The FICK equation as described assumes that one has normal blood values and lung function and indicates that there are both central (heart and lung) and peripheral (primarily muscles) components that contribute to your aerobic capacity.

Table 5.2 provides a list of many of the important adaptations in the central (torso—heart and lungs) and peripheral (limbs—working muscles) regions of the human body that are associated with performing aerobic activities for a minimum of six to eight weeks or longer. In general, these changes are associated with improved function of the cardiovascular and metabolic systems.

Obviously, $VO_2$ max varies from person to person due to factors such as age, gender, and genetics. Physical activity helps improve $VO_2$ max from sedentary baseline levels, and more training results in higher improvements as one moves from being sedentary to becoming physically active and achieving functional health (like meeting the Physical Activity Guidelines). Further improvements in $VO_2$ max can occur when individuals train to achieve higher levels of aerobic fitness (such as training to complete a 10 kilometer run in 70 minutes). And, for a few gifted people like Meb Keflezighi striving for peak performance, $VO_2$ max levels after years of training may be twice as high as those for average inactive individuals. Average resting and maximal values for the FICK equation for 20-year-old sedentary, physically active, and highly fit endurance athletic males are shown in Table 5.3.

The combination of the central and peripheral adaptations associated with participating in aerobic activities provides the basis for the variety of additional common physiologic, biomechanical, and behavioral responses to aerobic physical activity listed in Table 5.4.

**Table 5.3** | Average Resting and Maximal Cardiac Output, Stroke Volume, Heart Rate, and $VO_2$ Max for Sedentary, Trained, and Highly Trained Young Males

| | RESTING | | | MAXIMAL | | | |
|---|---|---|---|---|---|---|---|
| | CARDIAC OUTPUT (L/min) | STROKE VOLUME (mL) | HEART RATE (bpm) | CARDIAC OUTPUT (L/min) | STROKE VOLUME (mL) | HEART RATE (bpm) | $VO_2$ MAX |
| Sedentary | 5–6 | 68 | 74 | 20 | 100 | 200 | 42 ml · kg$^{-1}$ · min$^{-1}$ |
| Trained | 5–6 | 90 | 56 | 30 | 150 | 200 | 52 ml · kg$^{-1}$ · min$^{-1}$ |
| Highly Trained | 5–6 | 110 | 45 | 35 | 175 | 200 | 72 ml · kg$^{-1}$ · min$^{-1}$ |

Note: Values are shown in ml · kg$^{-1}$ · min$^{-1}$, which is based on oxygen consumption per unit of body weight.

*Source:* From Table 6.1 of W. Hoeger and S. Hoeger, *Lifetime Physical Fitness and Wellness* (Boston: Cengage Learning, 2015), 190.

**Table 5.4** | Common Physiologic, Biomechanical, and Behavioral Responses to Participating in Aerobic Physical Activity

| PHYSIOLOGICAL | BIOMECHANICAL |
|---|---|
| Reduced body fat<br>Reduced waist girth<br>Increased strength<br>Increased muscular endurance | Increased motor skill and confidence to engage further in physical activity and exercise<br><br>Improved proprioception, which helps coordination system response and balance |

| BEHAVIORAL | |
|---|---|
| Increased self-confidence<br>Improved self-efficacy<br>Decreased depression and anxiety<br>Experience with behavioral change<br>Improved stress management<br>Improved sleep patterns | |

*Source:* H. W. Kohl and T. D. Murray, *Foundations of Physical Activity and Public Health* (Champaign, IL: Human Kinetics, 2012).

## Beginning, Intermediate, and Advanced Aerobic Physical Activity and Exercise Programs

What do beginning, intermediate, or advanced aerobic physical activity programs look like? This is a question many kinesiology students hear from family, friends, and colleagues as they move through their undergraduate academic training. The following samples for adults demonstrate how the volume of training can be applied across the physical activity continuum based on individual and population aerobic outcome goals. Table 5.5 also includes examples of moderate and vigorous intensity aerobic physical activities for children and adolescents.

### Beginning Aerobic Activity Program

*Overall Goal*—Generally improve health for a 30-year-old healthy, sedentary adult

*Physical Activity or Exercise Mode*—Walk, cycle, swim, row, gardening, lawn maintenance, etc.

*Frequency*—3 to 5 days per week

*Intensity*—≥ 40% of maximum MET level (or $VO_2$ max)

*Duration*—Accumulate a minimum of 150 minutes per week (can be achieved by accumulating in a variety of ways, e.g., 10 to 15 minute bouts multiple times per day for most days of the week or 30 minutes per bout for 5 days per week)

### Intermediate Aerobic Activity Program

*Overall Goal*—Generally improve health-related fitness for a healthy, sedentary 19-year-old

*Physical Activity or Exercise Mode*—Walk, cycle, swim, row, etc.

*Frequency*—3 to 5 days per week and the accumulation of 30 to 60 minutes per bout

*Intensity*—60% to 80% of maximum MET level (or $VO_2$ max)

**Table 5.5** | Examples of Moderate- and Vigorous-Intensity Aerobic Physical Activities for Children and Adolescents

| TYPE OF PHYSICAL ACTIVITY | AGE GROUP | |
|---|---|---|
| | CHILDREN | ADOLESCENTS |
| Moderate-intensity aerobic | ▸ Active recreation, such as hiking, skateboarding, rollerblading<br>▸ Bicycle riding<br>▸ Brisk walking | ▸ Active recreation, such as canoeing, hiking, skateboarding, rollerblading<br>▸ Brisk walking<br>▸ Bicycle riding (stationary or road bike)<br>▸ Housework and yard work, such as sweeping or pushing a lawn mower<br>▸ Games that require catching and throwing, such as baseball and softball |
| Vigorous-intensity aerobic | ▸ Active games involving running and chasing, such as tag<br>▸ Bicycle riding<br>▸ Jumping rope<br>▸ Martial arts, such as karate<br>▸ Running<br>▸ Sports such as soccer, ice or field hockey, basketball, swimming, tennis<br>▸ Cross-country skiing | ▸ Active games involving running and chasing, such as flag football<br>▸ Bicycle riding<br>▸ Jumping rope<br>▸ Martial arts, such as karate<br>▸ Running<br>▸ Sports such as soccer, ice or field hockey, basketball, swimming, tennis<br>▸ Vigorous dancing<br>▸ Cross-country skiing |

*Source:* From "Physical Activity Guidelines Advisory Committee Report, 2008" (Washington, DC: U.S. Department of Health and Human Services, 2008), 18.

**Table 5.6** | Physical Activity Assessment Techniques

| TECHNIQUE | MEASURE(S) | STRENGTHS | WEAKNESSES |
|---|---|---|---|
| Caloric expenditure | Calories used during a period of time or during a specific physical activity. Can be laboratory- or field-based (like having a small group of individuals run the mile for time). | Precise. | Expensive; not practical for large groups of people. |
| Direct observation | Time spent at a certain intensity; type of physical activity. | Accurate; can be used in a field setting. | Can be expensive; difficult to measure over a period of time or with multiple people. |
| Electronic monitoring (e.g., accelerometers, heart rate, GPS, etc.) | Time spent at a certain intensity. | Can be used in a field setting; can be a useful motivating tool; can be used over many days. | Some tools do not capture non-walking or non-running physical activities very well. |
| Diaries | Time spent at a certain intensity; type of physical activity. | Helpful for assessing different types of activities. | Subject to memory recall; may affect the types of activities performed. |
| Questionnaires | Time spent at a certain intensity; type of physical activity. | Can be used in large population studies. | Subject to memory recall. |

*Duration*—Accumulate a minimum of 200 to 300 minutes per week (can be achieved by accumulating in a variety of ways, e.g., 20- to 30-minute bouts multiple times per day for most days of the week or 60 minutes per bout for 5 days per week)

### Advanced Aerobic Activity Program

*Overall Goal*—Improve maximal performance for a 25-year-old elite distance runner

*Physical Activity or Exercise Mode*—Running

*Frequency*—6 to 7 days per week (based on a progression program allowing appropriate rest (see Chapter 4), incorporating 2 bouts per day 3 to 5 times per week

*Intensity*—60% to $\geq$ 100% of maximum MET level (or $VO_2$ max), including intervals 2 to 3 times per week

*Duration*—Accumulate $\geq$ 300 minutes per week based on specific training regimen

## Measuring and Monitoring Aerobic Physical Activity and Fitness

Whether the physical activity is general movement or specific to exercise, there are many ways to measure the behavior. You will learn about many ways to measure and monitor aerobic physical activity and fitness in more detail in your future courses; therefore, we will provide you with just an overview of methods commonly used that link participation in physical activity and health. These methods range from precise assessment of caloric expenditure (like testing $VO_2$ max in an exercise physiology laboratory) to questionnaire measures designed to prompt a person to recall activities and exercise that they engaged in during a specific time frame. As you might imagine, these techniques each have strengths and weaknesses and several potential

sources of error. Key types of physical activity assessment techniques are highlighted in Table 5.6. The important point to remember is that they are all ways of measuring the behavior associated with physical activity and exercise.

An important distinction to make in this area is assessment of the actual behavior of physical activity (the movement) versus the physiologic consequences of that movement. The two outcomes, while related, have important distinctions. For example, consider two people walking at 3.5 miles per hour. One person is carrying a 35-pound backpack while the other has no load. Each is moving, but each may have a very different physiologic response. The person carrying the load is likely working harder, expending more calories, and has a higher heart rate response than the person with no load.

Directly measuring caloric expenditure is one of the more precise ways to assess physical activity (see Figure 5.6). Two

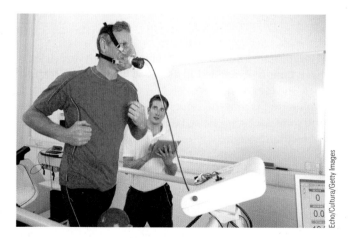

**Figure 5.6** | Measuring Oxygen Uptake and Caloric Expenditure during Exercise on a Treadmill

common techniques, the use of *portable oxygen consumption devices* and *doubly-labeled water*, are described here. Portable oxygen consumption devices directly measure the expiration of carbon dioxide during various physical activities and therefore can help to estimate energy expenditure. Doubly-labeled water is a technique that also relies on the use of oxygen and expiration of carbon dioxide to assess physical activity. With this technique, participants are asked to drink a dose of water that contains a stable isotope (form) of oxygen and one of hydrogen. Then, over the course of the next few days and weeks, the rate at which the two isotopes are excreted in the urine becomes directly proportional to physical activity behavior, and oxygen consumption (calories) can be estimated. The faster the isotope is excreted, the higher the dose of physical activity and caloric expenditure. While this procedure is very accurate, it requires very expensive equipment to perform.

Direct observation techniques require an observer (or a camera) to record physical activities and exercise that the person under observation performs in a defined time period. Note that this technique actually measures the movement. The type, frequency, intensity, and duration of the activity are recorded and stored for later analyses. Direct observation techniques are most frequently used in controlled settings (such as a park or physical education class) and can be very useful for assessing the effect of intervention studies designed to increase physical activity behaviors.

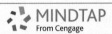

**A Tool for Physical Education Teachers**

**Go to your MindTap course** to learn more about SOFIT: System for Observing Fitness Instruction Time. The SOFIT tool assesses physical education classes by enabling the researcher to simultaneously collect data on student activity levels, the lesson context, and teacher behavior.

Electronic monitoring techniques for physical activity have rapidly expanded in the past years as our technologic society has evolved. The principle behind electronic monitoring is that the human body's movement in space and time can be measured objectively with these devices. Step counters (pedometers) and accelerometers are two popular devices, and new ones are emerging on the market all the time. Electronic devices can be used to estimate energy expenditure but have greater error than direct measures. Many can sync with smartphone applications to allow data collection and review as well as goal setting.

Sometimes the best way to measure a person's physical activity or exercise behavior is through a personal diary. Again, designed to measure the behavior, diary methods are especially useful in research studies of physical activity. With the physical activity diary method, a person is asked to keep an hour-by-hour record of every activity (even sitting, sleeping, watching television, etc.) in which he or she participates in a preselected period of time (usually randomly chosen). Assuming that the person has been adequately trained to recall these behaviors, researchers have a fairly complete picture of the subject's physical activity (and inactivity) behaviors.

Questionnaires are the most frequently used technique for assessing physical activity behaviors in the scientific literature. With questionnaires, large groups of people can be surveyed regarding their physical activity habits. Many different types of questionnaires are available, but the better ones attempt to assess recreational exercise and physical activity, occupation-related physical activity, transport-related physical activity, and other forms (such as household chores). Questionnaires can also be used to assess the types of activity as well as their intensity, frequency, and duration. Questionnaires have been frequently maligned because of recall bias—that is, because what a person reports on the survey may or may not represent an accurate recall of their behaviors. Can you remember what physical activities you have engaged in within the past week?

In contrast to physical activity and exercise, which are behaviors, **physical fitness** is a set of measurable physiological parameters.[12] Most people have their own views of what physical fitness looks like. What's yours? An Olympic-caliber weightlifter? A marathon runner? The fastest kid on the basketball court? How about grandparents who are happy and able to physically do everything they want to do without limitations? Although there are many possible conceptions of physical fitness, a useful list of parameters is shown in Table 5.7.

Physical fitness can be either health-related or skill-related. **Health-related fitness** attributes are related to improved health (e.g., reductions in chronic diseases, injury, disability). **Skill-related fitness** attributes are those that are the most important for successful movement and sports participation. Skill-related fitness parameters are also more likely to be determined by genes than by physical activity or exercise, although some can be improved with specific exercise training. However, they may or may not be related to health outcomes. For

**Table 5.7** | Physical Fitness Parameters

| HEALTH-RELATED FITNESS | SKILL-RELATED FITNESS |
|---|---|
| Aerobic capacity or aerobic fitness | Balance |
| | Agility |
| Muscular strength | Coordination |
| Muscular endurance | Power |
| Flexibility | Speed |
| Body composition | |

example, speed is an incredibly important fitness parameter in competition sports such as track and field. Speed can be improved with certain training techniques. People can be healthy, however, without being fast. Good balance, on the other hand, is important in gymnastics, but it is also critical for preventing falls among older people.

Aerobic physical activity and exercise are most closely tied to the fitness parameter of aerobic capacity. The purest measure of aerobic capacity is oxygen consumption ($VO_2$) during exercise. Aerobic fitness can be measured or estimated in the very tightly controlled setting of a laboratory or in field settings in which groups of people can be tested simultaneously. Many useful techniques to estimate oxygen consumption have been developed over the years. The unifying principle in all these methods is that aerobic physical activity uses oxygen, and a person who is better able to use oxygen during aerobic physical activity is more highly fit than another who is less able.

## Measuring Aerobic Capacity

A complete treatment of aerobic capacity assessment is beyond the scope of this text (you will get a complete treatment in your exercise physiology class). In brief, because aerobic capacity is an objective physiologic trait, many different laboratory and field tests have been devised with which to measure it. All are founded on the fundamental principle that physical activities and exercise all rely on processing oxygen.

### Laboratory or Clinical Methods

Laboratory or clinical methods to assess aerobic capacity can be classified as either maximal or submaximal. All require some form of physical activity or exercise to stimulate (overload) the individual. The common unit of measure of aerobic capacity is milliliters of oxygen, $ml \times min^{-1}$ when weight is supported (like in cycling) or (adjusting for body weight) $ml \times kg^{-1} \times min^{-1}$. Maximal tests (goal of reaching >85% of predicted maximal heart rate: 220 – age) titrate (slowly adjust) the "dose" of physical activity up to a point where the individual is working at or near her or his theoretical maximal limit. Respiration is measured using a device to collect expired air. The maximal amount of oxygen used at maximal exercise is the measure of aerobic capacity. Maximal tests can be done in a laboratory on a treadmill, on a cycle ergometer, or with any other type of equipment that allows a person to exercise to near maximal levels.

Submaximal tests (goal of testing at 70% to < 85% of predicted maximal heart rate) are somewhat easier to conduct, and results can be used to estimate maximal oxygen consumption using established equations that rely on the relationship between heart rate and oxygen consumption. In submaximal tests, the individual works below maximal effort, often for a fixed period of time. The heart rate response during the physical activity is observed and aerobic capacity is estimated using existing formulae. This type of test is frequently used in physicians' offices to aid in clinical diagnoses of the cardiovascular and/or pulmonary systems.

### Field Methods

Field methods to estimate aerobic capacity are all submaximal and are based on the same principles as laboratory-based measures. There is a known correlation between heart rate and oxygen consumption or time and oxygen consumption. Many different field tests to estimate aerobic capacity have been developed, but all function based on this relationship. For example, heart rate monitoring for a given exercise task can predict oxygen consumption (when age, gender, and body weight are known). Alternatively, with a fixed walking/running distance (20 meters, for example), observations of the heart rate response can be correlated with oxygen consumption. The lower an individual's heart rate response over the course of the exercise, the higher is her or his aerobic capacity. In addition, measuring the time it takes a person to travel a fixed distance (complete a 1-mile run, for example) without a measure of heart rate response is also a frequently used field test for aerobic capacity, particularly in military populations. The faster a person can complete a test, the higher his or her aerobic capacity is. Finally, there are progressive tests, such as a step test or the PACER (progressive aerobic cardiovascular endurance run) test, in which the activity required of the subject becomes increasingly difficult over time. The theory behind these field tests is that increasing the overload on the cardiovascular system allows a closer estimate of maximal oxygen consumption to be achieved. Such tests are popular in fitness centers and in physical education classes.

# EXAMPLES OF APPLYING AEROBIC PRINCIPLES IN KINESIOLOGY SUBDISCIPLINES

*In Lesson 1, you learned about the importance of understanding aerobic activities and the numerous health, physical fitness, and peak performance benefits associated with developing recommended and higher levels of aerobic fitness, including their contributions to increased longevity, improved quality of life, and optimized performance. In Lesson 2, you*

*will learn about examples of the application of aerobic physical activity principles to the subdisciplines of kinesiology and to the physical activity continuum.*

▸ Exercise Physiology
▸ Biomechanics

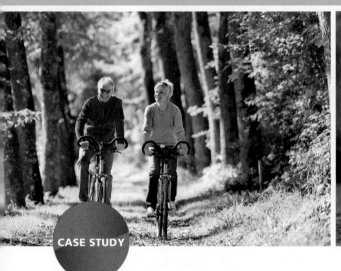

**CASE STUDY**

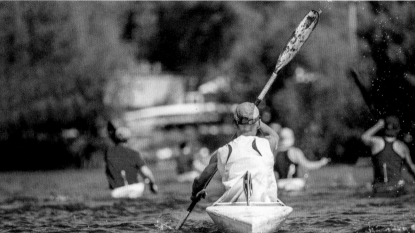

## In the real world . . .

As mentioned earlier, Dan and Beth are friends of Jerald Casey's family who plan to participate in a five-mile kayak charity fundraiser. Jerald asked Dan how he and Beth planned to complete the event successfully. Dan and Beth shared the following plan with Jerald and his pal James.

*Kayak Training Tips and Related Considerations*: Kayaking for five miles involves aerobic and anaerobic movements and successful training preparation that should include (1) regular steady aerobic training (30 to 60 minutes per session), (2) practicing anaerobic-type training (short 30-second to 2-minute steering and maneuvering skills), (3) completing some interval training including kayak work and resistance (such as weight lifting) work weekly, (4) practicing kayak stroke mechanics (biomechanically related), (5) developing at least a couple of aerobic pacing strategies based upon race day environmental data, (6) doing some mental preparation training (sports psychology; see Chapter 8 for more), and (7) learning more in practice about how factors such as kayak type

(flat bottom vs. v-shaped bottom), water levels, water currents, paddling skills, and wind resistance (both on the kayak and body surface area) can influence drag effects and how much effort is required to maintain the speed (about 12 minutes per mile) to finish the course within one hour.

*Dan and Beth's Kayak Training Plan*: After conducting a little independent research, Dan and Beth developed the following integrated plan that applied aerobic activity principles and other kayak-specific training principles to meet their goal within weekly preparation time limitations.

**Training Plan:**

For weeks 1–3, 2 days of steady aerobic paddling for 15–30 minutes at 12–14 minute/mile pace per session and performing 15–20 push-ups, 30 sit-ups.

For weeks 3–6, increase steady-state paddling to 30–40 minutes per session.

For weeks 1–6, 1 day of interval training including 30 seconds of paddling at 10 minute/mile pace focusing on proper stroke mechanics turning right and left and 30 seconds of

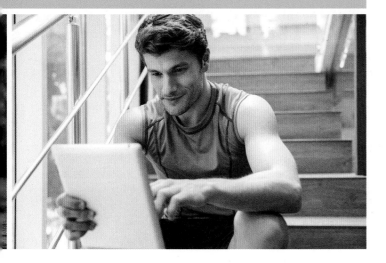

recovery repeated 5 times, followed by a five-minute slow paddle and then 5 bouts of 1 minute fast paddling at 10 minute/mile pace with 1 minute recovery; and, 1 additional day, when time allows, to perform light weight lifting (resistance work) such as 3 sets of 10 repetitions using 70%–85% of established maximum lifts for biceps curls, triceps extensions, overhead press, and squats.

Dan and Beth's proposed six-week kayak training plan should produce many of the central and peripheral physiological changes associated with performing aerobic activities that you learned about earlier in the chapter. The plan should also provide the strength and muscular conditioning that they will need to complete the five-mile kayak race within an hour. You will learn more about strength and muscle endurance principles in Chapter 6.

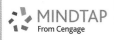

| | Go to your MindTap course to complete the Case Study activity for this chapter. |

# Exercise Physiology and Biomechanics

The following scenario provides an example of factors from the kinesiology subdisciplines of exercise physiology, biomechanics, and rehabilitation that influence distance running performance. The example demonstrates the integration of aerobic physical activity principles to promote high performance.

Quincy is a postcollegiate distance runner (age 26) who enjoys running 5K and 10K road races. He ran a best of 14:45 for the 5K and 30:30 for the 10K in college and remains very competitive, as he has won or finished in the top three in several recent road races ranging from the 5K to half-marathon distance. He currently is running daily, and on three or four days per week he runs for 30 minutes at 60% to 70% of his race pace in the morning and then performs intervals of various distances in the afternoon. His weekly mileage totals 70 to 90 miles per week.

Quincy began having pain in his left Achilles tendon about a month ago. The pain (on the medial aspect of the base of his left Achilles tendon) is very prominent when he awakes and first stands. The pain only dissipates slightly during the day, even when he applies ice to the site and doses with ibuprofen twice daily. After consulting with an athletic trainer (AT), a physical therapist (PT), and an orthopedic surgeon, Quincy found out that his injury was an overuse pronation injury (excessive inward movement of the foot as it roles to distribute the force of the ground strike when running). His injury was not responding effectively to traditional AT or PT therapies and it was not serious enough to warrant surgery, so he was referred to a podiatrist (foot and ankle specialist) by his orthopedic physician.

Quincy visited a local sports podiatrist a day after he was referred, and his diagnosis was confirmed. He further learned that his injury was very common in distance runners and that custom fitted orthotics (arch supports) usually corrected the excessive pronation and associated pain within a few weeks, after which he could return to his normal training.

During his podiatry visit, Quincy was casted and measured for rigid orthotics and was instructed to restrict his running to two to three miles per day as tolerated while applying ice twice daily to his tendon and continuing his anti-inflammatory meds (ibuprofen). When Quincy returned to pick up his new orthotics a week later, the podiatrist confirmed that the orthotics fit properly and instructed him to wear the orthotics in all shoes he used (daily and for running). He was also told to gradually increase his physical activities, as the orthotics would change his posture and movement biomechanics slightly, which might cause light to moderate muscle soreness for a week or so.

Quincy wore his orthotics for a full day after his office visit and began running the next day. He noticed that the orthotics helped support his arches (especially in his left foot) and his Achilles tendon felt better than it had in a long while, but he worried that the extra weight of the orthotics (about a half pound) would increase the energy required (oxygen cost) to run at his usual training paces. Quincy's collegiate coach verified that increased weight does increase the oxygen cost of running at any given pace (running economy). However, the biomechanical support of the orthotics allowed Quincy to control his pronation, and thus limit his Achilles tendon inflammation and pain, while returning to his vigorous aerobic training regimen. Therefore, even though the orthotics might have a slight negative impact (physiologically) on Quincy's high aerobic performance goals over time, they did allow him to return to his high aerobic training volume by positively influencing his running biomechanics and psychological confidence.

## Public Health ⚕

Maria works for a large banking corporation with offices all over the world. Her recent promotion has put her in charge of the worksite wellness program for the entire company. The company president and leadership are committed to having a healthy workforce. They assume that this will translate into more productivity and lower health care costs and ultimately help the company be more profitable and competitive. The vice president for human resources (Maria's boss) directs her to increase opportunities for all employees to increase their aerobic physical activity. Maria knows there are many company employees who are competitive runners; there is even a group of runners who compete for monthly mileage totals using a specially designed company intranet site. This represents only a small minority of the workforce, however, and Maria's job expectations are that she will increase participation such that 60% or more of the company employees are aerobically physically active at least 150 minutes each week (public health guidelines). Recent surveys suggest that only 25% of the employees are meeting these physical activity guidelines.

Being an expert in this area, Maria knows that simply building more company workout facilities isn't the answer to this problem. Building facilities is expensive and would more than likely induce most of the current exercisers to use company facilities rather than those they currently use. Maria sets out to develop a behaviorally based program designed to increase walking among employees who are not regular exercisers. She consults experts, who tell her that increasing access to places where employees can be physically active and creating social support structures (people who can help) are two highly recommended strategies for promoting physical activity, particularly walking.

Maria first negotiates with company management to implement a new policy allowing employees the flexibility to take 30-minute walking breaks during work time. This is paid time that employees can take throughout the day. She also travels to all the company offices around the world and maps out the nearest walking routes with varying distances. She trains local leaders at each office and gets the support of the local vice president of operations, knowing that leadership by example is incredibly important to increasing physical activity. Finally, she develops a social support system using the company intranet that allows people to record all of their walks, including the distance covered, and pairs people up in teams for monthly competitions. Financial incentives for monthly improvements and maintenance are built in to participants' paychecks and are attainable by virtually all participants if they meet physical activity guidelines. The first 12 months of the program are incredibly popular, and participation soars to over 75% of the employee base. The investments that the company has made for the program are far outweighed by the savings in terms of lower health care costs, reduced absenteeism, and increased productivity.

## Motor Learning and Sport/ Exercise Psychology 🏃 🏊

Steve is a consultant for a large investment group that purchases poorly performing companies and reorganizes them so that they become profitable. Steve's greatest passion, besides his job, is helping his son Joey become the best cross-country athlete in his high school. Steve wants to hire a personal coach for Joey during the off-season because he knows that a good coach can improve Joey's chances of success, but he is a bit hesitant to do so because of his previous bad experiences with running coaches when he was a competitive cross-country runner. Joey has developed a gait pattern similar to his father's, and Steve remembers all too well how coaches tried to change his running style to match the styles of Bill Rodgers, Steve Prefontaine, and Marty Liquori, who were all champion runners of the 1970s. Although Steve's style was best described by most people as awkward—something akin to a cross between a giraffe and a kangaroo—he was able to win more meets while running with his natural gait pattern than when he tried to adjust to match preeminent runners of his time. Steve does not want Joey to have the same painful experiences that he had as a high school athlete.

After reviewing numerous resumes, Steve decides to take Joey to Coach Ben's facility to see if Coach Ben can help improve Joey's performance. Coach Ben has studied both motor learning and exercise physiology and tries to combine the two fields of study whenever possible to improve athletic performance. Coach Ben also believes in evidence-based training, so he will collect data on Joey throughout the training period to document improvements. The first day of training for Joey includes videotaping Joey's natural running style while Joey's baseline submaximal $VO_2$ and $VO_2$ max are measured. Coach Ben realizes that, to help Joey to improve, he must enhance Joey's running economy by increasing Joey's aerobic capacity at submaximal speeds as well as his speed at $VO_2$ max. Coach Ben recognizes that coordinating specific motor recruitment activities such as intervals, plyometrics (bounding activities), and light resistance training within Joey's training routine should improve his performance. Coach Ben asks Steve to allow him to work with Joey for the next 12 weeks to see if they can prepare Joey for his senior year cross-country season.

Coach Ben begins training Joey and decides not to attempt to change his running style (e.g., shorten or lengthen stride length), which has been shown in biomechanical research studies to actually decrease running economy in trained runners. Rather, Ben starts by focusing on improving Joey's muscular recruitment patterns. Coach Ben decides to have Joey run regular interval sessions that require running at a faster-than-normal race pace (e.g., 800-meter race pace vs. 5K cross-country race pace), as well as race pace training, two to three times weekly. Interval training programs have been shown to increase $VO_2$ max and improve running economy, theoretically by helping runners recruit fewer muscle fibers (motor units) at the same speed, which implicates a motor learning/motor behavior effect. Ben also has Joey begin a resistance and plyometric training program, which has been shown in emerging research to improve endurance performance, likely due to changes in muscular recruitment patterns.[13]

Although changes in running economy are often small (1% to 3%) and therefore usually difficult to measure, they can be significant in improving running performance. In Joey's case, at the end of 12 weeks of training with Coach Ben, Joey had increased his $VO_2$ max by 5% and his running economy 1.5%, and he ran a personal best of 14:45 in a 5K time trial. While the post-training videotape of his running style did not look much different than his pre-training tape, Joey actually was able to increase his stride length slightly (one to two inches) at max race speed. (Remember, looks can be deceiving with regards to running economy; experienced runners adapt to their anatomy and develop an economical style relative to their biomechanics.)

## The Practice of Kinesiology

The Cooper Institute is an excellent example of the integration of a variety of kinesiology subdisciplines with evidenced-based principles of aerobic physical activity over several decades. The Cooper Institute, which as you have learned was established in 1970, initially included the Cooper Clinic, the Cooper Fitness Center, and the Cooper Research Center.

The Cooper Clinic was designed to promote preventive medicine and was focused on providing comprehensive physical examinations that included maximal aerobic capacity testing on a treadmill using standardized protocols like the Balke Protocol (laboratory $VO_2$ max measure) and the Cooper 12-minute or 1.5-mile run (field test estimating $VO_2$ max). Dr. Cooper and his colleagues have completed over 260,000 exams to date on over 110,000 people and the Cooper Center Longitudinal Study (CCLS) has become the primary research component that is recognized globally. The development and implementation of standardized testing procedures at the institute for more than 40 years have allowed researchers to generate databases that now allow comparisons of 3,000 aerobic physical activity and health variables among over 100,000 individuals.

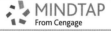

**Standardized Aerobic Capacity Testing**

**Go to your MindTap course** to learn more about the Balke Treadmill or Graded Exercise Testing Protocol.

The Cooper Fitness Center promotes physical activity and fitness through individual, family, and corporate memberships. In the early years, the fitness center was designed primarily for a variety of aerobic activities with some resistance training opportunities, but today it includes a 52,000-square-foot indoor multipurpose comprehensive fitness facility as well as outdoor physical activity paths (on 30 acres).

The Cooper Institute has become one of the most recognizable physical activity and health data-based programs in the world. The institute has produced numerous landmark kinesiology-related publications over the years, including "Physical Fitness and All-Cause Mortality: A Prospective Study of Healthy Men and Women"[14] and "Changes in Physical Fitness and All-Cause Mortality:

# People Matter Kerri Vasold, Doctoral Student in Kinesiology*

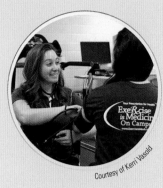

Courtesy of Kerri Vasold

**Q: Why and how did you get into the field of kinesiology?**

**A:** *I've always wanted to work in the health care field, and as an undergraduate student I bounced around with different career paths—first wanting to be a physician, then physical therapist, etc. Eventually, I found the field of kinesiology through the exercise science program at my university and immediately felt at home—I found a career path where I could help people through my love of physical activity and exercise.*

**Q: What was the major influence on you to work in the field?**

**A:** *Everyone has that goal of changing the world and making a difference in someone's life. For me, I wanted to reach everyone, not just someone. When I found kinesiology, I realized that physical activity could be a way to do that. I've always had a strong commitment to being physically active, playing sports as a child and incorporating activity into my daily life as an adult, and I wanted to help others do the same.*

**Q: What are your current research interests, and how do you translate your research results to practitioners?**

**A:** *My research interests center around the American College of Sports Medicine's Exercise is Medicine (EIM) initiative, specifically on university and college campuses (EIM-OC). Through this initiative, I promote the measurement of physical activity as a vital sign within our on-campus health care systems, and encourage*

*faculty, staff, and students to include physical activity in their daily schedules through a variety of events and opportunities offered on campus, including a physical activity mentoring program.*

**Q: How do you stay physically active yourself and promote good health to others directly around you?**

**A:** *Personally, I stay active through running and a variety of strength training/circuit training activities, group exercise classes, and community recreational sport leagues. I promote good health to others directly around me by encouraging that physical activity doesn't always have to take place in the gym or fitness studio—it can be something as simple as going for a walk.*

**Q: How have you had to integrate the sub-disciplines of kinesiology in your professional practice?**

**A:** *I work with a variety of individuals through my research efforts in EIM-OC including those in psychology of physical activity, exercise physiology, measurement of physical activity, and physical activity and public health. Multiple factors come into play when encouraging individuals to incorporate physical activity into their daily lives, so each of these subdisciplines makes it possible for this to happen.*

*Ms. Vasold is a Ph.D. student at Michigan State University. She earned a bachelor's degree in exercise science from Saginaw Valley State University. Her current research includes investigating the relationship between recreational sports participation and academic success in college students.

---

A Prospective Study in Healthy and Unhealthy Men."[15] Today the Cooper Aerobics Center includes the original components as well as the Cooper Spa, Cooper Hotel and Conference Center, Cooper Wellness, Cooper Complete, and Cooper Corporate Solutions. The institute provides kinesiology practitioners and other health-related professionals numerous opportunities for continuing education and certification.

The Cooper Institute model provides an excellent reference for professionals pursuing careers in kinesiology who are tasked with program development and management. Dr. Cooper founded the institute with a unique philosophy (at the time) focused on preventive medicine, helped maintain a long history of standardized protocols in testing and research, and sociologically promoted the evaluation of women and other understudied populations (who had been neglected previously) with regards to fitness research. By learning to develop standardized procedures and protocols like those at the institute, practitioners can more effectively implement programs and evaluate them over time.

---

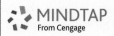
**MINDTAP** From Cengage

Now that you have completed this chapter, go to your MindTap course to complete all assigned activities. Check out the additional resources developed to help you apply the material in this chapter to your course and career goals.

# Chapter Summary

- Aerobic (oxidative) activities depend on good heart/lung (cardiorespiratory) function and heavily on metabolic reactions in muscle cells that require large amounts of oxygen (hence the word "aerobic") and that allow an individual to reach steady state.

- Regular participation in aerobic activities increases one's maximum capacity for using oxygen at higher intensities (maximal oxygen uptake or $VO_2$ max) and ability to maintain this rate of oxygen use for longer periods of time. Aerobic capacity (also known as aerobic fitness) is a broad measure of a human's ability to work for several minutes and is an indicator of how well the body is able to deliver oxygen and fuel to, and clear metabolic products from, working muscles.

- How much physical activity is necessary to improve health? For adults, the broad public health recommendation, based on scientific evidence, is at least 150 minutes per week of moderate-intensity aerobic physical activity, 75 minutes of vigorous-intensity aerobic physical activity, or an equivalent combination of both intensities for health promotion and disease prevention.

- Individuals who remain physically active, maintain their weight, and abstain from smoking as they age maintain their functional fitness levels (in this case cardiorespiratory or aerobic fitness) longer than those who do not.

- Participating in aerobic activities causes a combination of central and peripheral adaptations that provide the basis for common physiologic, biomechanical, and behavioral responses.

- Total volume is the physical activity parameter of most interest in discussions of physical activity and health. Total volume (an estimate of caloric expenditure) is the product of three individual physical activity parameters: frequency, intensity, and duration.

- Whether a physical activity is general movement or specific to exercise, there are many ways to measure the behavior. These methods range from precise assessment of caloric expenditure to questionnaire measures designed to prompt a person to recall activities and exercise that they performed during a specific time frame.

## Remember This

| | | | |
|---|---|---|---|
| aerobic | economy | (MHR) | steady state |
| aerobic capacity | FICK equation | maximal oxygen uptake | stroke volume (SV) |
| anaerobic | frequency | or $VO_2$ max | |
| arterial-venous oxygen | health-related fitness | metabolic equivalent of | |
| difference (A-$VO_2$ diff) | intensity | task (MET) | |
| cardiac output | intervals | physical fitness | |
| duration | maximal heart rate | skill-related fitness | |

## For More Information

Access these websites for further study of topics covered in the chapter:

- Find updates and quick links to these and other evidence-base practice related sites in your MindTap course.

- Search for further information about the physical activity continuum and aerobic physical activity principles at the Cooper Institute: www.cooperinstitute.org.

- Search for information and resources related to strategies to promote aerobic physical activity principles in the United States at the U.S. Physical Activity Guidelines webpage (www.health.gov/paguidelines) and the U.S. Physical Activity Plan webpage (www.physicalactivityplan.org).

- Search for more information about aerobic principles at the following commercial websites: www.exrx.net, www.brianmac.co.uk, and www.topendsports.com.

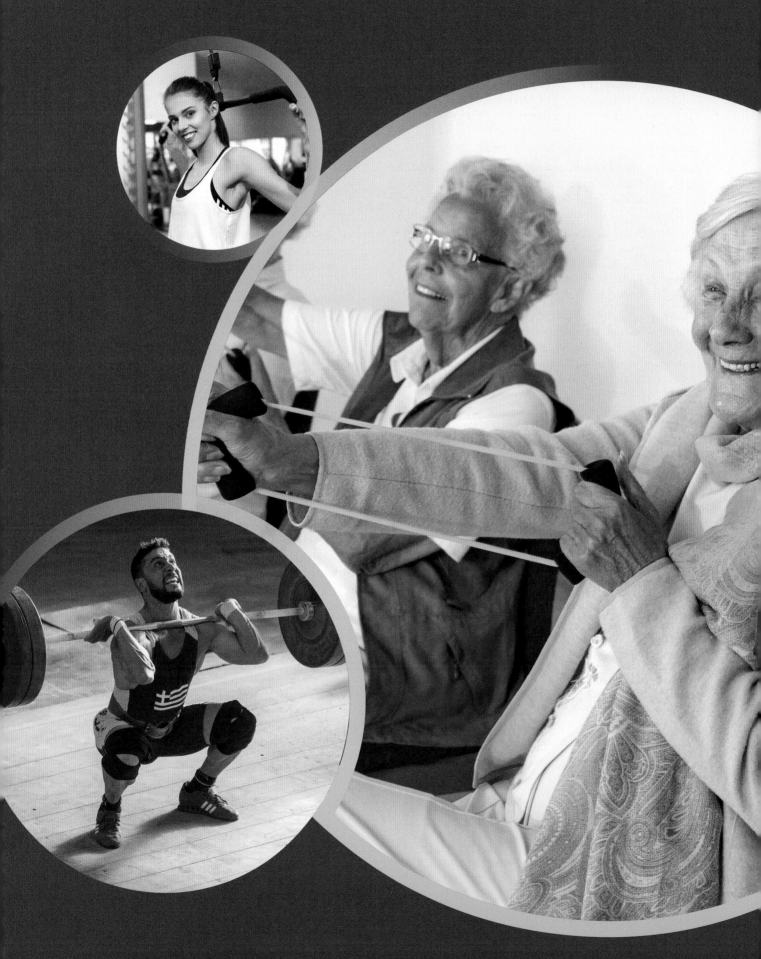

# The Physical Activity Continuum: Integration of Strength and Conditioning Principles

*What are strength and conditioning principles? How do they fit in the physical activity continuum?*

**LESSON 1** INTEGRATION OF STRENGTH AND CONDITIONING PRINCIPLES INTO KINESIOLOGY

**LESSON 2** EXAMPLES OF APPLYING STRENGTH AND CONDITIONING PRINCIPLES IN KINESIOLOGY SUBDISCIPLINES

## Learning Objectives

*After completing this chapter, you will be able to:*

**Define** the common terms associated with strength and conditioning physical activities.

**Explain** how strength and conditioning physical activities relate to the promotion of health and optimal human performance.

**Justify** the importance of understanding the relationship between strength and conditioning physical activity principles and the various subdisciplines of kinesiology.

**Describe** the specific health benefits of participating in strength and conditioning physical activities across the physical activity continuum.

**Explain** how the health benefits acquired through participation in strength and conditioning physical activities influence the prevention and management of chronic diseases and quality of life.

**Explain** common physiologic and biomechanical responses to participation in strength and conditioning physical activities.

**Describe** behavioral responses associated with increasing participation in strength and conditioning physical activities.

**Give** examples to show how overload, specificity, and adaptation are related to participation in strength and conditioning physical activities.

**Describe** various methods and measures by which strength and conditioning physical activities can be evaluated and monitored.

**Give** examples of application of strength and conditioning physical activity principles in kinesiology subdisciplines.

# INTEGRATION OF STRENGTH AND CONDITIONING PRINCIPLES INTO KINESIOLOGY

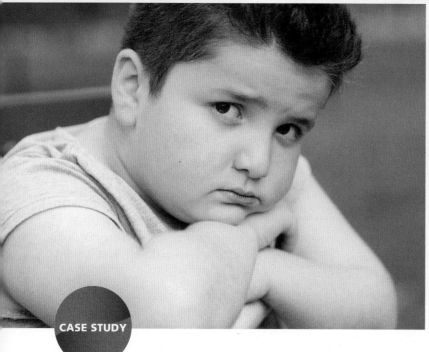

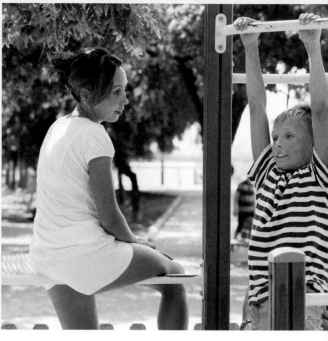

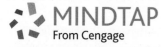

## In the real world...

As mentioned in Chapter 1, Eugene Casey is 10 years old and is very sedentary. He watches television and plays video games at least six hours each day in his bedroom and generally does not move much. Thus, Eugene comes nowhere near meeting the U.S. Physical Activity Guidelines for children and adolescents, which recommend participating in 60 minutes each day of moderate or vigorous-intensity physical activity, including muscle- and bone-strengthening activities on at least three days per week. Last month, Eugene's school physical education (PE) teacher, Mr. Daniels, introduced a four-week weight lifting unit that will require students who participate in the class to lift weights for 50 minutes on three days each week. Eugene is excited about weight lifting because he is considered obese (BMI > 95th percentile for his age and sex), is larger and stronger than his classmates, and performs poorly in PE when trying to play soccer or run a mile for time. In fact, many of his classmates make fun of him except when he lifts weights and gets a chance to show off his muscular strength, power, and endurance. Mr. Daniels has encouraged Eugene to focus on strength and conditioning activities in and out of PE class,

## MINDTAP
From Cengage

Go to your MindTap course now to answer some questions and discover what you already know about the physical activity continuum and integration of strength and conditioning principles for the musculoskeletal system.

## INTERACTIVE ACTIVITIES

### Research Focus
Go to your MindTap course to learn more about the history of strength and conditioning-related recommendations.

### Career Focus
Go to your MindTap course to learn more about drug testing policies in several sports.

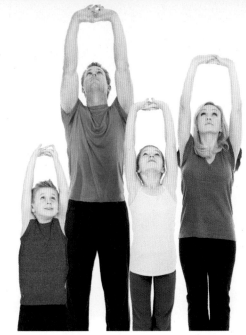

## Introduction: Strength and Conditioning and Kinesiology

What images come to mind when you think about strength and conditioning? Olympic-level weight lifters? College or professional football players? Body builders? Each of these groups of athletes certainly use strength training as an important part of their workout regimens. What about a grandmother who lifts hand weights during her exercise class? An adolescent girl who works out with weights and wants to improve her balance? A middle-aged man who climbs the stairs at his workplace to strengthen his legs after a knee replacement surgery? Each of these examples is as relevant as examples of strength training as the more traditional weight lifting examples in athletes.

**Muscular strength** is defined as the maximum force that a person can generate one time at a given speed (e.g., lifting a maximum amount for 1 repetition or **1 RM**) one time. Increases in strength are related to physiologic improvements in factors such as nerve recruitment, muscle synchronization, increases in the number of fibers in a muscle (**hyperplasia**), increases in the overall mass of a muscle (**hypertrophy**), and strength-to-body mass ratio. Improvements in strength generally occur with improved neuromuscular function and hypertrophy without hyperplasia—that is, more nerve recruitment with increases in muscle mass. In this chapter, **conditioning** refers to voluntary participation in various muscle-strengthening physical activities such as weight lifting, sprinting, calisthenics (moving your body weight), resistance band movement activities, plyometrics (bounding activities or other movements that focus on eccentric muscle contractions), and others that contribute to improvements in strength, bone health, coordination, balance, and muscle endurance (resistance to fatigue with multiple contractions).

**Flexibility** refers to the amount of movement (range of motion) around a joint that a person can achieve and involves muscles and connective tissue such as tendons and ligaments. Conditioning activities may also include activities to increase flexibility because flexibility generally decreases with aging and disuse. Although high levels of flexibility are important to maximizing peak performance in many skill sports (such as gymnastics, high jumping, and figure skating), flexibility does not seem to reduce the risk of musculoskeletal physical activity-related injuries, prevent low back pain, or prevent delayed onset of muscle soreness (24 to 48 hours post-exercise). Flexibility movements are traditionally included as part of warm-up activities prior to engaging in aerobic and musculoskeletal physical activities and exercise.

while gradually adding a few aerobic physical activities to his routine, and strive to meet the 60 minutes per day goal for physical activity. Eugene's parents are excited that he is trying to become more physically active, but they are worried that his participation may negatively affect his normal growth and development and perhaps even increase his risk of orthopedic injury. What do you think about the safety of regular resistance exercise for children 12 years old or younger? Does the scientific evidence show that resistance exercise is effective and safe at increasing strength and muscular endurance in children like Eugene? Can children and adolescents expect to gain muscle mass and increase muscle girth with resistance exercise over time? When did you first start lifting weights or participate in resistance exercise? Did you have quality instruction about how to participate in strength and conditioning physical activities, or did you learn on your own? What general guidelines would you recommend for youth who want to participate in strength and conditioning physical activities? We will follow up with Eugene's case story later in Lesson 2 of the chapter, after you have had a chance to learn about the integration of principles of strength and conditioning into the physical activity continuum.

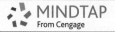
As you learned in Chapter 5, much research and scientific evidence support regular participation in aerobic physical activities to promote health and optimize cardiorespiratory performance. Strengthening and conditioning the musculoskeletal system has come to be recognized as just as important to health and human performance as the aerobic activities that were discussed in Chapter 5. Unfortunately, far fewer middle-aged and older adults participate regularly in strength and conditioning physical activities than in aerobic physical activities.[1]

Ever since ancient times, societies have been fascinated by physical feats related to strength and conditioning. As you learned in Chapter 1, understanding the philosophy, history, and sociology of strength and conditioning can help you better integrate musculoskeletal concepts in the practice of kinesiology. Records such as the most weight lifted in the Olympic Games for a variety of events or the greatest number of consecutive 225-pound lifts for the annual National Football League (NFL) draft combine tests continue to capture our imagination.

Historically, one example of someone who popularized strength and conditioning is Jack Lalanne. Jack Lalanne was known as the "godfather of fitness" (see www.jacklalanne.com/ for more information). He was born in 1914 and lived to the age of 96 (2011). He was inspired to improve his own lifestyle at the age of 15 and began practicing **physical culture** (or what we might term wellness today), which had its roots in the 1800s and consisted of the promotion of healthy living and exercise by using equipment such as medicine balls, hand wands, and dumbbells. Lalanne participated daily throughout his life in physical activities such as lifting weights and calisthenics, and in the promotion of healthy eating. He opened one of the first health and fitness clubs in Oakland, California, in 1936.

Jack hosted his own daytime television show for 34 years beginning in 1953 and was quite influential in encouraging women to become more active, which was novel for the time. At that time his promotion of fitness included workout albums, which were the forerunners of the exercise infomercials of today. Jack was lifting weights at a time when physicians advised against lifting weights because it was thought by many that it would make one muscle-bound and limit mobility. Of course, today we have much more scientific evidence that supports the importance of people of all ages participating in strength and conditioning activities.

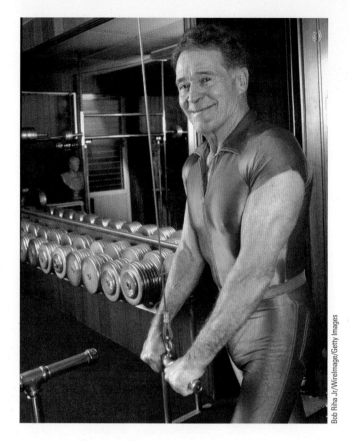

Bob Riha Jr/WireImage/Getty Images

Jack Lalanne was also known for his legendary strength and conditioning feats, which included:

- In 1959 (age 45): Performed 1,000 jumping jacks and 1,000 chin-ups in 1 hour and 22 minutes to promote his television show.

- In 1974 (age 60): Swam from Alcatraz Island to Fisherman's Wharf (San Francisco, California) with his hands and feet bound while towing a 1,000-pound boat.

- In 1984 (age 70): Swam and towed 70 rowboats one mile with his hands and feet bound.

Lalanne achieved many health and fitness honors in his lifetime, and in 2007 he was awarded the President's Council on Physical Fitness Lifetime Achievement Award for making significant contributions to the promotion of physical activity, fitness, and sports nationwide.

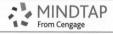

Strength and conditioning feats of performance and methods of training have been recorded throughout history, but interest in mass participation in strength and conditioning activities by the general public to promote health has lagged other forms of physical activity participation such as aerobic activities. For example, researchers have reported that only 8.7% to 21% of the U.S. adult population meets the national physical activity guideline of participating in muscle-strengthening activities on ≥ 2 days per week and only 6% meet the recommendation to engage all major muscle groups (shoulders, arms, back, chest, abdomen, legs, and hips). In comparison, it is reported that over 35% of the U.S. adult population engage in aerobic physical activities that meet recommendations.[2]

In this chapter, you will learn more about principles of strength and conditioning across the physical activity continuum and how to apply and integrate them. Regular participation in strength and conditioning activities affects and improves physiologic, biomechanical, psychological, motor behavior, and other factors of interest to practitioners of the subdisciplines of kinesiology. Likewise, physiologic, biomechanical, psychological, and other influences affect performance of strength and conditioning physical activities. For example, people with biomechanical limitations such as a knee joint that has been surgically replaced may be limited in some types of strength and conditioning activities they may be able to do. Specifically, much like Chapter 5, this chapter is designed to help all kinesiology students promote health and well-being through applying, monitoring, evaluating, and integrating strength and conditioning principles in practice. It is also designed to help you understand cultural, historical, and philosophical factors associated with participation in strength and conditioning activities—both your own participation and that of the individuals you will influence during your kinesiology career.

## Strength and Conditioning Basic Terms, Training Concepts, and the Physical Activity Continuum

Strength and conditioning physical activities consist of static and/or dynamic physical movements or exercise. **Static exercise** (or **isometric exercise**) activities rely primarily on the anaerobic pathways you learned about in Chapter 5 (Figure 6.1a). A static exercise muscular

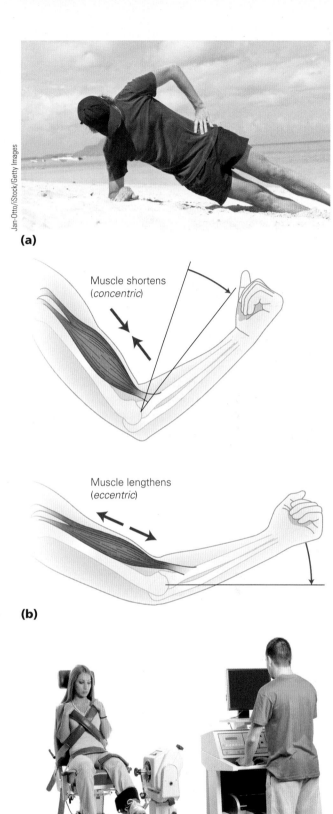

**Figure 6.1** | Examples of Static and Dynamic Exercise with Various Types of Muscle Contractions. (a) An example of static muscle contractions (b) An example of isotonic muscle contractions—Top: Muscle shortens (concentric). Bottom: Muscle lengthens (eccentric). The speed of the contractions is variable. (c) An example of isokinetic muscle contractions, dynamic, work-producing movements at a constant speed that include concentric and eccentric components.

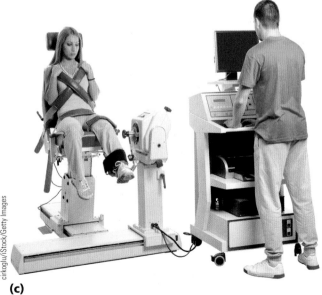

contraction includes an increase in force generated with no change in muscle length. Exercises such as pushing/stretching against a wall or pulling on a chain anchored to the floor are examples of static exercises. **Dynamic exercise** activities, in comparison, depend on both aerobic and anaerobic pathways and involve concentric (shortening) and eccentric (lengthening) through a large range of motion (ROM), as shown in Figure 6.1b. Lunges and leg swings are examples of dynamic exercises. Dynamic exercises can be either isotonic or isokinetic. Isotonic muscle contractions occur when the force exerted by the muscle includes concentric and eccentric movements at varying speeds throughout a large ROM. **Isokinetic** muscle contractions are dynamic, work-producing movements that include concentric and eccentric components at a constant speed and are performed through a large ROM (Figure 6.1c). By participating regularly in strength and conditioning physical activities, a wide variety of health and human performance benefits affecting muscles, bones, connective tissues, metabolic function, and mental health can be achieved.

Muscle contractions involve a complex series of events that include the central nervous system, muscle fibers, and metabolic pathways, as shown in Figures 6.2 and 6.3. You will learn much more about the specifics of muscles and movement in future courses including exercise physiology, biomechanics, and motor learning. However, the following section provides an overview of

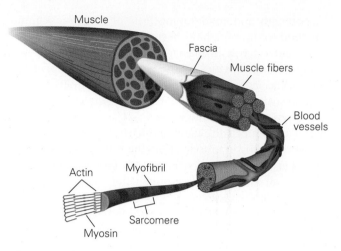

**Figure 6.3** | Components of Muscle Contraction from the Macro (Large) Scale to the Micro (Small or Molecular) Level. You will learn much more about the details of figures such as this in future kinesiology courses.

how movements that improve strength and conditioning are integrated. Understanding these movements involves basic knowledge of anatomy, physiology, biomechanics, motor learning, growth and development, aging, and other related kinesiology topics.

Muscle fibers are generally classified as **slow twitch** (primarily aerobic fibers and fatigue resistant) or **fast twitch** (primarily anaerobic fibers and highly related to speed and strength performance). An individual's percentage of slow and fast twitch fibers within various muscle groups helps determine his or her athletic performance abilities and is highly influenced by genetics. The average person has 50% slow twitch and 50% fast twitch fibers, whereas elite endurance athletes usually have > 80% slow twitch fibers and great sprinters and strength athletes usually have > 80% fast twitch fibers.

The **motor unit** is the basic unit of skeletal muscle contraction and includes a motor nerve and all the fibers that it controls (see Figure 6.4). Motor units can be

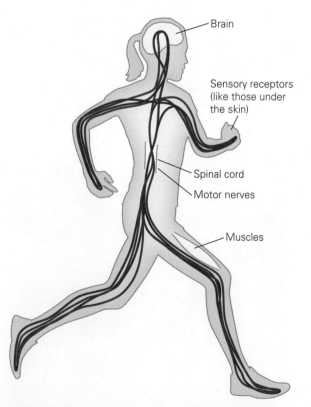

**Figure 6.2** | Components Involved in Integrated Neuromuscular Movement. You will learn much more about the details of figures such as this in future kinesiology courses.

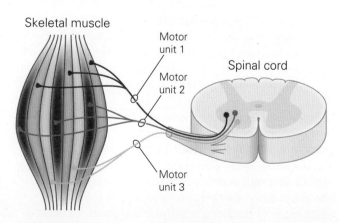

**Figure 6.4** | Motor Units in a Skeletal Muscle

small or large and the force and strength of skeletal muscle movements are directly related to the recruitment of motor units (see Figure 6.5). To stand at rest, we primarily recruit slow twitch muscle fibers (postural muscles); then, as we begin to walk and jog, we recruit more motor units (mostly slow twitch and a few fast twitch fibers); and to engage in maximal sprinting, we eventually recruit all slow and fast twitch fibers. Therefore, the energy cost of performing physical activities and exercise is directly related to the number of motor units or amount of muscle mass recruited.

Muscle contractions are coordinated and synchronized by nerves linked to your brain that innervate your muscles. The neuromuscular adaptations that occur with participation in strength and conditioning programs are closely integrated over time and include the adaptations of nerve reflexes and the muscle fibers recruited (specificity principle). The **proprioceptors** (body position receptors in the nervous system) help coordinate movements and are important for the maintenance or improvement of reaction time, balance, and movement economy (see Figure 6.6). Figure 6.6 shows a simple neuromusculoskeletal stretch reflex action and the factors involved in the knee jerk reflex. As you learned previously, placing regular physical demands on muscle fibers stimulates them to enlarge (hypertrophy); likewise, when we remain sedentary for many months or years we lose muscle strength and muscular endurance due to reduced muscle fiber size (**atrophy**). With aging, we can experience additional loss of muscle strength and endurance due to **sarcopenia** (loss of mainly fast twitch muscle fibers and reduced size of muscle fibers).

Measures of strength, **acceleration** (change in velocity over time), **work** (force × distance), and **power** (work per unit of time) are all important outcomes related to participation in strength and conditioning programs. As you learned in Chapter 5, the frequency, intensity, and duration of aerobic activities determine the resulting caloric expenditure across the physical activity continuum. The total volume for strength and conditioning activities is also related to frequency, intensity, and duration. Specifically, total volume can be impacted by factors such as:

**Exercise type:** including muscle mass required to perform an activity.

**Frequency:** number of days per week based on goals and abilities (beginner vs. advanced).

**Exercise order:** generally refers to starting with smaller muscle mass recruitment followed by recruitment of larger muscle mass groups to reduce the rate of muscular fatigue, especially for beginners.

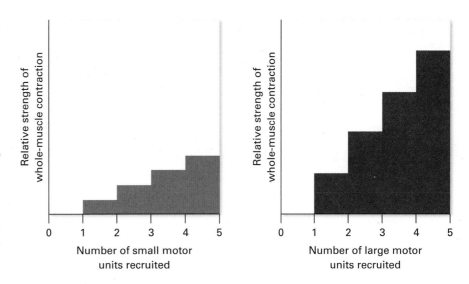

**Figure 6.5** | Comparison of Motor Unit Recruitment in Skeletal Muscles with Small Motor Units and Muscles with Large Motor Units. Generally the more motor units that are recruited, the greater the force of contraction.

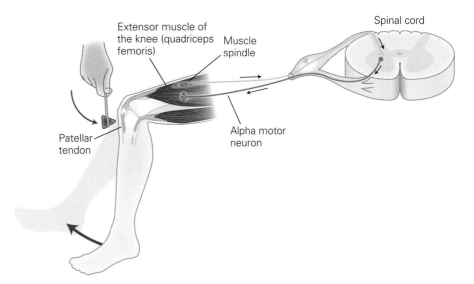

**Figure 6.6** | Simple Knee Reflex and the Components Involved in the Stretch Reflex. Notice nerve and musculoskeletal components are involved.

**Load (or intensity):** the amount of weight one lifts or resistance one moves against, the number of repetitions of the exercise performed, and the number of sets of the strength and conditioning activity performed—for example, the total amount of weight lifted or moved. A typical load might be described as 70% of 1 RM, for 10 reps, and performed for three sets separated by a rest interval between sets (a form of interval training).

**Duration:** largely determined by the number of repetitions and sets performed as well as the amount of rest between sets.

Remember, frequency, intensity, and duration factors that are components in strength and conditioning plans are similar to and need to be formulated using the overload, specificity, and adaptation principles you learned about in Chapters 4 and 5.

Strength and conditioning outcomes are also influenced by basic biomechanical and motor learning factors. It is important for you to understand the basic definitions of terms related to these areas of study and how they apply specifically to the physical activity continuum with regards to minimum recommendations and the avoidance of overtraining.

Some examples of biomechanical factors that directly affect changes in strength or muscular conditioning include the following:

*Motor unit recruitment and rate (frequency) of firing*—related to the types of movements performed and the total volume of strength and conditioning activities.

*Arrangement of muscle fibers*—basically angles of insertion and origin of muscles recruited for specific actions.

*Muscle length, length of the lever arm, joint angle*—all affect the strength, power, and work that can be performed effectively.

*Body size*—generally, the larger a person is the greater the muscle mass she/he has or can develop.

*Inertia and gravity*—the acceleration and velocity of muscular movements can vary based on the type of strength and conditioning activity performed and whether the activities involve, for example, free weights, weight machines, or elastic resistant bands.

Some examples of motor learning factors that directly affect changes in strength or muscular conditioning include the following:

*Open skill*—movement performed in an uncontrolled and unpredictable environment (e.g., agility drill in a team sport like basketball or football moves).

*Closed skill*—movement performed in a controlled and predictable environment (e.g., lifting weights in a gym or swinging a golf club).

*Reaction time and response time*—important variables related to balance and agility.

*Focus of attention and decision making under stress*—related to arousal levels and physical/mental readiness to perform physical activities.

*Vision and proprioception*—the ability to adjust physical effort and coordinate movements based on feedback.

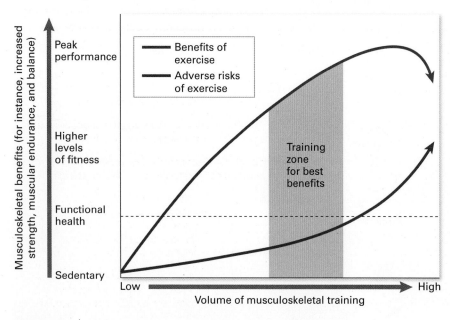

**Figure 6.7** | Training Continuum for Musculoskeletal Strength and Conditioning. The figure illustrates an optimal training zone for achieving better musculoskeletal benefits, but as explained in the text, benefits improve along the physical activity continuum based upon the volume of training.

A model for a training continuum for musculoskeletal strength and conditioning activities and their associated benefits is shown in Figure 6.7 and is similar to the model for aerobic training in Figure 5.2. Figure 6.7 shows the early and relatively large gains in musculoskeletal benefits due mostly to neural adaptations with low training volume, while later improvements are associated with greater gains in benefits due to hypertrophy and some further neural adaptations. The figure also reinforces the unifying training principles of overload, specificity, and adaptation that need to be applied appropriately for health promotion, higher fitness goals, or peak performance (also refer to Figure 4.10).

## Health and Quality of Life Benefits of Strength and Conditioning Physical Activities

Your skeletal muscles are fundamental to physical activity. The fuels they need to contract, carry out metabolism, and help you progress along the physical activity continuum are delivered by the cardiovascular system. Each type of physical activity—from typing on a keyboard to climbing stairs to moving heavy boxes to marathon running—requires muscles that are capable of creating force. Your skeletal muscles are attached to your bones in various ways and, through their contractions, allow you to move as directed by signals from your brain or sensory receptors in tissues (see a simple example of this concept in Figure 6.8).

Clearly, building and maintaining muscle strength is critical for all physical activity. Along the physical activity continuum, the amount of muscle strength necessary depends on the reason for physical activity. Regular participation in muscle strengthening and conditioning activities has been shown to be beneficial to the health of children and adolescents (ages 6–17 years), adults (ages

18–65 years), and older adults (ages > 65 years). Regular participation reduces the risk of **osteoporosis** (low bone density associated with loss of bone minerals); reduces the symptoms of **osteoarthritis** (a form of arthritis associated with lasting stiffness and swelling of joints); and preserves or increases skeletal muscle mass, strength, power, and neuromuscular (nerve and muscle) recruitment and activation. Higher levels of muscular strength may be necessary for other reasons, such as athletic performance or job requirements.

Regular participation in strength and conditioning activities throughout life, and across the physical activity continuum, helps improve balance and coordination and reduce the risk of falls. As you learned in Chapter 2, there is a close relationship between physical activity level and risk for functional/mobility limitations and falls. A summary of the health benefits of muscle strength and conditioning activities is shown in Table 6.1.

For children and adolescents to gain health benefits from strength and conditioning activities, engaging in muscle-strengthening and bone-strengthening activities on a minimum of three days per week is recommended (see Table 6.2 for examples). As mentioned earlier in the chapter, adults should participate in muscle-strengthening activities that engage all major muscle groups (shoulders, arms, back, chest, abdomen, legs, and hips) on two or more days per week for health benefits. Among older adults, performing specific muscle-strengthening

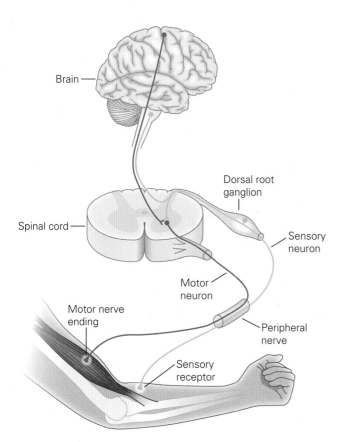

**Figure 6.8** | Simple Integration of the Brain, Nerves, Muscle, and Muscle Fibers That Can Produce Muscle Contractions

**Table 6.1** | Summary of Health Benefits of Participating in Strength and Conditioning Physical Activities

| |
|---|
| Associated with a lower risk of death due to any cause. |
| Risk reduction of hip fracture is 36% to 68% at the highest levels of physical activity. The magnitude of effect of physical activity on bone mineral density is 1% to 2%. |
| Risk reduction of osteoarthritis incidence (pain or disability) for various measures of walking ranges from 22% to 83%. |
| The magnitude of the effect of resistance types of physical activity on muscle mass and function is highly variable and dose-dependent. |
| Weight-bearing endurance and resistance types of physical activity (i.e., exercise training) are effective in promoting increases in bone mineral density (moderate-to-vigorous intensity; 3 to 5 days per week; 30 to 60 minutes per session). |
| Progressive, higher-intensity strength and conditioning activities (60% to 80% of 1 RM) can preserve or increase skeletal muscle mass, strength, power, and intrinsic neuromuscular function. |

*Source:* From "Physical Activity Guidelines Advisory Committee Report, 2008" (Washington, DC: U.S. Department of Health and Human Services, 2008), E10–E13. Available from health.gov/paguidelines/report/pdf/committeereport.pdf.

**Table 6.2** | Examples of Muscle- and Bone-Strengthening Activities for Children and Adolescents

| TYPE OF PHYSICAL ACTIVITY | AGE GROUP | |
| --- | --- | --- |
| | **CHILDREN** | **ADOLESCENTS** |
| Muscle-strengthening | ▸ Games such as tug-of-war<br>▸ Modified push-ups (with knees on the floor)<br>▸ Resistance exercises using body weight or resistance bands<br>▸ Rope or tree climbing<br>▸ Sit-ups (curl-ups or crunches)<br>▸ Swinging on playground equipment/bars | ▸ Games such as tug-of-war<br>▸ Push-ups and pull-ups<br>▸ Resistance exercises with exercise bands, weight machines, handheld weights<br>▸ Climbing wall<br>▸ Sit-ups (curl-ups or crunches) |
| Bone-strengthening | ▸ Games such as hopscotch<br>▸ Hopping, skipping, jumping<br>▸ Jumping rope<br>▸ Running<br>▸ Sports such as gymnastics, basketball, volleyball, tennis | ▸ Hopping, skipping, jumping<br>▸ Jumping rope<br>▸ Running<br>▸ Sports such as gymnastics, basketball, volleyball, tennis |

*Source:* From "Physical Activity Guidelines Advisory Committee Report, 2008" (Washington, DC: U.S. Department of Health and Human Services, 2008), 18. Available from health.gov/paguidelines/report/pdf/committeereport.pdf.

and balance activities based upon individual movement limitations can help reduce the risk of falls and provide additional health benefits. By encouraging regular participation in strength and conditioning activities, kinesiology professionals can help individuals and populations maintain and improve their quality of life and reduce the economic costs of premature disability related to reduced mobility.

## Health Benefits for All Ages of Participating Regularly in Strength and Conditioning Activities

It's never too late to gain strength along the physical activity continuum. In a 1994 research study, Dr. Maria Fiatarone and colleagues evaluated the muscular strength and muscle mass of 100 nursing home patients (average age of 87.3 years).[3] They randomized the patients into two groups: one that completed 10 weeks of weight training and a second, non-exercise group that received dietary supplements. The weight-training group significantly increased their muscular strength—by over 100% as compared to baseline measures—and they increased their bone mass by 2.7% as compared to the non-exercise group. The results of this study and others since have contributed to the body of evidence that supports the health benefits for all ages of participating regularly in strength and conditioning activities.

# Basic Physiological Responses and Benefits of Participation in Strength and Conditioning Activities

Regular participation in strength and conditioning activities produces neuromuscular and muscle tissue adaptations that promote good health and allow the attainment of higher-order fitness goals and peak performance. Tables 6.3 and 6.4 summarize these adaptations.

In addition to the general adaptations displayed in Tables 6.3 and 6.4, many physiological, biomechanical, and behavioral responses to regular participation in strength and conditioning activities are commonly observed. These are listed in Table 6.5.

**Table 6.3** | General Neuromuscular Adaptations to Strength (Resistance) Training

| |
| --- |
| ▸ Increases in motor cortex input that allows for greater neural control and increased force production |
| ▸ Increase in muscle recruitment (more motor units) increasing force production |
| ▸ Increases in neural firing rates and timing and coordination of recruitment that increase the rate of force production |
| ▸ Reduction in the inhibitory functions like the Golgi tendon organs allowing for increased force production, motor unit synchronization, and cross-training (education) that helps balance force production between both sides of the body |

**Table 6.4** | General Skeletal Muscle Adaptations to Strength (Resistance) Training

- Increases in muscle fiber size and cross-sectional size (muscle mass) that allows for increase in muscular strength
- Increases in myosin heavy chain protein and hypertrophy after early training changes associated with neural adaptations that allow for increases in muscular strength
- No change or decreases in capillary densities, and decreases in mitochondrial densities, which are associated with decreased oxidative capacity and reduced changes in aerobic power
- Increases in ATP, creatine phosphate, glycogen stores, fuel mobilization, and anaerobic enzyme activity that allow for improved energy utilization and muscular endurance
- Potential increases in ligament, tendon, collagen, and bone strength with decrease in body fat and increases in lean weight that can enhance functional health and may reduce falls (particularly in the elderly)

**Table 6.5** | Musculoskeletal Adaptations to Physical Activity and Exercise

| PHYSIOLOGICAL | BIOMECHANICAL |
|---|---|
| Increased muscular strength | Increased motor skill and confidence to engage further in physical activity and exercise |
| Increased muscular endurance | |
| Increased muscle fiber size (hypertrophy) | Improved proprioception, which helps coordination system response and balance |
| Increased neural recruitment | Improved economy |
| Increased anaerobic enzymes and energy stores | Improved mobility and ROM |
| Improved metabolic function | |
| Improved hormone-mediated bone remodeling | |
| Improved connective tissue function | |
| Increase in bone quality | |
| Maintenance or increase in lean muscle tissue | |
| Maintenance or loss of fat weight | |
| **BEHAVIORAL** | |
| Increased self-confidence | |
| Improved self-efficacy | |
| Possible reduction in depression and anxiety | |
| Experience with behavioral change | |
| Improved stress management | |
| Improved sleep patterns | |

*Source:* From H. W. Kohl and T. D. Murray, *Foundations of Physical Activity and Public Health* (Champaign, IL: Human Kinetics, 2012).

## Peak Performance and Strength and Conditioning Activities

Numerous factors affect the degree to which an individual or population can improve their muscle strength and muscle endurance along the physical activity continuum from physical inactivity to peak performance. Six factors that are commonly associated with optimal gains in strength and muscular endurance include genetics, nervous system adaptations, environmental factors, nutritional factors, the dose of physical activity, and exercise performed.

The National Football League (NFL) in the United States has an annual scouting combine (a series of peak performance tests) designed to evaluate and track the fastest, strongest, and most agile future professional players. The combine provides an excellent example of how athletes striving for peak performance can be compared to one another for future draft potential. The combine includes the following tests: the 40-yard dash, number of times a player can lift 225 pounds in the bench press, vertical jump, standing broad jump, three-cone drill, 20-yard shuttle, and 60-yard shuttle.

The overall best performances as of this writing for NFL Scouting Combine for speed, strength, and power events were as follows:

- 40-yard dash: Chris Johnson, East Carolina University (2008)—2.24 seconds
- Bench press repetitions: Stephen Paea, Oregon State University (2011)—49 repetitions
- Vertical jump: Chris Conley, University of Georgia (2015)—45 inches
- Standing broad jump: Byron Jones, University of Connecticut (2015)—12 feet, 3 inches

How would you compare to the maximal performances achieved for speed, strength, and power of the athletes listed above? Their results certainly represent the upper levels of peak human performance for speed, strength, and power. You can learn more and compare performances of players at different positions by performing a simple Internet search using key words "NFL Combine Results."

Unfortunately, in order to achieve peak performance in weight lifting, the NFL Scouting Combine, or activities such as power lifting and bodybuilding, some strength athletes have turned to illegal means to get stronger and more powerful. Arnold Schwarzenegger is an example of a former world-renowned body builder who admitted to using anabolic steroids, which were, and still are, illegal to use in sports participation. He later became famous as a movie star and as a politician perhaps due in part to his steroid-enhanced persona. His admission of steroid use tainted his weight lifting and body building accomplishments, as there is strong scientific evidence that steroids increase muscle strength and recovery from exercise. Anabolic steroids also cause serious health-damaging side effects. Unfortunately, no one will ever know if factors such as Arnold's hard training, genetics, and attention to nutrition could have enabled him to perform at the highest levels of strength and conditioning without drugs. Today, drug testing has become a regular part of screening at national and international sports competitions.

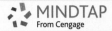

### Drug Testing in Sports

**Go to your MindTap course** to learn more about drug testing policies in several sports.

Three valuable resources for learning more about how to optimize strength and conditioning benefits for individuals and populations across the physical activity continuum are listed below. Links to each of the documents are included in the "For More Information" section at the end of this chapter and included in your MindTap course.

1. Physical Activity Guidelines Advisory Committee Report 2008
2. The American College of Sports Medicine (ACSM) Position Stand—*Quantity and Quality of Exercise for Developing and Maintaining Cardiorespiratory, Musculoskeletal, and Neuromotor Fitness in Apparently Health Adults: Guidance for Prescribing Exercise*
3. ACSM Position Stand—*Progression Models in Resistance Training for Healthy Adults.*[4]

These documents provide valuable evidence-based summaries of how best to achieve the health, physical fitness, and peak performance benefits of participating in strength and conditioning activities. An additional resource that is helpful for understanding the professional competencies related to strength and conditioning principles is the National Strength and Conditioning Association's *Strength and Conditioning Professional Standards and Guidelines.*[5]

## Beginning, Intermediate, and Advanced Strength and Conditioning Physical Activity and Exercise Programs

There has been quite a bit of scientific research on optimizing participating in strength and conditioning

activities for fitness. This section provides examples of how you might apply the strength and conditioning principles of total volume, overload, specificity, and adaptation when designing a beginning, intermediate, and advanced strength and conditioning program. The simple model provided uses only one exercise (the bench press as a weight-lifting activity). The goals for the programs provided include a beginner stage to increase overall strength, followed by an immediate stage to further increase strength and improve power, and an advanced stage to increase power and hypertrophy. If a novice were to start this program, he or she would start at the beginning level, with each week lifting four times: upper body exercise on day one, lower body exercise on day two, a rest period of no lifting on day three, upper body exercise on day four, lower body exercise on day five, and rest and repair on days six and seven. Once the novice has completed the beginning program, he or she can move into the intermediate program. The participant will test for new 1 RMs for their exercises of choice that they will complete in the intermediate program. The intermediate program will follow the same lifting and resting schedule as described in the beginning program, but the weekly volumes are increased as a percentage of 1 RM. Once the individual has completed the intermediate program, he or she moves into the advanced program. Prior to beginning the advanced program, the participant will again test for new 1 RMs for their exercises of choice that will be completed in the program. The advanced program will follow the same lifting and resting schedule as described in the beginning and intermediate programs, but the speed of the lifts is increased. In the advanced program, the participant attempts to lift the weights as fast as possible while remaining safe. Once participants have completed one full progression of levels, if they desire to increase strength and power further they can alternate between the intermediate and advanced level programs, always testing for new 1 RMs prior to starting the next level of the program.

Well-designed strength and conditioning programs for fitness and performance (at the upper end of the physical activity continuum) generally include multiple physical activities performed on at least two to three days per week that should be adjusted regularly to help meet individual or population goals. You can also find various commercial websites to learn more about designing beginning, intermediate, and advanced strength and conditioning programs for health, physical fitness, and peak performance.

**Sample Beginner Program**: Test for 1 RM prior to beginning this level. Remember to have a one-minute rest period between sets.

| BENCH PRESS | | | |
|---|---|---|---|
| | % 1 RM | SETS | REPS |
| Week 1 | 45 | 2 | 10 |
| | 50 | 2 | 10 |
| Week 2 | 45 | 2 | 10 |
| | 50 | 2 | 10 |
| Week 3 | 50 | 2 | 10 |
| | 55 | 1 | 10 |
| | 60 | 1 | 8 |
| Week 4 | 50 | 2 | 10 |
| | 55 | 1 | 10 |
| | 60 | 1 | 8 |
| Week 5 | 55 | 1 | 10 |
| | 60 | 2 | 10 |
| | 65 | 1 | 8 |
| Week 6 | 55 | 1 | 10 |
| | 60 | 2 | 10 |
| | 65 | 1 | 8 |
| Week 7 | 60 | 1 | 10 |
| | 65 | 1 | 10 |
| | 70 | 1 | 8 |
| | 75 | 1 | 6 |
| Week 8 | 60 | 1 | 10 |
| | 65 | 1 | 10 |
| | 70 | 1 | 8 |
| | 75 | 1 | 6 |
| Week 9 | 65 | 1 | 10 |
| | 70 | 1 | 10 |
| | 75 | 1 | 8 |
| | 80 | 1 | 6 |
| Week 10 | 65 | 1 | 10 |
| | 70 | 1 | 10 |
| | 75 | 1 | 8 |
| | 80 | 1 | 6 |
| Week 11 | 70 | 1 | 10 |
| | 75 | 1 | 10 |
| | 80 | 1 | 8 |
| | 85 | 1 | 6 |
| | 90 | 1 | 4 |
| Week 12 | 70 | 1 | 10 |
| | 75 | 1 | 10 |
| | 80 | 1 | 8 |
| | 85 | 1 | 6 |
| | 90 | 1 | 4 |

**Sample Intermediate Program:** Test for 1 RM prior to beginning the intermediate level. Remember to have a one-minute rest period between sets.

| BENCH PRESS | | | |
|---|---|---|---|
| | % MAX | SETS | REPS |
| Week 1 | 50 | 2 | 10 |
| | 65 | 2 | 10 |
| Week 2 | 50 | 2 | 10 |
| | 65 | 2 | 10 |
| Week 3 | 50 | 1 | 10 |
| | 65 | 2 | 10 |
| | 75 | 1 | 8 |
| Week 4 | 50 | 1 | 10 |
| | 65 | 2 | 10 |
| | 75 | 1 | 8 |
| Week 5 | 55 | 1 | 10 |
| | 70 | 1 | 10 |
| | 75 | 1 | 8 |
| | 85 | 1 | 6 |
| Week 6 | 55 | 1 | 10 |
| | 70 | 1 | 10 |
| | 75 | 1 | 8 |
| | 85 | 1 | 6 |
| Week 7 | 60 | 1 | 10 |
| | 75 | 1 | 10 |
| | 80 | 1 | 8 |
| | 85 | 1 | 6 |
| | 90 | 1 | 4 |
| Week 8 | 60 | 1 | 10 |
| | 75 | 1 | 10 |
| | 80 | 1 | 8 |
| | 85 | 1 | 6 |
| | 90 | 1 | 4 |
| Week 9 | 65 | 1 | 10 |
| | 80 | 1 | 8 |
| | 85 | 1 | 6 |
| | 90 | 1 | 4 |
| | 95 | 1 | 2 |
| Week 10 | 65 | 1 | 10 |
| | 80 | 1 | 8 |
| | 85 | 1 | 6 |
| | 90 | 1 | 4 |
| | 95 | 1 | 2 |
| Week 11 | 70 | 1 | 10 |
| | 85 | 1 | 8 |
| | 95 | 1 | 6 |
| | 100 | 1 | 4 |
| | 110 | 1 | 2 |
| Week 12 | 70 | 1 | 10 |
| | 85 | 1 | 8 |
| | 95 | 1 | 6 |
| | 100 | 1 | 4 |
| | 110 | 1 | 2 |

**Sample Advanced Program**: Test for 1 RM prior to beginning the advanced level. Remember all lifts are to be done as fast as possible and you need a one-minute rest period between sets. Once the individual has completed the advanced level program, he or she can alternate between the intermediate plan for twelve weeks and the advanced plan for eight weeks to improve both strength and power. Always test for new 1 RMs before starting any of the programs.

| BENCH PRESS | | | |
|---|---|---|---|
| | % 1 RM | SETS | REPS |
| Week 1 | 60 | 2 | 20 |
| | 70 | 2 | 20 |
| Week 2 | 60 | 2 | 20 |
| | 70 | 2 | 20 |
| Week 3 | 65 | 2 | 20 |
| | 75 | 2 | 20 |
| Week 4 | 65 | 2 | 20 |
| | 75 | 2 | 20 |
| Week 5 | 70 | 2 | 20 |
| | 75 | 2 | 20 |
| Week 6 | 70 | 2 | 20 |
| | 75 | 2 | 20 |
| Week 7 | 70 | 2 | 20 |
| | 80 | 2 | 20 |
| Week 8 | 70 | 2 | 20 |
| | 80 | 2 | 20 |

## Measuring Muscle Strength and Muscle Endurance

How do you measure a person's strength? This is a much more complicated question than it at first appears to be. In Chapter 5, multiple ways to measure aerobic performance and cardiovascular fitness, both in the laboratory and in field settings, were highlighted. What these tests all have in common is that they are each a broad measure of the same construct—maximal oxygen uptake ($VO_2$ max).

Measuring muscular strength is quite different in that strength depends on the training of individual muscles and groups of muscles. The principle of specificity is never clearer on the physical activity continuum than it is for muscular strength. For example, a volleyball athlete who is in a physical therapy program to strengthen the muscles around her knee after surgery to fix a ligament tear will indeed strengthen those muscles if she follows the protocol from her therapist. Unless she also focuses on other parts of her body, the only muscles that she will strengthen will be those around her knee. Thus, specificity is an important consideration when thinking about measuring muscle strength.

Musculoskeletal training results in a wide variety of specific health, physical fitness, and peak performance

adaptations (review Tables 6.1, 6.3, and 6.5). However, regular participation in muscle strength and muscle endurance physical activities usually does not produce significant gains in aerobic fitness ($VO_2$ max) like aerobic training, because these activities mostly stress anaerobic metabolic reactions (see Chapter 5). Some studies have shown that musculoskeletal training programs that include circuit training (multiple muscle strength/endurance stations where short bursts of exercises ~1 minute are performed with short rests ~15 seconds before the next burst of activities) have shown modest (~5%) improvements in $VO_2$ max. Therefore, if one wants cardiovascular and musculoskeletal health benefits from participating in physical activity, they are best served by performing a variety of aerobic and muscle strength and muscle endurance activities.

There is no universal summary measure of human strength as there is for cardiovascular fitness. As with cardiovascular fitness, however, the strength or power of a certain muscle or group of muscles can be measured in a laboratory or clinical setting or in a field setting.

### *Strength*

Laboratory and clinical tests of muscular strength are helpful ways to precisely assess the force that a muscle or group of muscles can produce. Applications of such tests include diagnostic and performance-related measures such as work performance and ergometry. Laboratory or clinical tests may use a tool known as a dynamometer. A handgrip dynamometer, the most frequently used tool, quantifies the maximum isometric strength that can be generated by the muscles in the forearm and hand. Persons being tested grip the device and squeeze at maximal effort for approximately five seconds. A gauge on the device allows quantification of the force generated during the test. Data generated from this kind of testing can help athletes who use their hands, such as tennis players and gymnasts, to improve their performance. Such testing is also helpful in occupational therapy settings, where improvements in hand strength among clients who use their hands frequently in their jobs can be measured before and after rehabilitation protocols have been implemented.

Field tests of muscular strength are convenient and low-cost approaches to measuring how strong a group of muscles is. They are more broadly applicable than laboratory tests in that more than one person can be tested at a time. They also allow for a broader range of muscles and groups of muscles to be tested than dynamometers. Such tests focus on dynamic strength and most often try to identify the maximum amount of weight that can be

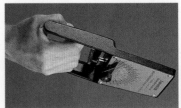
Werner Hoeger

lifted or moved at any one time. One dynamic (isotonic) test of muscle strength that is frequently used in the field is the 1-repetition maximum strength (1 RM) test. The 1 RM test is used to determine the maximum amount of weight a person can lift one time. For example, a 1 RM bench press test is used to determine the maximum amount of force that can be generated by an individual's chest and shoulder muscles. To conduct a 1 RM bench press test, the person being tested is first situated on the bench, lying on his or her back. With assistance, an achievable weight is loaded on the weight machine or bar. This weight is increased until the participant can no longer adequately push the weight to a fixed position. The final weight lifted is the 1 RM value. Such tests can be designed for muscles in the lower body as well, using squats or leg-press weight machines.

Although the 1 RM method for strength testing is acceptable in most situations, it may not be appropriate for novice lifters or adolescents learning to lift weights. Other measures used to estimate strength among novice lifters include the 5 RM or 10 RM methods. Both methods may underestimate strength among novice lifters; however, they are much safer to use when someone is first learning to lift weights. You can use online calculators available at www.exrx.net/Calculators/OneRepMax.html to estimate 1 RM using data from 5 RM and 10 RM performances.[6]

### Endurance

When assessing muscular strength, it is the maximal amount of force that can be generated that is of interest. In contrast, muscular endurance is the ability to generate adequate force to meet a demand over time. Muscular endurance is more applicable than maximal muscular strength when measuring the strength necessary to accomplish activities of daily living. For example, an elderly woman interested in maintaining healthy bones and reducing her risk of falling should focus on exercises that improve her muscular endurance throughout the day and that can also increase her maximal strength. She has no need to improve the peak strength of her muscles.

Similar tests for muscular endurance can be used in the laboratory or field setting, and these tests are commonly performed. (Once you complete the chapter conduct an Internet search for commercial strength and conditioning web sites as suggested by your instructor to learn more about specific field and lab tests to evaluate musculoskeletal performance.) For example, a sit-up test can measure muscular endurance in the abdomen and upper legs. An 80% maximum bench press test can be used to measure muscular endurance in the chest and shoulders. Another popular upper body test that can be used virtually anywhere is a push-up test. The flexed arm hang test is used to measure shoulder and arm endurance.

Two common threads link each of these muscular endurance tests. First, such tests typically measure muscle groups rather than specific muscles. For example, the muscle typically referred to as your hamstring is really four separate muscles. Tests that focus on that area of the body cannot isolate the strength of the individual muscles that make up the muscle group. Second, results from each test can be used quite effectively to measure change over time across the continuum. For example, the maximum number of push-ups that can be completed can be recorded before and after a muscle strengthening program has been implemented to measure how much the participants' endurance has improved. Therapists can use sit-up tests or other measures of trunk muscle endurance to set goals for patients to help reduce and control low back pain and discomfort.

# EXAMPLES OF APPLYING STRENGTH AND CONDITIONING PRINCIPLES IN KINESIOLOGY SUBDISCIPLINES

*In Lesson 1, you learned about the importance of understanding strength and conditioning activities and the numerous health and peak performance benefits associated with developing recommended and higher levels of strength and conditioning that contribute to health,* *improved quality of life, and optimizing performance. In Lesson 2, you will learn about examples of the application of strength and conditioning physical activity principles to the subdisciplines of kinesiology and to the physical activity continuum.*

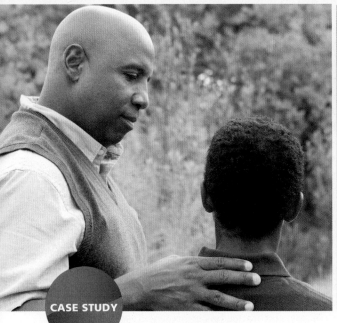

**CASE STUDY**

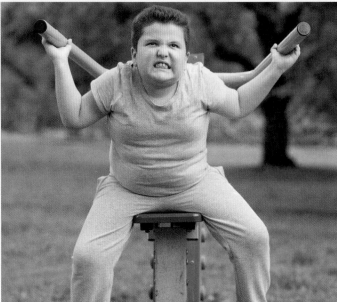

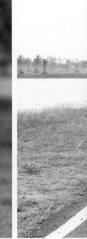

## In the real world . . .

Eugene Casey is excited about lifting weights and improving his strength and conditioning levels. However, his parents are concerned about how weight lifting might affect Eugene's growth and development patterns and about the potential risk for injuries. They are also interested in knowing whether lifting weights will effectively increase Eugene's strength and muscular endurance, since he is only 10 years old.

*Overview:* According to the U.S. National Strength and Conditioning Association (NSCA) 2009 Position Statement, *Youth Resistance Training*, for children (ages 7 to 8 up to age 11 for girls and 13 for boys based on sexual maturation) and adolescents (girls ages 12 to 18 and boys ages 14 to 18) the NSCA supports the following:[7, 8, 9]

1. A properly designed and supervised resistance training program is relatively safe for youth.

2. A properly designed and supervised resistance training program can enhance the muscular strength and power of youth.

3. A properly designed and supervised resistance training program can improve the cardiovascular risk profile of youth.

4. A properly designed and supervised resistance training program can improve motor skill performance and may contribute to enhanced sports performance of youth.

5. A properly designed and supervised resistance training program can increase a young athlete's resistance to sports-related injuries.

6. A properly designed and supervised resistance training program can help improve the psychosocial well-being of youth.

7. A properly designed and supervised resistance training program can help promote and develop exercise habits during childhood and adolescence.

In children, the gains in strength and muscular endurance associated with resistance training are primarily due to neural

- Exercise Physiology
- Biomechanics
- Public Health
- Sport/Exercise Psychology

- Motor Learning
- Practice of Kinesiology

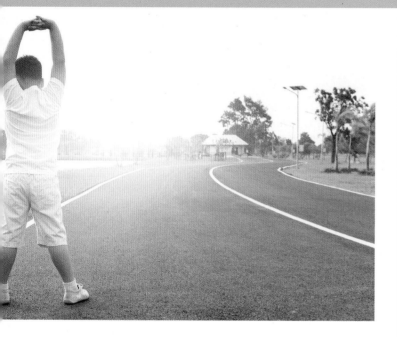

### Table 6.6 | General Resistance Training Guidelines for Children and Adolescents

- Provide qualified instruction and supervision
- Ensure the exercise environment is safe and free of hazards
- Start each training session with a 5- to 10-minute dynamic warm-up period
- Begin with relatively light loads and always focus on the correct exercise technique
- Perform 1–3 sets of 6–15 repetitions of a variety of upper- and lower-body strength exercises
- Include specific exercises that strengthen the abdominal and lower back region
- Focus on symmetrical muscular development and appropriate muscle balance around joints
- Perform 1–3 sets of 3–6 repetitions of a variety of upper- and lower-body power exercises
- Sensibly progress the training program depending on needs, goals, and abilities
- Increase the resistance gradually (5%–10%) as strength improves
- Cool down with less-intense calisthenics and static stretching
- Listen to individual needs and concerns throughout each session
- Begin resistance training 2–3 times per week on nonconsecutive days
- Use individualized workout logs to monitor progress
- Keep the program fresh and challenging by systematically varying the training program
- Optimize performance and recovery with healthy nutrition, proper hydration, and adequate sleep
- Support and encouragement from instructors and parents will help maintain interest

*Source:* A. D. Faigenbaum et al., "Youth Resistance Training: Updated Position Statement Paper from The National Strength and Conditioning Association," *Journal of Strength and Conditioning Research* 23, no. 5 (2009): S60–S79, S70.

(nerve and muscle firing, recruitment, and coordination) factors, while the strength gains in adolescents are associated with both neural factors (early in training) and hypertrophy (later in training and based on individual testosterone levels). Generally, resistance training programs for children should focus on fun activities that require them to move their body weight, develop general motor skills, and meet national physical activity guidelines related to a variety of physical activities (e.g., push-ups, curl-ups, jumping rope, pull-ups). For adolescents, resistance programs can be designed to minimally meet the national physical activity guidelines as well as goals for improved physical fitness levels and peak performance.

Table 6.6 contains general resistance training guidelines for children and adolescents, including specific exercises beyond those to meet the minimal national physical activity guidelines, from the NSCA.

Eugene became excited about physical activity through recognizing and practicing weight lifting to improve his strength and conditioning skills. By following guidelines like those provided by the 2008 Physical Activity Guidelines for Americans and the NSCA, he can continue to have fun lifting weights for a lifetime even as his specific strength and conditioning goals change over time.

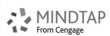

Go to your MindTap course to complete the Case Study activity for this chapter.

# Exercise Physiology ⬥

Do you remember the first time you (or someone you know) engaged in strength and conditioning physical activities to improve your health, physical fitness, or sports performance? How long did it take you to see a significant increase in your muscular strength? Probably four to six weeks. Did you see an increase in muscle size after four to six weeks of training? Most likely, you did not. So, how did you get stronger? Was it a combination of nervous stimulation (neural) and increase in muscle size (hypertrophy) integration?

As early as 1979, exercise physiologists studying strength and conditioning responses to training reported that the initial gains (first four to six weeks) in muscular strength were due to neural changes that affect muscle fiber recruitment (or motor unit recruitment), while increases in muscle size or hypertrophy require longer periods of time (> 6 weeks) and are dependent upon the further overloading of muscle groups and levels of testosterone. In long-term (1 ½ to 2 years) strength and conditioning programs it has been reported that further neural and hypertrophy changes also occur. The integration of neural and hypertrophy changes relative to strength (and use of illegal steroids) is shown in Figure 6.9.

## Strength and Conditioning Detraining

How long does it take to lose strength and conditioning benefits once one stops training? It is often difficult to conduct studies on detraining and physical activity or exercise because individuals do not like to stop physical activity programs once they have had success and significant improvements related to their outcome goals. However, good evidence indicates that if an individual stops a training regime completely, he or she will lose muscular strength and muscular endurance abilities at different rates. Let's consider someone with a 1 RM bench press of 140 pounds who is able to perform the following regime: 4 sets of 10 repetitions with 100 pounds, with one minute of rest between sets, four times per week. After about one month without training, this person would most likely still be able to perform a 1 RM of 140 pounds in the bench press, but after three weeks or so she or he would only be able to perform 3 sets lifting 100 pounds with one minute of rest.

Other physiological, biomechanical, and behavioral changes that occur with strength and conditioning would be reversed at varying rates based on their peak levels prior to detraining. The main point is that the benefits of strength and conditioning are integrated such that "if you don't use it, you lose it."

# Biomechanics ⬤

Rick, the CEO of Global Weightlifting, has read an article in a men's health magazine that implies loading of the contracting muscles during the eccentric phase of contraction improves the strength and power generation of the affected muscle group. Rick decides to task Doug, a product designer for Global Weightlifting, with using this newfound information to design a prototype biceps machine that will improve arm strength. Using the scientific method as his basis, Doug develops an arm curl machine that maximizes both concentric and eccentric forces during a lift. Upon careful review of related research, Doug decides that the machine must load 10% more force on the eccentric contraction as compared to the concentric contraction of the biceps.[10]

After several months of design development, Doug's machine is ready for beta testing. The machine consists of hydraulic cylinders mounted into a seated rack and attached to a curl bar. As the curl bar is moved toward the body in a seated curl, the cylinders produce an opposing force set by the user. Once the full range of motion of the concentric contraction of the curl is reached, the cylinders produce a 10% greater force to begin the eccentric contraction as the biceps lengthen and the curl bar moves away from the body. Doug uses two groups of test subjects to

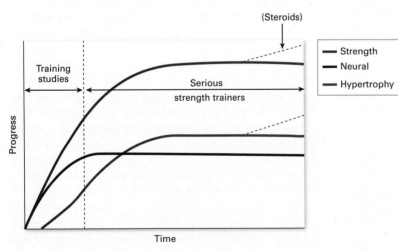

**Figure 6.9 | Relative Role of Neural and Muscular Adaptations to Resistance Training.** Initial gains (first four to six weeks) in muscular strength are due to neural changes that affect muscle fiber recruitment (or motor unit recruitment), while increases in muscle size or hypertrophy require longer periods of time (> 6 weeks) and are dependent upon the further overloading of muscle groups and levels of individual testosterone.

*Source:* Adapted from W. D. McArdle, F. I. Katch, and V. L. Katch, *Exercise Physiology: Energy, Nutrition and Human Development* (Philadelphia: Lippincot Williams & Wilkins, 2007), 541.

determine if use of the machine improves strength and power to a greater extent as compared to a traditional free weight curl. For six weeks, the control group lifts 80% of their 1 RM curl using free weights, while the experimental group lifts 80% of their 1 RM curl concentrically and 90% of their 1 RM curl eccentrically using the machine. Both groups lift four sets of five repetitions two days a week for six weeks. At the end of the six-week trial, Doug uses a strength dynamometer to determine arm curl strength of all the subjects. After analyzing the data, Doug reports to Rick that use of the machine has yielded significant improvements: 12% greater strength and 8% greater power as compared to free weight training. Doug also tells Rick, however, that the subjects using the new machine reported significantly higher amounts of muscle soreness (**delayed onset of muscle soreness** or **DOMS**) the day after using the machine as compared to the free weight group. Doug is concerned about not only the muscle soreness but also the desensitization of the Golgi tendon organ (sensory receptor organ that senses changes in muscle tension) in the biceps, which may increase risk of injury to the biceps over time. Doug suggests that the company complete further, long-term testing of the machine before marketing it to the public.

## Public Health

Yvette recently graduated with her bachelor's degree in kinesiology. For as long as she can remember, she has wanted to work with older adults, and right out of school she successfully landed a new job coordinating fitness programming for people living in a retirement community. Residents in the community range from people who are newly-retired and in their 50s to adults who are more than 100 years old. There is a broad spectrum of independence among the residents. Some people are fully functional and live fairly independently while others require constant monitoring and care due to conditions such as arthritis, Alzheimer's disease, and other forms of dementia.

Despite this range in independence, all the residents in the community share one common problem: the increasing risk of unexpectedly falling. When she hired Yvette, the general manager of the facility made it clear that preventing falls was one of the main goals of the community's staff. Yvette knew from her studies that falls can result from external causes (such as tripping over a loose rug) or internal causes (such as dizziness and/or a lack of balance). She also knew that falls can be extremely dangerous for older adults, who may sustain concussions and other neurologic trauma as well as broken bones (such as hips)—injuries that are very difficult for older people to recover from. Even minor trauma from a fall in an otherwise physically active older adult can lower his or her position along the physical activity continuum. This begins a cascade of loss of muscle mass followed by an increase in frailty.

Yvette set out to design a muscular strength and conditioning program for residents of the community to help them maintain muscle strength and prevent falls. To do this, she studied the scientific literature and developed an evidence-based program. She knew that people in their 90s were not the same as people in their 70s, but she also remembered from her studies that even 90-year-old people can increase their muscle mass and improve their strength. The program she developed could be individualized for specificity, overload, and adaptation so that people who were not as strong would begin the program with lower weights than others who were initially stronger. Her program focused on developing and maintaining core strength (strength of the torso) as well as limb strength to help people catch themselves prior to falling all the way to the ground. The core strength exercises consisted of chair squats and toe raises, and the limb strength conditioning exercises were various extension exercises of the arms and legs using elastic bands. Yvette personalized each program and kept track of residents' progress as well as the incidence of falls in the community. She also made it fun and focused on the social aspects of getting residents together to participate. In her first six months of work, she documented impressive gains in strength among participants, but just as important, the incidence of falls dropped substantially in the community as well.

## Sport/Exercise Psychology

Robyn has been hired as a strength and conditioning coach by a local school district to help prepare their junior high school athletes for the transition to high school athletics in future years. It seems that the transition from junior high to senior high athletics has been marred by numerous weight room accidents and injuries among freshmen at the high school in past years. Robyn's first order of business is to review the current resistance training programs and exercises to determine if they are age appropriate for junior high athletes. She discovers that the previous strength coach adhered to the suggested guidelines and policy positions of both the NSCA and ACSM concerning resistance training among adolescents, and all overloads and progressions of specific exercises meet the guidelines. Robyn then decides to observe the junior high school athletes in the weight room to determine if there is an issue with supervision or other environmental factors that may be affecting the injury rates.

After a week of observing both the girls' and boys' activities in the weight room, Robyn concludes that there is adequate supervision and initial training of proper lifting techniques. However, several of the students continue to use improper lifting form for the bench press, overhead press, and squats. Robyn remembers from her sport psychology class in college that one way to improve proper form and function of a task is to use imagery of that task in a controlled environment.[11]

Robyn decides to incorporate three new stations in the weight room. The stations will be imagery stations: a bench press imagery station located immediately prior to the bench press station, an overhead press imagery station located immediately prior to the overhead press station, and a squat imagery station located immediately prior to the squat station. Each of the imagery stations will be equipped with a dowel rod one and a half inches thick and the length of a weight bar. At each imagery station the students will be asked to close their eyes and imagine the perfect form for the lift. They will then hold the dowel rod in the position of the lift and slowly perform 10 reps of the proper form with their eyes closed to improve their kinesthetic awareness (sensory skill that your body uses to know where it is in space) of the bar while imagining and performing the lift. Finally, they will be asked to perform 10 additional repetitions of the lift with the dowel rod while they watch their form in a mirror. If the form observed in the mirror does not match their image of the perfect form, they must adjust accordingly. The students will be expected to do three sets of the imagery lifts at each station to reinforce the proper form. One year after the new imagery stations have been implemented in the junior high school, the high school coaches are reporting fewer accidents among the freshmen athletes.

## Motor Learning

Bill is an athletic trainer at a local community college. One of the college's star athletes has returned to the training room for rehabilitation after surgery to repair a torn anterior cruciate ligament (ACL). Bill finds that the athlete has developed a severe discrepancy in bilateral leg strength since the surgery. The affected leg has atrophied substantially compared to the one not subjected to the surgery, and the athlete is concerned that she will not be able to play in the upcoming season. Bill assures the athlete that, with the proper training regime, she will indeed be able to play in the upcoming season. He remembers from his kinesiology training that the main rehabilitation issue with surgery is neuromuscular deficit and the resulting need for neural recruitment strategies for the affected limb.[12]

Bill explains to the athlete that since her leg was immobilized and damaged, the muscles and neurons in the leg have regressed to an untrained state. He notes that this state is similar to that of a novice weight lifter, and thus the athlete will have to retrain the leg to restore the same recruitment and synchronization patterns that she had established pre-injury. Bill also points out to the

athlete that, because she had been engaged in leg conditioning prior to the injury, it will take her less time to recover than if she had not been in training. In fact, since the athlete maintained training of the uninjured leg pre- and post-surgery, some cross-limb innervation will help her regain the strength and neural response necessary to compete.[13]

Bill begins the athlete's rehabilitation with a leg-lifting regimen that consists of 50% of the athlete's 10 RM with four sets of 20 leg lifts and leg curls under slow and controlled contractions. After one week Bill increases the overload to 55%, and for the next six weeks he progresses the overload each week in 5% increments. At the beginning of the eighth week he has the student return to her normal weight-training program in preparation for the season.

## The Practice of Kinesiology

Have you ever noticed that individuals recovering from unexpected medical emergencies or surgery challenges such as an uncomplicated heart attack or ACL surgery are encouraged to get physically moving as soon as possible after their event and to limit their bed rest? This has not always been the case. As late as the mid-1960s, bed rest was often prescribed for several weeks after a heart attack or common orthopedic surgeries where the affected limb was usually casted for several weeks.

In 1968, Bengt Saltin, Ph.D., M.D. and colleagues at Southwestern Medical School in Dallas reported the results of what became known as the Dallas Bed Rest Study.[14] This group of investigators evaluated the effects of 21 days of complete bed rest on five men (two who were physically active and three who were sedentary). Following bed rest, all participants showed significant decreases in $VO_2$ max (~26%) and other worsening of other cardiovascular laboratory measures. The men then participated in 60 days (five days per week) of endurance exercise designed to restore their aerobic fitness levels. The sedentary men improved their $VO_2$ max levels by 40% while it took the active subjects a full 60 days just to return to their initial pre–bed rest levels (see Figure 6.10). Bed rest has also been associated with bone mineral losses and reductions in overall musculoskeletal strength.

The results of the original Dallas Bed Rest Study and a 2001 follow-up study[15] included the following important practical outcomes related to the practice of kinesiology:

1. Three weeks of bed rest in men at age 20 had a more significant negative effect on physical work capacity than 30 years of aging in these same men.
2. Recovery from surgery requires early ambulation instead of previously prescribed bed rest. The

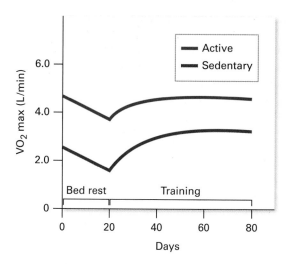

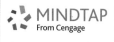

**Figure 6.10 | Bed Rest.** Bed rest is also associated with significant bone mineral losses and reductions in overall musculoskeletal health. The Dallas Bed Rest Study (21 days of complete bed rest) resulted in significant negative changes in cardiovascular and musculoskeletal function. In the 30-year follow-up Dallas study, it was concluded that three weeks of bed rest in men at age 20 had a more significant negative effect on physical work capacity than 30 years of aging in these same men.

maintenance of circulatory function is important for supplying nutrients to the working muscles to facilitate recovery.

3. The initial concepts developed in the late 1950s suggesting that individuals should return to physical activity very soon after a heart attack were confirmed.

4. It has become recognized that bed rest deconditioning is similar to the deconditioning associated with microgravity and spaceflight exposure. In fact, bed rest studies have been used regularly to examine the negative effects of microgravity on the cardiovascular system as well as those on bone and muscle.

Studies of astronauts who have spent many weeks in space (similar to physiological and biomechanical effects of bed rest) have shown:

a. Measurable bone loss—including loss of bone mass density and bone mineral content—that is not uniformly distributed across the skeleton.

b. Less vitamin D and calcium absorption, which negatively affects bone mass.

c. That it requires more time to replace bone mass upon return to earth than was required to lose it while in space.

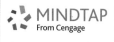

MINDTAP
From Cengage

Now that you have completed this chapter, go to your MindTap course to complete all assigned activities. Check out the additional resources developed to help you apply the material in this chapter to your course and career goals.

## Chapter Summary

▸ Strengthening and conditioning the musculoskeletal system is equally as important to health and human performance as the aerobic activities that were discussed in Chapter 5. Unfortunately, far fewer middle-aged and older adults participate regularly in strength and conditioning physical activities than in aerobic physical activities.

▸ Muscle contractions are coordinated and synchronized by nerves that innervate your muscles. The neuromuscular adaptations that occur with participation in strength and conditioning programs are closely integrated over time and involve the adaptations of nerve reflexes and the muscle fibers recruited (specificity principle).

▸ Strength and conditioning outcomes are also influenced by basic biomechanical and motor learning factors, and it is important to understand basic definitions of terms related to these areas of study and how they apply specifically to the physical activity continuum

with regards to minimum recommendations and the avoidance of overtraining.

▸ Regular participation in strength and conditioning activities produces neuromuscular and muscle tissue adaptations that promote good health and allow the attainment of higher-order fitness goals and peak performance.

▸ Specificity is an important consideration when assessing muscle strength. There is no universal measure of human strength as there is for cardiovascular fitness. Like cardiovascular fitness, the strength or power of a certain muscle or group of muscles can be measured in a laboratory or clinical setting or in a field setting.

▸ For children, the gains in strength and muscular endurance associated with resistance training are primarily due to neural (nerve and muscle firing, recruitment, and coordination) factors, while the strength gains in adolescents are associated with neural factors (early in training) and hypertrophy (later in training and based on individual testosterone levels). Generally, resistance

# People Matter Mike McFadden, Strength and Conditioning Coach*

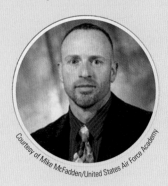

Courtesy of Mike McFadden/United States Air Force Academy

**Q: Why and how did you get into the field of kinesiology?**

**A:** *I was medically retired from the military after 15 years of service. I simply wasn't ready to quit. I knew that I would have to work harder and yet smarter to stay physically fit. Once I enrolled in my undergraduate program and began learning the basics of exercise physiology and biomechanics, I was hooked. I love that I'm able to train my athletes in hopes of keeping them safe and healthy, by training smarter than what I had growing up.*

**Q: What was the major influence on you to work in the field?**

**A:** *I am a combat veteran, served a few years in law enforcement, played a season of semi-professional football, and currently an avid outdoorsman. Staying physically fit and feeling I can still be prepared for any situation is what keeps me going. I emphasize that to my athletes. I believe that my past experiences, and the ways that I continue to train, help me to relate to them and to be an encouragement of what they can continue to do after the game is over.*

**Q: What are your current research interests, and how do you translate your research results to practitioners?**

**A:** *I have directed most of my research efforts toward understanding hamstring and ACL injury epidemiology, and applying training methods to mitigate those injuries. Recently, I have placed more emphasis on gaining a better understanding of applied sport psychology. I believe most of the work in the weight room should be focused on skill acquisition rather than putting up bigger numbers. I have presented at numerous conferences and workshops for strength coaches, athletic trainers, and physical therapists discussing these topics, and have witnessed a growing interest in the use of psychology in the training environment.*

**Q: How do you stay physically active yourself and promote good health to others directly around you?**

**A:** *I never do the same thing twice. I do not have set regimen or predetermined "body part" days. If I have a 30-minute window to get a workout in, then I will do a high-intensity interval training session. If I have more time, I will do multiple sets of structural exercises like squats, deadlifts, and farmer's carries with plenty of rest between sets. On a weekend, I love strapping on a pack and going for a hike up in the mountains of Colorado. I try to make sure that my athletes can see me doing all the things I ask them to do, such as mobility work, plyometrics, kettlebells, etc. While I may not push the amount of weight I once could, I make sure that I can effectively demonstrate proper technique on anything I program into a training session.*

**Q: How have you had to integrate the subdisciplines of kinesiology in your professional practice?**

**A:** *I believe that in order to be an effective strength coach, you must have a working knowledge of many subdisciplines: motor learning and human development, biomechanics/physics, basic and exercise physiology, and psychological theories as they apply to sports performance. I use all of these on a daily basis and in every training session. I cannot stop at thinking of the primary strength needs of a sport; but more so, the demands on the energy systems, potential mechanisms of injury, and motivational strategies needed for a sport that may have multiple positions and requirements. I develop at least two separate programs for my baseball team (pitchers vs. position players) throughout the year and often communicate to them differently. My personal philosophy is, as the coach, I have to be the one to adapt to the team/sport, not expecting each team to adapt to my training style.*

*Mike McFadden is assistant strength and conditioning coach at the U.S. Air Force Academy. He is currently the strength coach for water polo, men's swimming, baseball, and lacrosse, and oversees training for men's soccer, and assists with track and field.

---

training programs for children should focus on fun activities that require them to move their body weight, develop general motor skills, and meet national physical activity guidelines related to a variety of physical activities (e.g., push-ups, curl-ups, jumping rope, pull-ups).

▸ Prolonged bed rest is detrimental to bone, muscle, strength, muscular endurance, and aerobic measures like $VO_2$ max. Following adverse events like an uncomplicated heart attack or ACL knee surgery, it is important clinically that individuals return to physical activity quickly.

## Remember This

<table>
<tr><td>1 RM</td><td>exercise order</td><td>load (intensity)</td><td>sarcopenia</td></tr>
<tr><td>acceleration</td><td>exercise type</td><td>motor unit</td><td>slow twitch</td></tr>
<tr><td>atrophy</td><td>fast twitch</td><td>muscular strength</td><td>static exercise (isometric</td></tr>
<tr><td>conditioning</td><td>flexibility</td><td>osteoarthritis</td><td>   exercise)</td></tr>
<tr><td>delayed onset of muscle</td><td>frequency</td><td>osteoporosis</td><td>work</td></tr>
<tr><td>   soreness (or DOMS)</td><td>hyperplasia</td><td>physical culture</td><td></td></tr>
<tr><td>duration</td><td>hypertrophy</td><td>power</td><td></td></tr>
<tr><td>dynamic exercise</td><td>isokinetic</td><td>proprioceptors</td><td></td></tr>
</table>

## For More Information

Access these websites for further study of topics covered in the chapter:

- *Physical Activity Guidelines Advisory Committee Report 2008* (www.health.gov/PAGuidelines/Report/)

- The American College of Sports Medicine (ACSM) Position Stand—*Quantity and Quality of Exercise for Developing and Maintaining Cardiorespiratory, Musculoskeletal, and Neuromotor Fitness in Apparently Health Adults: Guidance for Prescribing Exercise* (www.acsm.org/access-public -information/position-stands)

- ACSM Position Stand—*Progression Models in Resistance Training for Healthy Adults* (www.acsm.org/access -public-information/position-stands)

- National Strength and Conditioning Association's Strength and Conditioning Professional Standards and Guidelines (www.nsca.com/uploadedFiles/NSCA /Resources/PDF/Education/Tools_and_Resources /NSCA_strength_and_conditioning_professional _standards_and_guidelines.pdf)

- Search for further information about the physical activity continuum and strength and conditioning physical activity principles at the National Strength and Conditioning Association: www.nsca.com.

- Search for information and resources related to strategies to promote strength and conditioning physical activities in the United States at the U.S. Physical Activity Guidelines webpage (www.health.gov/paguidelines) and the U.S. Physical Activity Plan webpage (www .physicalactivityplan.org).

- Search for information about strength and conditioning at the Research Digest page of the President's Council on Fitness, Sports, and Nutrition at www.fitness.gov.

- Search for more information about strength and conditioning principles at commercial websites by conducting an Internet search based upon your course instructor's recommendations.

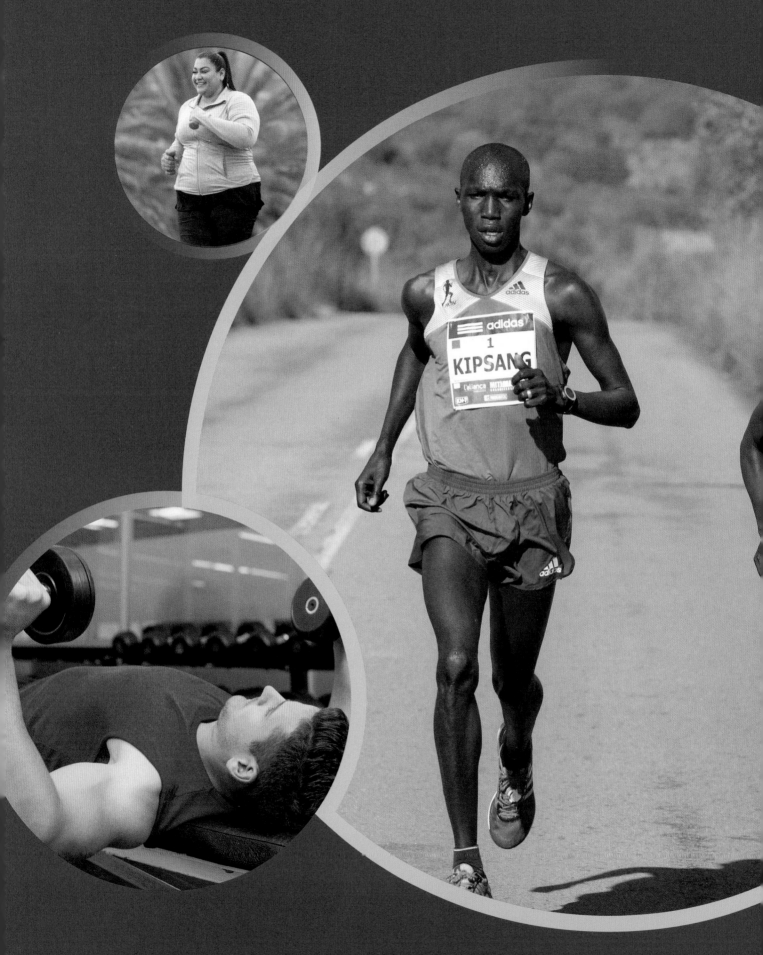

# The Physical Activity Continuum: Integration of Energy Balance and Body Composition

*What are energy balance and body composition principles? What role does the physical activity continuum play in weight management?*

**LESSON 1** INTEGRATION OF ENERGY BALANCE AND BODY COMPOSITION BASICS INTO KINESIOLOGY

**LESSON 2** EXAMPLES OF APPLYING ENERGY BALANCE AND BODY COMPOSITION BASICS IN KINESIOLOGY SUBDISCIPLINES

## Learning Objectives

*After completing this chapter, you will be able to:*

**Define** the common terms associated with energy balance and body composition.

**Explain** how energy balance and body composition relate to physical activity participation, health promotion, physical fitness, and optimal human performance.

**Justify** the importance of understanding energy balance, body composition, and their relationships with physical activity participation in the context of the various subdisciplines of kinesiology.

**Describe** the specific health benefits of energy balance and body composition as they relate to physical activity across the physical activity continuum.

**Explain** how the health benefits acquired through physical activities related to energy balance and body composition can influence the prevention and management of chronic diseases and quality of life.

**Explain** common physiologic and biomechanical influences that energy balance and body composition exert on successful participation in physical activities.

**Describe** behavioral responses associated with achieving energy balance and healthy body composition through participation in regular physical activities.

**Give** examples to show how overload, specificity, and adaptation in physical activities are related to achieving energy balance and healthy body composition.

**Describe** various methods and measures by which caloric balance and body composition can be evaluated and monitored.

**Give** and explain examples of application of caloric balance and body composition principles in successful participation in physical activities and in kinesiology subdisciplines.

# INTEGRATION OF ENERGY BALANCE AND BODY COMPOSITION BASICS INTO KINESIOLOGY

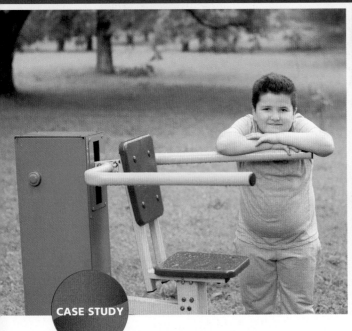

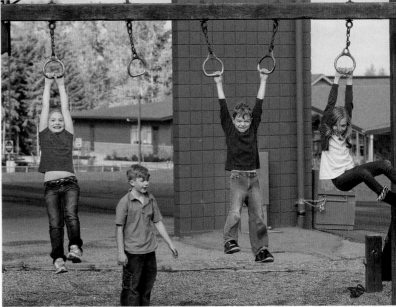

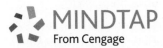

## In the real world . . .

As you may recall from Chapter 6, Eugene Casey is 10 years old and, though until recently very sedentary, is becoming more physically active. Eugene's PE teacher has him focusing on calisthenics and resistance exercises that require him to lift his own weight (like pushups and pull-ups) or a lower percentage of that weight (60% to 85%), which is within national recommendations for his age group, to improve his motor skills and motor performance, while helping him achieve energy balance and a healthier body composition. Eugene is trying to accumulate 60 minutes each day of a variety of moderate- or vigorous-intensity physical activities and exercises and is watching what he eats. He was considered obese based on his height and weight prior to beginning his weight-lifting program six months ago (BMI > 95th percentile level for his age and sex). However, he recently had his BMI measured again and discovered it had dropped to the 86th percentile. Eugene was excited that his BMI was much lower now that he had

## INTERACTIVE ACTIVITIES

### Research Focus

Go to your MindTap course to learn more about how prevalence of overweight, obesity, and diabetes (type 1, type 2, metabolic syndrome, and insulin resistance [IR]) are established and monitored globally and in the United States.

### Career Focus

Go to your MindTap course to learn more about the *2015 Dietary Guidelines for Americans*. The *Dietary Guidelines* provide important information related to achieving and maintaining a healthy body weight from a caloric intake perspective. Kinesiology professionals should use the regularly updated dietary guidelines to educate themselves about current nutrition-related scientific evidence.

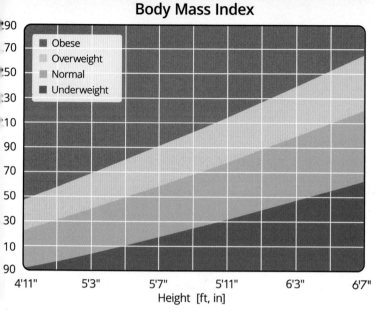

## Body Mass Index

Legend:
- Obese
- Overweight
- Normal
- Underweight

y-axis values (top to bottom): 290, 270, 250, 230, 210, 190, 170, 150, 130, 110, 90

x-axis: Height [ft, in] — 4'11", 5'3", 5'7", 5'11", 6'3", 6'7"

## Introduction: Energy Balance, Body Composition, and Kinesiology

Are you, or someone you know, trying to lose or gain weight? How many calories do you consume per day? How many calories do you need to maintain a healthy body weight at your age and physical activity level? Do you know someone who is overweight or obese, and do you understand how to differentiate between the two categories? What are effective physical activity strategies to lose or maintain weight and control the diseases associated with too much weight? What are the components of body composition? Do you currently have a body composition consistent with good health, your physical fitness goals, or peak performance? In order to answer each of these questions, you need to have a basic understanding of the principles of caloric balance and body composition.

Simply, **energy balance** describes the relationships among energy intake (the calories provided by the foods and beverages you eat and drink each day), energy expenditure (the calories you burn each day), and energy storage associated with the maintenance of body homeostasis (or balance). Many factors can influence the way the calories you take in are metabolized and include other physiologic, metabolic, environmental, and/or genetic influences as well.[1] Energy is usually expressed in units called **kilocalories (kcal)** or **Calories**. 1 kcal refers to the amount of energy required to raise the temperature of 1 kilogram (kg) of water 1 degree centigrade. (There are 2.2 pounds per kg.) **Moderate-intensity physical activity** has been defined as physical movements that require 3 to 5.9 kcal/min. **Vigorous-intensity physical activity** is defined as physical movements that require more than 6 kcal/min.[2] An example of moderate-intensity physical activity is a brisk walk; an example of vigorous-intensity activity could be a two-on-two basketball game. As you have learned in previous chapters, the 2008 Physical Activity Guidelines for Americans recommend that all adults engage in 150 minutes of moderate-intensity physical activity or 75 minutes of vigorous intensity physical activity weekly for good health. Energy expenditure can also be expressed in other ways such as METs, as you learned in Chapter 4. Light physical activity is consistent with 1 to 3 METs of physical activity intensity, moderate physical activities require 3 to 6 METs, and vigorous physical activities require greater than 6 METs (please review the Compendium of Physical Activities from Chapter 5).

A simple energy (caloric) balance equation is shown in Figure 7.1. Homeostasis is maintained when the energy you burn during daily life is replaced by a roughly equivalent amount of energy from the food you eat. If, on the other hand, someone wants to lose weight, he or she must take in fewer calories, expend more calories, or both. Although this appears easy, in reality, achieving and maintaining caloric balance and a healthy weight is an ongoing challenge

become more physically active, but he was disappointed that the 86th percentile still categorized him as being overweight. In fact, the physical fitness report card his parents, William and Maria, received from his PE class informed them that Eugene's BMI indicated that he was overweight for his age and sex. Although he has always been a big kid, Eugene's parents were alarmed because the PE report card stated that his BMI was too high and unhealthy—despite significant improvements over the previous six months on most fitness measures including the mile run, push-ups, curl-ups, and flexibility. What do you think? Is there scientific evidence that shows that a BMI in the 86th percentile is bad for the current or future health of a 10-year-old boy? Should BMI be measured in schools and the results sent to parents in the form of a standard report card? Can factors such as growth and development or physical activity levels affect BMI measures? How has Eugene's recent increased participation in physical activity and exercise influenced his health, physical fitness, and performance levels? How do you think Eugene's parents should respond to his PE report card? We will follow up with Eugene's case story in Lesson 2 of this chapter, after you have had a chance to learn about principles of energy balance, body composition, and their relationships with participation in physical activities.

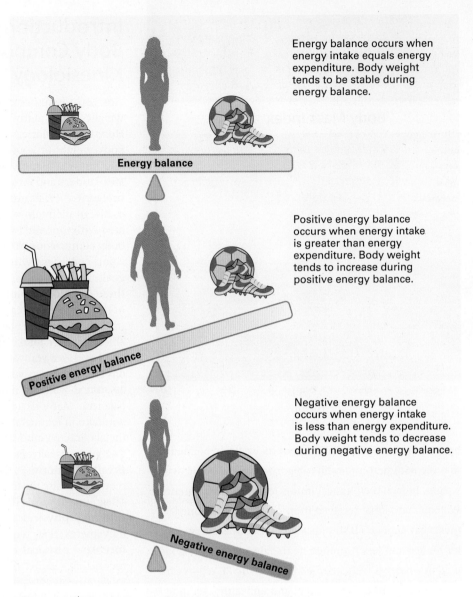

Energy balance occurs when energy intake equals energy expenditure. Body weight tends to be stable during energy balance.

Positive energy balance occurs when energy intake is greater than energy expenditure. Body weight tends to increase during positive energy balance.

Negative energy balance occurs when energy intake is less than energy expenditure. Body weight tends to decrease during negative energy balance.

**Figure 7.1** | Simple Energy (Caloric) Balance Equation

throughout life for most people. As you may have experienced in your own life, caloric intakes and expenditures often vary greatly, with alternating days of over- or undereating and days of little or no physical activity or plentiful exercise.

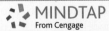
**MINDTAP**
From Cengage

### Physical Activity Guidelines

The 2008 Physical Activity Guidelines for Americans provide important information related to the role that physical activity plays in achieving and maintaining a healthy body weight. **Go to your MindTap course to** learn more about the scientific evidence related to energy balance and these recommendations.

Our bodies are composed of four general categories of substances: fat, lean tissue (muscle, bone, connective tissue,

and organs), water, and minerals. The distribution of these components varies from person to person. Some individuals have a great deal of fat mass and relatively little lean tissue whereas others have a roughly equal percentage of each. **Body composition** is a general term that refers to the distribution of these four components, usually presented as percentages. Importantly, body composition is different from body weight. In fact, two children with the same body weight and height may have vastly different body compositions. Fat and lean tissues have different densities, meaning that the weight of a person of a given body size (volume) varies based on body composition. Moreover, body fat and lean tissue have different metabolic demands and lean tissues "require" more calories to perform their functions.

The topics of caloric balance and body composition are most relevant to the global increases in the prevalence of obesity. **Obesity** is defined as the accumulation of excess fat mass that can be detrimental to health. Obesity can be identified in many ways, including measuring fat mass, calculating body fat percentage, and using other indicators such as waist circumference. Because it does not require any specialized equipment or tools, the most popular method of identifying obesity and overweight is the body mass index (BMI; BMI = [weight in kg]/[height in meters$^2$].)[3] Because taller people usually weigh more than shorter people, the BMI takes height into account. For adults (age > 18), obesity is defined as having a BMI > 30. **Overweight** for adults is a BMI of 25 to 29.9. A BMI of 18.5 to 24.9 is categorized as **healthy weight** and those with a BMI < 18.5 are considered **underweight**.

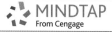
**MINDTAP** From Cengage

### Body Mass Index (BMI)

What is your BMI? There are several online calculators that you can use to quickly determine your BMI and to see how BMI varies with different heights and weights.

Because assessing relative BMI for children and adolescents is difficult, growth charts are typically used to place children among others their age and sex for comparison purposes. As you grew up, your pediatrician most likely used these growth charts to measure your progress. **Go to your MindTap course** to access charts to estimate your own BMI.

BMI is also used to assess obesity in children and adolescents, but it is a slightly more complicated application because these youth are still growing, developing, and maturing, like Eugene in our real world case study. Body composition changes with age in children and adolescents and gender plays an important part in these shifts. For this reason, when classifying a child's weight status it is more accurate to compare a child's BMI to that of others of her or his age and gender than to use a single set of standard ranges. These relative BMI comparisons help inform parents and doctors about how the child compares to other children. If a child is substantially underweight or overweight relative to similar children, his or her doctor may need to take corrective action working with the child and their parents. In Eugene's case, being at the 86th percentile indicates that he has a higher BMI than 85% of other 10-year-old male children.

The World Health Organization has estimated that worldwide obesity has doubled since 1980.[4] In the United States, the Centers for Disease Control and Prevention (CDC) has estimated that 35.7% of adults and 16.9% of children and adolescents were obese in 2009–2010.[5] Wang and colleagues have estimated that, if the current overweight and obesity trends continue into 2030, by that year 86.3% of adults will be overweight or obese and more than 30% of children and adolescents will be obese.[6] Figure 7.2 illustrates the increasing prevalence of obesity and diabetes among adults from 1994 to 2000 to 2014.

The basic concepts of energy balance are important for kinesiology practitioners to understand and to be able to

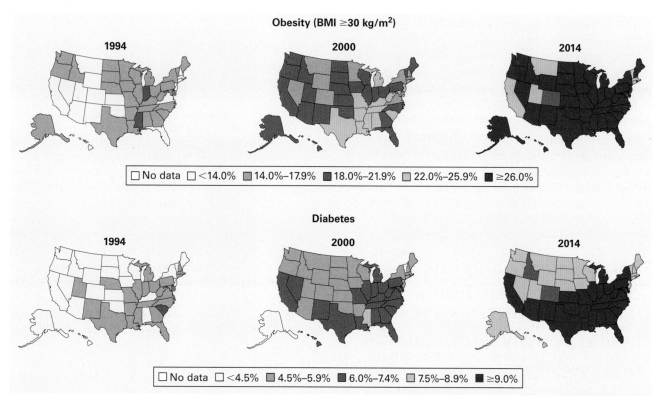

**Figure 7.2** | Prevalence of Obesity and Diabetes among Adults 1994 to 2000 to 2014

*Source:* From CDC, Division of Diabetes Translation, "Maps of Trends in Diagnosed Diabetes and Obesity," April, 2016, www.cdc.gov/diabetes/data/.

translate for others interested in achieving a healthy body composition. Overweight and obesity are linked to the **metabolic syndrome**, which includes combinations or clustering of factors like hypertension, abnormal blood lipids–fats, abnormal glucose or insulin levels, and increased waist girth that are associated with chronic diseases such as coronary heart disease and diabetes.

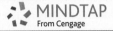

### Prevalence of Obesity, Overweight, and Diabetes

**Go to your MindTap course** to learn more about how prevalence (number of cases at a point in time relative to the population at risk of becoming a case) of overweight, obesity, and diabetes (type 1, type 2, metabolic syndrome, and insulin resistance [IR]) are established and monitored globally by the WHO and in the United States by the CDC.

As emphasized previously, energy balance and body composition are regulated by a complex physiological control system that is influenced by participation in physical activities and biomechanical, psychological, motor behavior, and other subdiscipline factors related to kinesiology. Likewise, physiologic, biomechanical, psychological, and other influences affect how we can regulate energy balance and body composition through regular participation in physical activities. Much like Chapters 5 and 6, this chapter is designed specifically to help all kinesiology students promote health and well-being through applying, monitoring, evaluating, and integrating energy balance and body composition principles in practice. It is also designed to help you understand cultural, historical, and philosophical factors associated with evaluating energy balance and body composition for yourself and for those you will influence during your kinesiology career. The chapter is not designed to provide you with all the specific details of a weight management program. However, it will provide you with the underlying kinesiology principles associated with participation in regular physical activity that help individuals achieve energy balance and healthy percentages of body composition.

## Energy Balance and Body Composition Basic Terms, Training Concepts, and the Physical Activity Continuum 🏃

### Energy Expenditure

Your daily **total energy** (caloric) **expenditure (TEE)** is composed of (1) your **resting metabolic rate (RMR;** for a 70-kg person, approximately 1 kcal/minute while sitting or about 1,440 kcal per 24 hours), (2) the **thermic effect of food (TEF;** energy required to absorb, digest, and metabolize food) for your diet, and (3) your **physical activity energy expenditure (PAEE)** that includes daily activities like bathing, as well as additional physical work you may do. Figure 7.3 shows the relative contributions of these components of TEE. **Basal metabolic rate (BMR)** is your absolute minimal metabolic rate and is measured under rigid, standardized conditions (including lying still following a five-hour fast; the avoidance of caffeine, nicotine, and alcohol for four hours; and abstinence from exercise for at least two hours). However, measures of RMR (sitting at rest) are more commonly used by researchers interested in energy balance questions.

The energy necessary to keep your heart pumping and all your other organ systems functioning is included in your RMR, which accounts for 60% to 70% of TEE. The energy you burn digesting and storing the food you eat each day is the TEF and accounts for about 10% of TEE. By simple subtraction, therefore, physical activity (such as standing, shivering, exercise, walking) can contribute from 20% to 30% of TEE. As you might surmise based on Figure 7.3, energy expended performing physical activity is the only easily changeable portion of TEE. If you are very sedentary, your PAEE might be only 100 kcal per day (the equivalent of three cheese and cracker snacks), whereas collegiate athletes, who are very physically active and sometimes train twice a day or more, often expend a total of 3,000 or more kcal per day. Your daily PAEE is the

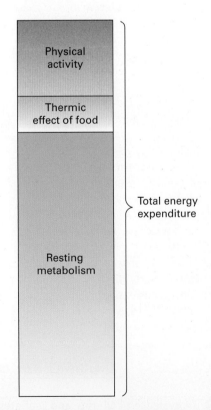

**Figure 7.3** | Components of Total Energy Expenditure (TEE)

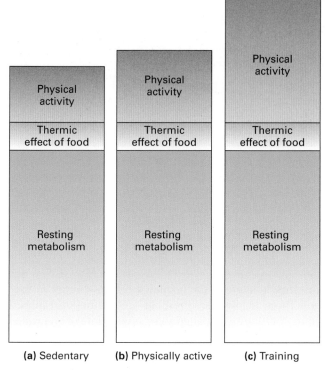

Figure 7.4 | Total Energy Expenditure for Three Different Levels of Physical Activity

(a) Sedentary    (b) Physically active    (c) Training

**Table 7.1** | Total Energy Requirements of Individuals at Varying Amounts of Exercise

| INDIVIDUAL | TOTAL DAILY CALORIES FOR ENERGY BALANCE |
| --- | --- |
| 25-year-old healthy sedentary man | ~2,400 kcal |
| 25-year-old healthy sedentary woman | ~2,000 kcal |
| 25-year-old healthy active man | ~3,000 kcal |
| 25-year-old healthy active woman | ~2,400 kcal |
| 25-year-old male professional boxer | ~5,000 kcal |
| 25-year-old female collegiate dancer | ~3,000 kcal |
| 25-year-old female elite marathoner | ~3,500 kcal |
| 25-year-old male elite marathoner | ~5,000 kcal |
| 25-year-old male Tour de France cyclist | ~9,000 kcal |

*Source:* From "Measurement of Moderate Physical Activity," *Medicine and Science in Sports and Exercise* 32, no. 9 (2000): S439–S516. Estimates from www.choosemyplate.gov.

primary and most important variable that is changeable with regards to energy balance (intake vs. expenditure), and Figure 7.4 shows examples of the energy expenditure required for three different levels of physical activity.

Another way to conceptualize the role that physical activity plays in energy balance is to consider the caloric requirements of different types of athletes compared to people who are inactive. Energy requirements differ by age, health status, and gender, but a rough estimate of daily total energy requirements of individuals (average age = 25 years) across the physical activity continuum is shown in Table 7.1. As Table 7.1 indicates, a mere 600 calories (roughly equivalent to a large order of french fries) separate the requirements of a healthy, sedentary 25-year-old man in energy balance from those of a healthy, active 25-year-old man in energy balance, but if the caloric needs are not balanced for the active person he will not be able to sustain his physically active lifestyle due to lack of energy or fatigue. The real jump in caloric requirements occurs with additional physical activity and exercise training (up to approximately 9,000 kcal per day for a Tour de France bicycle athlete). Therefore, in order to achieve caloric balance and achieve/maintain a healthy body composition, physically active individuals need to match their daily caloric intake needs with their caloric expenditure efforts as they change their dietary intake and energy expenditure.

## Achieving Energy Balance

It may be overly simplistic to assume that a calorie from ingested food is equal to a calorie expended. A more complex

version of the energy balance equation focused on specific factors related to physical activity and the study of kinesiology is shown in Figure 7.5. Recently, Hill and colleagues have suggested that, although it is often assumed that energy intake and energy expenditure can be independently modified, they are in fact interdependent upon one another and regulated by complex physiological control systems that involve automatic nerves (the autonomic nervous system), hormones, muscles, and body organs.[7, 8]

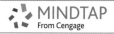

**Dietary Guidelines**

**Go to your MindTap course** to learn more about The *2015 Dietary Guidelines for Americans* (USDHHS, USDA). The *Dietary Guidelines* provide important information related to achieving and maintaining a healthy body weight from a caloric intake perspective. Kinesiology professionals should use the regularly updated dietary guidelines to educate themselves about current nutrition-related scientific evidence. This will allow practitioners to more effectively interact with professional nutrition experts, such as registered dietitians, in order to problem solve dietary issues related to caloric balance and body composition. While kinesiologists often provide basic nutritional advice and nutritional information to aid peak physical activity performance competitions and recovery from exercise (there is an entire specialty dedicated to sports nutrition), the majority of their academic training and expertise focuses more on energy expenditure topics. Although energy intake concepts are important to understand and apply, the role of energy expenditure has often been minimized as contributing to energy balance when dealing with overweight and obesity issues. Therefore, we have targeted energy expenditure as our main topic in this chapter.

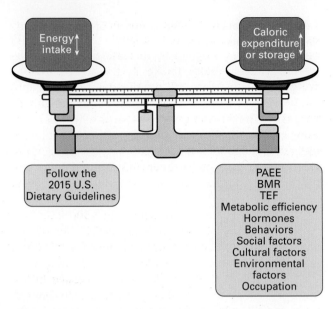

Figure 7.5 | A More Complex and Realistic Model of Energy Balance That Includes a Focus on Factors Related to Physical Activity Expenditure. Remember for effective weight management one should monitor caloric intake based on the 2015 U.S. Dietary Guidelines.

*Source:* Based on H. Kohl and T. Murray, *Foundations of Physical Activity and Public Health* (Champaign, IL: Human Kinetics, 2012), 100.

Societal changes in physical activity opportunities can also make achieving energy balance more difficult in today's world. Changes in average energy demands related to urbanization (more people moving to cities), industrialization (less manual labor), and transportation (less reliance on "active" modes of transportation) over recent years have contributed to a decrease in the required daily physical activity levels of most individuals. Think about your own life. How has your physical activity changed with "energy-saving devices"? These and other changes have made weight maintenance very challenging for sedentary individuals because more restriction of food is needed to match energy intake to already low and declining levels of energy expenditure. Failure to adequately restrict intake causes most individuals to gain weight (especially body fat) over time with aging (see Figure 7.6).

Figure 7.7 shows the results of a study in which positive weight gain of six men was measured over a period of seven days when their physical activity was purposely reduced. The participants in this study did not experience a decline in appetite or change their caloric intake in response to the reduction in activity, which resulted in weight gain (as measured as an increase in measured body fat).

Hill and colleagues further support the hypothesis that energy balance may be easier to achieve at higher levels of energy expenditure than at low or sedentary levels. Figure 7.8 shows a model of weight regulation based around a minimal physical activity threshold (which most likely varies among individuals). People with activity above

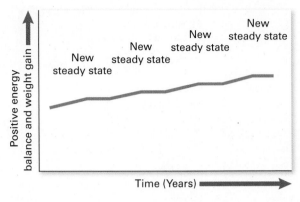

Figure 7.6 | Example of Adult Gradual Weight Gain Due to Caloric Imbalance (Intake vs. Expenditure)

*Source:* J. O. Hill, H. R. Wyatt, and J. C. Peters, "The Importance of Energy Balance," *U.S. Endocrinology* 9, no. 1 (2013): 27–31, 28.

this threshold are in the regulated zone of energy balance and those below the threshold are in the unregulated zone. Within the regulated zone, energy intake is elevated to meet the high energy needs and then energy intake and expenditure become very sensitive to each other—meaning that when one changes, the other is changed to match. In the unregulated zone, energy intake and energy expenditure become weakly sensitive (i.e., less responsive) to each other, and maintaining a healthy body weight requires sustained food restriction. In fact, becoming overweight or obese by storing extra calories consumed as fat

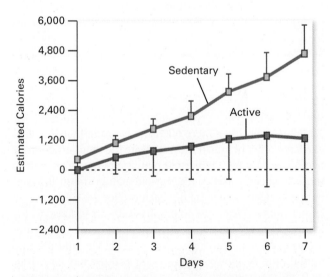

Figure 7.7 | Weight Gain (as Measured by Cumulative Fat Balance) over Seven Days When Physical Activity Was Purposely Reduced in Six Adult Men. Reduced physical activity resulted in net weight gain of about 4,776 kcals (or about one of pound of fat difference; 1 pound = 3,500 kcals) versus 1,194 kcals for the active regimen.

*Source:* J. O. Hill, H. R. Wyatt, and J. C. Peters, "The Importance of Energy Balance," *U.S. Endocrinology* 9, no. 1 (2013): 27–31, 30.

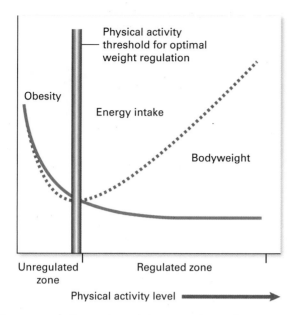

Physical activity
threshold for optimal
weight regulation

Obesity

Energy intake

Bodyweight

Unregulated
zone

Regulated zone

Physical activity level

**Figure 7.8** | Illustration of the Hypothesis That Energy Balance May Be Easier to Achieve at High Energy Expenditure, Which Represents the Regulated Zone. A sedentary individual is in the unregulated zone and will struggle to expend additional energy, therefore gaining weight and increasing the risk of obesity.

*Source:* J. O. Hill, H. R. Wyatt, and J. C. Peters, "Energy Balance and Obesity," *Circulation* 126 (2012): 126–132, 128.

may be the only way for physically inactive individuals to achieve energy balance in our food-abundant society.

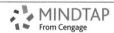

**MINDTAP**
From Cengage

**Energy Balance**

**Go to your MindTap course** to learn more about the energy balance from the National Institutes of Health.

## Body Composition and Physical Activity

Practitioners of kinesiology who hope to help individuals and populations achieve energy balance need to help others acquire the cognitive skills to match energy intake with energy expenditure and to counter the biological, sociological, and behavioral tendencies to overeat and be inactive. They should also help others recognize how changing factors like the built environment (the physical parts of where we all live, work, and play) can help individuals and populations make healthy choices to become and remain physically active more easily.

Everyone's body weight fluctuates over time—some of us cycle within a few pounds over the entire life span, while others gain and/or lose much larger amounts of weight. Some experience weight changes more frequently than others. It is difficult to know what

constitutes important changes, and particularly what to expect when you, a friend, or a family member embark on a weight-loss program by increasing physical activity and reducing caloric intake. A clinically meaningful **weight loss** (one that will positively influence health) has been defined as a loss of at least 5% of initial body weight.[9] A weight change of less than 3% (gain or loss) is indicative of **maintaining weight**. Once someone has lost a significant amount of weight (5%), that weight loss is considered successful (**prevention of weight re-gain**) if less than 5% of the weight loss is regained over a period of time.

A pound of fat stores approximately 3,500 kcal. That means that (roughly) a 350 kcal daily deficit over 10 days is needed to lose one pound of fat, although the 3,500 kcal estimation is rather imprecise (due to daily fluctuations in RMR and TEF). Fundamentally, those interested in losing weight must increase their physical activity enough to expend 350 additional kcal (this is roughly equivalent to briskly walking three miles each day), decrease daily caloric intake by 350 kcal, or (preferably) achieve a kcal deficit through some combination of both dietary restriction and energy expenditure. If a 200-pound person wants to achieve clinically meaningful weight loss (at least 5%), that means that she or he needs to lose 10 pounds (and probably more). That translates into at least 100 days of a caloric deficit of at least 350 calories. Moreover, as weight is lost fewer calories are needed for physical activity (heavier people need more calories to move their body) and thus more physical activity may be needed to continue to create the deficit. It is no wonder that weight loss is so difficult, particularly if one is not physically active!

Understanding and monitoring caloric intake and caloric expenditure are among the most challenging issues facing people trying to lose weight through dietary changes and physical activity. Was the bagel that you ate this morning small, medium, or large? Was the cream cheese you added to it light or full fat? How was it prepared? What would be the caloric "savings" from switching from a sugar-sweetened beverage to water with meals? All of these are important considerations for determining energy intake, and many people lack an awareness of the comparable caloric values of the foods they eat. For example, Figure 7.9 illustrates the differences between self-reported (what people say they ate or did) and actual (what was measured) daily caloric intake and caloric expenditure in obese individuals attempting to lose weight. These people underestimated their caloric intake by more than 100% and overestimated their caloric expenditure by 25%! Clearly there was a disconnect between their perceptions and reality about their achieved energy deficit. Given our current U.S. overweight and obese environment, kinesiology professionals need to teach people, especially children, cognitive skills learned in this chapter to help match energy intake with energy expenditure and to overcome current trends to overeat and be physically inactive.

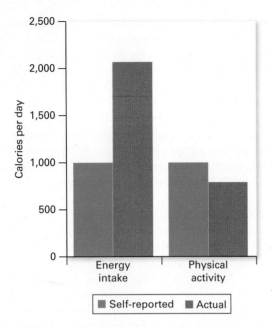

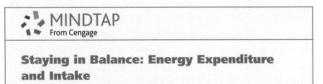

**Figure 7.9** | Differences between Self-Reported and Actual Daily Caloric Intake and Exercise in Obese Individuals Attempting to Lose Weight

*Source:* From S. W. Lichtman et al., "Discrepancy between Self-Reported and Actual Caloric Intake and Exercise in Obese Subjects," *New England Journal of Medicine* 327, no. 27 (1992): 1893–1898.

Can you lose weight without cutting back on the foods you eat? Certainly you are going to be hungrier when you exercise compared with when you don't because you are burning more calories. The approximate decrease in body weight based on total weekly minutes of physical activity without caloric restriction is shown in Figure 7.10. Although significant health benefits can be achieved by performing 150 minutes of physical activity per week, effective long-term weight maintenance often requires 300 minutes or more per week. As stated in the Physical Activity Guidelines, more than the minimum may be necessary to help achieve energy balance and weight loss. As you can see from Figures 7.9 and 7.10, individual perception and cognitive skills contribute to the lifelong challenges of energy balance and body composition related to the physical activity continuum.

---

### MINDTAP
From Cengage

**Staying in Balance: Energy Expenditure and Intake**

Do you know the calorie values of your favorite foods? Do you know the energy expenditure necessary to "burn" the foods you eat every day? If not, you may want to investigate these topics to better understand how much exercise is necessary to stay in homeostasis when you eat as you typically do. **Go to your MindTap course** to complete an activity on balancing energy expenditure and intake.

---

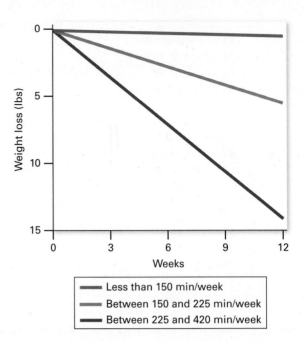

**Figure 7.10** | Approximate Decrease in Body Weight Based on Total Weekly Minutes of Physical Activity without Caloric Restrictions

Is all body fat bad? No, it is not—in fact, our bodies need fat to help with metabolism and other essential functions. **Essential fat** is the amount of fat necessary for normal body function and good health. Calories from any source (like carbohydrates, fats, or protein) that are consumed and not expended are stored as fat and are often called empty calories. Figure 7.11 illustrates the estimated lower limit of essential body fat: 3% for men and 12% for women. A healthy range of body fat for adults 20 to 30 years of age

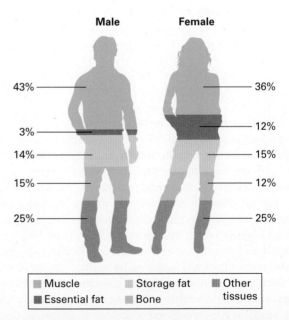

**Figure 7.11** | Typical Body Composition of an Adult Man and Woman

is 11% to 21% for men and 15% to 25% for women. The implications of these numbers are that it is possible to have too little fat as well as too much fat.

Fat may be distributed unevenly throughout the body. **Subcutaneous fat** is the layer of fat cells just under the skin (in your legs and arms, for example). **Visceral fat** surrounds vital organs, such as the stomach in the abdominal area (abdominal fat). Other terms used to describe fat distribution include central (located in the trunk region) versus peripheral (located in arms and legs). Not only is too much weight and fat deleterious to health, but the location of the fat on the body can also be a problem. Carrying too much abdominal fat is associated with a higher risk of some chronic diseases, particularly type 2 diabetes mellitus.

Slentz and colleagues studied the effects of physical activity and exercise on changes in visceral fat over an eight-month period.[10] One hundred and seventy-five sedentary, overweight men and women were randomly assigned to a control group; a low-volume, moderate-activity group (engaging in activity equivalent to walking about 12 miles per week); a low-volume, vigorous exercise group (equivalent to jogging slowly for about 12 miles per week); or a high-volume, vigorous exercise group (equivalent to jogging faster for 20 miles per week). The controls gained a significant amount of visceral fat over the study period whereas the moderate physical activity and exercise groups avoided significant visceral fat gain. The high-intensity joggers actually reduced their visceral fat significantly. The researchers concluded that a modest exercise program can control or reduce visceral fat accumulation.

## Health and Quality of Life

Although perhaps less important to college-age students, adverse body composition can affect health in many ways. There is debate, however, about where on the body composition continuum this risk begins. Premature morbidity and mortality (risk for disease and risk of death) are closely related to measures of body composition such as BMI (Figure 7.12), but in an unexpected fashion. Notice that those who are underweight (BMI $\leq$ 18) or extremely obese (BMI $\geq$ 35) are at increased health risk. Underweight individuals are at higher risk for immune deficiencies, certain cancers, and eating disorders. Excessively overweight individuals are at higher risk for type 2 diabetes, hypertension, cardiovascular disease, sleep disorders, osteoarthritis, some cancers, gallbladder disorders, and respiratory problems. Notice in Figure 7.12 that the overall health risks are not elevated much except in those who are excessively lean or substantially obese.

Participating in physical activity and exercise without increasing caloric intake, and thus creating an energy deficit, can help individuals and populations reduce total body fat, waist circumference, and intra-abdominal fat; maintain or increase lean muscle mass; and prevent the regain of lost

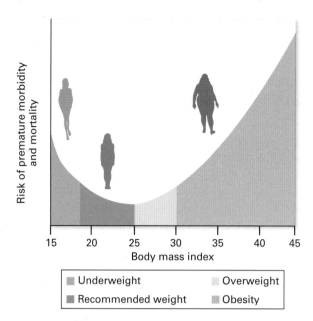

Figure 7.12 | Mortality Risk versus Body Mass Index

weight. Physical activity and exercise are also closely associated with decreased risks for chronic disease processes such as those associated with metabolic syndrome, type 2 diabetes, and cardiovascular disease, as well as orthopedic problems linked with obesity and overweight. Table 7.2 summarizes some of the health benefits associated with achieving energy balance and a normal body composition.

**Table 7.2 | Summary of Health Benefits of Achieving Energy Balance and Body Composition Considerations in Relationship to Participating in Physical Activities**

- Aerobic physical activity is associated with achieving weight maintenance. Resistance training can be helpful with weight control but may increase muscle mass; usually, smaller training volumes that may not provide enough caloric expenditure for effective weight maintenance are used.

- Higher volumes of physical activity are required for weight loss (> 5%), particularly if caloric intake is not controlled, but results are consistent with those achieved through dietary interventions alone. Effective weight loss of at least 5% should include caloric intake control.

- The maintenance of physical activity reduces weight regain after a period of significant weight loss. Abdominal obesity is reduced with aerobic physical activity; less is known regarding the effects of resistance training.

- There is no dose-response evidence that physical activity affects weight maintenance, but 150 minutes of physical activity per week can help with weight control and 300 minutes per week has been recommended to achieve weight maintenance after weight loss (> 5%) and to control abdominal obesity.

- The accumulation of physical activity is important for weight maintenance, weight loss, weight maintenance following weight loss, and reduction of abdominal obesity.

*Source:* From *Physical Activity Guidelines Advisory Committee Report, 2008* (Washington, DC: U.S. Department of Health and Human Services, 2008).

## Basic Physiologic Responses of Participation in Physical Activities Affecting Energy Balance and Body Composition

Participating in regular physical activity and exercise provides integrated physiological, biomechanical, and behavioral benefits that improve energy balance and body composition. It is important to remember that physical activity and exercise create many positive changes in a multitude of kinesiology-related factors. Table 7.3 contains a list of adaptations associated with physical activity, energy balance, and body composition.

Physiologically, physical activity increases caloric expenditure, which can help people lose weight (if they control their caloric intake), achieve a healthier body composition, and move toward energy balance. Physical activity and exercise increase muscular endurance, which in turn improves functional health, increases lean muscle mass, and allows people to do more physical work before they fatigue.

Biomechanically, physical activity may help improve economy of movement (the amount of energy it takes to perform a certain motion, such as jogging). Movement economy is directly related to body weight and body composition, particularly in weight-bearing activities. Thus, more physical activity may improve movement economy and result in the need for fewer calories to accomplish the same activity. Carrying excess body weight and body fat reduces the range of motion for many physical activities and negatively affects peripheral proprioception (i.e., sense of space and movement), which can reduce one's ability to balance and prevent falls.

Self-confidence and self-esteem are two very important concepts in exercise psychology and behavioral science perspectives of physical activity. **Self-confidence** can be defined as one's self-assurance regarding one's personal judgments. **Self-esteem** is one's response to others and what one hears from those in one's social network (e.g., low or high self-esteem). **Self-efficacy** can be defined as one's confidence in performing specific skills (like various physical activities). Psychologically, physical activity and exercise associated with weight loss and weight maintenance may help increase self-confidence, self-esteem, and self-efficacy for some people, while reducing the risk of depression and anxiety. Weight loss and the achievement of a healthy body composition through participation in physical activities can improve self-confidence and often facilitate the improvement in motor skills for many that can further promote movement activities across the lifespan.

## Energy Balance and Body Composition for Peak Performance

Body composition and body weight are clearly important issues for all of us, but they are especially critical to athletes. Even small changes in body composition (lower percentage of body fat) are associated with improved performance, specifically in weight-bearing sports such as gymnastics, dance, long-distance running, wrestling, and others. In some sports such as football, it is important to increase muscle mass and weight to improve performance. However, having too much weight gain (fat weight) or increases in percentage of body fat can slow athletes down, leave them less agile, and adversely affect performance. Therefore, it is important to develop a healthy balance between lean muscle mass and fat weight based upon sport specificity.

To achieve peak performance among athletes, it is important to match high caloric expenditure levels with equally high intakes, or else the athletes will lack the energy they need to perform. As you learned from Table 7.1, the energy needs of those who are sedentary are much lower than those of competitive athletes. It is

**Table 7.3** | Adaptations to Fitness Programming Related to Body Composition

| PHYSIOLOGICAL | BIOMECHANICAL | PSYCHOLOGICAL AND BEHAVIORAL |
|---|---|---|
| Increased muscular endurance | Improved economy | Increased self-confidence |
| Increased VO$_2$ max | Improved balance | Increased self-efficacy |
| Improved caloric balance | Improved mobility | Decreased depression and anxiety |
| Improved metabolism | Improved proprioception | Increased motor skill |
| Lower percentage of body fat | | Experience with behavioral change and increased confidence to engage further in physical activity and exercise |
| Smaller waist circumference | | |
| Less intra-abdominal fat | | |
| Maintenance of or increased lean muscle mass | | |
| Maintenance of or loss of weight | | |

important for those with lofty exercise performance goals to recognize that although often being leaner helps improve their performance, losing too much weight is associated with behavioral disorders (e.g., body image issues and eating disorders) and negative physiological adaptations (e.g., lowered immune function, lower glycogen stores, and overtraining syndrome).

For example, Jeanette is a 22-year-old dance major who is on the university dance performance team, the Dazzling Diamonds. Jeanette is one of the best of 20 dancers on the team, and the Diamonds have won numerous state and national competitions. The team usually practices two to three hours per day during the week with competitive and demonstration performances on the weekends. Jeanette and her teammates recently had their body compositions measured, and Jeanette was determined to have a BMI of 17 and a percent body fat of 12%.

Many of Jeanette's friends and competitors have asked her if she is anorexic because she looks so skinny. Anorexia nervosa is a compulsive eating and/or exercise disorder (overtraining), in which the individual is too lean for good health. She has become concerned about all the questions she has gotten about her physique, and although she feels fine and is performing well, she wants to seek advice from a kinesiology professional about her current body composition.

What advice would you give Jeanette? One way to evaluate Jeanette's low percentage of body fat is to remind her that high-performing female dancers are usually leaner than average college-age female nondancers and carry much less weight than an average college-age female. It would also be helpful to remind her that while being leaner can help improve performance, it can also lead to increased risk of upper respiratory infections

due to suppressed immune function and the negative effects of potential disordered eating behaviors, secondary amenorrhea/abnormal menstruation due to a high dose of physical activity, and osteoporosis (declining bone quality).

As you have learned, Jeanette's BMI of 17 classifies her as underweight, and her percentage of body fat represents the minimal level of essential fat. Although she is probably at or very close to her optimal performance weight and body composition, depending on measurement errors, she is also very close to being too lean. It would be important to encourage her to maintain energy balance by matching her caloric needs to her high energy expenditure levels, and she should be discouraged from losing more weight. It would also be important to determine if she is menstruating regularly because if she is not, she may have abnormal hormonal function, which may require follow-up with her physician and other health care professionals.

# Basic Strategies for Achieving Energy Balance and a Healthy Body Composition

Effective strategies to achieve energy balance and a healthy body composition involve several factors including current body composition, and current dietary and physical activity behaviors. Influences on these factors including the built environment, personal goals, mental stress, occupation, leisure time pursuits, resting metabolic rate, genetics, self-esteem, body image, and peer influences. Table 7.4 contains basic strategies that kinesiology practitioners can use to help individuals and populations

**Table 7.4** | Possible Caloric Intake and Caloric Strategies for Weight Management

| | UNDERWEIGHT BMI <18.5 | NORMAL BMI 18.5–24.9 | OVERWEIGHT BMI 25–29.9 | OBESE BMI >30 |
|---|---|---|---|---|
| **Caloric Intake** | Use Dietary Guidelines for Americans (2015 DGA)<br><br>Increase intake 200–500 kcal/day | Use 2015 DGA | Use 2015 DGA and reduce intake 200–300 kcal/day* | Consult physician and registered dietitian<br><br>Follow 2015 DGA<br><br>Reduce intake by 500 calories per day* |
| **Caloric Expenditure** | Become or remain physically active<br><br>Use 2008 Physical Activity Guidelines for Americans (2008 PAGA)<br><br>Do not try to lose more weight! | Become or remain physically active<br><br>Follow 2008 PAGA | Become or remain physically active<br><br>Follow 2008 PAGA Guidelines<br><br>Expend 200–300 kcal per day minimum in exercise | Become or remain physically active<br><br>Follow 2008 PAGA Guidelines<br><br>Go slowly and try to expend 500 kcal/day in exercise |

*Should not reduce dietary intake to less than 1400–1500 calories per day unless under medical supervision.

achieve energy balance for varying body composition levels (based on BMI measures).

In addition, the following realistic and health-promoting tips can help in achieving a healthy body composition:

- Have contacts interact with a health care professional (such as a physician) to verify that their body composition goals are realistic and not extreme or unhealthy.

- Measure BMI, waist circumference, and percentage of body fat to help identify a healthy goal weight.

- Use the 2015 Dietary Guidelines for Americans for healthy eating.

- Adjust caloric intake and caloric expenditure depending on individual needs and interpretations of BMI, waist circumference, and percentage of body fat.

- Set a goal to initially engage in 150 minutes of physical activities per week and increase this to 200 to 300 minutes/week over the course of six weeks to six months.

- Allow plenty of time (20 to 30 weeks) for long-term results; educate individuals to be prepared for potential relapses (weight gain) and to prepare re-adoption (energy balance) strategies for continued success.

- Retest BMI, waist circumference, and percentage of body fat every three months.

- Develop incentives and encourage individuals to log their physical activity and exercise minutes so they can reevaluate themselves every three to six months.

## Measuring and Monitoring Basal Metabolism, Body Composition, and Physical Activity Outcomes

Kinesiology professionals have been interested in the measurement of resting metabolism, energy expenditure, and body composition for more than 100 years and have developed laboratory and field methods that you will learn about in detail during some of your future course work (such as exercise physiology courses). Laboratory methods require controlled laboratory settings (e.g., regulation of temperature, control of participant activities, and detailed standardized testing protocols). Field methods are less controlled than laboratory measures but allow measurement of larger numbers of participants. Field methods are usually validated to ensure their accuracy against laboratory measures.

Both laboratory and field measures can provide valuable information; however, it is important to consider factors such as the accuracy required, ease of use for the test, time required for the test, cost of testing, subject comfort and effort, and requirements of training for testing personnel when choosing the best approach for test selection.

### Laboratory Measurement of RMR

The most common method of measuring and monitoring energy expenditure at rest (RMR) in the laboratory is indirect calorimetry. In the laboratory, it is fairly straightforward to measure the components of energy expenditure. Figure 7.13 shows one application of the indirect calorimetry technique, which measures the amount of oxygen consumed at rest or during physical activity. In another version of indirect calorimetry for measurement BMR, a person rests in a controlled room for a period of time. Energy expenditure is assessed based on measurements of air samples that are taken while the person is in the room. The air supply is constant and measured, and calibrated gas collection devices are used to measure and analyze oxygen and carbon dioxide changes in the room.

Because carbon dioxide is a by-product of energy metabolism, it is a very good indicator of total energy expenditure in this kind of controlled setting. Someone who burns more energy (through exercise, for example) is easily differentiated from someone who is sedentary and not burning any additional calories through physical activity. With the assistance of a diary or observation by study personnel, it is possible to quantify the amount (frequency, intensity, and duration) and type

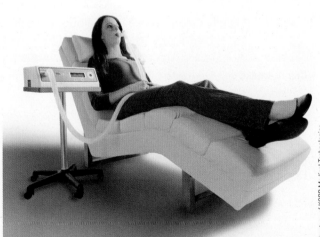

**Figure 7.13** | Example of the Measurement of Resting Metabolic Rate Sitting Quietly at Rest

Courtesy of KORR Medical Technologies

of physical activity in which study participates engage. Thus, PAEE can be measured as well. These data, coupled with careful measurements of the food a person eats and wastes she or he produces, can give a very accurate measure of TEE.

Resting metabolism can increase over time with greater caloric expenditure through physical activity and exercise, but as you have already learned, these changes are small—not nearly as significant as changes to the total caloric expenditure that occur with daily EEPA.

## Field Measures of BMR

Most field measures of BMR are based on prediction equations that estimate caloric expenditure at rest and during various physical activities. The Harris-Benedict equations are one commonly used method to calculate BMR.[11] You can estimate your BMR by using either of the following formulas (or see websites for electronic calculators). There are two key steps to using the Harris-Benedict equations.

In step one, you estimate your BMR based on your gender, height (in either centimeters or inches), weight (in either kilograms or pounds), and age:

**Women**: BMR = 655 + (4.35 × weight in pounds) + (4.7 × height in inches) − (4.7 × age in years)

**Men**: BMR = 66 + (6.23 × weight in pounds) + (12.7 × height in inches) − (6.8 × age in years)

**Women**: BMR = 655 + (9.6 × weight in kg) + (1.8 × height in cm) − (4.7 × age in years)

**Men**: BMR = 66 + (13.7 × weight in kg) + (5 × height in cm) − (6.8 × age in years)

In step 2, you can determine your total daily calorie needs by multiplying your BMR by the appropriate activity factor, as follows:

1. If you are sedentary (little or no exercise): TEE= BMR × 1.2

2. If you are lightly active (light exercise/sports 1–3 days/week): Calorie-Calculation = BMR × 1.375

3. If you are moderately active (moderate exercise/sports 3−5 days/week): Calorie-Calculation = BMR × 1.55

4. If you are very active (hard exercise/sports 6−7 days a week): Calorie-Calculation = BMR × 1.725

5. If you are extra active (very hard exercise/sports & physical job or 2 times per day training): Calorie-Calculation = BMR × 1.9

The Harris-Benedict equations and other BMR equations can also be found on various websites that offer mathematical calculators for you to use.

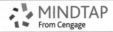

**MINDTAP**
From Cengage

**Calculating Caloric Expenditure**

**Go to your MindTap course** to learn more about the use of caloric expenditure calculators.

## Laboratory or Clinical Methods of Measuring Body Composition

Over the years, measurement of body composition in the laboratory or clinical setting has become very precise. It is possible to separate fat from lean tissue and water and quantify the location of the fat throughout the body. Some frequently used laboratory and clinical methods for measuring body composition are magnetic resonance imaging (MRI), computer tomography (CT), dual energy x-ray absorptiometry (DXA), underwater or hydrostatic weighing, air displacement plethysmography (measurement of change in volume) using devices like the Bod Pod, and bioelectrical impedance analysis (BIA). The MRI and CT techniques are the most accurate methods for measuring body composition, but they are very costly and used mainly in medical research studies; therefore, kinesiology professionals generally rely on hydrostatic weighing, the Bod Pod, DXA, or BIA as body composition lab methods. Descriptions of the hydrostatic weighing, air displacement plethysmography, DXA, and BIA body composition techniques are shown in Figure 7.14.

## Field Methods of Measuring Body Composition

Common field methods of assessing body composition include measurement of BMI, body circumferences (waist and hip), and skinfolds. You have already learned about BMI and its calculation. Table 7.5 summarizes adult

**Table 7.5** | Weight Classifications Using Body Mass Index (BMI)

| BODY MASS INDEX (KG/M²) | CLASSIFICATION |
|---|---|
| < 18.5 | Underweight |
| 18.5–24.9 | Healthy weight |
| 25.0–29.9 | Overweight |
| 30 | Obese |

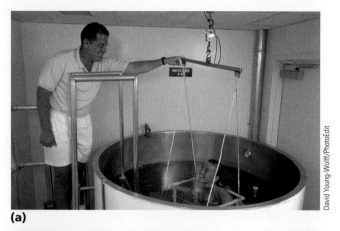

(a)

David Young-Wolff/PhotoEdit

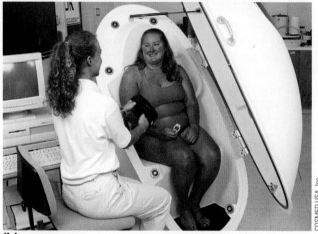

(b)

COSMED USA, Inc.

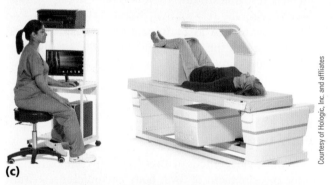

(c)

Courtesy of Hologic, Inc. and affiliates

**Figure 7.14** | Examples of Laboratory or Clinical Measures of Body Composition. (a) Hydrodensitometry measures body density by weighing the person first on land and then again while submerged in water. The difference between the person's actual weight and underwater weight provides a measure of the body's volume. A mathematical equation using the two measurements (volume and actual weight) determines body density, from which the percentage of body fat can be estimated. (b) Air displacement plethysmography estimates body composition by having a person sit inside a chamber while computerized sensors determine the amount of air displaced by the person's body. (c) Dual-energy x-ray absorptiometry (DXA) uses two low-dose x-rays that differentiate among fat-free soft tissue (lean body mass), fat tissues, and bone tissue, providing a precise measurement of total fat and its distribution in all but extremely obese subjects.

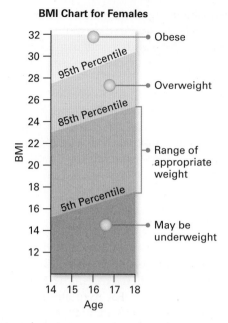

**BMI Chart for Females**

- 95th Percentile
- 85th Percentile
- 5th Percentile

Obese
Overweight
Range of appropriate weight
May be underweight

**Figure 7.15** | Body Mass Index Chart for 14- to 18-Year-Old Females

*Source:* Based on CDC values at nccd.cdc.gov/dnpabmi/calculator.aspx.

BMI classifications, and Figure 7.15 presents a representative example of BMI classification for children and adolescents.

Figure 7.16 shows the waist-to-hip ratio measurement commonly used to estimate body composition. Table 7.6 shows how to estimate disease risk using just the adult waist circumference and Table 7.7 shows an example of the percentiles for waist circumference for a sample of children and adolescents ages 2 to 18.

An example of skinfold measures and a description of how this method can be used by kinesiology professionals

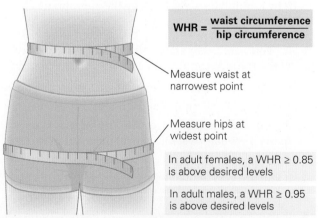

$$WHR = \frac{waist\ circumference}{hip\ circumference}$$

Measure waist at narrowest point

Measure hips at widest point

In adult females, a WHR ≥ 0.85 is above desired levels

In adult males, a WHR ≥ 0.95 is above desired levels

**Figure 7.16** | General Illustration of Obtaining Waist and Hip Circumference Measures with a Tape Measure to Determine Waist-to-Hip Ratio Circumference

**Table 7.6** | Disease Risk According to Waist Circumference in Inches

| MEN | WOMEN | DISEASE RISK |
|---|---|---|
| < 35.5 | < 32.5 | Low |
| 35.5–40.0 | 32.5–35.0 | Moderate |
| > 40.0 | > 35.0 | High |

to estimate body composition is shown in Figure 7.17. Table 7.8 provides one example (for women) of how body composition can be estimated by collecting data for sex, age, and the sum of three skinfold measures.

## Body Composition Interpretation and Monitoring

So, there are many ways to measure body composition, but which is the best method? The answer to this question is, "It depends!" For example, Table 7.9 shows a comparison of methods to estimate body composition. The best method for you to use is the one that best fits your measurement skills and resources.

The interpretation and monitoring of body composition are important skills that kinesiology professionals

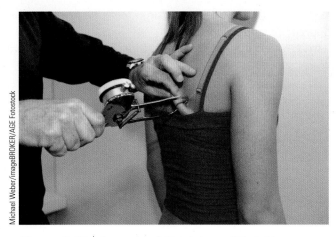

Michael Weber/imageBROKER/AGE Fotostock

**Figure 7.17** | Example of Obtaining a Skinfold Measurement. Skinfold measures like the Subscapular measurement shown here can be used with other measures like age and gender to help predict body composition.

should acquire to help individuals and populations achieve their energy balance and body composition goals through proper educational messaging. For example, when BMI is

**Table 7.7** | Estimated Values for Waist Circumference (in inches) by Percentile for European American Children and Adolescents, According to Sex

| AGE (y) | PERCENTILE FOR BOYS | | | | | PERCENTILE FOR GIRLS | | | | |
|---|---|---|---|---|---|---|---|---|---|---|
| | 10TH | 25TH | 50TH | 75TH | 90TH | 10TH | 25TH | 50TH | 75TH | 90TH |
| 2 | 16.88 | 18.46 | 18.54 | 19.13 | 19.92 | 16.96 | 17.75 | 18.66 | 19.52 | 20.66 |
| 3 | 17.59 | 19.21 | 19.37 | 20.15 | 21.25 | 17.59 | 18.42 | 19.40 | 20.43 | 21.81 |
| 4 | 18.30 | 19.92 | 20.19 | 21.18 | 22.59 | 18.22 | 19.09 | 20.15 | 21.33 | 22.91 |
| 5 | 19.01 | 20.66 | 20.98 | 22.24 | 23.93 | 18.85 | 19.76 | 29.90 | 22.24 | 24.05 |
| 6 | 19.72 | 21.27 | 21.81 | 23.26 | 25.27 | 19.48 | 20.39 | 21.65 | 23.14 | 25.19 |
| 7 | 20.43 | 22.12 | 22.63 | 24.29 | 26.61 | 20.11 | 21.06 | 22.40 | 24.05 | 27.08 |
| 8 | 21.14 | 22.87 | 23.46 | 25.31 | 27.95 | 20.74 | 21.73 | 23.14 | 24.96 | 27.44 |
| 9 | 21.85 | 23.58 | 24.29 | 26.37 | 29.25 | 21.37 | 22.40 | 23.89 | 25.86 | 28.58 |
| 10 | 22.55 | 24.33 | 25.07 | 27.40 | 30.59 | 22.00 | 23.07 | 24.60 | 26.77 | 29.72 |
| 11 | 23.26 | 25.03 | 25.90 | 28.42 | 31.92 | 22.63 | 23.70 | 25.35 | 27.67 | 30.82 |
| 12 | 23.97 | 25.78 | 26.73 | 29.48 | 33.62 | 23.26 | 24.37 | 26.10 | 28.58 | 31.96 |
| 13 | 24.68 | 26.53 | 27.55 | 30.51 | 34.60 | 23.89 | 25.03 | 26.85 | 29.48 | 33.11 |
| 14 | 25.39 | 27.24 | 28.38 | 31.77 | 35.94 | 24.52 | 25.70 | 27.59 | 30.39 | 34.21 |
| 15 | 26.10 | 27.99 | 29.17 | 32.59 | 37.28 | 25.15 | 26.37 | 28.24 | 31.29 | 35.35 |
| 16 | 26.81 | 28.70 | 29.99 | 33.62 | 38.62 | 25.78 | 27.00 | 29.09 | 32.20 | 36.49 |
| 17 | 27.51 | 29.44 | 30.82 | 34.64 | 39.96 | 26.41 | 27.67 | 29.84 | 33.11 | 37.59 |
| 18 | 28.22 | 30.19 | 31.65 | 35.66 | 41.29 | 27.04 | 28.34 | 30.59 | 34.01 | 38.74 |

*Source:* From J. Fernandez, D. Redden, A. Pietrobelli, and D. Allison, "Waist Circumference Percentiles in Nationally Representative Samples of African-American, European-American, and Mexican-American Children and Adolescents," *Journal of Pediatrics* 145 (2004): 439–444.

**Table 7.8** | Skinfold Thickness Technique: Percent Fat Estimates for Women Calculated from Triceps, Suprailium, and Thigh

| SUM OF 3 SKINFOLDS | AGE AT LAST BIRTHDAY | | | | | | | | |
|---|---|---|---|---|---|---|---|---|---|
| | 22 OR UNDER | 23 TO 27 | 28 TO 32 | 33 TO 37 | 38 TO 42 | 43 TO 47 | 48 TO 52 | 53 TO 57 | 58 AND OVER |
| 23–25 | 9.7 | 9.9 | 10.2 | 10.4 | 10.7 | 10.9 | 11.2 | 11.4 | 11.7 |
| 26–28 | 11.0 | 11.2 | 11.5 | 11.7 | 12.0 | 12.3 | 12.5 | 12.7 | 13.0 |
| 29–31 | 12.3 | 12.5 | 12.8 | 13.0 | 13.3 | 13.5 | 13.8 | 14.0 | 14.3 |
| 32–34 | 13.6 | 13.8 | 14.0 | 14.3 | 14.5 | 14.8 | 15.0 | 15.3 | 15.5 |
| 35–37 | 14.8 | 15.0 | 15.3 | 15.5 | 15.8 | 16.0 | 16.3 | 16.5 | 16.8 |
| 38–40 | 16.0 | 16.3 | 16.5 | 16.7 | 17.0 | 17.2 | 17.5 | 17.7 | 18.0 |
| 41–43 | 17.2 | 17.4 | 17.7 | 17.9 | 18.2 | 18.4 | 18.7 | 18.9 | 19.2 |
| 44–46 | 18.3 | 18.6 | 18.8 | 19.1 | 19.3 | 19.6 | 19.8 | 20.1 | 20.3 |
| 47–49 | 19.5 | 19.7 | 20.0 | 20.2 | 20.5 | 20.7 | 21.0 | 21.2 | 21.5 |
| 50–52 | 20.6 | 20.8 | 21.1 | 21.3 | 21.6 | 21.8 | 22.1 | 22.3 | 22.6 |
| 53–55 | 21.7 | 21.9 | 22.1 | 22.4 | 22.6 | 22.9 | 23.1 | 23.4 | 23.6 |
| 56–58 | 22.7 | 23.0 | 23.2 | 23.4 | 23.7 | 23.9 | 24.2 | 24.4 | 24.7 |
| 59–61 | 23.7 | 24.0 | 24.2 | 24.5 | 24.7 | 25.0 | 25.2 | 25.5 | 25.7 |
| 62–64 | 24.7 | 25.0 | 25.2 | 25.5 | 25.7 | 26.0 | 26.2 | 26.4 | 26.7 |
| 65–67 | 25.7 | 25.9 | 26.2 | 26.4 | 26.7 | 26.9 | 27.2 | 27.4 | 27.7 |
| 68–70 | 26.6 | 26.9 | 27.1 | 27.4 | 27.6 | 27.9 | 28.1 | 28.4 | 28.6 |
| 71–73 | 27.5 | 27.8 | 28.0 | 28.3 | 28.5 | 28.8 | 29.0 | 29.3 | 29.5 |
| 74–76 | 28.4 | 28.7 | 28.9 | 29.2 | 29.4 | 29.7 | 29.9 | 30.2 | 30.4 |
| 77–79 | 29.3 | 29.5 | 29.8 | 30.0 | 30.3 | 30.5 | 30.8 | 31.0 | 31.3 |
| 80–82 | 30.1 | 30.4 | 30.6 | 30.9 | 31.1 | 31.4 | 31.6 | 31.9 | 32.1 |
| 83–85 | 30.9 | 31.2 | 31.4 | 31.7 | 31.9 | 32.2 | 32.4 | 32.7 | 32.9 |
| 86–88 | 31.7 | 32.0 | 32.2 | 32.5 | 32.7 | 32.9 | 33.2 | 33.4 | 33.7 |
| 89–91 | 32.5 | 32.7 | 33.0 | 33.2 | 33.5 | 33.7 | 33.9 | 34.2 | 34.4 |
| 92–94 | 33.2 | 33.4 | 33.7 | 33.9 | 34.2 | 34.4 | 34.7 | 34.9 | 35.2 |
| 95–97 | 33.9 | 34.1 | 34.4 | 34.6 | 34.9 | 35.1 | 35.4 | 35.6 | 35.9 |
| 98–100 | 34.6 | 34.8 | 35.1 | 35.3 | 35.5 | 35.8 | 36.0 | 36.3 | 36.5 |
| 101–103 | 35.2 | 35.4 | 35.7 | 35.9 | 36.2 | 36.4 | 36.7 | 36.9 | 37.2 |
| 104–106 | 35.8 | 36.1 | 36.3 | 36.6 | 36.8 | 37.1 | 37.3 | 37.5 | 37.8 |
| 107–109 | 36.4 | 36.7 | 36.9 | 37.1 | 37.4 | 37.6 | 37.9 | 38.1 | 38.4 |
| 110–112 | 37.0 | 37.2 | 37.5 | 37.7 | 38.0 | 38.2 | 38.5 | 38.7 | 38.9 |
| 113–115 | 37.5 | 37.8 | 38.0 | 38.2 | 38.5 | 38.7 | 39.0 | 39.2 | 39.5 |
| 116–118 | 38.0 | 38.3 | 38.5 | 38.8 | 39.0 | 39.3 | 39.5 | 39.7 | 40.0 |
| 119–121 | 38.5 | 38.7 | 39.0 | 39.2 | 39.5 | 39.7 | 40.0 | 40.2 | 40.5 |
| 122–124 | 39.0 | 39.2 | 39.4 | 39.7 | 39.9 | 40.2 | 40.4 | 40.7 | 40.9 |
| 125–127 | 39.4 | 39.6 | 39.9 | 40.1 | 40.4 | 40.6 | 40.9 | 41.1 | 41.4 |
| 128–130 | 39.8 | 40.0 | 40.3 | 40.5 | 40.8 | 41.0 | 41.3 | 41.5 | 41.8 |

*Note:* Body density is calculated based on the generalized equation for predicting body density of women developed by A. S. Jackson, M. L. Pollock, and A. Ward and published in *Medicine and Science in Sports and Exercise* 12 (1980): 175–182. Percent body fat is determined from the calculated body density using the Siri formula.

*Source:* From Table 4.1 by W. W. K. Hoeger and S. A. Hoeger, *Lifetime Physical Fitness and Wellness* (Belmont, CA: Cengage Learning, 2010).

**Table 7.9** | Comparison of Methods Used to Estimate Body Composition

| METHOD | ACCURACY | PRACTICALITY AND PORTABILITY | EASE OF USE | TIME | COST | SUBJECT COMFORT AND EFFORT | TECHNICIAN TRAINING |
|---|---|---|---|---|---|---|---|
| Underwater (hydrostatic) weighing | SEE = ±2.7% | Practical in exercise physiology laboratories or large fitness centers; not portable | Requires subject to submerge, exhale, and hold breath | ~30 minutes because the procedure should be repeated 5 to 10 times | Initial purchase of equipment is expensive | Subject may be uncomfortable wearing a bathing suit, submerging in water, and exhaling air | Training is needed but is not difficult |
| Plethysmography | SEE = ±2.7–3.7% | Requires 8' × 8' space; can be moved with proper equipment, but takes effort | Requires subject to sit quietly | ~5 minutes | Initial purchase of equipment is expensive | Subject may be uncomfortable wearing a bathing suit and cap and sitting in an enclosed space | Minimal training needed |
| Skinfold measurements | SEE = ±3.5% | Practical in settings that have a private area; very portable | Requires subject to be still; measurement sites must be determined and marked | <5 minutes | Initial purchase of equipment is relatively inexpensive | Subject may be uncomfortable partially disrobing; some skinfolds are difficult to grasp | Training and consistency are critical; technique improves with experience |
| Bioelectrical Impedance Analysis (BIA) | SEE = ±3.5% | Practical in most settings; very portable | Easy to use | <5 minutes | Initial purchase of equipment is moderately expensive | Procedure is simple but pre-measurement guidelines require substantial subject compliance | Minimal training needed |
| Dual-Energy X-ray Absorptiometry (DXA) | SEE = ±1.8%; more research needed to verify SEE | Practical in imaging centers, physicians' offices, or research facilities; not portable | Easy to use | ~5 to 10 minutes | Initial purchase of equipment is very expensive | Simple procedure; subject is exposed to a very small amount of radiation; use prohibited during pregnancy | Training is needed; license to operate is required |
| Computed Tomography Scans (CT) and Magnetic Resonance Imaging (MRI) | Not yet established | Practical in imaging centers and research facilities; not portable | Requires subject to be still throughout the entire procedure | ~30 minutes | Initial purchase of equipment is very expensive | Procedure is relatively simple with some subject discomfort | Training is needed; license to operate is required |

*Note:* SEE = Standard Error of the Estimate

*Source:* From Table 11.1 by M. Dunford and J.A. Doyle, *Nutrition for Sport and Exercise* (Belmont, CA: Cengage Learning, 2007).

measured, the units are kg/m² and errors involved with predicting percentage of body fat from BMI are large (~6% error) because BMI does not take lean muscle mass into account (many physically active people have more lean muscle mass than their sedentary counterparts). Also, when professionals measure skinfolds, which is one of the most practical/portable/cheap options for most applied situations, they are obtaining an estimate of percent body fat that is different from BMI measures and more accurate (~3% error). Table 7.10 provides common standards for evaluating body composition of adults and health-related interpretations of body composition categories.

**Table 7.10** | Standards for Evaluating Body Composition of Adults

| BODY COMPOSITION CATEGORY | AGE | | | |
|---|---|---|---|---|
| | <30 | 30–39 | 40–49 | OVER 50 |
| **Men** | | | | |
| High | >28% | >29% | >30% | >31% |
| Moderately high | 22–28% | 23–29% | 24–30% | 25–31% |
| Optimal range | 11–21% | 12–22% | 13–23% | 14–24% |
| Low | 6–10% | 7–11% | 8–12% | 9–13% |
| Very low | ≤5% | ≤6% | ≤7% | ≤8% |
| **Women** | | | | |
| High | >32% | >33% | >34% | >36% |
| Moderately high | 26–32% | 27–33% | 28–34% | 29–35% |
| Optimal range | 15–25% | 16–26% | 17–27% | 18–28% |
| Low | 12–14% | 13–15% | 14–16% | 15–17% |
| Very low | ≤11% | ≤12% | ≤13% | ≤14% |

**High**—Percentage fat at this level indicates the person is seriously overweight to a degree that can have adverse health consequences. The person should be encouraged to lose weight through diet and exercise. Maintaining weight at this level for a long period places the person at risk for hypertension, heart disease, and diabetes. A long-term weight-loss and exercise program should be initiated. **Moderately high**—It is likely that the person is significantly overweight, but the level could be high, in part, because of measurement inaccuracies. It would be wise to carefully monitor people in this category and encourage them not to gain additional weight. People in this category may want to have their body composition assessed by the underwater weighing method. **Optimal range**—It would be highly desirable to maintain body composition at this level. **Low**—This is an acceptable body composition level, but there is no reason to seek a lower percentage body fat level. Loss of additional body weight could have health consequences. **Very low**—Percentage fat level at this range should be reached only by high-level endurance athletes who are in training. Being this thin may carry its own additional mortality risk. Individuals, especially females, this low are at risk for having an eating disorder such as anorexia nervosa.

*Source:* From Tables 4.2 and 4.7 by A.S. Jackson and R. M. Ross, *Understanding Health and Fitness,* 3rd ed. (Dubuque, IA: Kendall Hunt Publishing, 1997).

# EXAMPLES OF APPLYING ENERGY BALANCE AND BODY COMPOSITION BASICS IN KINESIOLOGY SUBDISCIPLINES

*In Lesson 1, you learned about the importance of understanding the basics of energy balance and body composition along with the numerous health and peak performance benefits associated with achieving energy balance and a healthy body composition. In Lesson 2, you will learn about examples of the*

*relationships among energy balance, achieving or maintaining a healthy body composition, physical activity principles, and the subdisciplines of kinesiology across the physical activity continuum.*

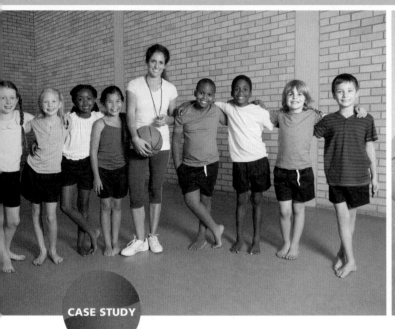

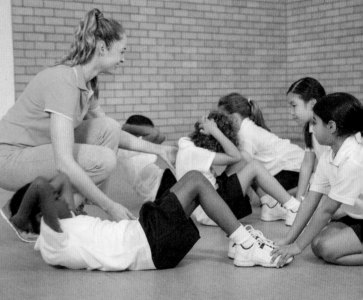

**CASE STUDY**

## In the real world . . .

As described earlier in this chapter, Eugene Casey has lost weight and improved his BMI to the 86th percentile for his sex and age. However, his parents have received a PE report card showing that while he improved his fitness levels for the mile run, push-ups, curl-ups, and flexibility, his BMI indicates he is overweight and considered unhealthy.

BMI is considered one of the best ways to estimate body composition in large populations such as school-age children because it is simple and does not require participants to remove clothing or be touched except for normal measurements of height and weight (generally performed by school nurses). High BMI scores among children (> 85th percentile for sex and age) are associated with a high risk for becoming overweight and obese as adults

compared with lower BMI scores, particularly if they are and remain sedentary. However, BMI measures do not take into account the amount of lean tissue mass one carries as compared to fat tissue mass. Therefore, a physically active and growing boy like Eugene may have increased his muscle mass through weight training and may be healthier than he was prior to beginning training, when his BMI was at the > 95th percentile level.

Several states in the United States require that schools or school districts measure student height and weight for the calculation of BMI, and the majority require parent notification. Arkansas was the first state to require school BMI measurement in 2007. BMI screening and surveillance were initiated with the goal of helping combat obesity in children and adolescents. If BMI report cards encourage parents to help their children achieve energy balance and a healthier body composition (e.g., adjusting

▸ Exercise Physiology
▸ Biomechanics
▸ Public Health
▸ Sport/Exercise Psychology
▸ Motor Learning
▸ Practice of Kinesiology

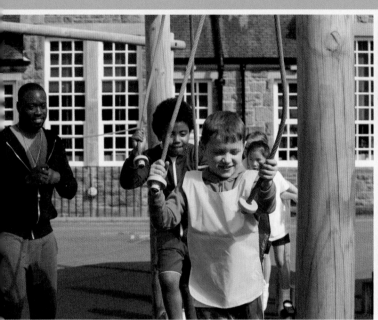

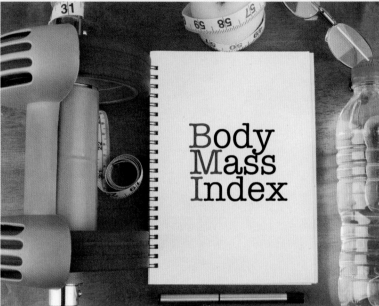

caloric intake, increasing physical activity levels, and reducing screen time), then BMI reporting is meaningful. However, parents like William and Maria are often concerned that BMI report cards put too much pressure on students and may lead to bullying if a student is underweight, overweight, or obese. Some kinesiology experts also wonder whether this popular state legislation policy may lead to an increase in eating disorders for those with higher BMIs. It will be interesting to see how the controversy over BMI report cards will play out over time.

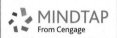 Go to your MindTap course to complete the Case Study activity for this chapter.

# Exercise Physiology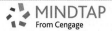

For extremely obese individuals (BMI> 40 or > 35 with pre-existing medical issues such as type 2 diabetes), bariatric surgery, also called gastric surgery, is an option. Bariatric procedures are aggressive weight loss strategies that are performed as a last alternative for adolescents and adults who cannot lose weight through normal behavioral change strategies or medication. Figure 7.18 shows examples of two gastric surgery procedures: gastric bypass and gastric banding. Even when they successfully promote weight loss, bariatric procedures often produce many side effects, and weight regain can occur. Nonetheless, those who enjoy success with the procedures and avoid their preprocedure behaviors (high energy intake and low physical activity expenditure) can achieve long-term weight loss ( $\geq 5$ years) that, based on limited data, approaches 50% to 60% of initial weight. Some individuals with type 2 diabetes and those at high risk for diabetes due to metabolic syndrome experience normalization of their blood glucose levels as well.

If a person is candidate for bariatric surgery, he or she will undergo intensive screening and be interviewed prior to the procedure, as well as followed throughout the whole process (presurgery, postsurgery, and after discharge) by a multidisciplinary team that includes a kinesiology-related subdiscipline professional (e.g., exercise physiologist, physical therapist, or occupational therapist). Other bariatric team members usually include professionals such as surgeons, nurses, dietitian nutritionists, social workers, and psychiatrists. An integrated approach to bariatric surgery is essential if the patient is to succeed in achieving negative energy balance, significant weight loss, and healthier body composition.

Obviously, the kinesiology professional's role in bariatric surgery is to evaluate the physical activity and exercise history of the patient to ensure that she or he can increase and maintain engagement in physical activities and exercise following the procedures. Patients are also evaluated and educated regarding behavioral theories that can help them adopt successful physical activity strategies.

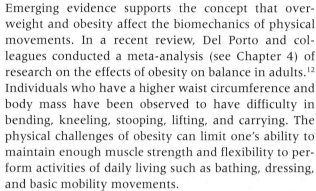

**MINDTAP**
From Cengage

**Surgical Treatment for Obesity**

**Go to your MindTap course** to learn more about the gastric bypass and gastric banding surgical procedures.

# Biomechanics

Emerging evidence supports the concept that overweight and obesity affect the biomechanics of physical movements. In a recent review, Del Porto and colleagues conducted a meta-analysis (see Chapter 4) of research on the effects of obesity on balance in adults.[12] Individuals who have a higher waist circumference and body mass have been observed to have difficulty in bending, kneeling, stooping, lifting, and carrying. The physical challenges of obesity can limit one's ability to maintain enough muscle strength and flexibility to perform activities of daily living such as bathing, dressing, and basic mobility movements.

The increased body mass that accompanies obesity changes the way the body moves, and that modifies

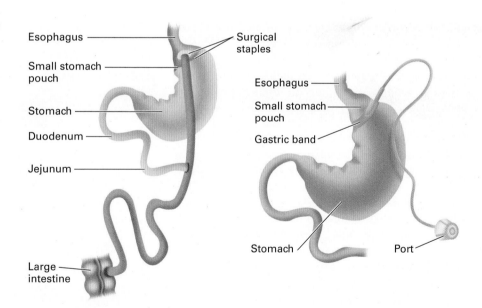

In gastric bypass, the surgeon constructs a small stomach pouch and creates an outlet directly to the small intestine, bypassing most of the stomach, the entire duodenum, and some of the jejunum. (Dark areas highlight the flow of food through the GI tract; pale areas indicate bypassed sections.)

In gastric banding, the surgeon uses a gastric band to reduce the opening from the esophagus to the stomach. The size of the opening can be adjusted by inflating or deflating the band by way of a port placed in the abdomen just beneath the skin.

**Figure 7.18** | Gastric Procedures to Treat Severe Obesity

how the limbs react to forces, which can negatively affect functional capacity and postural balance. Increases in abdominal fat shift the body's center of mass (COM) toward the front of the body, out of line of the body's base of support. Obese individuals adjust to their increased body weight by reductions in gait speed, cadence, and stride. These adaptations are associated with reduced muscle coordination, force production, and resistance to fatigue.

Overweight, abdominal obesity, and low levels of muscular strength are strongly associated with balance deficiencies, particularly in the elderly. Obesity requires more muscle recruitment and more cognitive attention to maintain postural stability, which is a significant challenge to individuals who have gained weight rapidly without significant increases in muscle strength over time to maintain postural control. Obesity makes it even more difficult to recover balance once someone loses postural stability. Limited evidence from the research literature suggests that weight loss can help improve or restore muscular strength, muscular endurance, and postural stability, although the dose of physical activity or balance training required is currently not known.

# Public Health

Angela is a wellness manager at a large worksite that serves as the headquarters of a computer hardware manufacturer. She has developed a weight-loss challenge program for employees who work at the company headquarters. For this program, she has helped people to join teams in a competition to lose the highest percentage of body weight over a 24-week period. Because of her kinesiology training, Angela knows that energy balance is the key determinant of obesity and overweight. She is interested in helping company employees to create a negative energy balance through an increase in physical activity (caloric expenditure) and a decrease in caloric intake, and plans to award the first prize to the team that loses the highest combined percentage of their initial body weight. Her initial challenge for the 24 weeks is a contest to see how many steps each team can take each day (the total of all team members). She has purchased pedometers—small step counters—and has distributed them to all employees who have signed up for the challenge program. The total number of steps each employee achieves each day are recorded using a company intranet site.

With a good knowledge of human behavior, Angela helps participants to set weekly goals, monitor their behavior, and use the inherent social support of the team-building process to create an environment in which each team is trying to outdo the other to see who can accumulate the most steps and lose the most weight in the 24-week

period. Although Angela knows that caloric restriction is the other important component of weight loss, she also knows that physical activity has health benefits beyond its role in weight control. Thus, she is really hoping to see positive changes due to the pedometer challenge.

After 24 weeks, she evaluates her results. Although the final numbers were close, the team that reported the most weight loss only came in second place in the total number of steps they recorded (10,238 steps per day). However, the team with the highest number of recorded steps (average of 12,304 steps per day) did report very clear increases in mood, outlook, and productivity in the workplace. These results help Angela to set specific target goals for all employees to accumulate 10,300 steps each day for weight loss.

# Sport/Exercise Psychology

Behavioral theories and **logic models** (frameworks that provide an integrated approach with which to plan, implement, evaluate, and report interventions requiring accountability) help kinesiology practitioners explain and predict changes in energy balance and body composition for individuals and populations. Table 7.11 lists and describes some of the most popular behavioral theories related to physical activity interventions.

One of the behavioral theories from Table 7.11 most commonly used by kinesiology professionals assisting clients to achieve energy balance and a healthy body composition is the **Transtheoretical model** (or **Stages of Change model**), which you first learned about in Chapter 4. Figure 7.19 shows the steps of the stages of

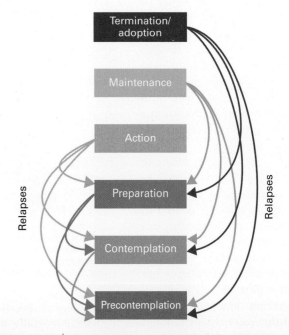

**Figure 7.19** | The Transtheoretical Model or Stages of Change Model

**Table 7.11** | Popular Behavioral Theories and Theoretical Models for Physical Activity Behavior

| THEORY OR MODEL | KEY BEHAVIORAL CONSTRUCTS | EXPLANATION |
| --- | --- | --- |
| Health Belief Model[13] | Perceived susceptibility, perceived severity, perceived benefits, perceived barriers, cues to action, self-efficacy | People become physically active if they feel at risk for a negative health outcome (i.e., perceived susceptibility and severity), expect that by being physically active they will prevent that negative health outcome (i.e., perceived benefits), and believe that they can intiate and maintain the physical activity (i.e., perceived barriers, self-efficacy). |
| Theory of reasoned action-theory of planned behavior[14] | Attitudes, subjective norms, behavioral control, behavioral intention | People's intentions to be physically active depend on their beliefs about physical activity weighted by evaluations of these beliefs (i.e., attitudes), the beliefs of other people about physical activity weighted by the value attributed to these opinions (i.e., subjective norms), and the perceived ease or difficulty of being physically active (i.e., perceived behavioral control). People who intend to become physically active are likely to do so. |
| Social cognitive theory[15] | Reciprocal determinism, environment, outcome expectancies, observational learning, reinforcement, self-efficacy | Reciprocal relationships exist among the environment, personal factors (e.g., beliefs), and physical activity. Beliefs (i.e., outcome expectancies, self-efficacy) can influence actions, and vice versa. Beliefs are molded by structures within the social and physical environment. Physical activity can influence the environment and is determined by that environment. These processes occur through observational learning and reinforcement. |
| Self-determination theory[16] | External regulation, introjected regulation, identified regulation, integrated regulation, intrinsic motivation | Actions vary in the degree to which they are volitional, without any external influence. Motivation to be physically active occurs along a continuum from external regulation (i.e., rewards, others' demands), to introjected regulation (i.e., moral reasons), to identified regulation (i.e., useful outcomes), to integrated regulation (i.e., important for personal growth), to intrinsic motivation (i.e., mastery, enjoyment). |
| Transtheoretical model[17] | Stages of motivational readiness for change, processes of change | People progress through five stages of change on the way to being physically active: precontemplation, contemplation, preparation, action, and maintenance. Processes of change are activities that people use to move through the stages: consciousness raising (increasing awareness), dramatic relief (emotional arousal) environmental reevaluation (social reappraisal), social liberation (environmental opportunities), self-reevaluation (self-reappraisal), stimulus control (reengineering), helping relationship (supporting), counter conditioning (substituting), reinforcement management (rewarding), and self-liberation (committing). |

*Source:* Adapted from G. F. Dunton, M. Cousineau, and K. D. Reynolds, "The Intersection of Public Policy and Health Behavior Theory in the Physical Activity Arena," *Journal of Physical Activity and Health* 7, no. 21 (2010): S91–S96.

change model plus two additional outcome steps, which include the following:

▸ **Precontemplation** means an individual or population is not even thinking about being physically active relative to achieving energy balance and a healthy body composition.

▸ **Contemplation** means an individual or population is starting to think about being physically active to achieve energy balance and a healthy body composition, but has not started the process.

▸ **Preparation** means an individual or population has started making small changes in behavior toward becoming physically active to achieve energy balance and a healthy body composition.

- **Action** means an individual or population has become physically active at a minimum threshold (such as 150 minutes per week) in an attempt to achieve energy balance and a healthy body composition.

- **Maintenance** means an individual or population has remained physically active for at least six months to achieve energy balance and a healthy body composition.

- **Termination/adoption** means an individual or population is successful at adopting regular physical activity or terminates the behavior.

- **Relapse** means an individual or population has stopped participating in physical activity after starting, which is commonly due to factors such as illness, injury, or vacations, but may also be due to other, preventable barriers.

Figure 7.20 shows an example of a logic model for a research study (The HEALTHY Study) that was designed to provide interventions focused on reducing diabetes risk in middle school students. The figure suggests that the multiple interventions of increasing physical activity, improving nutritional intake, and reducing sedentary behaviors in sixth grade adolescents will result in better energy balance and cardiovascular fitness. As students continue to improve, they will reduce their percent of body fat (adiposity) and improve their regulation of insulin and glucose levels, thus reducing metabolic syndrome and diabetes risk. As you can see,

logic models can provide kinesiology professionals with a road map regarding relationships that can help individuals and populations become and stay physically active to achieve energy balance and a healthy body composition.

## Motor Learning

As you learned previously, adult obesity negatively affects biomechanics relative to gait and postural stability. Adult obesity may also negatively affect cognition or the ability to develop a motor plan.[18] Motor planning refers to the ability to plan a movement before it is executed. Obese individuals have poorer motor planning skills than non-obese individuals, which is associated with poor performance on movement tasks. In obese populations, poor motor planning could contribute to more frequent losses of balance or the inability to recover from unavoidable losses of balance.

The area of study linking obesity and cognition is relatively new, but preliminary research comparing obese to non-obese individuals shows that obese adults perform significantly worse on tests of motor planning and mental flexibility related to executing movement tasks. While the reasons for these research observations are not well understood, they may be related to impaired brain metabolic function or cerebellum (structure at the back of the brain that regulates balance) function. It remains to be determined whether the application of motor learning principles can help obese individuals improve their adaptive abilities during physical activities.

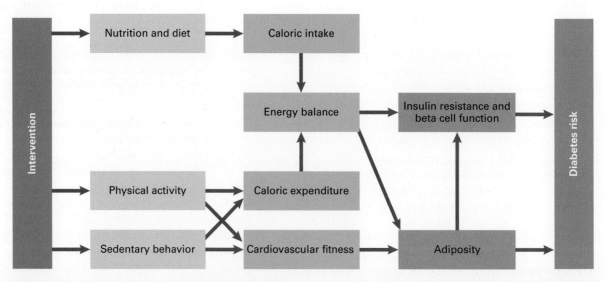

**Figure 7.20** | Logic Model for the HEALTHY Middle School Diabetes Intervention and Prevention Study

*Source:* From the National Institute of Diabetes and Digestive and Kidney Diseases, The HEALTHY Study, www.healthystudy.org.

# The Practice of Kinesiology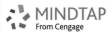

Colin is a 25-year-old college student who has a BMI of 29. His percentage of body fat, as measured in the exercise physiology laboratory with three-site skinfolds, is 24%. How you would you interpret his body composition data based on his primary goals of becoming more physically active and maintaining good health? What body composition goals can you provide Colin to reduce his future health risks?

One way to evaluate Colin's body composition measures is to recognize that both his BMI and percentage of body fat are higher than they should be for good health (see Table 7.5 and Table 7.10). If his percentage of body fat were lower (in the optimal range), this might suggest he is carrying a lot of muscle mass, which is not identified by BMI measures. At 24% body fat, it is likely that Colin is significantly overweight, but also possible that his fat percentage has been somewhat overestimated through measurement error (see interpretation information with Table 7.10). It would be important for Colin to have his percentage of body fat monitored, and he should be encouraged to avoid gaining more weight.

For good health, Colin should try to lower his BMI into the 18.5 to 25 range (Table 7.5). He should try to reduce his percentage of body fat to a level between 11% and 21% (Table 7.10).

---

MINDTAP
From Cengage

Now that you have completed this chapter, go to your MindTap course to complete all assigned activities. Check out the additional resources developed to help you apply the material in this chapter to your course and career goals.

---

## Chapter Summary

- Energy balance is the relationship among energy intake, energy expenditure, and energy storage associated with the maintenance of body homeostasis. It is influenced by caloric intake (eating) and caloric expenditure (physical activity).

- Body composition refers to the distribution of fat and lean mass (muscle and bone, water, and minerals) in the body. In this chapter, weight control refers to how participating in regular physical activity interacts with the kinesiology science subdisciplines (exercise physiology, biomechanical, behavioral) and environmental challenges to influence the ability of individuals or populations to achieve and maintain a healthy body composition.

- Body fat is unevenly distributed throughout the body, and there are certain patterns of fat distribution that may increase a person's risk of certain chronic diseases.

- Resting metabolic rate accounts for 60% to 70% of TEE, while TEF accounts for about 10%. Therefore, participating in daily physical activities such as standing, shivering, exercising, or walking can contribute from 20% to 30% of TEE. Your daily PAEE is the primary and most important variable that is changeable with regards to energy balance (on the energy expenditure side of things). Certainly, energy intake is very important and can be modified by using the recommendations from the 2015 Dietary Guidelines.

- Participating in physical activity and exercise can help individuals and populations reduce total body fat, waist circumference, and intra-abdominal fat; maintain or increase lean muscle mass; and prevent the regain of lost weight.

- It is important for those with high exercise performance goals involving weight-bearing activities such as gymnastics, dance, long-distance running, wrestling, and others to recognize that although being leaner helps improve their performance, losing too much weight is associated with behavioral disorders (e.g., body image issues and eating disorders) and negative physiological adaptations (e.g., lowered immune function, lower glycogen stores, and overtraining syndrome).

- Common field methods of measuring body composition include BMI, body (waist and hip) circumferences, and skinfolds. The interpretation and monitoring of body composition are important skills that kinesiology professionals should acquire to help individuals and populations achieve their energy balance and body composition goals through proper educational messaging.

- Overweight and obese conditions can negatively affect physiological, biomechanical, and behavioral factors relative to the physical activity continuum and across the lifespan.

# People Matter Ali Brian, Professor of Physical Education*

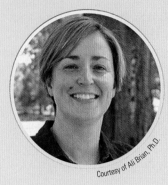
Courtesy of Ali Brian, Ph.D.

**Q:** **Why and how did you get into the field of kinesiology?**

**A:** *I wanted to pursue a career that would enable me to help children learn the tools necessary to choose to be physically active throughout their lifespan. I understood the value of motor competence as it relates to physical activity and obesity. Many young children from socioeconomically disadvantaged environments present delays with their motor skills. I wanted the chance to help them remediate these delays and learn their motor skills.*

**Q:** **What was the major influence on you to work in the field?**

**A:** *When I was in high school, I worked at sport camps for children as a counselor. Many children who attended seemed to struggle with performing basic movement skills. I wanted to learn how to teach physical education with hopes that all young children would have the chance to develop the confidence and competence to choose to be physically active later on in life. Possessing degrees in kinesiology enables me to do just that.*

**Q:** **What are your current research interests, and how do you translate your research results to practitioners?**

**A:** *My research situates within providing young children who are socioeconomically disadvantaged with gross motor skill and physical activity interventions at their preschool centers. The purpose of our program is to lower children's risk for obesity through motor competence and physical activity. I translate this research for practitioners as preschool teachers themselves receive training from me to deliver our intervention.*

**Q:** **How do you stay physically active yourself and promote good health to others directly around you?**

**A:** *I enjoy riding my road bike throughout the parks in South Carolina as much as possible. I love hiking with my miniature schnauzer, Henry, as it is healthy for both of us. I am also lucky to live near a small lake and four rivers where I can swim and kayak.*

**Q:** **How have you had to integrate the subdisciplines of kinesiology in your professional practice?**

**A:** *I consistently integrate motor development, physical education, adapted physical education, and exercise science into the development, delivery, and assessment of our intervention programming. In addition, I teach courses such as motor development, adapted physical education, and elementary physical education methods to undergraduates and graduates majoring in kinesiology.*

*Dr. Brian's research interests are working in socioeconomically disadvantaged communities promoting perceived and actual motor skill development of children with and without disabilities through engaging with early childhood teachers and parents. In addition, Dr. Brian explores and assesses associations among motor competence, perceived motor competence, and physical activity for young children with and without disabilities within the context of preventing childhood obesity.

# Remember This

action
basal metabolic rate (BMR)
body composition
contemplation
energy balance
essential fat
healthy weight
kilocalories (kcal) or Calories
logic models
maintaining weight

maintenance
metabolic syndrome
moderate-intensity physical activity
obesity
overweight
physical activity energy expenditure (PAEE)
precontemplation
preparation
prevention of weight re-gain

relapse
resting metabolic rate (RMR)
self-confidence
self-efficacy
self-esteem
subcutaneous fat
termination/adoption
thermic effect of food (TEF)
total energy expenditure (TEE)

Transtheoretical model (Stages of Change model)
underweight
vigorous-intensity physical activity
visceral fat
weight loss

# For More Information

Access these websites for further study of topics covered in the chapter:

▸ Find updates and quick links to these and other evidence-based practice-related sites in MindTap.

▸ Search for further information about the relationships among physical activity, energy balance, and body composition at the Centers for Disease Control and Prevention (CDC): www.cdc.gov.

▸ Search for information and resources about the relationships among physical activity, energy balance, and body composition in the United States at the 2008 U.S. Physical Activity Guidelines webpage (www.health.gov/paguidelines) and the U.S. Physical Activity Plan webpage (www.physicalactivityplan.org).

▸ Search for information about the relationships among physical activity, energy balance, and body composition at the American College of Sports Medicine webpage: www.acsm.org.

▸ Search for more information about the relationships among physical activity, energy balance, and body composition at the National Institute of Diabetes and Digestive and Kidney Diseases website: www.niddk.nih.gov.

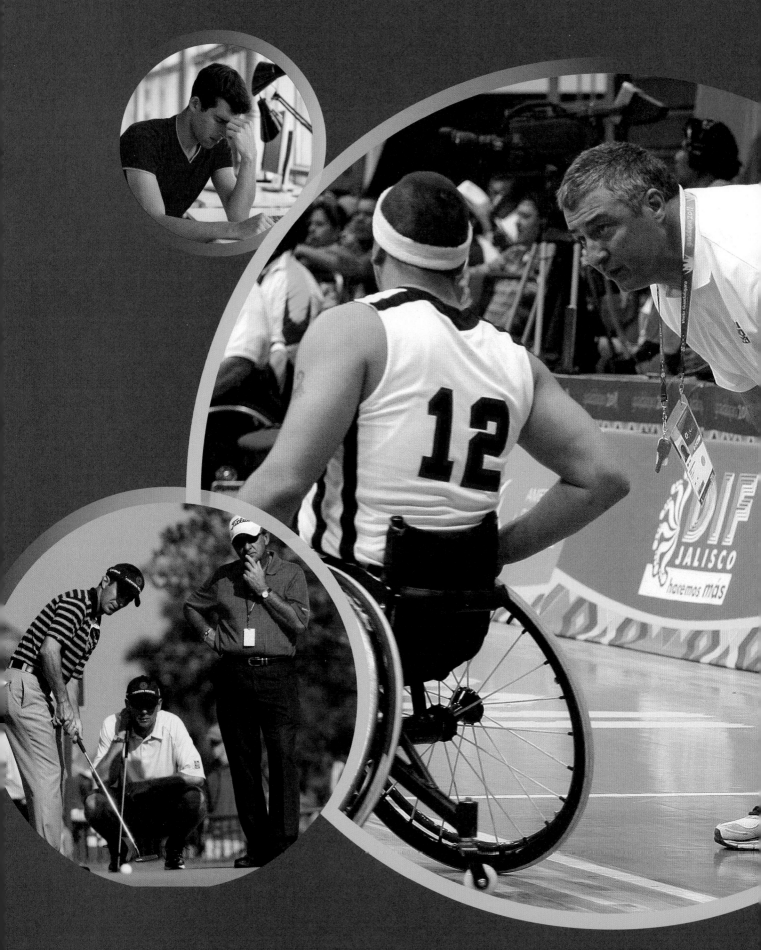

# Integration of Mental Health, Psychology, and the Physical Activity Continuum

*What are common aspects of mental health that affect health status and/or might limit participation in physical activity?*

**LESSON 1** INTEGRATION OF MENTAL HEALTH, PSYCHOLOGY, AND THE PHYSICAL ACTIVITY CONTINUUM

**LESSON 2** EXAMPLES OF APPLYING MENTAL HEALTH, PSYCHOLOGY, AND PHYSICAL ACTIVITY BASICS IN RELATIONSHIP TO THE KINESIOLOGY SUBDISCIPLINES

## Learning Objectives

*After completing this chapter, you will be able to:*

**Define** the common terms associated with mental health and physical activity.

**Explain** the relationship between mental health, physical activity, and the promotion of health, physical fitness, and optimal human performance.

**Justify** the importance of understanding mental health and its relationship to participation in physical activities in the context of the various subdisciplines of kinesiology.

**Describe** the specific reported health benefits of physical activity for people with mental health disorders.

**Explain** the psychosociological influences of physical activity on people with mental disorders across the physical activity continuum.

**Explain** how the health benefits acquired through physical activity can influence the prevention and management of mental health disorders and the quality of life.

**Explain** how successful participation in physical activity exerts physiologic and biomechanical influences on mental health.

**Describe** common psycho-behavioral responses associated with participation in regular physical activities for people with mental health concerns.

**Give** examples of modifications of overload, specificity, and adaptation in relation to mental health through participation in physical activity.

**Explain** how sport/exercise psychology improves overall health, physical fitness, and peak performance in people with mental health concerns.

**Describe** common assessment methods and measures that are used to evaluate and monitor the mental health of individuals and populations.

**Give** and explain examples of the application of mental health principles that affect successful participation in physical activity in relation to the kinesiology subdisciplines.

# INTEGRATION OF MENTAL HEALTH, PSYCHOLOGY, AND THE PHYSICAL ACTIVITY CONTINUUM

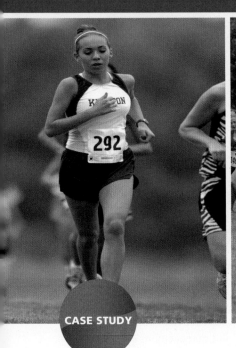

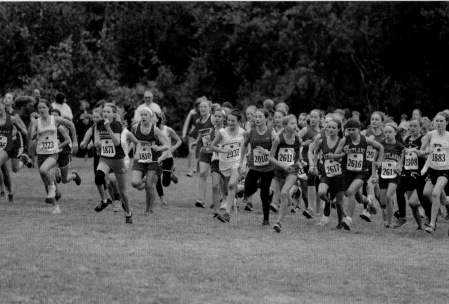

**CASE STUDY**

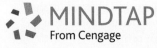

## In the real world . . .

As you remember from Chapter 1, Cara Casey (age 14) is a healthy eighth grader, does well in school, and enjoys physical activity. She played basketball and baseball when she was younger and now participates in club dance six evenings a week. She is considering trying out to be a high school cheerleader or a dancer, but her friend Amy is trying to talk her into trying out for the cross-country team next year as a freshman in high school. Amy is a year older than

Cara, enjoys running, and really likes her coach, who was previously an assistant cross-country coach at the local university. Coach Glenn encourages his runners (girls and boys) to train smart and uses mental preparation techniques such as goal setting, record keeping, motivation, self-talk cues, relaxation techniques, and precompetitive routines to optimize their training and competitive experiences.

Amy tells Cara about how Coach Glenn learned to prevent overtraining among runners by using a strategy that focused on more than just observing the negative physical

## MINDTAP
### From Cengage

Go to your MindTap course now to answer some questions and discover what you already know about the integration of mental health, psychology, and the physical activity continuum.

## INTERACTIVE ACTIVITIES

**Research Focus**

Go to your MindTap course to learn more about the Americans with Disabilities Act of 1990 (ADA). The ADA prohibits discrimination against people with physical disabilities and ensures equal opportunity for persons with disabilities in employment, state and local government services, public accommodations, commercial facilities, and transportation.

**Career Focus**

Go to your MindTap course to learn more about the coaching profession and the physical activity continuum.

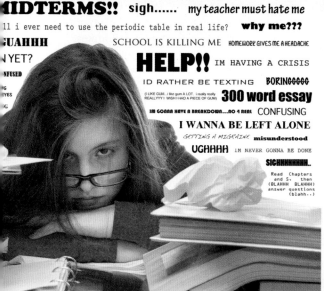

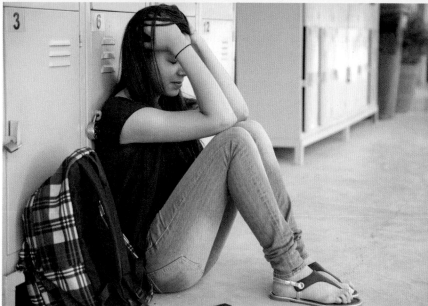

changes that can result from running too much. He said physical symptoms such as always being tired (chronic fatigue), inability to get a good night's sleep (insomnia), and abnormal upper respiratory infections provide helpful information but don't tell the whole story about how to manage a team of elite runners. The mental aspects of being an athlete are important as well. In fact, he claimed that the insight he gained had helped his team win the men's and women's conference championships in his first year of coaching. Coach Glenn used the **Profile of Mood States (POMS)**[1,2] when he coached his college runners to monitor their feelings of tension-anxiety, depression-dejection, anger-hostility, vigor, fatigue-inertia, and confusion-bewilderment (see p. 184 later in this chapter for more about the POMS). Coach Glenn had learned from running experts at workshops that the POMS could provide insight about the mental aspects of overtraining (review Chapter 4 for more on overtraining) among runners, particularly in relationship

to negative addiction and loss of vigor (joy and drive of participating).

What do you think? Is there scientific evidence behind coaching techniques such as mental training intended to improve or help monitor progress in high-performance athletes? If you are or were an athlete, what kinds of mental training have you experienced? Why would coaches trying to optimize training benefits for their athletes also benefit from integrating mental health strategies into their training programs? How might the monitoring of mood states of athletes help a coach modify the principles of overload, specificity, and adaptation in relationship to mental health to improve peak performance? We will follow up with Coach Glenn and the specific mental health strategies he used that helped his runners excel in Lesson 2 after you have had the opportunity to learn more about mental health, psychology, and the physical activity continuum.

# Introduction: Mental Health, Physical Activity, and Kinesiology

An integrated model of kinesiology and subdisciplines was introduced in Chapter 2. As shown in Figure 2.3, multiple factors should be considered by kinesiologists to help individuals and populations achieve and/or maintain health. Mental health (part of the kinesiology subdiscipline of sport/exercise psychology discussed throughout this chapter) can affect physical health and thus can influence place and progress across the physical activity continuum. For example, how does a physical activity and exercise program affect individuals who have depression, anxiety, or mental stress? What health benefits, if any, does regular participation in physical activities confer on those with mental health disorders? How can specific mental health strategies or specific adaptations affect optimal performance among athletes? Whether you are working to help someone begin a physical activity program, meet the U.S. physical activity guidelines, or reach peak performance, the application of health behavior and psychology concepts is fundamental for success.[3]

In this chapter, we will explore and emphasize the scientific evidence connecting physical activity with mental health. Three key focus areas are (1) known health, physical fitness, and peak performance benefits for those with selected mental health disorders; (2) mental and adaptive strategies to enhance physical fitness and performance; and (3) integrated strategies that can provide therapeutic, physical fitness, or peak performance benefits to a diversity of individuals that need mental health support commonly delivered by kinesiology professionals. The chapter has not been designed to be a complete overview of the subdiscipline of sport/exercise psychology. However, you will be introduced to a variety of psychosocial factors that can influence successful participation along the physical activity continuum.

The World Health Organization (WHO)[4] defines **health** as, "A state of complete physical, mental and social well-being, and not merely the absence of disease." **Mental health** refers to a state of well-being in which every individual realizes his or her own potential, can cope with the normal stresses of life, can work productively and fruitfully, and is able to make a contribution to her or his community (WHO).[5] Multiple social, psychological, and biological factors determine an individual's level of mental health at any point in time. For example, ongoing socioeconomic influences such as poverty and low levels of education negatively affect the mental health of individuals and communities. Poor mental health is also associated with rapid social change; stress at work, at school, or at home; gender and sexual discrimination; social exclusion; unhealthy lifestyles; risks of violence and physical illness; and human rights violations.[6] This chapter will introduce the role that physical activity plays in promoting mental health and the different aspects of mental health along the physical activity continuum.

The prevalence and societal economic costs of mental health disorders are difficult to determine due to recognition and acceptance issues, cultural stigmas associated with mental health problems, wide variations in the availability and costs of treatment, and the severity and duration of mental disorders. In the United States, it has been estimated that more than one in four—that is, over 70 million people—have a mental health problem. The economic burden of mental health disorders totals tens of billions of dollars each year, and common mental health disorders like depression and anxiety significantly decrease work productivity.[7]

Many distinct mental health disorders have been recognized and described based on emotional and behavioral symptoms.[8] The role of physical activity in the prevention or treatment of many of these disorders has received increasing attention in recent years as research in this area has advanced. The most common mental health problems studied in relation to physical activity are mood, anxiety, psychological distress, and well-being cognitive function, sleep, and adverse psychological events.[9] Although not a panacea, participation in physical activity does seem to help with several disorders.

Psychology plays an important part in the physical activity continuum. In kinesiology, current links with psychology as a discipline include interactions with physical activity, mental health, and sport/exercise psychology. A conceptual model that integrates psychosocial influences across the physical activity continuum is shown in Figure 8.1. In the center of the figure is the physical activity continuum indicating changes in physical activity behavior, from remaining sedentary to achieving functional health by meeting or exceeding the U.S. physical activity guidelines, goal-oriented physical fitness outcomes (e.g., lose weight, run a 10K, bench press 150 pounds), and peak performance.

In the middle of the figure, the psychosocial influences of aging and mental and physical challenges are included across the entire continuum. These are important factors that can affect the levels of success (positively and negatively) for individuals and populations in reaching their physical activity goals.

Surrounding the continuum are several psychosocial influences covered in this chapter that may positively affect the adoption or present barriers to achieving higher levels of physical activity by individuals or populations along the continuum. It is important to recognize that not every psychosocial variable shown will influence every level of the continuum, while some may. Research has helped to identify specific health behavior strategies that effectively assist people who are sedentary to become physically active and even to meet the minimal physical activity guidelines for health. As a person or a population

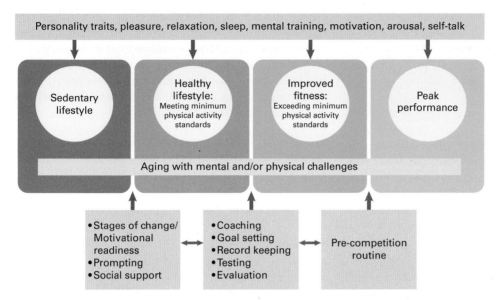

Figure 8.1 | Psychosocial Health and the Physical Activity Continuum. The figure illustrates possible psychosocial influences on physical activity participation and successful participation along the continuum. In this chapter, you will learn how the possible psychosocial factors can act positively and negatively on physical activity success at all levels of the physical activity continuum.

of people moves toward goal-oriented physical fitness or peak performance, specialized psychological techniques that sport/exercise psychologists frequently use are available to help recreational athletes and elite athletes (particularly professional and world-class athletes) reach their peak performance. Therefore, taken together, psychological principles underpin behavior change all the way along the physical activity continuum.

# Mental Health and Physical Activity: Basic Terms, Training Concepts, and the Physical Activity Continuum

## Common Mental Health Disorders

The following common mental disorders or problems have been studied in relation to physical activity and exercise:[10]

▸ Mood disorders
▸ Anxiety disorders
▸ Psychological distress
▸ Age-related changes in cognitive function
▸ Sleep disorders
▸ Low self-esteem
▸ Eating or exercise-related disorders

**Mood disorders** include depression, bipolar or manic–depressive disorders, medical conditions related to mood changes, and substance-induced mood disorders.[11] Depression can be classified as mild (also known as dysthymia) or as major depressive disorder (MDD). **Dysthymia**, which has been estimated to affect approximately 1.5% of the U.S. adult population, is defined as mild depression symptoms that persist for at least two years. MDD, on the other hand, is a manifestation of depressive symptoms that are much more severe—bad enough to negatively affect daily functioning—and last two weeks or more. An estimated 6.7% of U.S. adults have MDD. Adolescents (ages 13 to 18) in the United States have a lifetime combined prevalence of 11.2% for dysthymia and MDD.[12]

**Depression** is a popular term in today's society. The symptoms of depression are diverse and can include difficulty concentrating and making decisions, loss of interest in hobbies and activities, feelings of hopelessness and helplessness, insomnia, and even thoughts of suicide. The worries that are accompanied by depressive symptoms can also lead to physical symptoms such as fatigue, headaches, muscle tension and aches, difficulty swallowing, trembling, twitching and irritability, sweating, and hot flashes. Depression may be related to other factors such as abuse of alcohol or drugs, phobias, obsessions, and preoccupation with physical challenges. Periodic feelings of mild depression are normal for us all and can be caused by grief due to a significant loss or a current medical condition. However, depression or mood disorders that persist beyond two months may indicate major mood change problems.

**Anxiety** can be broadly defined as a condition of nervousness, uneasiness, or apprehension about a future event or events. Anxiety, although a predictable part of everyday life, can become a mental disorder that hinders daily functioning. Anxiety is usually classified as either state anxiety or trait anxiety. **State anxiety** refers to a person's existing or current emotional state, which can be situational and can change quickly. Trait anxiety refers to a broader pattern that reflects a person's personality, which is more long term and usually more stable.

An individual's trait anxiety can be described in general as either type A (aggressive, high-stress personality) or type B (low-key, low-stress personality). Chronic anxiety disorders can lead to specific phobias, social phobias, panic disorders, obsessive-compulsive disorder, or posttraumatic stress disorders.

**Psychological distress** refers to mental stressors that are not congruous with good health or well-being. The negative feelings you may have when you are sick or facing medical procedures such as surgery are examples of distress. In exercise studies, psychological distress is often measured by assessing the participants' subjective feelings of a lack of well-being. Higher reported levels of well-being are usually associated with a higher quality of life.

Do you know anyone, perhaps a grandparent or a great aunt or uncle, who gets confused easily? **Age-related decline in cognitive function** refers to gradual decreases in the ability to process, select, manipulate, or store information over time; it affects both behavior and functional ability. Seemingly straightforward routines such as putting away the clean dishes can become difficult and confusing as cognitive function worsens. Central nervous system (CNS) disorders associated with genetics and aging that have been linked to mental disorders include dementia (i.e., a loss of brain function that affects memory, thinking, language, judgment, and behavior), multiple sclerosis, Parkinson's disease, and Alzheimer's disease.

**Self-esteem** refers to feelings of self-worth and value that can positively influence mental health. In short, it is one's opinion of oneself. High self-esteem can influence many relevant outcomes such as academic or job performance, athletic success, and satisfaction with relationships. Studies show that people who begin an exercise program may experience higher self-esteem than nonexercisers. Further, more experienced exercisers may maintain higher levels of self-esteem over time if they continue to exercise compared to people who stop exercising. If adverse events such as injury or the adoption of addictive behaviors (e.g., compulsive running,

exercise addiction, disordered eating) occur, self-esteem may be reduced or become inconsistent with good mental health. Other addictive behaviors that are associated with poorer mental health are anorexia nervosa (limiting food intake and becoming excessively lean), **bulimia** (bingeing and purging), and **muscle dysmorphia** (a preoccupation with muscularity).

## Health and Quality of Life Benefits of Participation in Physical Activities for Those with Mental Health Disorders

Whether participating in physical activity (short-term or long-term) prevents mental health disorders is unknown. However, since the 1980s, scientific evidence demonstrating that physical activity lowers the risk for anxiety symptoms, anxiety disorders, depression symptoms, major depressive disorder, and age-related decline in cognitive function has mounted. Research also suggests that physical activity enhances psychological well-being and can delay the psychological effects of dementia.[13]

A framework showing three ways in which physical activity and exercise can be used and evaluated over time is shown in Figure 8.2. The framework can help kinesiology practitioners and clinicians understand the specific effects of physiological and behavioral changes associated with physical activity and exercise on mental health for people with mental disorders. Along a time continuum, the parameters used are acute (8 to 12 weeks), continuation (4 months to 1 year), and maintenance (greater than 1 year periods). Physical activity treatment modalities include (1) **monotherapy** (only treatment), (2) as an **augmentation** (in addition to therapies such as medications), and (3) as an **adjunct therapy** (providing health benefits other than treating the disorder). Currently, research supports physical activity only as an adjunct therapy because other mental health treatment modalities appear more effective.[14]

### Physical Activity and Cognitive Function

Do individuals who are physically active have better cognitive function compared to those who are inactive? Or, do school children who are more physically fit do better academically? Emerging scientific evidence suggests that the answer may be "Yes." Researchers investigating the brain function outcomes shown in Figure 8.3 in relationship to physical activity and exercise have reported many positive associations. The popular media often promote sound bites implying a cause and effect relationship between

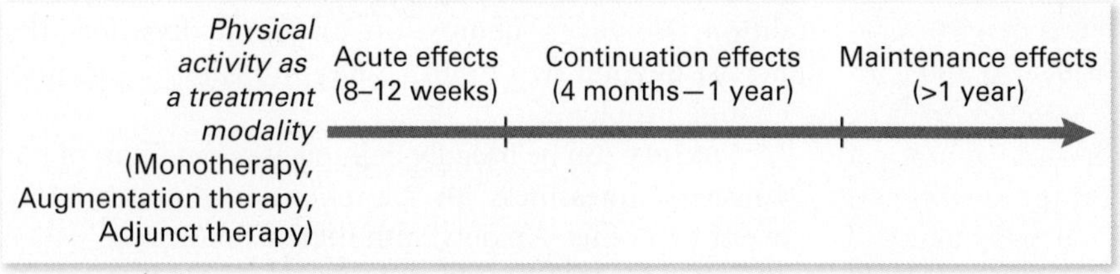

| Physical activity as a treatment modality (Monotherapy, Augmentation therapy, Adjunct therapy) | Acute effects (8–12 weeks) | Continuation effects (4 months—1 year) | Maintenance effects (>1 year) |

**Figure 8.2** | Framework for Ways in Which Physical Activity and Exercise Can Be Used and Evaluated over Time for People with Mental Disorders

*Source:* Adapted from A. L. Dunn and J. S. Jewell, "The Effects of Exercise on Mental Health," *Current Sports Medicine Reports* 9 (2010): 202–207.

regular exercise participation and improved brain function when describing these findings. However, definitive conclusions about the effects of physical activity and exercise on brain function cannot yet be drawn.

### Physical Activity and Feelings of Psychological Distress

A summary of research findings of several studies regarding the relationships between low, moderate, and vigorous levels of physical activity and feelings of distress is shown in Figure 8.4. Participation in moderate-intensity physical activities is related to a significantly lower risk of feelings of distress than maintaining a low level of physical activity. An interesting additional observation from this figure is that, while reported feelings of distress are lower at the highest level of physical activity, the more dramatically lower level of distress is between those who do very little activity and those who do a moderate amount. Thus, the mental health benefits of physical activity appear to be attainable with a moderate level of physical activity—they aren't reserved for those who are the most active.

### Physical Activity and Sleep

Sleep is that necessary time when we recharge our minds and our bodies. As a college student, you may identify with the nearly one third of adults in the United States who suffer from insomnia yearly, or the many who are sleep deprived.[15] Although sleep has been recognized as essential to good mental health since the time of the ancient Greeks, researchers have only recently begun to systematically study the relationships among sleep, physical activity, and exercise. Insufficient sleep is associated with many chronic diseases and conditions such as diabetes, cardiovascular disease, obesity, and depression. Currently, the U.S. National Heart, Lung, and Blood Institute recommends that adults sleep seven to eight hours per night.[16] Emerging evidence suggests that those who participate in regular physical activity have better quality of sleep compared to those who are sedentary. Conversely, a sufficient amount and quality of sleep have also been found to be important for effective post-training recovery among those working daily at high performance levels (e.g., athletes).

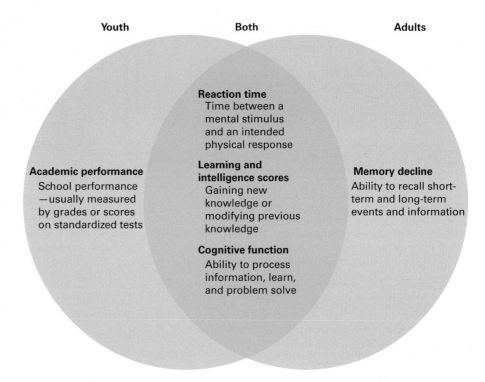

**Figure 8.3** | Brain and Cognitive Function Outcomes in Youth and Adults That Have Been Studied for Associations with Physical Activity and Exercise

Source: From H. Kohl and T. Murray, *Foundations of Physical Activity and Public Health* (Champaign, IL: Human Kinetics, 2012), 160.

Some of the documented health benefits associated with mental health and physical activity are summarized in Table 8.1.

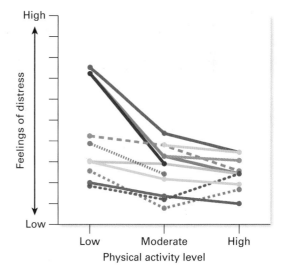

**Figure 8.4** | Physical Activity and Feelings of Distress (Studies Conducted from 1995–2007). The figure represents the research findings of several studies.

*Source:* Adapted from *Physical Activity Guidelines Advisory Committee Report, 2008* (Washington, DC: U.S. Department of Health and Human Services, 2008), available from health.gov/paguidelines/report/pdf/committeereport.pdf, G8–G22.

**Table 8.1** | Summary of Mental Health Benefits of Participating in Physical Activities

> There is clear evidence that physical activity reduces the risk of depression and cognitive decline in adults and older adults. There is some evidence that physical activity improves sleep. There is limited evidence that physical activity reduces distress and anxiety.

> Compared with inactive people, people who are physically active have a 20% to 30% lower risk of depression, distress, and dementia.

> There appears to be a positive dose-response relationship between physical activity and mental health. Moderate and high levels of physical activity are similarly associated with lower risk of depression and distress, compared to low levels of physical activity exposure, which is nonetheless more protective than inactivity or very low levels of physical activity.

> There is insufficient evidence to determine whether there is a dose-response relationship between physical activity and anxiety, cognitive health, or sleep.

> The physical activity dose associated with mental health benefits is a program of three to five days per week, 30 to 60 minutes per session, and moderate to vigorous intensity.

> However, the minimal or optimal type or amount of exercise for mental health is not yet known.

*Source:* Physical Activity Guidelines Advisory Committee, *Physical Activity Guidelines Committee Report, 2008* (Washington, DC: U.S. Department of Health and Human Services, 2008).

## Basic Physiological Responses and Movement Benefits of Participation in Physical Activities for Those with Mental Health Disorders

The basic physiologic and movement benefits of physical activity that improve mental health are difficult to quantify. They are probably unlike the other health benefits you have learned about thus far, which demonstrate a dose-response relationship associated with physical activity participation (e.g., aerobic, strength, and energy expenditure). Important questions can include: Is there a specific pattern of physical activity that optimizes stress management? Is one type of activity more effective in controlling depression? Is such activity, but done at a different intensity, also helpful in maintaining cognitive function? The answers to these questions are unknown but most likely would vary between individuals. Although specific dose-related effects have not been established, a theoretical relationship between the dose of physical activity and stress can be described, as shown in Figure 8.5. The point at which individuals or populations move from normal stress (**eustress**) and an optimal level of stress to distress is highly variable and unique to each individual or population.

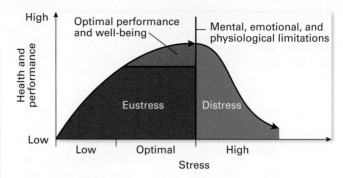

**Figure 8.5** | A Theoretical Relationship between the Dose of Physical Activity and Stress. Specific dose-related effects have not been established, and optimal levels of stress to distress are highly variable and unique to each individual or population.

The unifying principle of overload (Chapter 4) suggests that a system must be stressed (overloaded) for a physical training effect to occur. Is there, similarly, a minimum intensity of exercise or physical activity that is needed to trigger mental health benefits? According to the best scientific evidence, there is a threshold for attaining these benefits, and it cannot be reached through light-intensity activity. Based on neurobiology studies, it does not appear that engaging in light physical activities (< 3 METS), such as slow walking or strolling and performing basic activities of daily living, is enough to produce positive mental health benefits. Most physiological, biomechanical, and behavioral benefits of physical activity on mental health are tied to changes in brain and nervous system function. These changes may best be observed and evaluated by using the framework described previously in Figure 8.2.

A list of the adaptations associated with physical activity and related to mental health is shown in Table 8.2.

**Table 8.2** | Mental Health-Related Adaptations to Physical Activity

| | |
|---|---|
| **PHYSIOLOGICAL** | Improved cerebral capillary growth and development |
| | Improved brain blood flow and oxygenation |
| | Hypothesized increased cerebral nervous activation |
| | Improved regulation of neurotransmitters (promoting hormone function) |
| | Increased growth and maintenance of brain nerve cells and nervous transmission |
| **BIOMECHANICAL** | Improved movement economy |
| | Improved balance, stability, and mobility |
| | Improved peripheral proprioception |
| **BEHAVIORAL/PSYCHOLOGICAL** | Increased self-esteem |
| | Increased well-being |
| | Increased self-efficacy |

*Source:* Physical Activity Guidelines Advisory Committee, *Physical Activity Guidelines Committee Report* (Washington, DC: U.S. Department of Health and Human Services, 2008).

# Mental Health Strategies for Achieving Physical Fitness and Peak Physical Activity Performance

In addition to the role that exercise and physical activity play in promoting mental health, researchers have devoted substantial attention to the mental aspects of training and sports competition. Sport/exercise psychologists have identified a variety of science-based strategies from the fields of motor learning, motor behavior, motor development, sociology, and psychology that can help kinesiology practitioners improve their clients' specific goal oriented physical fitness and peak physical activity performance. By effectively applying the strategies related to the specific psychosocial influences in Figure 8.1, you can help people become more physically active along the physical activity continuum based upon their goals (e.g., functional health and meeting guidelines, physical fitness, or peak performance). Key concepts or strategies include coaching, personality traits, goal setting and record keeping, motivation, arousal regulation, mental practice and coaching, pleasure, self-talk cues, relaxation, sleep, social support, stage of change motivational readiness, and prompting.

## Coaching

We have all probably had a coach help us improve our physical activity performance in sports or in a school extracurricular activity (e.g., band, drill team, or choir) as a child or adolescent. Coaching is important at every level of the physical activity continuum and helps us integrate all the physical and mental aspects of improvement in physical activities and exercise outcomes (see Figure 8.1). For example, a wellness coach can help those who are sedentary achieve functional health and personal goal-oriented levels of physical fitness. Personal trainers (see Chapter 10 to learn more about personal training) and sports coaches (see Chapter 12 to learn more about coaching) specialize in helping individuals achieve their peak performance goals.

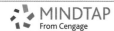

**Coaching**

**Go to your MindTap course** to learn more about the coaching profession and the physical activity continuum.

## Personality Traits

Individual and population personality traits influence thoughts, feelings, and behaviors related not only to becoming and remaining physically active, but also to achieving physical fitness and high levels of performance. A good coach understands how to identify personality types and tailor individualized physical activity programming using various psychosocial influences for success. Scientific evidence supports the notion that certain personality traits are associated with higher levels of participation and success in physical activity and exercise. These traits include greater self-confidence, better coping skills, increased ability to focus, greater capacity to redirect feelings of anxiety into positive prompts, and more drive or willpower to succeed.

## Goal Setting and Record Keeping

Goal setting and record keeping are two strategies coaches and sport/exercise psychologists use to improve physical activity performance. Quite simply, if there is no training goal, you won't know when you have succeeded. Moreover, if you don't keep track of your progress toward a goal you have set, you will never know if you reach it. Goal setting and record keeping are fundamental behavioral strategies that have been used by coaches and their high-performance athletes for many years. Major George Corbari, the former executive officer of the Center for Enhanced Performance at the United States Military Academy at West Point, has recommended seven goal-setting steps for practitioners trying to assist individuals with improving their performance.[17]

1. Have the individual define his or her performance dream
2. Assess the individual's ability to achieve the dream
3. Develop subgoals (4–5) based on barriers to achieving the dream
4. Make a plan of action based on these subgoals
5. Set and pursue short-term goals that help achieve subgoals
6. Commit to the goals set
7. Continually log and monitor progress using a journal or spreadsheet

Numerous social media (e.g., texting and social messaging) and other electronic aids (e.g., cell phone and stand-alone devices) are readily available to allow kinesiology practitioners to help clients with goal setting and record keeping. While social media and other electronic aids have become globally popular, there is currently insufficient evidence to show that they are in and of themselves effective in helping individuals become more physically active.[18] Emerging evidence does suggest that many researchers feel they will have significant influences on increasing individual and population physical activity in the near future, as new strategies are developed that further link technology and behavior.

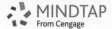
## Motivation

Although it makes practical sense that high-performance athletes would be motivated to achieve success, stimulating and nurturing motivation for physical activity is complex. Motivation as a concept includes **extrinsic motivation** (external input, e.g., encouragement from a coach or kinesiology practitioner or incentives such as a trophy or cash) and **intrinsic motivation** (internal input that provides feelings of pleasure and success). Relative to the physical activity continuum, extrinsic motivation with incentives is probably the most effective approach for motivating a sedentary person to become physically active. To successfully achieve the maintenance level (see behavioral change model discussion in Chapter 7) or peak performance level,

individuals typically need to acquire higher levels of intrinsic rather than extrinsic motivation.

## Arousal

**Arousal** refers to the drive or willpower to engage in physical activity or exercise at peak levels (competition) and is related to the trait and state anxiety of competitors. As shown in Figure 8.6, conflicting theories regarding the association of arousal with peak performance include the drive, inverted U, individual point, and other theories.

**Drive theory** suggests that the more a coach or kinesiology practitioner motivates a competitor, the higher that competitor's arousal and, therefore, the better her or his performance will be. Do you think this is true? Or can athletes become too psyched up to compete and then perform poorly (choke)? The **inverted U theory** suggests that individuals reach an optimal level of arousal, beyond which their arousal levels drop off and their peak performance decreases. The optimal arousal for an individual is dependent upon how an individual perceives the intensity of a specific task and how it creates a low, medium, or high level of anxiety. Viewing anxiety as generally positive leads to better performance. However, too much anxiety may cause too much stress and can be associated with poor performance. Do you think arousal levels affect confidence levels during competition? The **individual point theory** suggests that a coach or kinesiology practitioner needs to tailor motivation and feedback to the needs of each individual he or she works with to optimize arousal levels for peak performance. Therefore, like the arrows to the right and left shown on the inverted U theory graph, there is a continuum (or sliding scale) of arousal levels that are consistent with optimizing an individual's peak performance.

## Mental Practice/Imagery

Mental practice refers to the practicing of mental skills that can enhance physical activity performance. These mental techniques promote both future positive peak performance and learning from past positive and negative experiences. One of many examples of mental practice is **imagery**, the ability to create or recreate a physical activity or exercise experience. The ability to visualize and reflect on physical activity performances has been found to improve physical fitness levels and maximum performance. Good coaches are effective at teaching mental imagery skills.

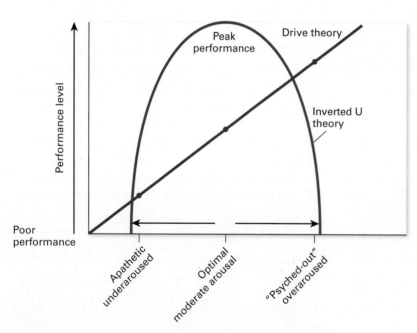

**Figure 8.6** | Example of Theories Associated with Maximizing Arousal for Physical Activity and Especially for Peak Performance. To optimize arousal, one needs to focus a variety of strategies to help develop the drive and willpower to engage in regular physical activity (arrows in the figure pointing left and right on inverted U indicates there may be individual point fluctuation in optimal arousal for peak performance). See the text for more details about arousal theories.

*Source:* Based on R. Pate, B. McClenaghan, and R. Rotella, *Scientific Foundations of Coaching* (Philadelphia: Saunders College Publishing, 1984).

## Pleasure

It seems simplistic to acknowledge the fact that achieving physical fitness and peak levels of performance are associated with intense pleasure for average and elite performers. However, the pleasure and displeasure associated with physical activity and exercise have recently been shown to affect the maintenance of intensity levels all across the physical activity continuum.[19] Coaches and kinesiology practitioners should remember that pleasure (e.g., fun and play) is an important variable that affects the ability to achieve the maintenance stage (in the stage of change model), achieve peak performance, and avoid long periods of relapse all across the physical activity continuum.

## Self-Talk Cues: Attentional Focus

Elite physical performers possess a greater ability to focus on specific cues that improve peak performances than do less active individuals. Attentional focus refers to one's ability to concentrate on what is important for peak performance while ignoring or minimizing the attention paid to negative cues (like high levels of state anxiety and being overanxious). Elite physical activity performers also have better-developed mental skills (inherent and learned) such as **self-talk cues**. Appropriate self-talk cues allow them both to **associate**—that is, to focus on their body's feedback (e.g., breathing, heart rate, muscle pain) during exercise and adjust their movements accordingly—and to **disassociate**—that is, to ignore or suppress their body's feedback during exhaustive exercise (e.g., running a marathon).

## Relaxation

Relaxation techniques help to reduce competitive stress in athletes as well as the daily distress resulting from situations we all face as individuals. The combined use of imagery and attentional focus techniques that revolve around the pleasure of participating or competing in physical activities have been advocated by sport/exercise psychologists to reduce anxiety and distress. A variety of stress management techniques, including meditation, breathing techniques, yoga, and Tai Chi, can be used to promote relaxation and reduce distress for individuals and populations across the physical activity continuum.

## Pre-Competitive Routines

Pre-competitive routines and practice (repetition of training) are important factors that affect all levels of physical activity performance. Pre-competition routines are more than rituals (like wearing your lucky socks); they include preparing nutritionally, hydrating, mental focusing, and being prepared for varying conditions (e.g., hot weather, practice game vs. championship game, varying intensity or pacing). Pre-competition routines often include a physical warm-up, focusing on competitive tactics, mental imagery, and equipment checks. Regularly scheduled practice sessions (regular, but not so frequent as to cause overtraining and burnout) and the use of motor learning techniques such as appropriate feedback help shape peak performance and can help individuals prepare their pre-competitive routines. **Feedback** is knowledge about the results of an individual's movements; this includes both intrinsic feedback (information from within) and extrinsic (external) feedback based on observations by a coach, by a crowd, or through video. Feedback can be classified as **knowledge of performance** (**KP**, e.g., how a movement felt or what observers said about it) and **knowledge of results** (**KR**, e.g., personal interpretation or official ruling). Feedback helps those at all skill levels learn and move more effectively. Pre-competitive routines (rituals) are often used by coaches to help athletes warm up, increase attentional focus, achieve appropriate arousal levels, visualize their physical activity performance, and prepare for peak performance.

## Sleep

The process of recovery (or **restoration**) from performing physical activities at high intensities requires athletes and coaches to consider and account for a variety of factors. For example, the amount of time individuals need to recover from peak levels of physical activity sufficiently to perform at high levels again is dependent upon:

1. *Age.* Older individuals usually recover more slowly.
2. *Experience.* More experienced individuals usually recover more quickly.
3. *The environment.* For example, hot weather conditions can increase the time needed for the recovery process.
4. *The volume of physical activity or exercise.* Recovery is complicated (delayed) by several days of high intensity and long durations of training.
5. *Nutrition and fluids.* The slower the rate at which calories, water, and electrolytes are replaced, the slower the recovery.
6. *Sleep.* Lack of sleep inhibits or slows recovery. Competitive athletes often need 9 to 10 hours of sleep nightly to optimize their training. Sleep is one of the most overlooked aspects of training schedules.

Lack of sleep has become a recognized factor associated with poorer mental and physical performances.[20] About one-third of the U.S. adult population suffers from sleep disorders, sleep deprivation, and excessive daytime sleepiness.[21] There is also emerging evidence that many children and adolescents do not get enough quality sleep time to focus well in school and other daily activities.

Sleep in relationship to physical activity has only been a focus of serious study since 2007, but the current evidence from a small number of research studies shows that people who are more physically active report better sleep (less insomnia) than inactive people There is also limited evidence that active people have better quality of sleep than those who are inactive. Clearly, much more research is needed to provide individual dose/response recommendations to optimize sleep in relationship to physical activity participation.

# Behavioral Theories and Theoretical Models of Behavior Change for Physical Activity Promotion

Behavioral scientists rely on theories and theoretical models to explain and predict health behaviors, behavioral changes, and the maintenance of behaviors. These theories and theoretical models are important guides for individual-focused programs and promotion projects for physical activity. Typically, theoretical models are used to determine what outcomes can be expected when helping individuals adopt the skills they need to begin or continue physical activity.

Some people remain regular exercisers for their entire adult lives, whereas others have never exercised even once. What psychological principles differentiate these two types of people? Is it possible to predict who will be active and who won't? Behavioral scientists often rely on theories of human behavior to try to make such predictions. Five popular behavior theories and theoretical models that you first learned about in Chapter 7 (review Table 7.11) have been used to explain and predict the physical activity behavior of individuals.

Although a complete treatment of each aspect of these theories and models is beyond the scope of this textbook, it is important to be familiar with them and with the constructs they are designed to influence. Different scientists prefer different behavior change theories or models. Unfortunately, no single theory or model has proven to excel in its ability to predict behavior change and maintenance. Each has strengths and weaknesses based on, many believe, the varying effects of the environment on individual behavior. Chapter 13 provides a more in-depth discussion of environmental influences on physical activity behavior.

**Decisional balance** refers to a person's ability to weigh the pros and cons of being physically active and to take action based on that balance. For example, in the transtheoretical model of behavioral change (also see Chapter 7), the cons are perceived as outweighing the pros in the precontemplation and contemplation stages, whereas the pros should outweigh the cons in the action and maintenance stages.

**Self-efficacy** in physical activity behavior refers to a person's confidence in his or her ability to be physically active and deal with the external threats and barriers that could slow, stop, or reverse progress. Research has identified self-efficacy as a key construct of several of the health behavior theories in Table 7.11. Strategies appropriate for each stage of motivational readiness incorporate some form of skills training to enhance self-efficacy for becoming and remaining physically active.

## Barriers to Physical Activity

What keeps us from being physically active? Not enough time is the number one reason people don't exercise at levels recommended for health enhancement. Individually adapted behavior change programs for physical activity promotion frequently incorporate strategies for helping people identify and overcome barriers. Barriers are the real or perceived factors that hinder or prevent increases in physical activity. Identifying barriers can help people prioritize physical activity. Once the barriers are identified, strategies can be developed to overcome them.

A short quiz that is useful in identifying barriers to physical activity is shown in Table 8.3. Do any of these barriers apply to you? What strategies might be useful in overcoming the barriers and making physical activity a priority in your life?

## Social Support for Health Behavior Change

Related to, but distinct from, theories of behavior change is the concept of social support. **Social support** refers to the degree to which people perceive that they are receiving assistance to overcome health challenges. Social support is thought to be key to promoting physical activity, either integrated into the existing health behavior theories and models reviewed earlier or as a stand-alone strategy.

Social support has been foundational to attempts to understand health behavior change and maintenance for years. The value placed on social support stems from observations that people with shared experiences and goals benefit from the support they receive from others. This support can take many forms: two people who want to become more physically active begin to walk together in the mornings before work; a wife encourages her husband to restart a physical activity program; or a mother enables her child to participate in a sport league after school. Each of these examples (and others) constitutes some form of social support for physical activity.

The three basic types of social support are perceived, received, and connected.[22] Perceived support refers to the perception that one is adequately supported. For example, a woman who knows she can count on a church friend or friends to walk with her when she needs company

**Table 8.3** | Barriers to Being Physically Active

| HOW LIKELY ARE YOU TO SAY? | VERY LIKELY | SOMEWHAT LIKELY | SOMEWHAT UNLIKELY | VERY UNLIKELY |
|---|---|---|---|---|
| 1. My day is so busy now, I just don't think I can make the time to include physical activity in my regular schedule. | 3 | 2 | 1 | 0 |
| 2. None of my family members or friends like to do anything active, so I don't have a chance to exercise. | 3 | 2 | 1 | 0 |
| 3. I'm just too tired after work to get any exercise | 3 | 2 | 1 | 0 |
| 4. I've been thinking about getting more exercise, but I just can't seem to get started. | 3 | 2 | 1 | 0 |
| 5. I'm getting older so exercise can be risky. | 3 | 2 | 1 | 0 |
| 6. I don't get enough exercise because I have never learned the skills for any sport. | 3 | 2 | 1 | 0 |
| 7. I don't have access to jogging trails, swimming pools, bike paths, etc. | 3 | 2 | 1 | 0 |
| 8. Physical activity takes too much time away from others commitments—time, work family, etc. | 3 | 2 | 1 | 0 |
| 9. I'm embarrassed about how I will look when I exercise with others. | 3 | 2 | 1 | 0 |
| 10. I don't get enough sleep as it is. I just couldn't get up early or stay up late to get some exercise. | 3 | 2 | 1 | 0 |
| 11. It's easier for me to find excuses not to exercise than to go out to do something. | 3 | 2 | 1 | 0 |
| 12. I know of to many people who have hurt themselves by overdoing it with exercise. | 3 | 2 | 1 | 0 |
| 13. I really can't see learning a new sport at my age. | 3 | 2 | 1 | 0 |
| 14. It's just too expensive. You have to take a class or join a club or buy the right equipment. | 3 | 2 | 1 | 0 |
| 15. My free time during the day are too short to include exercise. | 3 | 2 | 1 | 0 |
| 16. My usual social activities with family or friends do not include physical activity. | 3 | 2 | 1 | 0 |
| 17. I'm too tired during the week, and I need the weekend to catch up on my rest. | 3 | 2 | 1 | 0 |
| 18. I want to get more exercise, but I just can't seem to make myself stick to anything. | 3 | 2 | 1 | 0 |
| 19. I'm afraid I might injure myself or have a heart attack. | 3 | 2 | 1 | 0 |
| 20. I'm not good enough at any physical activity to make it fun. | 3 | 2 | 1 | 0 |
| 21. If we had exercise facilities and showers at work, then I would be more likely to exercise. | 3 | 2 | 1 | 0 |

Follow these instructions to score yourself:

1. Enter the circled number from each of the 21 items in the Barriers to Being Active Quiz above in the numbered spac provided below, putting together the number for statement 1 on line 1, statement 2 on line 2, and so on.

2. Add the three scores on each line. Your barriers to physical activity fall into one or more of seven categories: lack time, social influences, lack of energy, lack of willpower, fear of injury, lack of skill, and lack of resources. A score of 5 or above in any category shows that this is an important barrier for you to overcome.

| — + — + — = _____ | | | — + — + — = _____ | |
|---|---|---|---|---|
| 1   8   15 | Lack of time | | 5   12   19 | Fear of injury |
| — + — + — = _____ | | | — + — + — = _____ | |
| 2   9   16 | Social influence | | 6   13   20 | Lack of skill |
| — + — + — = _____ | | | — + — + — = _____ | |
| 3   10   17 | Lack of energy | | 7   14   21 | Lack of resources |
| — + — + — = _____ | | | | |
| 4   11   18 | Lack of willpower | | | |

*Source:* U.S. Department of Health and Human Services, Public Health Service, Centers for Disease Control and Prevention, National Center for Chronic Disease Prevention and Health Promotion, Division of Nutrition and Physical Activity, *Promoting Physical Activity: A Guide for Community Action* (Champaign, IL: Human Kinetics, 1999), 100–101.

experiences perceived support for physical activity. Received support is more direct and measurable; it refers to the amount of support a person can rely on. An example of this is a basketball team that must have five members to play. Each member trusts the others to show up at the designated time and place so the team can play. Finally, connected support refers to the degree to which a person is socially integrated. Social integration provides implicit social support as a result of the connections made through participation. Examples of sources of connected support include clubs, communities, community events such as fun runs, the workplace, and family and friends. Connected support is thought to be helpful in physical activity promotion because of the experiences that can be shared through a social network.

Behavioral and social approaches for physical activity promotion involve two basic strategies. First, people can be instructed in behavior change and management skills according to one of the health behavior theories or theoretical models in Table 7.11. Second, supportive social and physical environments conducive to physical activity behaviors can also be constructed. These strategies are complementary. Behavioral approaches give people the skills to be physically active and to overcome barriers to being active. Social approaches make it easier to use those skills.

Behavioral and social approaches increase physical activity participation as part of leisure, occupation, transportation, or at-home activities. Like informational approaches, behavioral and social approaches to increase physical activity are based on the theory that when people are told to engage in specific health behaviors that are generally perceived as being good for them (e.g., improving health), they will change their behavior.

### Point-of-Decision Prompting

Prompting (a visual or audio cue or reminder) is a technique typically used to increase physical activity in an individually adapted behavior change program, but can be aimed at larger groups of people as well. **Point-of-decision prompting** is a scientifically proven strategy for physical activity promotion that is similar to other individually based prompting strategies. At a point of decision (e.g., to make an active choice or a sedentary choice), the prompt is placed to encourage selection of the active choice. These strategies have most often been used at elevators and escalators in buildings where choosing to walk the stairs is a reasonable and convenient alternative. Evidence suggests that up to 10% more people take the stairs up rather than riding the escalator when influenced by point of decision prompts.

## Common Testing and Monitoring of Mental Health and Physical Activity Outcomes

Tests that are used to evaluate, diagnose, and treat mental disorders are used by physicians and sport/exercise psychologists with research interests in studying physical activity and exercise behavior. Mental health screening tests include self-administered questions (see the targeted learning activities at end of the chapter), in-person interviews and counseling sessions, and observational studies. It is important for kinesiology professionals to understand that mental health screenings can help encourage positive physical activity and exercise behaviors among individuals and populations. However, the tests should not be abused or used to stereotype behaviors or promote barriers to participation. Also, the tests are best used by trained professionals.

An extensive review of the numerous mental health assessments related to participating in physical activity and exercise is beyond the scope of this text. However, one example of a commonly used assessment of mood disorders is described here to provide you with insight into how sport/exercise psychologists might use such tools to predict peak performance. The Profile of Mood States (POMS) is a based on responses to a questionnaire that was initially designed to evaluate mood disorders among college students. The POMS includes a series of questions and includes key markers such as tension-anxiety, depression-dejection, anger-hostility, vigor, fatigue-inertia, and confusion-bewilderment (see Figure 8.7). All the POMS markers except vigor are negative relative to mood states.

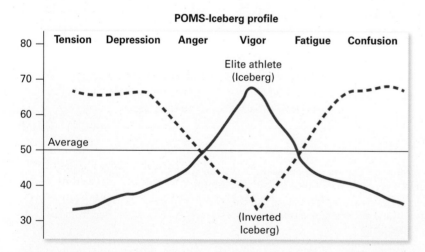

**Figure 8.7 | The Profile of Moods.** This shows an "iceberg" profile for an elite athlete who is primed for peak performance due to low levels of tension, depression, anger, fatigue, and confusion, but high levels of vigor. The inverted iceberg profile shows someone with an opposite profile and is consistent with poor physical performance.

*Source:* Adapted from W. P. Morgan and M. L. Pollock, "Psychological Characterization of the Elite Distance Runner," *Annals of the New York Academy of Science* 301 (1977): 382–403; W. P. Morgan, "Negative Addiction in Runners," *The Physician and Sports Medicine* 7, no. 2 (1979): 56–63, 67–69.

In the 1970s, William P. Morgan, Ph.D. became the first sport/exercise psychologist to use the POMS to compare high-level performing athletes (such as elite runners and winter Olympics competitors) with average college students. In a series of studies, Morgan and colleagues found that athletes reported significantly higher levels of vigor and received lower mood state scores for tension, anger, depression, fatigue, and confusion, which they termed the "Iceberg Profile."[23,24] Morgan also demonstrated that athletic POMS scores that changed over time were associated with an inverted Iceberg Profile, which indicated overtraining and staleness. Both the Iceberg Profile and its inversion are depicted in Figure 8.7.

## Physical Disabilities

Although physical disabilities are not explicitly associated with poor mental health, people with physical disabilities can experience the same types of mental health disorders as able-bodied people. And athletes who compete with a physical disability face similar performance issues as able-bodied athletes. Individuals with physical disabilities are among the **understudied populations**—groups who have not been scientifically studied as extensively as others.[25] This is an unfortunate situation throughout health and medicine disciplines, and the field of kinesiology is no different. For example, oftentimes solid scientific evidence regarding physical activity and exercise patterns and outcomes for individuals of a certain sex and/or race/ethnicity, of low social economic status, or with certain physical disabilities is limited. Behavioral strategies that successfully promote physical activity among children with disabilities are probably very different from those that have proven useful for able-bodied children. Likewise, coaching techniques that work for professional golfers may or may not be transferrable to wheelchair athletes.

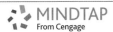

### The Americans with Disabilities Act

**Go to your MindTap course** to learn more about The Americans with Disabilities Act of 1990 (ADA). The ADA prohibits discrimination against people with physical disabilities and ensures equal opportunity for persons with disabilities in employment, state and local government services, public accommodations, commercial facilities, and transportation. Much progress has been made in the United States since the original ADA of 1990 was passed. The ADA regulations were updated in 2010.

Individuals with physical disabilities may also experience underlying mental challenges such as depression, anxiety, and chronic pain, all of which you have learned about. However, all individuals with physical disabilities

must face the mental challenge of regaining as much mobility and functional health as possible, and staying as physically active as possible for health's sake.

Physical disabilities related to physical activity that have been commonly studied include lower limb loss, cerebral palsy, multiple sclerosis, mood, anxiety, Parkinson's disease, spinal cord injury, stroke, and traumatic brain injury. Commonly promoted kinesiology subdiscipline strategies related to achieving higher levels of physical activity, physical fitness, and peak performance for those with physical disabilities include adapted physical education (see Chapter 11 for more), physical therapy, occupational therapy, athletic training, and transitional programming such as the Warrior Games that help wounded veterans return to sports, the Special Olympics, and the Paralympics.

Physical activity is important to health for all people, regardless of their physical or mental capacity. It is important for kinesiology professionals to understand how to adjust physical activity programming not only for people with mental health disorders, but also for those with physical disabilities, because they are at higher risk for developing additional serious health problems if they become or remain sedentary. Table 8.4 shows that adults with physical disabilities in the past have been found to be significantly less physically active than their nondisabled counterparts, and that they participate in less regular, and less vigorous, physical activities. It has also been reported that those with physical disabilities have more secondary problems such as fatigue, weight gain, deconditioning, and pain, which are associated directly or indirectly with their disability.[26]

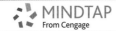

### Healthy People 2020: Disability and Health

**Go to your MindTap course** to learn more about Healthy People 2020 and the physical activity objectives for those with disabilities.

Table 8.4 | Comparison of Physical Activity Prevalences for Adults with Disabilities and without Disabilities

| | WITH DISABILITIES | WITHOUT DISABILITIES |
|---|---|---|
| No leisure time activity | 56% | 36% |
| 30 minutes activity 5 + days per week | 12% | 16% |
| 20 minutes vigorous physical activity for cardiorespiratory fitness 3+ days per week | 13% | 25% |

*Source:* Physical Activity Guidelines Advisory Committee, *Physical Activity Guidelines Committee Report* (Washington, DC: U.S. Department of Health and Human Services, 2008), Table G11.1.

# EXAMPLES OF APPLYING MENTAL HEALTH, PSYCHOLOGY, AND PHYSICAL ACTIVITY BASICS IN RELATIONSHIP TO THE KINESIOLOGY SUBDISCIPLINES

*In Lesson 1, you learned about the basics of integrating mental health, psychology, and the physical activity continuum. You learned about some of the basic mental health concepts and strat-* *egies that can be used when working with individuals and populations to acquire health, physical fitness, or peak performance benefits. In Lesson 2, you will learn through real-life examples*

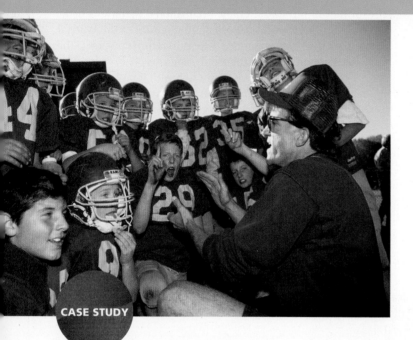

CASE STUDY

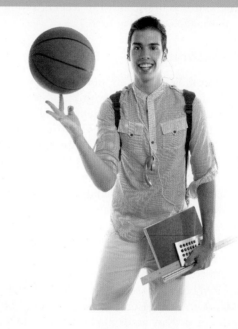

## In the real world . . .

As you will recall from earlier in this chapter, Cara Casey is being encouraged by her friend Amy to think about trying out for cross-country in high school, because Amy thinks very highly of her coach for including mental preparation in his training program. Coach Glenn had previously coached cross-country at the local university, and he had been successful at winning conference championships and preventing overtraining and burnout in his runners. He first used the POMS questionnaire (assisted by a colleague of his who was a sport psychologist) with his college runners to evaluate their mood states in relation to their psychological vigor (or drive) to perform.

In his first year of collegiate coaching, Glenn was told by the previous coach that the cross country team from the last three years had the talent to potentially win a conference title, but many of the runners got injured or burned out between August and the championship meet in the first

week of November. Coach Glenn wondered if these runners simply became over-trained, or if they were just not ready to give their best performances at the championship meet.

In his first season of coaching, Coach Glenn decided to monitor his runners' mental states by administering the POMS questionnaire to them at the beginning of the school year (August), at mid-term (October), and during the week before conference championships (November). He knew that the normal POMS results for elite athletes showed significantly higher levels of vigor and lower mood state scores for tension, anger, depression, fatigue, and confusion. Though not all his athletes were necessarily elite, as a group they showed similar POMS results as better runners (a little lower on vigor than reported for elite athletes; please review Figure 8.7) in August. By October, the athletes reported significantly increased levels of tension, anger, depression, fatigue, and confusion, while vigor had significantly dropped. Coach Glenn speculated that the runners were getting over-trained due to the normal mid-term challenges

*how mental health and sport/exercise psychology concepts are related to physical activity principles and the subdisciplines of kinesiology across the physical activity continuum.*

▶ Exercise Physiology
▶ Biomechanics
▶ Public Health
▶ Sport/Exercise Psychology
▶ Motor Learning
▶ Practice of Kinesiology

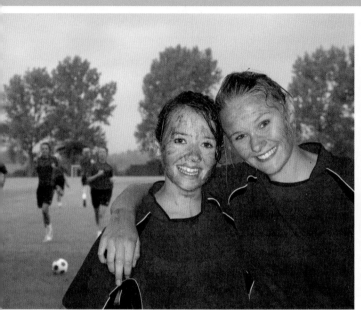

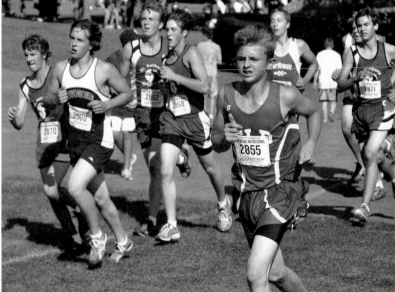

of collegiate athletes in training (e.g., lack of sleep, stress of mid-term tests, training regimen), so he decided to modify the overload aspects of their weekly training (reduce the volume of training; see Chapter 4) and encouraged his runners to employ effective strategies to optimize recovery from training.

When the runners completed the POMS in November, Coach Glenn was excited because his runners' vigor had increased back to the August levels and the scores for tension, anger, depression, fatigue, and confusion had fallen. At the conference meet a few days later, both his women's and men's teams triumphed. Coach Glenn was voted "Coach of the Year" by his coaching peers because they were impressed not only by his running knowledge but also his skill at monitoring the moods of his athletes. While

he was proud of his runners and happy for the recognition, Coach Glenn knew that the POMS was not a magic bullet that guaranteed success. Rather, like many mental health assessments, the POMS is an effective tool to provide insight about mood states and help identify when it is appropriate to modify physical activity to improve performance. Effective mental health training for athletes can help maximize performances while reducing the risks of adverse events like overtraining and burnout.

| 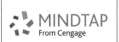 | Go to your MindTap course to complete the Case Study activity for this chapter. |

## Exercise Physiology 🌐

A common psychobiological tool used by many exercise physiologists during exercise testing (and sometimes training) is the Borg Ratings of Perceived Exertion (RPE) Scales, shown in Figure 8.8. The scale on the left with ratings of 6–20 is the original scale that Dr. Gunnar Borg developed by exercise testing subjects and questioning them regarding their overall feelings of bodily responses with respect to various variables like heart rate, breathing, sweating, and leg pain. The participants reported a number that best reflected how they felt at each stage of the test through the verbal anchors (e.g., very, very light; very light; and so on). Dr. Borg found that a rating of 6

was consistent with the physiological markers of sitting, whereas a rating of 20 was associated with maximal exercise effort. This 6–20 scale is appropriate to use when evaluating continuous exercise testing. The 10-point plus scale on the right side of Figure 8.8 is a revised scale that Dr. Borg developed to assess exertion associated with work tasks such as shoveling sand or carrying heavy objects. On this 10-point plus scale, a rating of 0 for a task is associated with rest and a 10 or greater reflects maximal physical effort.

Researchers often use RPE to evaluate exercise intensity. RPE is also useful in predicting work performance to exhaustion. Clinically, RPE can serve as a valuable exercise prescription cue for intensity once individuals learn to accurately assess their bodily feedback.

| CATEGORY SCALE | CATEGORY– RATIO SCALE | |
|---|---|---|
| 6 | 0 Nothing at all | "No intensity" |
| 7 Very, very light | 0.3 | |
| 8 | 0.5 Extremely weak | Just noticeable |
| 9 Very light | 0.7 | |
| 10 | 1 Very weak | |
| 11 Fairly light | 1.5 | |
| 12 | 2 Weak | Light |
| 13 Somewhat hard | 2.5 | |
| 14 | 3 Moderate | |
| 15 Hard | 4 | |
| 16 | 5 Strong | Heavy |
| 17 Very hard | 6 | |
| 18 | 7 Very strong | |
| 19 Very, very hard | 8 | |
| 20 | 9 | |
| | 10 Extremely strong | "Strongest intensity" |
| | 11 | |
| | Absolute maximum | Highest possible |

**Figure 8.8 | The Borg Perceived Exertion Scales.** These scales are psychophysiological in nature and use numbers and verbal anchors to describe overall physical exertion during participation in physical activity or exercise. See text for further description.

*Source:* From G. Borg, "Psychological Bases of Physical Exertion," *Medicine and Science in Sports and Exercise* 14 (1982): 377–381.

## Biomechanics ⚫

One of the most difficult biomechanical challenges an athlete may face is to change her or his sport technique or move from one position to another in a team sport (e.g., offense to defense in football). Have you ever been asked to move to a new position or a new event in a sport or physical activity? How did you feel? You probably felt uncoordinated as you engaged in the activity and awkward when you tried to attend to feedback from your body (proprioception). Coaches need to understand that asking athletes to change position really means asking them to try to change their biomechanics. Often this makes the athlete's movements less economical (or less efficient) instead of more economical, which probably was the coach's initial goal.

As you learned in Chapter 2, individual efficiency like that for running economy includes many factors:

▸ Psychomotor factors: motivated or tried, over-trained

▸ Physiological factors: trained or untrained, maximal heart rate or stroke volume

▸ Biomechanical factors: gait movements, muscle and joint geometry

▸ Biochemical factors: lactate threshold, glycogen depletion, or number of muscle fibers recruited at a given speed

▸ Other factors: training level, gender, experience, age

It has been reported that when coaches try to change an experienced athlete's stride length, it initially causes an increase in energy cost. In other words, there is a loss in efficiency initially and that loss may adversely affect performance. Although the athlete may become more economical (efficient) over time, the time-response for these changes is highly variable and unpredictable. This does not mean one cannot improve biomechanical techniques, but it suggests that a coach or mentor should consider the mental challenges and muscle memory (past motor patterns) involved as well as the new physical movements to be implemented when integrating changes.

## Public Health

Marion is a middle-aged mother of two daughters. She and her husband Andre both work at a university and have each gained a substantial amount of weight in the past 10 years. Although neither has exercised regularly, Marion has been thinking for some time that they both need to increase their weekly exercise and lose weight. One day, Marion noticed an advertisement for a weight-loss study being conducted in the Psychology Department. She convinced Andre to enroll in the 12-week study with her. The essence of the study was that two different behavioral strategies for increasing physical activity were to be tested. She was randomized to a strategy designed to match the person's stage of motivational readiness and help her to become more active by helping her identify and overcome obstacles that are getting in the way of her exercise time. Andre was randomized to the other strategy: providing a health club membership to make it easier to get to the gym during the week.

Because Marion had already been thinking about increasing her exercise time, the research study staff was able to tailor her behavioral strategy to help her problem solve to overcome barriers to exercise. She did not have to be convinced of the importance of exercising; she was already contemplating making a change. However, she thought that she didn't have enough time while working full time and running the household. The behavioral intervention was targeted to this stage of readiness, and Marion was able to exceed the target of 150 minutes per week of moderate-intensity physical activity during 10 out of the 12 study weeks. Combined with dietary restriction, this increase in activity enabled Marion to lose 15 pounds in that time period.

Andre started off very strong in the 12-week study—a free health club membership removes a significant barrier (cost) for many people. He got up each morning and was at the gym by 6:00 a.m., working this visit into his daily routine. After three weeks of regular attendance, however, he started to slow down and miss a few days. Work or other obligations got in the way and he had no tools with which to cope with the barriers. He kept saying to himself that he would resume the next week. Like many people who join gyms as a New Year's resolution, Andre drifted away and by the end of the twelfth week had stopped going altogether. Although he lost weight initially, by the end of the twelfth week he had only lost a total of three pounds.

Because behavioral theories were employed to match Marion's needs and stage of motivational readiness through her behavioral intervention, she was able to initiate and stick with her exercise program. In contrast, Andre, who was not equipped to handle life's barriers because he had no behavioral training, ended up where he began.

## Sport/Exercise Psychology

Jack T. Daniels, Ph.D. has described a model that explains sport/exercise psychology traits (including personality factors) associated with achievement of high levels of running performance.[27] Although Daniels designed his model for evaluating sport psychology factors for runners, the model may also be applied to other situations like predicting academic achievement or career success. In his simple model, Daniels describes four major factors that contribute to running success as (1) opportunity (physical and social environment that encourages one to run); (2) direction or coaching that hopefully is positive, but might be negative or neutral in relationship to performance; (3) inherent ability/genetics or potential; and (4) intrinsic motivation or motive from within. Daniels further suggests that opportunity and direction are not unique to any individual personality; therefore, practitioners can focus on observing potential and intrinsic motivation levels to build strategies to improve running performance based on the scenarios displayed in Table 8.5.

Table 8.5 shows that individuals might present any of four different scenarios regarding their potential and intrinsic motivation. Practitioners can devise strategies to move individuals toward higher levels of physical activity/sport achievement based on the categories they fall into. Individuals rated as level 1 from Table 8.5 are usually champions (peak performers) and can challenge even the best coach or sport/exercise psychologist to develop new strategies to promote further success. Individuals rated as level 2 are capable of high levels of performance but are unenthused about the process (practice or competition), and therefore frustrate

**Table 8.5** | A Simple Personality and Genetic Sport/Exercise Psychology Performance Model

| |
| --- |
| 1 – High potential, high motivation |
| 2 – High potential, lower motivation |
| 3 – Lower potential, high motivation |
| 4 – Lower potential, lower motivation |

*Source:* Adapted from J. Daniels, *Daniels' Running Formula*, 3rd ed. (Champaign, IL: Human Kinetics, 2013).

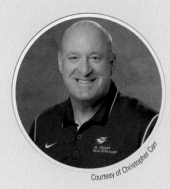
Courtesy of Christopher Carr

**Q:** **Why and how did you get into the field of kinesiology?**

**A:** *I have an undergraduate major in Psychology with a Communications minor; I played DIII college football and did my Masters in Counseling Psychology while working as a GA FB coach and class instructor in the Counseling Psychology department. I then worked four years in adolescent substance abuse treatment and prevention, and during this time learned more about sport psychology. I decided I was most interested in working with injured athletes and wanted to work as a sport psychologist, so I did my Ph.D. in Counseling Psychology but worked with the Chair of the School of Physical Education (Dr. Richard Cox, whose major research/teaching was in sport and exercise psychology) to develop a doctoral minor in Sport Psychology (taking courses in exercise science, motor learning, sociology of sport, and sport psychology). I did my undergraduate at Wabash College and both MA/Ph.D. at Ball State University. I then did the third year of my doctoral program at the U.S. Olympic Training Center (in the sport psychology department) in Colorado Springs, where I had been accepted as a clinical research assistant in Sport Psychology (part of USOC Sport Science Department).*

*My pre-doctoral internship was at The Ohio State University Counseling and Consultation Services; at this time I knew I wanted to work as a counseling sport psychologist and prepared to do so in my future career.*

**Q:** **What was the major influence on you to work in the field?**

**A:** *Having been an athlete in college, and having some experience in coaching, I knew that my passion was in helping athletes to overcome adversities, challenges, and other emotional/mental issues. I knew that if psychologists could be employed in the military and other performance areas, then I could develop a career as a psychologist working with athletes. At the same time, I knew that the field of kinesiology/exercise science would provide me invaluable graduate education into the sport psychology realm and thus I pursued this training in my doctoral degree.*

**Q:** **What are your current research interests, and how do you translate your research results to practitioners?**

**A:** *I am more practitioner than researcher, so my practice is mostly applied work. I*

---

coaches and sport/exercise psychologists. They can usually earn a spot on a sports team and play regularly, but until they become more intrinsically motivated they will probably not reach the performance level of a champion.

Individuals rated as level 3 are excited to do whatever the coach or mentor wants them to do to improve physical activity achievement, but their lower potential can prevent them from doing as well as the level 1 performer. They can make a strong contribution to an athletic team, but they tend to over-train and have unrealistic expectations for success. Individuals on a sports team that have low potential and that are unmotivated (level 4) are usually cut (released) or quit soon. However, kinesiology professionals should recognize that while sports may not appeal to the level-four category person, who shares many characteristics with sedentary individuals, he or she should still be encouraged and educated to be physically active for good health.

## Motor Learning

Sport/exercise psychologists not only work with athletes with psychological training but also work with them to improve their motor skills performance. For example, many professional golfers depend upon sport/exercise psychologists to fine-tune their motor skills because success in golf is very dependent upon repeating movement skills (the golf swing) within a small margin of error. If you have played golf or watched someone play, what were the differences between average and better golfers? Were they all physical in nature (body size, strength, or power) or were some related to mental factors such as concentration, attitude, and personality? What mental skills best enable a competitive golfer to play championship golf?

Most professional golfers would probably agree that to be competitive they need to be able to focus on various cues that allow them to select the correct club, set up a proper stance, initiate and complete a synchronous

*currently work as a consulting sport psychologist to two NCAA Division I athletics departments on a weekly basis, another DI school on a monthly basis, and am the team performance psychologist with an NBA team (sixth year). I work with academic faculty at these institutions to help facilitate relevant research as well as provide supervision for students seeking experience in the counseling sport psychology field.*

**Q:** **How do you stay physically active yourself and promote good health to others directly around you?**

**A:** *I exercise (walk/cardiovascular/weight training) at least three to four times a week, and because I'm around active/athletic clients, I believe this is part of my job (maintaining health/fitness). I also find that exercise is a mental process and allows time for refocus, reflection, and re-evaluation of program plans and current practice.*

**Q:** **How have you had to integrate the subdisciplines of kinesiology in your professional practice?**

**A:** *I believe that my experiences in exercise science (academic/coursework/collaborative*

*training at USOTC w/biomechanics and exercise physiology) have given me a solid foundation to understand the science of sport movement, sports medicine, and sport science. As a psychologist, I believe an integrated and collaborative performance team (e.g., sport psychologists, sports medicine physicians, sports nutritionists, sport science experts) is the most optimal model of care for athletes at all levels of participation, from youth sports to elite competitors.*

*Chris Carr, Ph.D., HSPP, CC-AASP is a Sport and Performance Psychologist at St. Vincent Sports Performance in Indianapolis, IN. He is the consulting performance psychologist for the Indiana Pacers and provides consulting counseling sport psychology services for the Purdue University and Butler University Athletics departments. He also provides sport psychology consulting services for Central Michigan University athletics and consults with other collegiate athletics departments on sport psychology and psychological health care for student-athletes. He is on the U.S. Olympic Committee Sport Psychology Registry (since 1992) and is a licensed psychologist in both Indiana and Michigan. Dr. Carr has been a U.S. team sport psychologist in the 2002 Winter Olympic Games (U.S. Men's Alpine Team) and 2008 Summer Games (U.S. Diving); he has attended over 35 World Championships/World Cups as a team sport psychologist. Dr. Carr has a Ph.D. in Counseling Psychology with a minor in Sport Psychology from Ball State University. A former collegiate football student-athlete, Dr. Carr lives with his wife in Westfield, IN, and his daughter is a senior student-athlete (gymnast) at Central Michigan University.

swing, and follow through properly. Sport/exercise psychologists help golfers learn to master the skills of motor learning such as attentional focus, timing, relaxation, practice and pre-competitive routines, and feedback. They also depend upon using the integrated skills of motor behavior, motor development, and motor control to optimize golf performance.

## The Practice of Kinesiology

What kinds of mental health challenges do you think kinesiology professionals might face when supervising in-patient and out-patient cardiac rehabilitation? Some obvious mental health obstacles that inpatients would face include anxiety, depression, anger, and denial. Cardiac rehabilitation specialists are trained to recognize that anxiety and depression may be prominent in cardiac patients due to concerns about their heart health and future. The effective cardiac rehabilitation specialist

will focus on returning patients quickly to physical activity (based on their clinical status) and helping them learn more about how personally managing their heart health can reduce anxiety and depression. Most inpatients will also express anger and denial as part of their mental healing process. These patients typically wonder why this bad thing (e.g., heart attack or partially blocked artery) happened to them. Eventually, some patients will act as though they did not or do not have a heart problem, or try to demonstrate that they are affected minimally by the event. When cardiac patients experience denial, they may try to do too much physical activity for their clinical condition or ignore the warning signs of heart disease (such as chest pain and shortness of breath) that will increase their chances of another life-threatening event.

Outpatients in cardiac rehabilitation also face a variety of mental challenges and have questions about their heart health such as "Is it safe for me to have sex with my loved one, and if so, when will that be? Is it safe for me to go back to work, and if so, when can I go back? I've never been very physically active before, so how do I stay active to manage my future heart health and reduce my risk for future cardiac events?" As you may have guessed, cardiac specialists are trained to integrate kinesiology principles to provide their patients with specific strategies for returning to normal life (having sex, returning to work, and maintenance of physical activity) appropriate for their various cardiac clinical conditions.

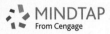 **MINDTAP** From Cengage

Now that you have completed this chapter, go to your MindTap course to complete all assigned activities. Check out the additional resources developed to help you apply the material in this chapter to your course and career goals.

## Chapter Summary

▸ In the United States it has been estimated that more than one in four—over 70 million people—have a mental health problem. The economic costs of mental health disorders total tens of billions of dollars each year, and common mental health disorders like depression and anxiety significantly reduce work productivity.[28]

▸ The mental health problems most commonly studied in relation to physical activity are mood disorders, anxiety, psychological distress and lack of well-being, cognitive function, sleep, and adverse psychological events. Although not a panacea, participation in physical activity seems to help with several disorders.

▸ An emerging body of scientific evidence shows that physical activity lowers the risk for anxiety symptoms, anxiety disorders, depression symptoms, major depressive disorder, and age-related decline in cognitive function. There is also evidence that physical activity enhances psychological well-being and can delay the psychological effects of dementia.

▸ Based on neurobiology studies, it does not appear that engaging in light physical activities (< 3 METS, like slow walking or strolling and performing the basic activities of daily living) is sufficient to produce positive mental health benefits. The physiological, biomechanical, and behavioral benefits of physical activity on mental health are mostly tied to brain and nervous system changes.

▸ The following psychosocial influences can be used to help others meet guidelines and move toward peak performance: personality traits, goal setting, record keeping, motivation, arousal, mental practice/imagery, pleasure, self-talk cues, relaxation, pre-competitive routines, and sleep.

▸ Behavioral scientists rely on theories and theoretical models to explain and predict health behaviors and changes in and maintenance of those behaviors. These theories and theoretical models guide individual-focused programs and promotion projects for physical activity.

## Remember This

adjunct
age-related decline in cognitive function
anorexia nervosa
anxiety
arousal
associate
augmentation
bulimia
decisional balance
depression

disassociate
drive theory
dysthymia
eustress
extrinsic motivation
feedback
health
imagery
individual point theory
intrinsic motivation
inverted U theory

knowledge of performance (KP)
knowledge of results (KR)
mental health
monotherapy
mood disorders
muscle dysmorphia
point-of-decision prompting
Profile of Mood States (POMS)

psychological distress
restoration
self-efficacy
self-esteem
self-talk cues
social support
state anxiety
trait anxiety
understudied populations

# For More Information

Access these websites or Twitter sites for further study of topics covered in the chapter:

- Find updates and quick links to these and other evidence-based practice-related sites in your MindTap course.

- Search for further information about mental health and physical activity at MENPA on Twitter: MENPA @GuyFaulkner.

- Search for information and resources related to the relationships among physical activity, mental health, and understudied populations in the United States at the U.S. Physical Activity Guidelines webpage (www.health.gov/paguidelines) and the U.S. Physical Activity Plan webpage (www.physicalactivityplan.org).

- Search for information about adapted physical education at the Adapted Physical Education National Standards webpage: www.apens.org.

- Search for more information about sport and understudied populations at the Special Olympics website: www.specialolympics.org/.

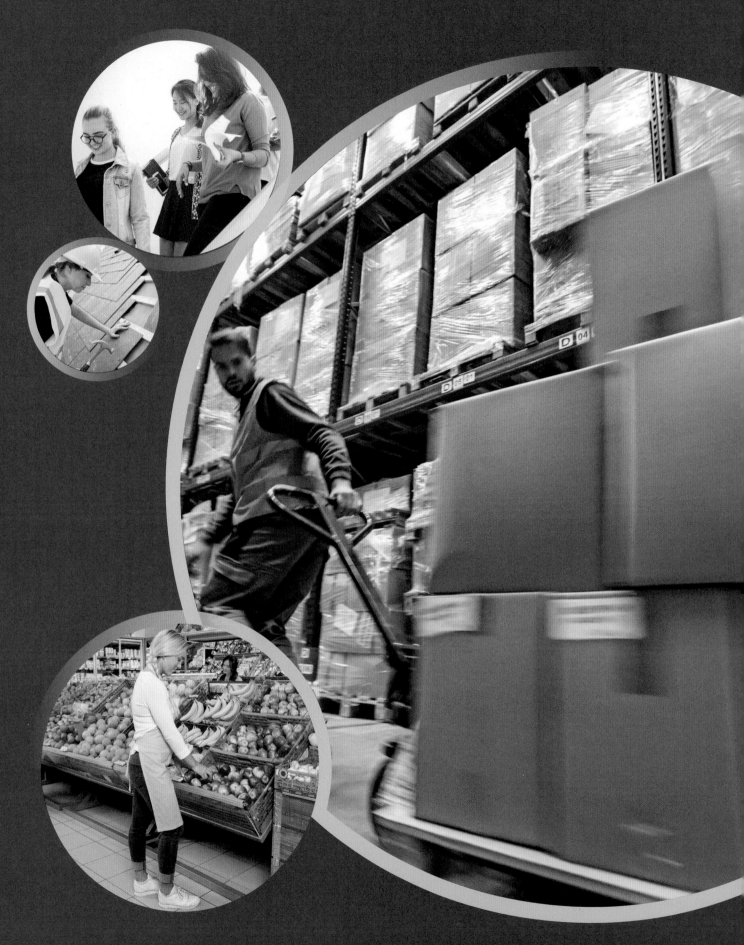

# Integration of Kinesiology and Physical Activity into the Workplace

*What knowledge, skills, and abilities do kinesiology majors need to acquire and use to pursue careers in business and industry?*

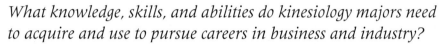

**LESSON 1** INTEGRATION OF BUSINESS AND INDUSTRY WITH THE PRINCIPLES OF PHYSICAL ACTIVITY AND KINESIOLOGY

**LESSON 2** EXAMPLES OF APPLYING BUSINESS AND INDUSTRY PRINCIPLES OF PHYSICAL ACTIVITY IN RELATIONSHIP TO THE KINESIOLOGY SUBDISCIPLINES

## Learning Objectives

*After completing this chapter, you will be able to:*

**Define** the common terms associated with business and industry (workplace) physical activity principles.

**Explain** how workplace physical activity principles promote health, physical fitness, and optimal human performance.

**Justify** the importance of business and industry participation in the promotion of physical activities.

**Explain** how the promotion of physical activities in the workplace can integrate the various subdisciplines of kinesiology.

**Describe** the specific health benefits of participating in physical activity programs in the workplace with regards to the physical activity continuum.

**Explain** how the health benefits acquired through participation in workplace physical activity programs can positively influence worker productivity, health care costs, health outcomes, and organizational change.

**Explain** the essential elements of effective workplace programs.

**Explain** a systematic process for building a workplace health promotion program that includes assessment, planning, implementation, and evaluation.

**Give** examples of modifications of overload, specificity, and adaptation in the workplace that improve overall health, physical fitness, and peak performance through participation in physical activity.

**Describe** common methods and measures used in business and industry settings for evaluating and monitoring individuals and populations.

**Explain** a variety of examples of the application of business and industry concepts to participation in physical activity in the context of kinesiology-related subdisciplines.

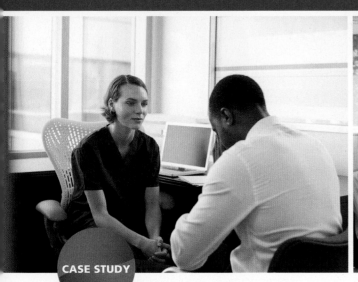
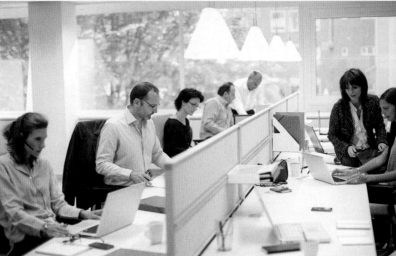

**CASE STUDY**

## In the real world . . .

When he arrived home from work one day last week, William Casey told his wife Maria that his company was starting a new comprehensive, multicomponent worksite program that places a major emphasis on physical activity and exercise. His company had supported an informal volunteer program for the past several years, but now company leadership had made an executive decision to implement organizational change based on "lean thinking" (reducing waste and doing more with less) to reduce health care costs and increase employee productivity.

William told Maria that he was excited about the new worksite health program because he knew he

needed more physical activity, but he was worried that since he has a lot of health risks already (see Chapter 1 case study) he might be singled out by the company as someone who was perhaps expendable because of his higher health care costs. As you may remember, William has hypertension and chest pain (controlled with medications), and he has depended heavily on the company's insurance carrier to help pay medical costs for himself and his family in the last two years. In addition, the new worksite program coordinator has already distributed a health risk appraisal questionnaire to all employees, and the top leadership of the company sent a memo requiring them to complete this questionnaire within one week. William and Maria had already

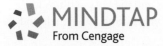

**From Cengage**

Go to your MindTap course now to answer some questions and discover what you already know about the integration of kinesiology and physical activity into the workplace.

## INTERACTIVE ACTIVITIES

### Research Focus

Worksite health promotion isn't just an economic and health issue in the United States. Go to your MindTap course to learn more about the historical, philosophical, and cultural aspects of health promotion in the workplace.

### Career Focus

Go to your MindTap course to learn more in-depth information about the Centers for Disease Control and Prevention (CDC) workplace health promotion toolkit.

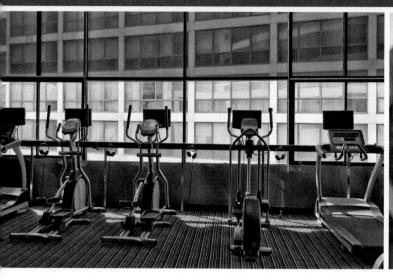
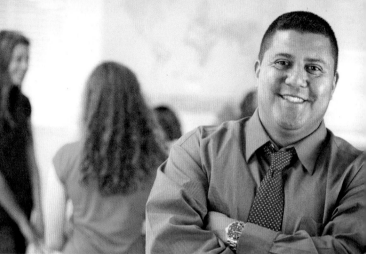

discussed the changes to U.S. health care resulting from the implementation of the Affordable Care Act (2010) but did not completely understand if or how new health care insurance laws would affect them health-wise or economically.

Now in 2017, national debate continues concerning potential changes to future health care insurance coverage.

What do you think? Should William be worried that he will be singled out and his family will lose their health care? Will he have to pay more money, or can the new worksite health program help control their personal costs as well as costs to the company? What available evidence shows how a worksite health program can reduce health care costs for employees as well as employers? How do you think worksite health programs can increase worker productivity, positive health outcomes, and organizational change? How can William's company leadership develop a social-ecological model that supports individual and group success for the adoption and maintenance of physical activity? What can the company do to develop interpersonal, organizational, community, and business policy factors that support and maintain unhealthy behaviors? How can the worksite health promotion leadership alter the social environment to produce changes in individuals and support population change within the organization?[1] How would you evaluate William's health risk appraisal results and develop strategies for successful physical activity changes within the company worksite plan? We will follow up with William and his specific worksite experiences in Lesson 2, after you have had the opportunity to learn more about the integration of business and industry with the principles of physical activity and kinesiology.

# Introduction: Business and Industry (the Workplace), Physical Activity, and Kinesiology

The costs of providing health care (or, as some refer to it, "disease care") in the United States have accelerated to over 15% of the gross domestic product (GDP) and are forecasted to approach 20% of the GDP by 2020 (see Figure 9.1). These numbers alone are staggering—they reveal the dramatic rise in U.S. health care expenses to be much faster than the rate of inflation. Moreover, this rate of increase is much more marked in the United States compared to other countries around the world (see Figure 9.2).

Traditionally in the US, health insurance has been available through employers, although there is no mandate to do so. Thus, people who are unemployed or work at jobs where no insurance is available to purchase have been at a disadvantage. Largely due to the costs associated with health care delivery, a major overhaul of the U.S. health care system was initiated in 2010. The passage of federal health care reform (**Affordable Care Act of 2010**) prioritized the quality and efficiency of health care for all Americans, while improving attention to preventing chronic diseases and improving public health. The legislation included unprecedented funding for health promotion, wellness, and prevention that extends specifically to the workplace. Although changes are inevitable in the future, this legislation provided incentives for workplaces as a key area for disease prevention and health promotion.

Just as schools serve as sites for health promotion in children, business and industry settings provide logical sites at which to promote healthy lifestyles for adults, as the vast majority of the adult population is employed, at least part time. The ready access to hundreds of thousands of workers theoretically enables worksite programs to have a broad reach. An extra motivation is that worksite health promotion can be implemented in diverse settings at various population levels (e.g., federal, state, and local) and can include individuals from various cultural strata (e.g., blue collar, agricultural, white collar) and economic strata (e.g., minimum wage, low wage, and high wage). Moreover, recent advances in technology and research into program effectiveness allow implementation of such programs in small workplaces (< 50 people) or among workforces that are dispersed over a large geographic area.

Health promotion programs that encourage physical activity and other positive health behaviors have been a part of the workplace for over 100 years. For example, the Pullman Company, a major producer of railroad cars between the 1860s and the 1960s, had a recreation and fitness program for employees that promoted exercise and athletic competition beginning in 1879.[2] The emergence of labor unions helped to usher in the idea of workplace insurance and health care as benefits of employment. By the mid- to late twentieth century, many such programs had been expanded as "executive health and fitness" programs designed as a benefit or perk for employees in a leadership role within the company and thus not available to other employees.

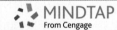

## MINDTAP
From Cengage

### The History of Worksite Health Promotion

Worksite health promotion isn't just an economic and health issue in the United States. **Go to your MindTap course** to learn more about the historical, philosophical, and cultural aspects of health promotion at the workplace.

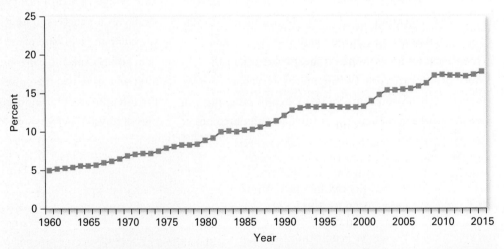

**Figure 9.1** | U.S. National Health Expenditures as a Percent of the Gross Domestic Product (GDP) by Year. The costs of providing health care are forecasted to approach 20% of the GDP by 2020.

*Source:* Centers for Medicare & Medicaid Services, Office of the Actuary, National Health Statistics Group; U.S. Department of Commerce, Bureau of Economic Analysis; and U.S. Bureau of the Census.

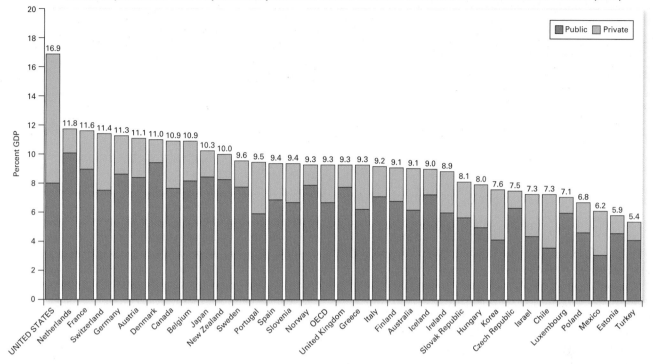

**Health Expenditures in 2012, public and private, in various countries as a share of Gross Domestic Product (GDP)**

**Figure 9.2** | Health Expenditures, Public and Private, in Various Countries as a Share of Gross Domestic Product (GDP), 2012

*Source:* Data from the Organisation for Economic Co-operation and Development (OECD), 2014, available at www.oecd.org.

Why is workplace health promotion an issue of importance to kinesiology professionals? In today's workplace, an unintended consequence of "lean thinking" in business and industry settings has been prolonged periods of sitting and physical inactivity for many employees. Low levels of occupational physical activity have been associated with musculoskeletal problems, pain, increases in sick leave, absenteeism, lower work productivity, excess health care costs, and other ill-health effects.[3] There is also emerging evidence that prolonged sitting, which is typical of many occupations (many employees sit for at least half of the working day), has negative influences on blood fats (triglycerides and cholesterol) and glucose (blood sugar) transport.[4] Figure 9.3 illustrates just how much the daily occupational energy expenditure among workers in the United States has decreased since 1960, which has been suggested as one factor that has contributed to population increases in overweight and obesity. Promoting physical activity and other important positive health behaviors in business and industry settings is consistent with many of the acquired kinesiology knowledge, skills, and abilities

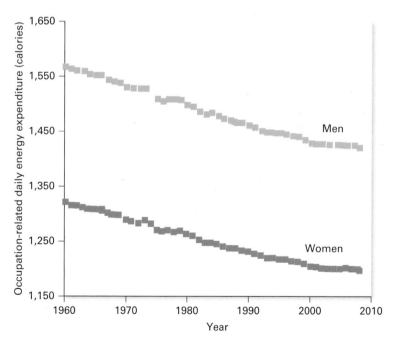

**Figure 9.3** | Reduction in Daily Occupational Energy Expenditure among Workers in U.S. Private Industry since 1960. Strong scientific evidence supports the negative health effects associated with prolonged sitting. Decreases in daily energy expenditure at work have also been suggested as one factor that has contributed to population increases in overweight and obesity.

*Source:* T. S. Church et al., "Trends over 5 Decades in U.S. Occupation-Related Physical Activity and Their Associations with Obesity," *PLOS One*, May 25, 2011, doi: 10.1371/journal.pone.0019657.

(KSAs) and job opportunities you will learn about in your major courses of study.

Pronk defines the **business** sector as, "a subdivision of the economic system comprised of organizations designed to provide goods and/or services to consumers, governments, or other businesses."[5] **Industry**, "a separate economic subdivision, is involved in activities related to the creation of finished products as the result of the manufacturing of raw materials into goods and products." Together business and industry form the workplace (or worksite) discussed in this chapter. Health promotion in the workplace is a viable career opportunity for many kinesiology majors and an important area that can impact health care and public health policies.

In this chapter, we will explore the scientific evidence related to physical activity and kinesiology principles for business and industry settings. Several models from the research and popular literature that promote physical activity and other positive health behaviors for the workplace will be covered in later sections of the chapter. The primary focus of this chapter will be the model for workplace health promotion developed by the Centers for Disease Control and Prevention (CDC). We will also cover related resources that can help kinesiology professionals prepare effectively to promote physical activity and healthy lifestyles at the worksite. The CDC workplace health promotion model emphasizes four main steps: assessment, a planning process, program implementation, and an evaluation process.

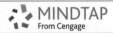

### The CDC Workplace Health Promotion Model

**Go to your MindTap course** to learn more in-depth information about the Centers for Disease Control and Prevention workplace health promotion model.

Why are employers interested in health promotion? The fundamental assumption is that healthier employees have lower health care costs (of which employers pay an estimated 30%), are more productive, are absent less frequently, and are happier than employees who are not as healthy. Physical activity promotion efforts (along with interventions related to other positive health behaviors such as smoking cessation, stress reduction, and health screening) can influence individuals and populations within the workplace, organizational policies, families, and communities. Sick leave costs

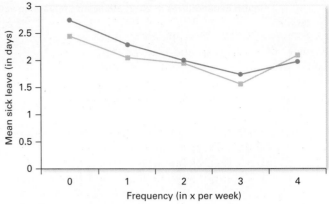

**Figure 9.4** | Dose-Response Relationship between Vigorous Physical Activity Participation and the Frequency of Sick Leave in Dutch Workers. Those workers that did not participate in vigorous-intensity physical activities had more sick days than those who participated in three days of vigorous-intensity physical activities. The authors found that sick leave benefits appear to diminish with more than three days of participation in vigorous-intensity physical activity.

*Source:* K. Proper and W. van Mechelen, "Effectiveness and Economic Impact of Worksite Interventions to Promote Physical Activity and Healthy Diet," World Health Organization, 2012, accessed May 19, 2016, www.who.int.

an employer a substantial amount in both real dollars and lost productivity. Recent research suggests that physical activity may actually lower the risk of workplace absenteeism. The dose-response relationship between vigorous physical activity participation and the frequency of sick leave (measured every four months) for three years in a large sample of Dutch workers is shown in Figure 9.4. The two lines graphed in the figure represent the data from two cross-sectional databases. As is evident, those individuals who did not participate in vigorous-intensity physical activity had the highest average sick leave versus those who participated in three days of vigorous-intensity physical activity.[6] Workers who had been vigorously active one to two times per week had on average seven days less sick leave over three years than those who did not perform such activities. The authors found that sick leave benefits appear to diminish with more than three days of participation in vigorous-intensity physical activity.

Do worksite physical activity programs save money for the employer? The economic impact of worksite physical activity-based health promotion programs is difficult to determine for a variety of reasons, including a lack of well-controlled studies. However, Pronk reported the **cost-benefit ratios** (ratios that represent the dollars saved—or "earned"—for each dollar spent) of company-sponsored fitness programs to be between $1.07 and $5.38.[7] Thus, for every dollar spent by an employer in promoting physical activity, a return on investment of 7% to 438% might be expected. In general, the social costs and health care costs of physical inactivity are substantial, and integrating physical activity into a comprehensive program is a sound strategy to generate positive health and economic impacts.[8]

Chenoweth reported that more than 50% of corporate health care costs are due to modifiable risk factors such as low levels of physical activity, tobacco use, and obesity.[9] Table 9.1 shows an example of the direct and indirect economic costs of physical inactivity and other modifiable health risk factors that have been reported by others.

Reportedly, 50% of American worksites with more than 750 employees provide *some type* of health promotion program (at minimum, using at least one type of healthy initiative such as supporting smoking cessation), but an average of only 33% to 38% of smaller companies (250–749 and < 49 persons) have established programs.[10] It has also been estimated that only about 6.9% of U.S. worksites offer comprehensive health promotion programs, which can have greater overall impact on health-related economic markers.[11] Workplace health promotion programs with a major focus on increasing and maintaining physical activity levels for employees and their families can create a positive culture for business and industry that can translate into healthier communities.

In the *Steps to Wellness: A Guide to Implementing the 2008 Physical Activity Guidelines for Americans in the Workplace*, business leaders were asked to respond to the question,

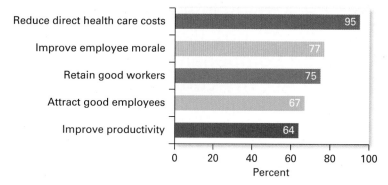

**Figure 9.5** | Primary Reasons Business Leaders Invest in Workplace Health Promotion

*Source:* Centers for Disease Control and Prevention, *Steps to Wellness: A Guide to Implementing the 2008 Physical Activity Guidelines for Americans in the Workplace* (Atlanta: U.S. Department of Health and Human Services, 2012), 11.

"Why do I invest in worksite wellness?"[12] Their responses, shown in Figure 9.5, target five important economic markers: direct health costs, employee morale, retention, recruitment, and productivity. By far, the most frequent motivation was reduction of direct health care costs.

Worksite health promotion programs commonly include combinations of programming that focus on educational, physical, organizational, and/or environmental activities. In the 2008 Employee Benefits Survey, conducted by the Society for Human Resource Management (SHRM) at its 60th annual convention, companies reported offering the components listed in Table 9.2 within their wellness programs.

Although many companies currently offer one or two of the components listed in Table 9.2, few offer a comprehensive worksite health promotion program that is consistent with promoting a positive and consistent culture of health and physical activity promotion.

**Table 9.1** | Examples of Direct and Indirect Costs Associated with Physical Inactivity and Other Unhealthy Behaviors

|  | INSIDE HEALTH CARE | OUTSIDE HEALTH CARE |
|---|---|---|
| **Direct Costs** | Visits to physician<br>Medications<br>Home care<br>Physical therapy<br>Surgery<br>Hospitalization | Out-of-pocket expenses<br>Travel expenses<br>Informal care<br>Costs of devices |
| **Indirect Costs** | Health care costs during life years gained | Productivity losses due to absenteeism, disability, or death |

*Source:* Modified from K. Proper and W. van Mechelen, "Effectiveness and Economic Impact of Worksite Interventions to Promote Physical Activity and a Healthy Diet" (background paper prepared for the WHO/WEF Joint Event on Preventing Noncommunicable Diseases in the Workplace, Dalian, China, September 2007).

**Table 9.2** | Common Wellness Programming Components (shortened version)

| COMPONENT | PROGRAMS INCLUDING COMPONENT |
|---|---|
| Wellness resources and information | 72% |
| On-site voluntary vaccination | 69% |
| Health care premium discount for annual employee health risk assessment | 11% |
| Health care premium discount for participation in wellness program | 9% |
| Health care premium discount for abstinence from using tobacco products | 8% |
| Fitness equipment subsidies | 6% |
| Nap room | 5% |

*Source:* Society for Human Resource Management, "2008 Employee Benefits Survey Results" (from report released at the SHRM 60th Annual Conference and Exposition in Chicago, IL, June 2008).

# Physical Activity in Business and Industry Settings: Basic Terms, Common Components, and the Physical Activity Continuum 🏃

Table 9.3 contains definitions of a variety of common terms used in worksite health promotion programming that have been modified and adapted for use in this text. You should become acquainted with each of these terms in order to be able to effectively communicate with the business and industry health promotion culture.

As you learned in previous chapters, the physical activity continuum represents a pathway for moving from sedentary behaviors (or nonparticipation in physical activities or other health-promoting activities, for example) to achievement of health by meeting the 2008 U.S. Physical Activity Guidelines across the lifespan, and individual progress is related to physical and mental challenges. Those with higher-order physical activity or health promotion goals must focus on making adjustments using the principles of overload, specificity, and adaptation to achieve higher levels of physical activity performance, health promotion, or peak performance.

For example, in the business and industry sectors, employers often offer health promotion programming to increase the physical activity and fitness of their employees—or at least to move them from sedentary patterns toward achieving functional health. In many corporate settings, employers now offer company challenges designed to provide competitive experiences that encourage employees to achieve positive change in health-related behaviors (e.g., employee competitions

**Table 9.3 | Common Terms Related to Worksite Health Promotion***

**Worksite health care costs:** health care costs for the workplace associated with modifiable unhealthy behaviors such as low levels of physical activity, tobacco use, and obesity.

**Worksite health promotion or wellness program:** various education and participation activities that a worksite implements to promote healthy lifestyles for employees and their families and produce a healthier workforce.

**Comprehensive worksite health promotion program:** includes health-related programming, implementation of health-related policies, health benefits package (insurance plus other services or discounts regarding health), and environmental supports that promote health and physical activity.

**Wellness:** a concept redesigned in the 1980s to describe the constant and deliberate efforts to stay healthy in the following domains: physical, emotional, mental, social, environmental, occupational, and spiritual.

**Business and industry or corporate culture:** norms or "how things get done" within a company. A particular set of attitudes or behaviors that define a company and how its employees work together.*

**Culture of health and physical activity:** norms regarding how a company promotes health and physical activity to its employees and recognizes the benefits of a healthy workplace.

**Absenteeism:** missing work due to minor ailments associated with unhealthy behaviors such as low levels of physical activity.

**Presenteeism:** nonproductivity due to covering job responsibilities and/or tasks for other workers who are not performing up to normal levels of performance due to their unhealthy behaviors.

**Accessibility:** worksite availability to positive health promotion education and experiences.

**Aging workforce:** current trend in which U.S. employees are working longer than ever prior to retirement and the older employee population is at higher risk for work-related injuries (e.g., falls) and chronic diseases.

**Employee retention:** retention of current employees in the workforce. Worksite health promotion can provide perks that help to keep productive employees as well as maintain and improve their health.

**Employee recruitment:** recruitment of new employees. Worksite health promotion is good for business and industry as a positive element of public relations and is attractive to potential employees.

**Employee health insurance:** employer-subsidized health insurance. Health insurance is commonly provided by companies, but the costs have spiraled higher and higher in the past decade, sparking national controversy (both for and against) for business and industry with the passage of the Affordable Health Care Act in 2010.

**Business and industry or corporate image:** the public's perception of a company. Worksite health promotion is consistent with good business practices, is positive for workers and the local community, and can have national and global influences.

**Productivity:** effective employee performance associated with a healthy and motivated individual.

**Worker's compensation costs (WCC):** costs of work-related injuries or incidences that are preventable (not all are) and due to unhealthy behaviors. Many companies also have worker's comp programs that help employees improve work skills or return to work after injury.

*See the following resource for more information: Centers for Disease Control and Prevention, *Steps to Wellness: A Guide to Implementing the 2008 Physical Activity Guidelines for Americans in the Workplace* (Atlanta: U.S. Department of Health and Human Services 2012).

**Table 9.4** | Strategies to Increase Physical Activity in Business and Industry Settings

| | |
|---|---|
| STRATEGY 1 | Businesses should provide opportunities and incentives to adopt and maintain a physically active lifestyle. |
| STRATEGY 2 | Businesses should engage in cross-sectional partnerships to promote physical activity within the workplace, and such efforts should extend to local communities and geographic regions. |
| STRATEGY 3 | Professional and scientific societies should create and widely disseminate a concise, powerful, and compelling business case for investment in physical activity promotion. |
| STRATEGY 4 | Professional and scientific societies should develop and advocate for policies that promote physical activity in workplace settings. |
| STRATEGY 5 | Physical activity and public health professionals should support the development and deployment of surveillance systems that monitor physical activity in U.S. workers and physical activity promotion efforts in U.S. workplaces. |

*Source:* National Physical Activity Plan Alliance (NPAPA), www.physicalactivityplan.org

based on weight loss success, miles walked or run, or daily steps completed). In some cases, usually in larger business and industry settings, competitive sports leagues (e.g., softball and kickball) have been organized by employers to provide improved worksite morale, employee camaraderie, and company image.

The U.S. National Physical Activity Plan was developed and promoted by the National Physical Activity Plan Alliance and suggests five strategies to consider for targeting business and industry for the promotion of increased physical activity levels among employees. The five strategies are listed in Table 9.4.

## Health Care Costs, Work Productivity, Health Outcomes, and Organizational Benefits of Participation in Physical Activities in Business and Industry Settings

The benefits of promoting physical activity and other positive health behaviors at the workplace generally include increased effective disease prevention behaviors, improved worker productivity, reduced health care costs, improved health, and organizational policy change. Some of the specific benefits of participating in workplace physical activity health promotion for employers and employees as summarized by the CDC are shown in Table 9.5. Typically, the effectiveness of physical activity programs at the workplace depends upon the dose and volume of activity introduced, but often effectiveness is also enhanced when multiple interventions are included in a campaign or package and implemented together.

**Table 9.5** | Summary of Benefits of Participating in Physical Activities in Business and Industry Settings

- Reduced feelings of depression
- Improved stamina and strength
- Lower risk of obesity
- Reduced risks of cardiovascular disease (blood pressure and cholesterol), stroke, and type 2 diabetes
- Lower absenteeism
- Lower health care costs related to disease risks (cardiovascular, musculoskeletal, stroke, and type 2 diabetes)
- Increases in physical activity and physical fitness
- Improved employee morale and positive work environment changes that increase productivity, retention, and recruitment

The U.S. Preventive Services Task Force (Community Guide) has summarized worksite policies and programs that can provide a variety of health promotion benefits and positive worksite change.[13] The Community Guide categorizes potential interventions as recommended, meaning they are strongly supported by evidence from the research literature; not recommended, meaning they are harmful or there is no evidence available; or insufficient, meaning there is not enough evidence to determine if the strategy is effective or not (it might be in some cases). The task force recommendations and findings for worksite health promotion are shown in Table 9.6.

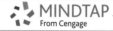

**Developing Health Promotion Programs**

A complete review and listing of all considerations and benefits for developing health promotion programs for the workplace is beyond the scope of the text. However, **go to your MindTap course** for more information, including more detailed information on the Steps to Wellness program and specific corporate wellness programs.

# Essential Elements of Effective Workplace Health Promotion Programs

The *Essential Elements of Effective Workplace Programs and Policies for Improving Worker Health and Wellbeing* is a resource document developed by the National Institute for Occupational Safety and Health (NIOSH). The document

**Table 9.6** | Task Force Recommendations and Findings—Worksite Health Promotion

| INTERVENTIONS TO PROMOTE SEASONAL INFLUENZA VACCINATIONS AMONG HEALTH CARE WORKERS | |
|---|---|
| Interventions with On-Site, Free, Actively Promoted Vaccinations | Recommended June 2008 |
| Interventions with Actively Promoted, Off-Site Vaccinations | Insufficient Evidence June 2008 |
| **INTERVENTIONS TO PROMOTE SEASONAL INFLUENZA VACCINATIONS AMONG NON-HEALTH CARE WORKERS** | |
| Interventions with On-Site, Reduced Cost, Actively Promoted Vaccinations | Recommended June 2008 |
| Interventions with Actively Promoted, Off-Site Vaccinations | Insufficient Evidence June 2008 |
| **ASSESSMENT OF HEALTH RISKS WITH FEEDBACK (AHRF) TO CHANGE EMPLOYEES' HEALTH** | |
| AHRF Used Alone | Insufficient Evidence June 2006 |
| AHRF Plus Health Education with or without Other Interventions | Recommended February 2007 |
| **PREVENTING CHRONIC DISEASE** | |
| Skin Cancer Prevention: Interventions in Outdoor Occupational Settings | Recommended August 2013 |
| Diabetes Prevention and Control: Self-Management Education at the Worksite | Insufficient Evidence September 2000 |
| Obesity Prevention: Worksite Programs to Control Overweight and Obesity | Recommended February 2007 |
| **PROMOTING PHYSICAL ACTIVITY** | |
| Point-of-Decision Prompts to Encourage Use of Stairs | Recommended June 2005 |
| Creation of or Enhanced Access to Places for Physical Activity Combined with Informational Outreach Activities | Recommended May 2001 |
| **REDUCING TOBACCO USE AND SECONDHAND SMOKE EXPOSURE** | |
| Smoke-Free Policies | Recommended November 2012 |
| Incentives and Competitions to Increase Smoking Cessation | |
| Incentives and Competitions When Used Alone | Insufficient Evidence June 2005 |
| Incentives and Competitions When Combined with Additional Interventions | Recommended June 2005 |

*Source:* Community Preventive Services Task Force, *Community Guide,* available at www.thecommunityguide.org/topic/worksite-health

is a part of the Total Worker Health strategy and highlights 20 components that promote comprehensive health promotion in the workplace for business and industry to consider. These 20 components are listed in Table 9.7 and are divided into four categories: organizational culture and leadership, program design, program implementation, and program evaluation.

## Assessment, Planning, Implementation, and Evaluation of Workplace Health Promotion Programs

Building a comprehensive worksite health promotion program should be a systematic process based upon models like those promoted by the CDC that includes consideration of the essential elements from Table 9.7. Figure 9.6 shows a CDC workplace health promotion development model that focuses on four main steps: assessment, planning, program implementation, and evaluation. Step 1, *assessment,* involves three components: organizational, individual, and community assessment. Step 2, *planning/workplace governance,* involves five components: leadership support, management, a workplace health improvement plan, dedicated resources, and communications and informatics. Step 3, *implementation,* involves four components: programs, policies, health benefits, and environmental support. Finally, Step 4, *evaluation,* involves four components: worker productivity, health care costs, improved health outcomes, and organizational change or "creating a culture of health." Underlying these four steps are *contextual factors* such as the size of the company or industry sector that need to be considered when building a workplace health promotion program.[14]

**Table 9.7** | Essential Elements of Effective Workplace Programs (based on Total Worker Health™)

### ORGANIZATIONAL CULTURE AND LEADERSHIP

1. **Develop a "human-centered culture."** Effective programs thrive in organizations with policies and programs that promote respect throughout the organization and encourage active worker participation, input, and involvement. A human-centered culture is built on trust, not fear.

2. **Demonstrate leadership.** Commitment to worker health and safety, reflected in words and actions, is critical. The connection of workforce health and safety to the core products, services, and values of the company should be acknowledged by leaders and communicated widely.

3. **Engage mid-level management.** Supervisors and managers at all levels should be involved in promoting health-supportive programs. They are the direct links between the workers and upper management and will determine if the program succeeds or fails. Mid-level supervisors are the key to integrating, motivating, and communicating with employees.

### PROGRAM DESIGN

4. **Establish clear principles.** Effective programs have clear principles to focus priorities, guide program design, and direct resource allocation. Prevention of disease and injury supports worker health and well-being.

5. **Integrate relevant systems.** Program design involves an initial inventory and evaluation of existing programs and policies relevant to health and well-being and a determination of their potential connections. In general, better-integrated systems perform more effectively. Integration of diverse data systems can be particularly important and challenging.

6. **Eliminate recognized occupational hazards.** Changes in the work environment (such as reduction in toxic exposures or improvement in work station design and flexibility) benefit all workers. Eliminating recognized hazards in the workplace is foundational to Total Worker Health™ principles.

7. **Be consistent.** Workers' willingness to engage in worksite health-directed programs may depend on perceptions of whether the work environment is truly health supportive. Individual interventions can be linked to specific work experience. Change the physical and organizational work environment to align with health goals.

8. **Promote employee participation.** Ensure that employees are not just recipients of services but are engaged actively to identify relevant health and safety issues and contribute to program design and implementation. Barriers are often best overcome through involving the participants in coming up with solutions. Participation in the development, implementation, and evaluation of programs is usually the most effective strategy for changing culture, behavior, and systems.

9. **Tailor programs to the *specific* workplace and the diverse needs of workers.** Workplaces vary in size, sector, product, design, location, health and safety experience, resources, and worker characteristics such as age, training, physical and mental abilities, resiliency, education, cultural background, and health practices. Successful programs recognize this diversity and are designed to meet the needs of both individuals and the enterprise. One size does *not* fit all—flexibility is necessary.

10. **Consider incentives and rewards.** Incentives and rewards, such as financial rewards, time off, and recognition, for individual program participation may encourage engagement, although poorly designed incentives may create a sense of "winners" and "losers" and have unintended adverse consequences. Vendors' contracts should have incentives and rewards aligned with accomplishment of program objectives.

11. **Find and use the right tools.** Measure risk from the work environment and baseline health in order to track progress. Optimal assessment of a program's effectiveness is achieved through the use of relevant, validated measurement instruments.

12. **Adjust the program as needed.** Successful programs reflect an understanding that the interrelationships between work and health are complex. New workplace programs and policies modify complex systems. Interventions in one part of a complex system are likely to have predictable and unpredictable effects elsewhere.

13. **Make sure the program lasts.** Design programs with a long-term outlook to assure sustainability. Short-term approaches have short-term value. Programs aligned with the core product/values of the enterprise endure. There should be sufficient flexibility to ensure responsiveness to changing workforce and market conditions.

14. **Ensure confidentiality.** Be sure that the program meets regulatory requirements (e.g., HIPAA, state law, ADA) and that the communication to employees is clear on this issue. If workers believe their information is not kept confidential, the program is less likely to succeed.

### PROGRAM IMPLEMENTATION AND RESOURCES

15. **Be willing to start small and scale up.** Although the overall program design should be comprehensive, starting with modest targets is often beneficial if they are recognized as first steps in a broader program. For example, target reduction in injury rates or absence. Consider phased implementation of these elements if adoption at one time is not feasible. Use (and evaluate) pilot efforts before scaling up. Be willing to abandon pilot projects that fail.

16. **Provide adequate resources.** Identify and engage appropriately trained and motivated staff. If you use vendors, make sure they are qualified. Take advantage of credible local and national resources from voluntary and government agencies. Allocate sufficient resources, including staff, space, and time, to achieve the results you seek.

*(Continued)*

**Table 9.7** | (Continued)

| |
|---|
| 17. **Communicate strategically.** Effective communication is essential for success. Everyone (workers, their families, supervisors, etc.) with a stake in worker health should know what you are doing and why. The messages and means of delivery should be tailored and targeted to the group or individual and consistently reflect the values and direction of the programs. Communicate early and often, but also have a long-term communication strategy. Provide periodic updates to the organizational leadership and workforce. |
| 18. **Build accountability into program implementation.** Accountability reflects leadership commitment to improved programs and outcomes and should cascade through an organization starting at the highest levels of leadership. Reward success. |
| **PROGRAM EVALUATION** |
| 19. **Measure and analyze.** Develop objectives and a selective menu of *relevant* measurements, recognizing that the total value of a program, particularly one designed to abate chronic diseases, may not be determinable in the short run. Integrate data systems across programs and among vendors to enable both tracking of results and continual program improvement. |
| 20. **Learn from experience.** Adjust or modify programs based on established milestones and on results you have measured and analyzed. |

*Source:* DHHS (NIOSH), "Essential Elements of Effective Workplace Programs and Policies for Improving Worker Health and Wellbeing," October 2008, www.cdc.gov/niosh/docs/2010-140/pdfs/2010-140.pdf.

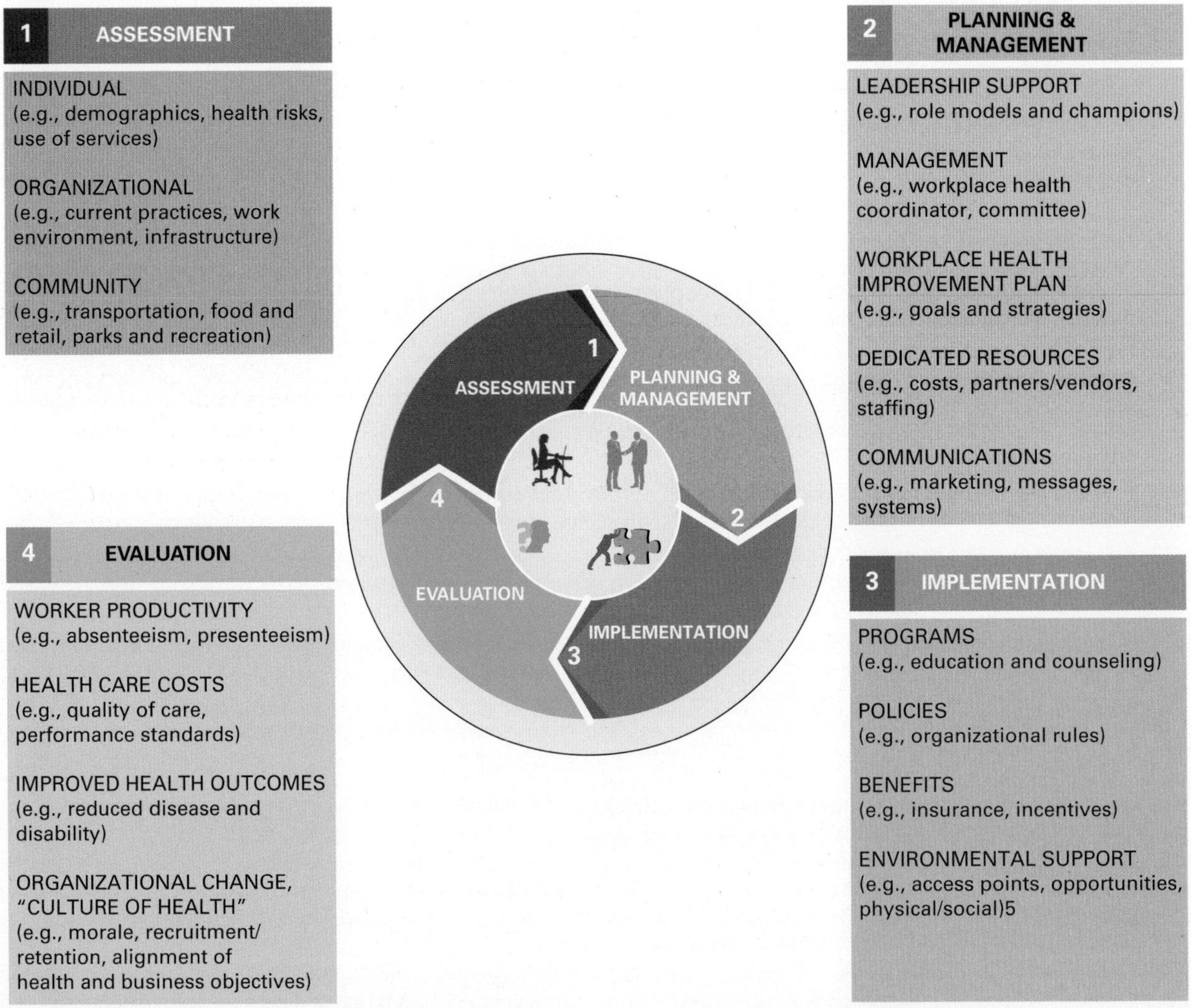
1 ASSESSMENT
INDIVIDUAL (e.g., demographics, health risks, use of services)
ORGANIZATIONAL (e.g., current practices, work environment, infrastructure)
COMMUNITY (e.g., transportation, food and retail, parks and recreation)
2 PLANNING & MANAGEMENT
LEADERSHIP SUPPORT (e.g., role models and champions)
MANAGEMENT (e.g., workplace health coordinator, committee)
WORKPLACE HEALTH IMPROVEMENT PLAN (e.g., goals and strategies)
DEDICATED RESOURCES (e.g., costs, partners/vendors, staffing)
COMMUNICATIONS (e.g., marketing, messages, systems)
1 ASSESSMENT
PLANNING & MANAGEMENT
2
IMPLEMENTATION
3
EVALUATION
4
3 IMPLEMENTATION
PROGRAMS (e.g., education and counseling)
POLICIES (e.g., organizational rules)
BENEFITS (e.g., insurance, incentives)
ENVIRONMENTAL SUPPORT (e.g., access points, opportunities, physical/social)5
4 EVALUATION
WORKER PRODUCTIVITY (e.g., absenteeism, presenteeism)
HEALTH CARE COSTS (e.g., quality of care, performance standards)
IMPROVED HEALTH OUTCOMES (e.g., reduced disease and disability)
ORGANIZATIONAL CHANGE, "CULTURE OF HEALTH" (e.g., morale, recruitment/retention, alignment of health and business objectives)

**Figure 9.6** | The CDC Workplace Health Model

*Source:* Centers for Disease Control and Prevention, "Workplace Health Model," 2016, available at www.cdc.gov/workplacehealthpromotion/model/.

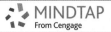
## Assessment

The process of assessment is dependent upon a variety of worksite data sources. The CDC website describes a variety of potential data sources that kinesiology professionals can consider when performing the assessment phase of workplace health promotion development. These sources may include:

1. Site visits to the workplace that involve observations and interviews of employees and employers about health and physical activity beliefs, attitudes, current policies, and worksite challenges to implementation.

2. Employee surveys such as health risk appraisals (HRAs), biometric measures (e.g., height, weight, bloodwork values), job satisfaction inventories, and others.

3. Analysis and review of health benefits employees receive as part of their health/insurance plans, including vacation and personal use days.

4. Other data sources, which might include statistics related to attendance, worksite injuries, participation in current health promotion programming, and incentives (if any) for participation, as well as other information.

## Planning/Worksite Governance

The process of planning and governance at the worksite includes identifying strategies for successful direction, leadership, and organization. The CDC Workplace Health Promotion website provides a variety of tactics and strategies that kinesiology professionals can consider when performing the planning/governance phase of workplace health promotion development. Some of the CDC recommendations include:

1. Use multiple opportunities and methods to help employees learn about and participate in workplace health promotion activities.

2. Identify and develop leadership (senior level support) that includes a program role model (or champion) that can be sustained over time.

3. Identify a worksite coordinator and committee for oversight of the program.

4. Develop a worksite improvement plan that includes data collection, while ensuring and maintaining employee confidentiality.

5. Plan for appropriate resources to develop and maintain the program. Focus on effective communication strategies to promote the program to employees.

6. Develop and complete an evaluation plan for the worksite health promotion program that includes systematic reevaluation over time.

## Implementation

The process of implementing the worksite health promotion program should only begin after steps 1 and 2 have been addressed and at least a basic evaluation plan for the program has been considered and designed. The CDC Workplace Health Promotion website also provides intervention strategies for a variety of health topics (including physical activity) that kinesiology professionals can use when implementing workplace health promotion programs.

## Evaluation

Kinesiology professionals should recognize that the evaluation phase of workplace health promotion is critical because it provides evidence to business and industry leaders that a specific workplace health program model is effective and should be continued. Ideally, evaluation plans should be developed as part of the initial planning process and before implementation of programming. The CDC Workplace Health Promotion website provides evaluation strategies including baseline, process, and outcome measures that are applicable to physical activity and a variety of other health topics.

Figure 9.7 shows a CDC framework for evaluation of workplace health promotion programs, which consists of a cycle with six steps:

### Step 1: Engage stakeholders

People who stand to benefit as well as those who are not supportive are stakeholders. Engage them early.

### Step 2: Describe the program

Communicate early and often with goals and objectives, and strategies that will be used to achieve them.

### Step 3: Focus the evaluation design

Evaluating and measuring the effectiveness (or lack of effectiveness) of a program is key. What gets measured gets changed.

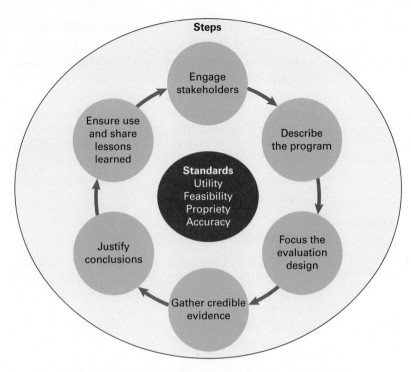

**Steps**

Engage stakeholders

Describe the program

Focus the evaluation design

Gather credible evidence

Justify conclusions

Ensure use and share lessons learned

**Standards**
Utility
Feasibility
Propriety
Accuracy

**Figure 9.7** | CDC Framework for Workplace Program Evaluation

*Source:* Centers for Disease Control and Prevention, "Framework for Program Evaluation in Public Health," *Morbidity and Mortality Weekly Report 1999*, available at www.cdc.gov/workplacehealth promotion/model/evaluation/index.html.

### Step 4: Gather credible evidence

Data are key.

### Step 5: Justify conclusions

Interpret the data cautiously and objectively.

### Step 6: Ensure use and share lessons learned

Evaluation without communication is useless.

# Examples of Implementation of Physical Activity Interventions in Business and Industry

The CDC Workplace Health Promotion website has links to specific health topics such as physical activity interventions for business and industry workplace health promotion programs. There are several examples of program implementations with evaluations based upon baseline, process, and outcome measures. One specific example that is provided includes the determination of increasing work productivity by evaluating the physical activity and absenteeism of employees. This example is as follows:

*Baseline*

- Determine the average number of sick days per employee over the previous 12 months for health conditions related to physical inactivity such as hypertension. This measure may be less useful if there has been a large increase or decrease in numbers of employees over the past 12 months.
- Determine the costs of worker absenteeism, including costs of replacement workers, costs in training replacement workers, and loss of and delay in productivity.
- Determine the time employees spend during working hours participating in physical activity-related worksite programs.

*Process*

- Reassess the average number of sick days per employee for physical inactivity-related conditions at the first follow-up evaluation.
- Conduct periodic repeats of other baseline measures.

*Outcome*

- Assess changes in the average number of sick days per employee for physical inactivity-related conditions in repeated follow-up evaluations.
- Assess changes in the time employees spend during working hours participating in physical activity–related worksite programs.
- Assess changes in costs from baseline.

Pronk produced a list of worksite-based interventions to promote physical activity based on a social-ecological model and a review of the research literature.[15] A proposed framework that stakeholders may have in physical activity and the level of influences by which physical activity might be promoted in the workplace are shown in Figure 9.8. The CDC and other national and international groups support the social-ecological model approach for implementing business and industry workplace promotion programs. Table 9.8 contains Pronk's compilation of the physical activity interventions that have been attempted in the workplace.

# Business and Industry Worksite Health Promotion Measures and Monitoring Processes in the Workplace

Generally, a best practices approach to measuring and monitoring the success of health promotion programs in the workplace would include a variety of employee and

**Table 9.8** | Worksite-Based Interventions to Promote Physical Activity Organized According to a Social-Ecological Model

| SOCIAL-ECOLOGICAL DIMENSION | INTERVENTION EXAMPLE |
|---|---|
| Individual | Printed motivationally tailored physical activity intervention materials |
| | Standard and motivationally tailored Internet-based messages to promote physical activity |
| | E-mail intervention using messaging to promote physical activity |
| | Internet-based counseling for physical activity, nutrition, and weight management |
| | Telephone-based coaching or counseling for physical activity change |
| | Use pedometers or other wearables to increase physical activity |
| | Individual face-to-face counseling to increase physical activity levels |
| Inter-individual, group-based | Integrate 10-minute exercise breaks into daily routines conducted individually or in a group setting |
| | Incentive-based online physical activity intervention using a team-based format |
| | Light physical exercise interventions (resistance training and guidance) focused on headache, neck and shoulder symptoms |
| | Health fairs and worksite-wide events that include biometric and behavioral self-assessments with feedback |
| | Walking groups and buddy systems to create supportive social networks at work |
| | Facilities and signs aimed at helping workers meet recommended levels of physical activity (point-of-decision prompts) |
| Organizational | Implementation of an all-employee health assessment or health risk appraisal including physical activity assessment and feedback integrated with educational outreach and follow-up |
| | Use of incentives to promote physical activity among employees and their families, e.g., subsidize health club memberships, pay mileage costs for employee transport by bicycle, use insurance benefits–integrated incentives to promote physical activity (e.g., reduction in copays or deductibles), and/or reduce health insurance premiums |
| | Policies designed to support employee physical activity, e.g., permission to conduct business meetings during walks, create and/or enhance access to places for physical activity (painted, well-lit stairs, etc.) |
| | Informational outreach activities and campaigns to promote physical activity |
| Environmental | Provide secure parking for bicycles |
| | Install showers and changing rooms for workers' use |
| | Advocate and support the introduction and passage of legislation that supports active commuting to work |
| | Provide tax breaks for companies that implement comprehensive worksite health promotion programs |
| | Provide onsite fitness facilities and/or a physical activity–friendly campus, including the distribution of walking maps and easy access to walking/running routes |
| | Companies participate in community-based worksite exercise competitions |
| | Community-wide physical activity campaigns |

*Source:* N. Pronk, "Worksite-Based Interventions to Promote Physical Activity Organized According to Social-Ecological Model," *Journal of Physical Activity and Health* 6, no. 2 (2009): S229.

| | | Make physical activity... | | | | | | |
|---|---|---|---|---|---|---|---|---|
| | | Possible | Simple | Socially rewarding | Financially rewarding | Personally relevant | Organizationally relevant | Community connected |
| **Level of influence** | Individual | | | | | | | |
| | Inter-individual | | | | | | | |
| | Organizational | | | | | | | |
| | Environmental | | | | | | | |

**Figure 9.8** | A Physical Activity Framework Model for Physical Activity Promotion in the Workplace: Interaction between Social-Ecological Factors and the Level of Various Worksite Health Promotion Influences

*Source:* N.P. Pronk, "Physical Activity Promotion in Business and Industry: Exercise, Context, and Recommendations for a National Plan," *Journal of Physical Activity and Health*, 6, Suppl. 2 (2009): S230.

employer measurements and analyses over time for the following areas:[16]

» Engagement metrics (e.g., quality measures of active participation rates and drop-out rates)

» Satisfaction metrics (e.g., specific program feedback from all involved)

» Health behavior change (e.g., increase or decrease in physical activity behaviors)

» Biometric health and clinical inputs (e.g., physical characteristics like height, weight, blood pressure, blood cholesterol, and others)

» Health risk reduction (e.g., changes in behaviors or evaluation of health care claims and costs)

» Productivity impacts (e.g., absenteeism, workers' comp claims)

» Health care cost impacts (e.g., employee utilization of health care services)

» Return on investment (e.g., ratio of benefits to cost—difficult to measure)

(All measures described above may be obtained in a variety of ways, such as administering questionnaires, telephone surveys, using human resource data sources, and/or gathering social media information.)

Specifically, some of the most commonly used measures and monitoring instruments found in today's worksite health promotion programs that target physical activity and health risk reduction include:

**Health risk appraisals (HRAs):** HRAs help identify health risks and can be used for baseline data and reviewed over time to track reductions in health risks. HRAs come in a variety of forms, and you can find many examples online. Good examples of a population-based HRA is the CDC's Behavioral Risk Factor Surveillance System (BRFSS).

**Biometric tests/health screenings:** Many companies provide employees opportunities to have clinical measures such as blood pressure, body composition, blood cholesterol, blood glucose, skin cancer risk, and others evaluated at the worksite.

**Fitness tests:** Although fitness testing is sometimes included with biometric tests, the level of fitness assessment can vary based on the physical activity continuum and the worksite population. For example, a company might pay for executive physical exams (conducted by a physician) and graded exercise testing (treadmill test with electrocardiogram monitoring) for their leadership (just a few executives), while other employees in the same company may only be asked to submit to simple, inexpensive assessments.

**Wearables:** Commonly used in the workplace to encourage employees to begin to increase their physical activity. They are useful for tracking steps per day in order to monitor physical activity over time and are often used as incentives for challenges among different subgroups of workers.

Many more methods to assess physical activity at the workplace are available, but no one tool can be recommended for every situation. Usually it is best to combine approaches to measuring physical activity or health-related outcomes in the workplace and develop a surveillance database at the workplace of interest. **Surveillance** has been defined as the ongoing, systematic collection, analysis, and interpretation (e.g., regarding physical activity, risk factors, or health events) essential to planning, implementation, and evaluation of public health.[17]

# EXAMPLES OF APPLYING BUSINESS AND INDUSTRY PRINCIPLES OF PHYSICAL ACTIVITY IN RELATIONSHIP TO THE KINESIOLOGY SUBDISCIPLINES

*In Lesson 1, you learned about the integration of business and industry with the principles of physical activity and kinesiology. You learned about why physical activity and other positive health behaviors are promoted at the workplace to help develop a corporate culture of health. Effective physical activity and health promotion at the workplace can positively*

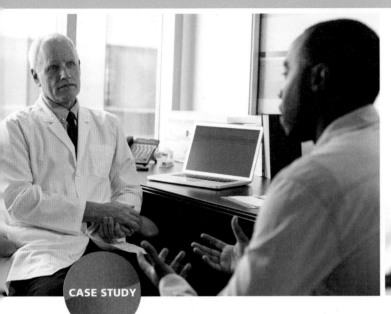

**CASE STUDY**

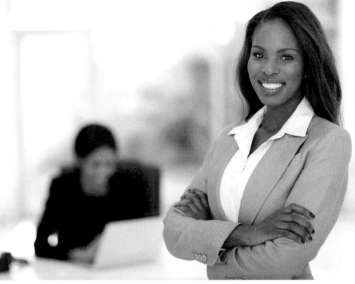

## In the real world . . .

As you may recall from earlier in this chapter, William Casey's company announced the implementation of a comprehensive health promotion program at the workplace. William was worried that the new mandatory program might increase his health care costs (insurance premiums) or, in a worst-case scenario, his high blood pressure and chest pain history might get him fired or forced out of his job. As things turned out, the health promotion director at work, Marsha, met with William and provided him with a plan to help him maintain or improve his current health status, while targeting improvements in his productivity, controlling his health care costs, stabilizing his health status, and effectively changing health behavior policies at work.

Based on William's responses to an initial HRA and brief interview with Marsha, he was asked to undergo testing focusing on his heart disease risks (regular measures of blood pressure, blood cholesterol, chest pain episodes), complete a clinical graded exercise test (GXT) to screen for heart disease (covered by the company's new health insurance package as an incentive), and follow up once a month with a company wellness coach. As you might expect based on what you learned in Lesson 1, the results of William's tests helped Marsha develop a comprehensive plan for him and helped control health care costs for other individuals and the company.

Completing the HRA reminded William of job and health factors that affected his hypertension and chest pain episodes. His GXT results will be interpreted by his personal physician to determine if he actually has heart disease and/or needs clinical follow-up tests to further manage his condition. The concept of wellness coaching is commonly incorporated as part of worksite health promotion and is a frequent area in which kinesiology majors find employment. Wellness coaches build relationships with employees and give them individual attention and feedback to help them achieve health and physical activity goals. In William's case, his company wellness coach helped him further understand how to manage his

*influence disease prevention behaviors, improve worker productivity, reduce health care costs, improve health, and inspire organizational policy change.*

*As you learned in Chapters 1 and 2, there are a variety of career options for kinesiology majors including jobs in business and industry promoting worksite health, fitness, performance, and safety. In Lesson 2, you will learn about examples of how workplace physical activity and health concepts*

*are related to the subdisciplines of kinesiology and how to integrate them into effective programming strategies.*

- Exercise Physiology
- Biomechanics
- Public Health
- Motor Learning
- Practice of Kinesiology

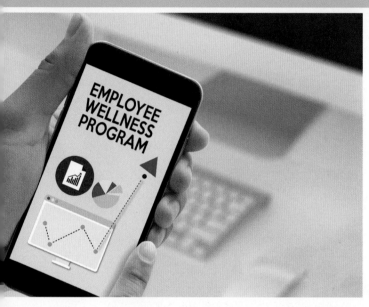

health conditions and how to achieve more regular physical activity, reduce his stress, and be more compliant in taking his hypertension and chest pain medications. He also became more focused on enjoying his daily work.

Marsha and her staff hope to build a culture of health and evaluate employee progress over four to five years in a best practices approach to worksite health promotion. As part of her job duties, Marsha was asked to implement, through her administrative leadership, a best practices workplace health promotion framework focused on eventually determining the health and economic impacts of program implementation. The evaluation framework chosen by company executives was based on components shown in Figure 9.9. The framework in Figure 9.9 includes an initial process evaluation phase, an impact evaluation phase, and an outcomes evaluation phase. The program is currently in the initial phase, but William and the company leadership like what they have experienced thus far.

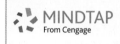 Go to your MindTap course to complete the Case Study activity for this chapter.

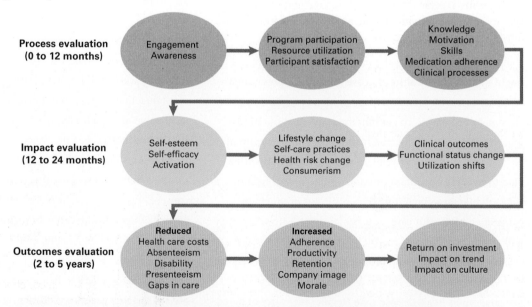

**Figure 9.9** | Best Practices in Evaluating Worksite Health Promotion Evaluation Programs

*Source:* Adapted from J. Grossmeier et al., "Best Practices in Evaluating Worksite Health Promotion Programs," *American Journal of Health Promotion* 24, no. 3 (Jan/Feb 2010): 4.

## Exercise Physiology

Exercise as a stimulus to the human body has helped scientists and physicians understand physiologic responses and potential disease risks for many years. In controlled settings, treadmills and cycle ergometers are frequently used to test how a person responds physiologically to a "dose" of exercise. **Graded exercise testing (GXT)** has been used for job-related heart disease screening and high-risk employees in many different workplace settings, including the U.S. Army, since the 1970s (the Over-40 Army Physical Fitness Test [APFT] or Cardiovascular Screening Program).[18] If a soldier has significant cardiovascular risks (e.g., hypertension, high cholesterol, chest pain) and is over 40 years of age, he or she will receive a diagnostic GXT, usually performed on a treadmill using the Bruce protocol. The Bruce treadmill protocol starts at 1.7 mph with a 10% grade and increases in speed and grade every three minutes. During the test (review Figure 5.6), a physician evaluates subject responses such as heart rate, blood pressure, symptoms, 12-lead electrocardiogram (ECG), time completed, and reasons for stopping. The Bruce GXT protocol is often used to help screen soldiers who may not be fit for duty due to cardiovascular health conditions or who appear to be at higher health risk. The test provides a clinically safe alternative to the Army's standard two-mile run evaluation.

Based on the observations from the GXT, a physician can determine, from the over-40 APFT protocol, whether the soldier has a positive test (indicates probable heart disease and need for further follow-up), a negative test (normal), or an equivocal test (suspected heart disease and need for further follow-up) with regards to cardiovascular disease. The clinical data collected during the test can also indicate the soldier's cardiovascular fitness level. For example, to meet the age-40 Army cardiovascular fitness requirements, women must achieve a minimum workload equivalent to a $VO_2$ max (see Chapter 5) of about 24.7 $ml \cdot kg^{-1} \cdot min^{-1}$ (equal to completing about six minutes on the Bruce protocol) and men, a $VO_2$ max equivalent of about 32 $ml \cdot kg^{-1} \cdot min^{-1}$ (equal to completing about eight minutes on the Bruce protocol). For soldiers with documented physical challenges, there are alternate tests (such as cycle, swim, walk) to determine cardiovascular fitness.

## Biomechanics

In the workplace, kinesiology practitioners (e.g., athletic trainers, physical therapists, occupational therapists; see Chapter 1) often apply biomechanics and **ergonomic** (scientific study of people at work) principles to promote effective physical activity, health, and safety in the workplace. For example, if you, as a kinesiology professional, were employed at a large oil and gas refinery, how would you determine the following?

1. What are the critical physically demanding tasks or repetitive motions related to muscular strength (e.g., lifting, carrying, and twisting/turning) required for common jobs at the worksite?

2. What tests might you use to evaluate and promote the development of adequate employee strength to safely perform critical job tasks?

3. How could you use effective strength testing and follow-up over time to promote effective worksite health promotion?

One model that you might consider to solve this challenge is to implement (based on leadership review and approval) an overall job task analysis at the worksite. Then, based on the outcomes of a battery of isometric strength test evaluations, you could determine minimum scores that are consistent with being able to successfully perform critical job tasks safely and effectively. Dr. Andrew S. Jackson and colleagues (1990) evaluated workers at a large refinery plant and found that valve cracking and valve turning were two of the most physically demanding tasks in terms of strength. Based on their worksite evaluations, Dr. Jackson measured the sum of three isometric (static) strength measures (grip, arm curl, and back extension) to determine the probability of being able to crack and turn valves in a safe and comfortable manner. Figure 9.10 shows a prediction curve that suggests workers at the plant had a 100% probability of performing common valve cracking if they had an isometric strength sum score of between 350 and 400 pounds of force. Once these criteria were established, strategies could be developed to regularly test new employees (once hired) to determine if they could perform strength-related critical

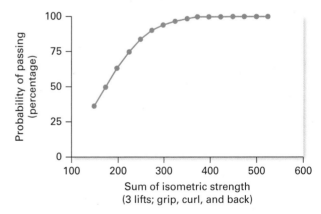

**Figure 9.10** | Probability of Cracking a Valve in a Refinery Workplace Setting Based upon the Sum of 3 Isometric (Static) Strength Measures (Grip, Arm Curl, and Back Extension). The graphic shows the importance of ergonomic testing to promote effective physical activity, health, and safety in the workplace.

*Source:* A. S. Jackson et al., "Strength Test for the Texas City Plant – Union Carbide Corporation, Center of Applied Psychological Services" (Houston, TX: Rice University, 1980).

job tasks safely and effectively. The testing could also be used in job-related strength and conditioning worksite programs to help workers who do not meet the minimum requirements (i.e., 300 to 400 pounds of force or sum of isometric/static strength) become stronger and eligible for such job tasks in the future.

## Public Health 🩺

The Take-a-Stand Project, 2011 is a good example of a public health and physical activity initiative that focused on reducing prolonged sitting time at the workplace.[19] As you learned in Lesson 1, prolonged sitting is associated with increased health risks, including premature development of chronic diseases.

Pronk and colleagues designed a study in partnership with a sit–stand work station device manufacturer. These devices (WorkFit S or WorkFit C) encourage workers to stand and move about more (e.g., walking). A total of 34 employees (24 in an intervention group, 10 in a comparison group) from the Health Promotion Department at Health Partners in Minneapolis, MN, were evaluated to determine the effects of reduced sitting on health-related outcomes, mood states (POMS; see Chapter 8), and indicators of work and office behavior. While working, the subjects were asked to respond to text messages regarding whether they were sitting (scored as a 0), standing (scored as 1), or walking (scored as 2). The study lasted 7 weeks: week 1 was used for baseline data collection (no intervention) for all subjects; weeks 2 to 5 were intervention periods with installed sit–stand work stations; and weeks 6 and 7 were post-intervention periods without sit-stand work stations.

Mean scores for sitting, standing, and walking among employees for each period of the study are shown in Figure 9.11. As Figure 9.11 indicates, the intervention significantly reduced sitting time (scored as 0) during the intervention compared to baseline and post-intervention. The authors reported that the intervention reduced sitting time by 224% (66 minutes per day), reduced self-reported upper and lower neck pain by 55%, and improved the mood states (see Chapter 8) of workers. This research represents one of the first intervention trials to actually provide evidence that sedentary behavior in the workplace can be reduced while conferring health benefits.[20] More studies using additional strategies are needed to learn more about how to reduce prolonged sitting in the workplace.

## Motor Learning 🏃

Each year, about 800,000 individuals in the United States suffer a stroke (interruption of blood flow to the brain), and many are of working age. Only about 30%

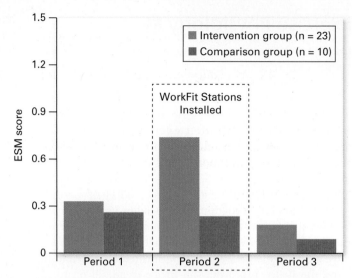

**Figure 9.11** | Average Experience Sampling Methodology (ESM) Scores (0 = Sitting, 1 = Standing, 2 = Walking) for Intervention (Reduced Sitting Time) with a Sit to Stand Device versus Comparison (No Intervention) Group

*Source:* N. Pronk et al., "Reducing Occupational Sitting Time and Improving Worker Health: The Take-a-Stand Project, 2011," *Preventing Chronic Disease* 9 (2012): 4.

of workers who have a stroke return to work and of those who do, 15% leave six months after returning. More and more often, occupational therapists (many with kinesiology backgrounds) are being asked (via employee assistance programs and health insurance providers) to help rehabilitate workers who have suffered a mild stroke.

Occupational therapists treating individuals who have suffered a stroke assess a variety of factors, including body functions, performance skills, and physical activities. Colleen Fowler proposed a working framework for understanding the person, the environment, and occupational factors that should be considered when rehabilitating those who have experienced a mild stroke for return to work.[21] The following list contains some of the common categories of measures that occupational therapists use to assess and evaluate stroke victims who return to work:[22]

### Individual Factors

*Sensory factors*—such as visual, auditory, and proprioception deficits

*Motor function*—fine and gross motor movement abilities and overall movement skills

*Physiology*—overall fitness and fatigability

*Cognition*—ability to plan, organize, perform sequencing behaviors, understand concepts, and adjust to new situations

*Psychosocial*—symptoms of stress, irritability, emotionalism, anxiety, and depression

*Culture*—expectations of self and family caregivers

**Environmental Factors**

*Workplace culture*—workplace health promotion support, acceptance, and programming

*Social support*—stroke education of colleagues in the workplace

*Physical environment*—work space factors and technology assistance considerations

*Social policies*—health insurance coverage and laws affecting those with physical/mental disabilities

**Occupational Factors**

*On-site evaluation*—analysis of job requirements and possible adjustments to maintain/improve work safety and productivity

## The Practice of Kinesiology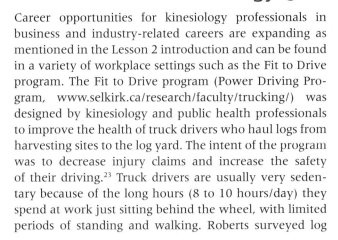

Career opportunities for kinesiology professionals in business and industry-related careers are expanding as mentioned in the Lesson 2 introduction and can be found in a variety of workplace settings such as the Fit to Drive program. The Fit to Drive program (Power Driving Program, www.selkirk.ca/research/faculty/trucking/) was designed by kinesiology and public health professionals to improve the health of truck drivers who haul logs from harvesting sites to the log yard. The intent of the program was to decrease injury claims and increase the safety of their driving.[23] Truck drivers are usually very sedentary because of the long hours (8 to 10 hours/day) they spend at work just sitting behind the wheel, with limited periods of standing and walking. Roberts surveyed log haulers and heavy equipment operators for the Weyerhaeser Company regarding injury and accident rates and found the following:[24]

- 75% of workers tested were obese
- 37% had undiagnosed pre-diabetes (blood glucose levels 100–120 mg/dL) and 11% were fully diabetic (glucose > 120 mg/dL)
- 95% suffered from chronic joint or muscle pain

The *Fit to Drive Program: Integrated Injury Prevention, Health, and Wellness for Truck Drivers* is linked specifically to strategies 1 and 3 of the *National Physical Activity Plan* in the business and industry sector (see Table 9.4). Results from the first three months indicated that 50% of the truckers participating in the program lost significant amounts of weight and were increasing their daily physical activity levels. The 80% of drivers participating who had serious health problems (e.g., hypertension, diabetes) all reported that they had been able to reduce their reliance on prescription medications. Lessons learned from implementation of the program included:

- An understanding of the culture of truck driving and personnel characteristics.
- Management must be willing to commit to intervention programming and sustain those efforts (in this case for at least four years) before it becomes part of the worksite culture.
- The implementation success and sustainability of the programming are dependent upon its being culturally specific and customizing elements to meet individual needs.

---

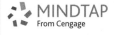 From Cengage

Now that you have completed this chapter, go to your MindTap course to complete all assigned activities. Check out the additional resources developed to help you apply the material in this chapter to your course and career goals.

---

## Chapter Summary

- The passage of federal health care reform (Affordable Care Act of 2010) prioritized the quality and efficiency of health care for Americans, while emphasizing preventing chronic diseases and improving public health. The legislation included unprecedented funding for health promotion, wellness, and prevention that extends specifically to the workplace.

- In today's workplace, an unintended consequence of "lean thinking" (less human effort, less equipment, less space, while exceeding customer expectations) in business and industry settings has been prolonged periods of sitting and physical inactivity for many employees. Low levels of occupational physical activity have been associated with musculoskeletal problems, pain, increases in sick leave, absenteeism, lower work productivity, excess health care costs, and other ill-health effects.

- Employers are interested in health promotion because of their fundamental assumption that healthier employees have lower health care costs (of which employers pay an estimated 30%), are more productive, are absent less frequently, and are happier than employees who are not as healthy. Physical activity interventions (along with other positive health behavior interventions like smoking cessation, stress reduction, and health screens) can influence individuals, populations within the workplace, organizational policies, families, and communities.

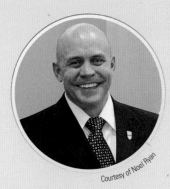

Courtesy of Noel Ryan

**Q: Why and how did you get into the field of kinesiology?**

**A:** *I grew up in Australia where our culture was focused on being outdoors, as well as sporting. I enjoyed playing many sports including soccer, cricket, and rugby during my adolescence and early adult life. My first job out of college was a high school health and physical education teacher in Australia. I was very interested in motor learning, skill acquisition, and fitness.*

**Q: What was the major influence on you to work in the field?**

**A:** *I came to the United States to study at the University of Houston and complete a master's degree in kinesiology and was amazed by the various areas of concentration a student could pursue. I gravitated toward exercise physiology, exercise testing, motor learning, and measurement and evaluation. I was fortunate to work on a number of grants that looked at solutions for obesity rates for women in minority populations and elementary school children. My master's thesis chair, Dr. James Morrow, Jr., was also a personal inspiration for both his research and for living a healthy lifestyle.*

**Q: What are your current research interests, and how do you translate your research results to practitioners?**

**A:** *My current concentration is related to the delivery of health and wellness resources to workers in remote populations. I work for Chevron, a company that is truly committed to health and wellness and to programs that enable fitness for duty in offshore oil workers in the Gulf of Mexico. We support the workforce in building individual skills and through health programs, healthy meals, and education about benefits resources. To make this program sustainable we are hoping to embed a culture of health by encouraging proper eating habits, educating chefs on how to cook*
healthier meals and snacks, and adding healthy choice requirements for catering contracts.

**Q: How do you stay physically active yourself and promote good health to others directly around you?**

**A:** *We are lucky at Chevron that we have access to an on-site gym and a walking trail through the campus. I schedule time to utilize these resources throughout the week and am able to complete longer workouts over the weekends utilizing the paths along the beautiful Lake Pontchartrain. Additionally, over the past 10 years I have scheduled annual physical exams with my physician to track my cardiovascular numbers and monitor my health. We have developed a program in our location to encourage annual physicals.*

**Q: How have you had to integrate the subdisciplines of kinesiology in your professional practice?**

**A:** *My roles during my career at Chevron have been related to Health, Productivity, and Fitness for Duty. My studies in exercise physiology, exercise testing, and exercise prescription have been vital for understanding the critical work tasks an employee must perform and quantifying the physical demand of the job. This is especially important in developing fitness programs and providing health resources to ensure that our workforce can safely perform these roles throughout the duration of their employment. My measurement and evaluation studies have instilled the need to quantify the outcomes of the programs that we put in place. It is vital in our company to show the value of the investment toward maintaining health to our leaders.*

*Noel Ryan is the Occupational Health Supervisor with Chevron's Gulf of Mexico Business Unit in Covington, LA. He leads a team of specialists who are responsible for programs related to fitness for duty, industrial hygiene, ergonomics, and health promotion.

• Workplace health promotion programs that include a major focus on increasing and maintaining physical activity levels for employees and their families can create a positive culture for business and industry that can translate into healthier communities.

• Worksite health promotion programs commonly include combinations of programming that focus on educational, physical, organizational, and/or environmental activities.

• The essential elements of effective workplace wellness programs can be classified into four categories: organizational culture and leadership, program design, program implementation, and program evaluation.

• The CDC workplace health promotion development model focuses on four main steps: assessment, planning, program implementation, and evaluation. Kinesiology professionals should consider using the essential elements of effective programs and the CDC model to develop effective workplace health promotion strategies focusing on physical activity and health outcomes.

## Remember This

absenteeism
accessibility
Affordable Care Act of 2010
aging workforce
biometric tests/health screenings
business
business and industry or corporate culture
business and industry or corporate image
comprehensive worksite health promotion program
cost-benefit ratios
culture of health and physical activity
employee health insurance
employee recruitment
employee retention
ergonomic
fitness tests
graded exercise testing (GXT)
health risk appraisals (HRAs)
industry
presenteeism
productivity
surveillance
wearables
wellness
worker's compensation costs (WCC)
worksite health promotion or wellness program
worksite health care costs

## For More Information

Access these websites for further study of topics covered in the chapter:

▸ Find updates and quick links to these and other evidence-base practice related sites on your MindTap course.

▸ Search for further information about physical activity in business and industry settings using the NCCDPHP toolkit at www.cdc.gov/workplacehealthpromotion.

▸ Search for information and resources about the effectiveness of physical activity in business and industry settings in *The Guide to Community Preventive Services* at www.thecommunityguide.org.

▸ Search for information about worksite health promotion strategies for practitioners at the International Association for Worksite Health Promotion: www.acsm-iawhp.org.

▸ Search for more information about physical activity in business and industry settings provided by the National Institute for Occupational Safety and Health (NIOSH) at www.cdc.gov/niosh/TWH/essentials.html.

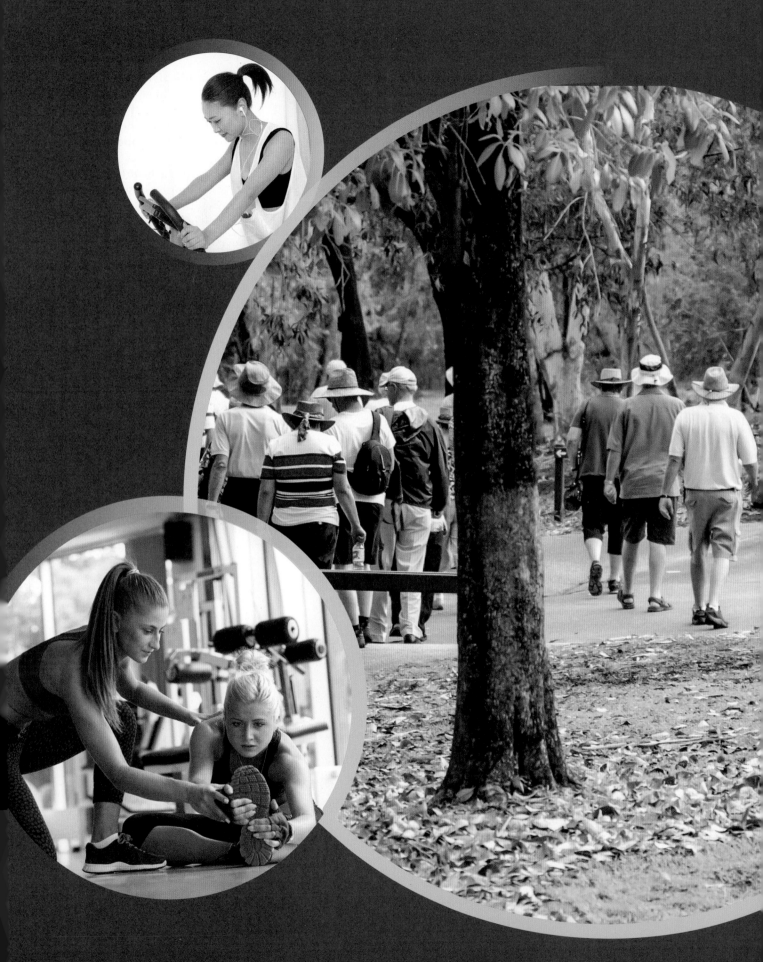

# Integration of Kinesiology with Leisure Time, Recreation, and Career Personal Training

*What knowledge, skills, and abilities do kinesiology majors need to have and use to pursue careers in leisure and recreation settings, as well as in career personal training opportunities?*

**LESSON 1** INTEGRATION OF LEISURE TIME, RECREATION, AND PERSONAL TRAINING WITH THE PRINCIPLES OF PHYSICAL ACTIVITY AND KINESIOLOGY

**LESSON 2** EXAMPLES OF APPLYING LEISURE TIME, RECREATION, AND PERSONAL TRAINING PRINCIPLES OF PHYSICAL ACTIVITY IN RELATIONSHIP TO THE KINESIOLOGY SUB-DISCIPLINES

## Learning Objectives

*After completing this chapter, you will be able to:*

**Define** the common physical activity principles and terms associated with leisure time, recreation, and personal training.

**Explain** how leisure time, recreation, and personal training physical activity principles promote health, physical fitness, and optimal human performance.

**Explain** the importance of physical activities within leisure time, recreation, and personal training settings in relation to the various subdisciplines of kinesiology.

**Describe** the specific health benefits of participating in physical activity programs in leisure time, recreation, and personal training settings with regards to the physical activity continuum.

**Explain** how the health benefits acquired through participating in physical activity programs in leisure time, recreation, and personal training settings can positively influence communities.

**Explain** the essential elements of effective leisure time, recreation, and personal training programs.

**Explain** a systematic process for building partnerships, promotions, and policies that increase physical activity.

**Give** examples of modifications of overload, specificity, and adaptation in leisure time, recreation, and personal training settings that improve overall health, physical fitness, and peak performance through participation in physical activity.

**Describe** common methods and measures used to evaluate and monitor individuals and populations in leisure time, recreation, and personal training settings.

**Explain** a variety of examples of the application of leisure time, recreation, and personal training concepts to participation in physical activity in the context of kinesiology-related subdisciplines.

# INTEGRATION OF LEISURE TIME, RECREATION, AND PERSONAL TRAINING WITH THE PRINCIPLES OF PHYSICAL ACTIVITY AND KINESIOLOGY

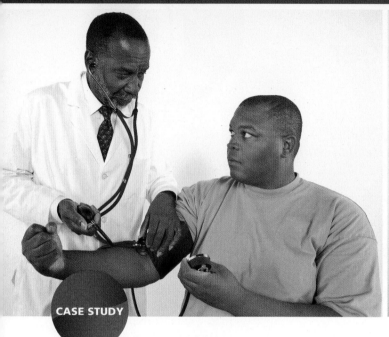

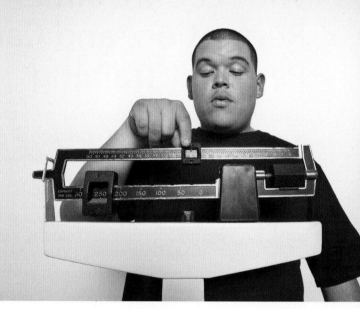

**CASE STUDY**

## In the real world . . .

Jerald Casey is a busy young man: he is going to college and working to help pay for school, while living at home. As you learned in Chapter 1, Jerald is physically inactive and overweight, but he wants to become active and start losing weight—if he can somehow work it into his busy schedule. He is excited about returning to school in two weeks because of the recent completion of the Bulldog Trail (named after the school mascot), a multiuse trail three miles long that runs around and through campus. The trail was built as part

of a health promotion project to encourage all students to be "active Bulldogs."

Jerald plans on getting up a little bit earlier each day prior to classes and walking, jogging, or cycling regularly on the trail. He is hoping that his new time management plan will allow him to restructure his school days so that he can pursue more leisure physical activity in his discretionary time (the time that is up to individual choice). Do you think Jerald will improve his health and lose weight just by using the trail regularly? What evidence is available that shows that building trails in parks and at schools

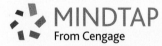

**From Cengage**

Go to your MindTap course now to answer some questions and discover what you already know about the integration of kinesiology with leisure time, recreation, and career personal training.

## INTERACTIVE ACTIVITIES

**Research Focus**

Go to your MindTap course to compare the physical activity levels of adults in your state with the U.S. national averages.

**Career Focus**

Go to your MindTap course to learn more about future trends and recent or past fads in personal training. You can also track future trends and recent or past fads by following the annual ACSM survey results.

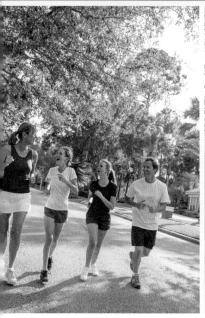 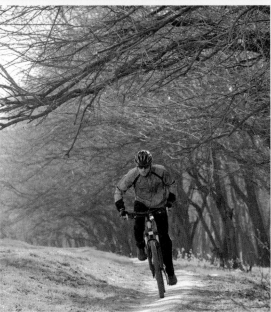 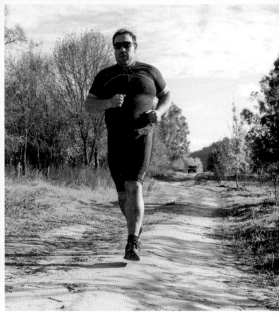

can increase physical activity levels of visitors or students and improve their health? How do factors such as age, education level, income level, trail accessibility, type of trail, and safety issues affect how frequently the Bulldog Trail will be used by Jerald and others? Does your college or university have a multiuse trail, or is there one close to your campus? Would you use the trail if you had one, or do you use one that already exists? How could trails

be used as a resource to promote physical activity during leisure time, as part of recreation, and with the aid of personal trainers? We will follow up with Jerald to see what barriers and successes he encounters in using the Bulldog Trail later in Lesson 2, after you have had the opportunity to learn more about the integration of leisure time, recreation, and personal training with the principles of physical activity and kinesiology.

# Introduction: Leisure Time, Recreation, Career Personal Training, Physical Activity, and Kinesiology

The US National Physical Activity Plan (refer to Chapter 9) contains several strategies for targeting physical activity promotion in community recreation, fitness, and park settings. In this chapter, we focus primarily on promotion of physical activity to individuals and groups during leisure time, recreation, and integrating career personal training experiences. Our approach, although a bit different than that of the National Physical Activity Plan methodology, includes specific knowledge, skills, and abilities (KSA) materials for kinesiology professionals in training who might seek careers in these various settings. We have included details about career personal training in this chapter, as compared to the workplace or other topics because most individuals or populations using personal trainers do so during their discretionary leisure time. Personal trainers can help people increase their physical activity and fitness, particularly during leisure time. In Chapter 13, we will focus more specifically on sport and related career opportunities for kinesiology professionals (also see Chapter 11 for more about school sports). The specific National Physical Activity Plan community recreation, fitness, and parks strategies are listed in Table 10.1.

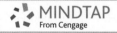

## Promoting Physical Activity in Community Recreation, Fitness, and Parks

Go to your **MindTap course** to learn more about specific strategies for implementing the PRFS strategies in Table 10.1.

Discretionary or leisure time is sometimes difficult to define and ever more difficult to find. With obligations to school, family, work, and others, any leisure time we have is usually realized in the form of small breaks, and much of it is often spent in sedentary activities involving screen time (phones, computers, television, and videos).[1] U.S. economic studies show that spending is higher for goods/services associated with sedentary activities such as media and spectator sports than for those related to more physically active behaviors such as sporting goods equipment and fitness facility memberships.[2] The opportunities and potential to promote physical activity and kinesiology-related subdiscipline concepts for leisure time, recreation, and career personal training to large populations are considerable. The career opportunities for kinesiology professionals who wish to work with individuals and populations during leisure time, recreation, and personal training are expanding rapidly, and that expansion is forecast to continue.[3]

## Physical Activity in Leisure Time Settings: Basic Terms, Common Components, and Influencing Factors

**Leisure time physical activity** includes participation during discretionary time in exercise, recreation, or hobbies that are not part of essential activities such as one's job, school or household work, or transportation.[4] How Americans spend their leisure time on an average day is illustrated in Figure 10.1, and time spent in leisure and sports activities each day by age is shown in Figure 10.2.[5] As the data in Figures 10.1 and 10.2 clearly indicate, most Americans spend their leisure time in sedentary behaviors. The television continues to dominate our leisure time while sports and exercise contribute only a small amount.

How many people in the United States are physically active? Are there trends? How do we get such information? In the United States, multiple sources of survey data contribute to our understanding of physical activity behaviors.

**Table 10.1** | Strategies for Promoting Physical Activity in Community Recreation, Fitness, and Parks

| STRATEGY 1 | Communities should develop new, and enhance existing, community recreation, fitness, and park programs that provide and promote healthy physical activity opportunities for diverse users across the lifespan. |
|---|---|
| STRATEGY 2 | Communities should improve availability of and access to safe, clean, and affordable community recreation, fitness, and park facilities to support physical activity for all residents. |
| STRATEGY 3 | Community recreation and park organizations, the fitness industry, and private business should recruit, train, and retain a diverse group of leaders, staff, and volunteers to promote, organize, lead, and advocate for initiatives that encourage physical activity in their communities. |
| STRATEGY 4 | Community recreation and park organizations, the fitness industry, and private business should advocate for increased and sustainable funding and resources to create new, or enhance existing, physical activity facilities and services in areas of high need. |
| STRATEGY 5 | Community recreation and park organizations and the for- and not-for-profit fitness industry should improve monitoring and evaluation of participation in community-based physical activity programs to gauge their effectiveness in promoting increased levels of physical activity for all. |

*Source:* National Physical Activity Plan Alliance (NPAPA), www.physicalactivityplan.org.

For example, data about physical activity behaviors among adults have been gathered on an ongoing basis through the National Health Interview Survey (NHIS). State-specific data are gathered by telephone and Internet-based surveys and can be assessed electronically via the Behavioral Risk Factor Surveillance System (BRFSS).[6] Periodic surveys like the National Health and Nutrition Examination Survey (NHANES) also provide valuable data to help researchers understand trends in leisure time physical activity.[7] The Youth Risk Behavior Surveillance System (YRBSS) provides physical activity behavior data for high school students (grades 9 through 12), but for younger adolescents or children, very few data are available. An example of the variety of national US survey data available on physical activity is shown in Table 10.2. Although key

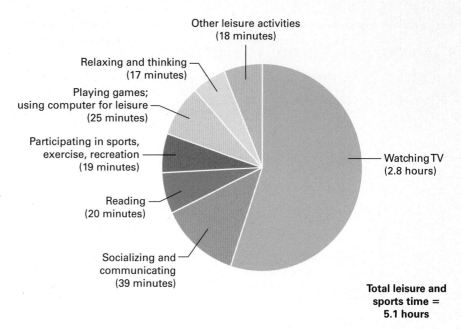

**Figure 10.1** | How U.S. Individuals Age 15 and Over Spend Leisure Time on an Average Day

Note: Data include all persons age 15 and over. Data include all days of the week and are annual averages for 2012.

*Source:* Bureau of Labor Statistics, *American Time Use Survey* (Washington, DC: U.S. Department of Labor, 2013).

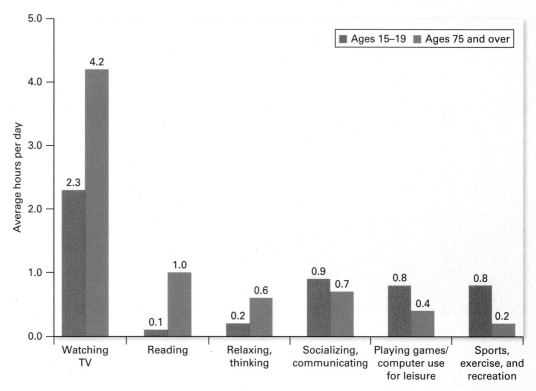

**Figure 10.2** | Average Hours Spent per Day in Leisure and Sports Activities, by Youngest and Oldest Populations

Note: Data include all days of the week and are annual averages for 2012.

*Source:* Bureau of Labor Statistics, *American Time Use Survey* (Washington, DC: U.S. Department of Labor, 2013).

**Table 10.2** | Characteristics of US National Physical Activity Surveys, 1998–2007.

| CATEGORY | NHIS | NHANES | BRFSS |
|---|---|---|---|
| Survey years physical activity data were collected[a] | 1998–2007 | 1999–2006 | 2001, 2003, 2005, 2007 |
| Recall period | Respondent selects recall period[b] | Past 30 days[c] | Usual week[d] |
| Self-reported | Yes | Yes | Yes |
| List of specific activities | No | Yes | No |
| Assesses moderate-intensity physical activity | Yes, but includes light intensity | Yes | Yes |
| Assesses vigorous-intensity physical activity | Yes | Yes | Yes |
| Which intensity level is asked about first? | Vigorous | Vigorous | Moderate |
| Definition of moderate-intensity physical activity | Light sweating or a slight to moderate increase in breathing or heart rate | Light sweating or a slight to moderate increase in breathing or heart rate | Small increases in breathing or heart rate |
| Definition of vigorous-intensity physical activity | Heavy sweating or large increases in breathing or heart rate | Heavy sweating or large increases in breathing or heart rate | Large increases in breathing |

Abbreviations: BRFSS, Behavioral Risk Factor Surveillance System, NHIS, National Health Interview Survey, NHANES, National Health and Nutrition Examination Survey.

[a] Includes years in which the same physical activity question was asked of respondents, NHIS asked a slightly different physical activity question in the first half of 1997, which included a minimum duration of "at least 20 minutes." This changed midyear in 1997 to "at least 10 minutes" and has remained unchanged ever since.

[b] NHIS physical activity questions allow respondents to select the recall period. To define physical activity levels, the average number of times per week (rounded to the nearest time) was calculated for those respondents who selected monthly or yearly time periods.

[c] NHANES has separate questions about active transportation and moderate household activities that are not included as part of this analysis.

[d] BRFSS has a separate question about monthly participation (yes or no) in any physical activities or exercises such as running, calisthenics, golf, gardening, or walking for exercise that was not included as part of this analysis.

*Source*: From S.A. Carlson et al., "Differences in Physical Activity Prevalence and Trends from 3 U.S. Surveillance Systems," *Journal of Physical Activity and Health* 6, no. 1 (2009): S18–S27.

characteristics can change each year of survey operation, it is instructive to compare the sources. For the most current approaches in each of these surveys, visit their websites. Physical activity surveillance data systems also exist for other countries, including Australia, Canada, and Brazil.

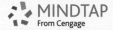

**MINDTAP**
From Cengage

**Physical Activity Levels and Trends in the United States**

**Go to your MindTap course** to compare the physical activity levels of adults in your state with the U.S. national averages.

Moore at al. studied the 23-year trends for no leisure time physical activity among adults by using responses to a single "yes" or "no" question from the BRFSS. The question was: "During the past month, other than your regular job, did you participate in any physical activities or exercise such as running, calisthenics, golf, gardening, or walking for exercise?"[8] The percentage of U.S. adults engaging in no leisure time physical activity from 1988 to 2010 is shown in Figure 10.3. As you can see, a slight improvement in no leisure time physical activity has occurred, yet in 2010 about 1 in 4 Americans still reported that they do not engage in *any* leisure time physical activity.

As with many other health indicators, leisure time physical activity participation in the United States is related to several demographic characteristics of the populations (and subpopulations) under observation. Such factors include sex, age, race/ethnicity, and education levels. For example, the data in Figure 10.3 clearly show sex differences in reported no leisure time physical activity, with 5% more women reporting no leisure time activity than men in 2010. Why might that be? Does the male/female difference seem to be getting larger over time? Do women have less leisure time than men?

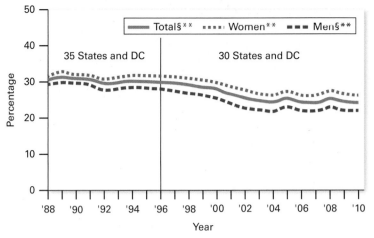

§Significant linear trend for 35 states and Washington, DC, 1988–1995 (p < 0.01) across all years.

**Significant linear trend for 50 states and Washington, DC, 1996–2010 (p < 0.01) across all years.

**Figure 10.3** | Prevalence of No Leisure Time Physical Activity by Adults from 1988–2010 Based on Behavioral Risk Factor Surveillance and System Data

*Source:* L. Moore et al., "Trends in No Leisure-Time Physical Activity—United States, 1988–2010," *Research Quarterly for Exercise and Sport* 83, no. 4 (2012): 588.

Age and race/ethnicity are other demographic factors linked to differences in physical activity. For example, the data in Figure 10.4 separate the sex-specific data into age groupings as well. Notice that nearly 50% of younger adult males (age 18 to 24) reported participation in leisure time physical activity while only about 25% of older adult men (age 75+) were physically active in their leisure time. Considering older adults likely have more discretionary time than younger people, does this seem counterintuitive? What other patterns do you see in Figure 10.4?

Even after accounting for the sex and age differences in physical activity participation illustrated

above, race/ethnicity is a powerful predictor of leisure time physical activity participation. Taking into account different ages and combining men and women, the percentage of adults aged 18 years and over who engaged in regular leisure time physical activity, by race/ethnicity is shown in Figure 10.5.[9] Clearly Hispanic adults and non-Hispanic black adults have much lower participation (about 27%) than white adults (nearly 40%). Can you think of reasons why these disparities may exist? Do white adults have more opportunities for leisure time than other race/ethnicity groups?

For high school–aged students, the YRBSS provides physical activity data focused on meeting the 2008 Physical Activity Guidelines for Americans (60 minutes per day of moderate and vigorous physical activity daily with three days of muscle-strengthening activities).[10] For example, when students were asked if they were physically active at least 60 minutes per day for all seven days in the last week, 48.3% of the total sample reported that they did not meet guidelines (58.4% of females and 38.2% of males). When students were asked if they participated in muscle-strengthening activities on three or more days, 72.9% of the total sample reported that they did not meet guidelines (82.3% of females and 63.4% of males). Based on the available YRBSS data, adolescents are much less physically active than recommended for good health, which encourages children and adolescents to acquire 60 minutes or more of moderate or vigorous physical activity including muscle-strengthening and bone-strengthening activities.[11]

Educational attainment is another demographic factor that frequently predicts health and positive

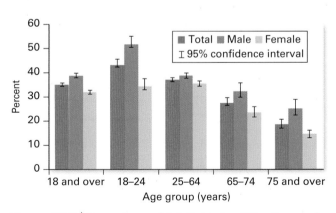

**Figure 10.4** | Percentage of Adults by Age Who Engaged in Regular Leisure Time Physical Activity in 2010

*Source:* Centers for Disease Control and Prevention National Health Interview Survey (Washington, DC: U.S. Department of Health and Human Services, March 11, 2011), www.cdc.gov/nchs/data/nhis/earlyrelease/201103_07.pdf

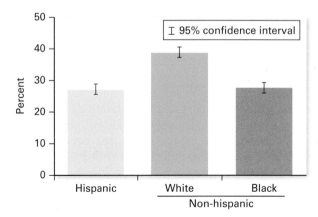

**Figure 10.5** | Percentage of Adults by Race/Ethnicity Who Engaged in Regular Leisure Time Physical Activity in 2010

*Source:* Centers for Disease Control and Prevention, *National Health and Nutrition Examination Survey* (Washington, DC: U.S. Department of Health and Human Services, 2011), www.cdc.gov/nchs/data/nhis/earlyrelease/201103_07.pdf

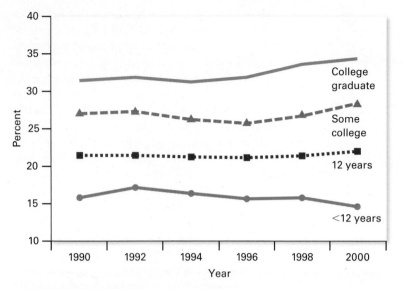

**Figure 10.6** | Trends for US Adults Meeting Recommended Physical Activity Levels* by Education

*Three or more METs, >30 minutes accumulated total, >5 days per week.

Source: Centers for Disease Control and Prevention, Behavioral Risk Factor Surveillance System (Washington, DC: U.S. Department of Health and Human Services, 2011), www.cdc.gov/brfss/.

health behaviors. An example of physical activity-related trends over time (1990–2000) based on the respondent's educational level is seen in Figure 10.6.[12] As shown, those who report completing a four-year college degree are approximately 20% more likely to report meeting physical activity recommendations than those who have not completed 12 years (high school graduation) of education. Why might educational attainment be related to physical activity participation?

An additional factor that might affect the evaluation of leisure time physical activity trends is changes over time in the level of physical activity considered adequate to meet guidelines/recommendations. As our understanding of the health benefits of physical activity has improved with more science, recommendations have changed and been refined. Schoenborn and colleagues reviewed the NHIS data for physical activity and compared trends for success in meeting Healthy People 2010 objectives (2000–2009) and the 2008 Physical Activity Guidelines.[13] The Healthy People 2010 criteria for aerobically active adults (developed prior to the 2008 Physical Activity Guidelines) were ≥30 minutes of moderate-intensity activity, five days per week and ≥20 minutes of vigorous-intensity activity for five days per week. The 2008 Physical Activity Guidelines criteria included ≥150 minutes of moderate-intensity activity per week, or ≥75 minutes of vigorous-intensity activity, or

≥150 minutes of an equivalent combination of moderate and vigorous physical activity.

Based upon their study definitions, Schoenborn and colleagues showed that, compared with estimates based on Healthy People 2010 criteria, prevalence estimates shifted upward by more than 10 percentage points when the 2008 guidelines were applied (see Figure 10.7).[14] They also found differences (see Figures 10.8 and 10.9) in activity level based on sex, age, race/ethnicity, and educational levels similar to those described by Moore and colleagues, the CDC, and Brownson and Boehmer when data were analyzed using both sets of physical activity recommendations.[15]

By monitoring and following the trends of leisure time physical activity over time, kinesiology professionals can gain a better understanding about how to develop integrated strategies to increase physical activity levels of individuals and populations. Tracking physical activity trends also helps professionals evaluate the progress of specific physical activity interventions such as those delivered in recreation or personal training settings.

## Physical Activity in Recreation Settings: Basic Terms, Common Components, and Influencing Factors

**Recreation** has been defined as part of the time spent in leisure and is associated with fun, enjoyment, and pleasure.[16] Obviously, most recreational experiences (such as walking, cycling, picnicking, sports, and camping) can

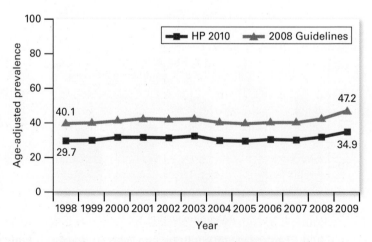

**Figure 10.7** | Trends in Aerobic Activity 1998–2009: Healthy People 2010 versus 2008 U.S. Physical Activity Guidelines

Source: CDC/NCHS, National Health Interview Survey, 2011.

include participation in a variety of physical activities. Common career opportunities in recreation-related fields that require a strong kinesiology preparation include directors of aquatics, directors of youth camps/sports programs, physical fitness resort/park coordinators, university fitness centers employees, home and fitness equipment supply, and recreational therapists. As with all kinesiology subdisciplines, career opportunities in this area are developing as interest in physical activity, health, physical fitness, and peak performance increases. Further, many new career opportunities will involve addressing barriers and facilitators of the built environment (such as development and renovation of parks, greenbelts, and trails).

Clearly gyms and fitness centers have traditionally been the "place" for leisure physical activity. Recently, other parts of the built environment, such as sidewalks, bicycle lanes, parks, and even empty parking lots have been leveraged as ways to promote physical activity. Parks are places that can be frequently overlooked. Parks have been classified into five categories: mini-parks, neighborhood parks, community parks, district parks, and regional parks.[17] The most common type is the neighborhood park, which provides local social and movement opportunities for residents. State and national parks also provide numerous opportunities for self-directed and organized outdoor physical activity experiences (e.g., hiking, sightseeing, and swimming).

Although parks have traditionally been thought of as places to relax and unwind, emerging research suggests that they are becoming popular settings for participating in common aerobic activities such as walking, cycling, and swimming. Spending time in parks has been found to help adults reduce mental stress and improve mood, and parks provide a healthy place in which to escape and rejuvenate.[18] One study reported that adults who used parks in the past month were over four times as more

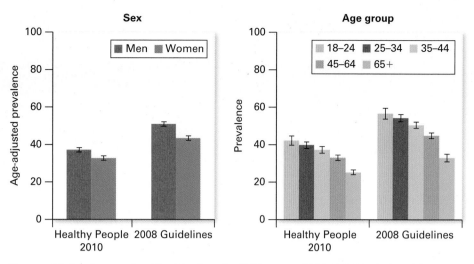

**Figure 10.8** | Comparing Healthy People 2010 versus 2008 U.S. Physical Activity Guidelines Criteria for Aerobic Activity, by Sex and Age
*Source:* CDC/NCHS, National Health Interview Survey, 2011.

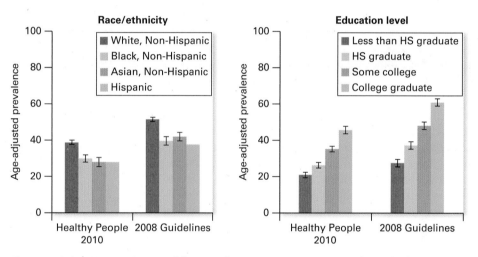

**Figure 10.9** | Comparing Healthy People 2010 versus 2008 U.S. Physical Activity Guidelines Criteria for Aerobic Activity, by Race/Ethnicity and Education
*Source:* CDC/NCHS, National Health Interview Survey, 2011.

likely to meet public health recommendations for engaging in physical activity as those who did not. The majority of research indicates that living closer to parks is associated with greater levels of physical activity for adults.

Godbey and Mowen reported that when the public was surveyed about the top three perceived benefits of using park and recreation facilities, exercise, enjoyment, and improving health were the most frequent responses, which are similar results as noted by others.[19] The survey results that Godbey and Mowen cite in their literature review and the survey of Cleveland Metroparks use by middle age and older users that support these conclusions are shown in Table 10.3.

Local park and recreation services use by adults over age 50 in one study are shown in Tables 10.3 and 10.4. The

**Table 10.3** | Benefits Ascribed to Use of Cleveland Metroparks by Middle Age and Older Users

| BENEFIT | PERCENTAGE |
|---------|-----------|
| Exercise | 48 |
| Renewal | 21 |
| Nature | 16 |
| Health | 6 |
| Other | 9 |

Source: From. L. Payne, B. Orsega-Smith, G. Godbey, and M. Roy, "Local Parks and the Health of Older Adults," *Parks and Recreation* 33, no. 10 (October 1998): 64–70.

study found that 85% of the total sample had visited a local park in the last 12 months.[20] In addition, over 50% of the respondents used the local park regularly, indicating that these individuals valued park and recreation use and nearly half (48%) of the respondents used the park for exercise.

Interestingly, broad economic trends seem to predict park use. Park use seems to increase during times of economic downturns. The data in Table 10.5 are from a survey of park use by families with children during an economic downturn year (2009). The data suggest that families with children use parks to entertain their children, perhaps substituting for other costlier options. This park use most likely increases the children's physical activity levels. Although no one is advocating for an economic downturn, the utility of parks as a low-cost alternative for places to be physically active has substantial potential to increase physical activity behaviors.

Family-based approaches to promote physical activity such as park and recreation activities are important strategies that can shape the future physical activity levels of children and adolescents.[21] Parents can positively influence the physical activity levels of their children in several ways:

1. Increase the number and diversity of opportunities for their children to be physically active.

2. Support and encourage physical activity for children by placing value on participation.

3. Model physical activity experiences and share in the fun and enjoyment.

**Table 10.4** | User Percentages of Local Park and Recreation Services (Age 50 and Older)

| USAGE | PERCENTAGE |
|-------|-----------|
| Once a week | 38 |
| One to three times per month | 21 |
| Less than once per month | 25 |
| Never | 15 |

Source: G. Godbey, L. Payne, and B. Orsega-Smith, "Examining the Relationship of Local Government Recreation and Park Services to the Health of Older Adults," Grant Research Results (Washington, DC: Robert Wood Johnson Foundation, 2004). www.rwjf.org/content/dam/farm/reports/program_results _reports/2007/rwjf15773.

**Table 10.5** | Greater Use of Parks and Playgrounds in 2009

| PARK USERS WITH CHILDREN IN THE HOUSEHOLD | Greater use: 30% |
| | Same use: 60% |
| | Less use: 10% |
| PARK USERS WITH CHILDREN UNDER AGE 6 IN THE HOUSEHOLD | Greater use: 38% |
| | Same use: 51% |
| | Less use: 10% |

Source: Trust for Public Land, available at www.tpl.org.

4. Help shape children's abilities necessary for and perceptions of their own competence in performing and participating regularly in physical activities.

Integrated approaches connecting families with social settings found in parks, trails, schools, churches, and neighborhoods can provide kinesiology professionals excellent opportunities to promote and increase physical activity.

Mowen and colleagues reported that a variety of factors can affect individuals' and groups' use of parks.[22] For example, it has been found that a park with paved walking trails is 27 times more likely to be used for physical activity than a park with no trails. Parents choose to visit parks that have water attractions, shade, and swings, and that are relatively clean. Starnes and colleagues reviewed the research on trail use to promote physical activity from the perspective of the public health, leisure sciences, urban planning, and transportation fields.[23] They found a growing research interest among professionals in studying trail use and physical activity, but the available evidence is limited.

Some of the correlates between intrapersonal and environmental variables that are related positively to, or related negatively to, or that have no effect on trail use by participants based on 13 reviewed studies are shown in Table 10.6.[24] The various relationships among the numerous intrapersonal and environmental correlates/considerations can have positive, negative, or neutral effect on trail use. This means that kinesiology professionals interested in the promotion of physical activity through trail development should evaluate specific factors (e.g., using neighborhood and community surveys) that should promote trail use in their unique situation. They can then determine how to focus on positive trail use factors while minimizing the local negative or neutral influences. For example, trails that are perceived as clean, safe, and easily accessible would likely be used more often than trails that are not well maintained, have limited access in terms of hours of operation, or are perceived as unsafe. Also, in some cases various intrapersonal and environmental correlates/considerations can be rated as neutral by potential trail users based upon individual/population opinions, judgments, and perceptions. How do you think each of the intrapersonal and environmental correlates/considerations listed in Table 10.6 might affect trail use in your local area?

**Table 10.6** | Intrapersonal and Environmental Correlates/Considerations That Can Affect Trail Use

| INTRAPERSONAL |
|---|

**Demographic**

Age

Race or ethnicity

Education

Income

Gender

Employment status

Marital status

Number of children in household

Home ownership

Membership in environmental group

**Behavioral and physiological**

Regularly active or not

Body mass index

Physical activity limitations

Psychological characteristics

Importance of activity to user

Place attachment to the trail (months of association)

| ENVIRONMENTAL |
|---|

**Trail**

Greater parking lot area

Type of trail

Trail surface (gravel versus paved or asphalt)

Mixed views

Surface condition

Litter and noise

Vegetation density along trail

Drains and tunnels

Length of trail (1/4–1/2 mile vs. longer and shorter trails)

**Neighborhood characteristics**

Distance from home to trail

Land use mix

Population density

Greenness

Length of street segments near trail

County is perceived as an easy place to be active

Accessibility of trail

Safety of the county

Midsized community

Lack of busy street and steep hill barriers

**Policy**

Support for creating public spaces for people to exercise

Willingness to pay taxes to build more parks and trails

Willingness to pay taxes to support government-funded campaigns to promote healthy eating and exercise

| Temporal and Weather |
|---|

Weekend days and particular months

Temperature, sunshine, daylight hours

Precipitation (rain and snow)

*Source:* From H. A. Starnes et al., "Trails and Physical Activity: A Review," *Journal of Physical Activity and Health* 8 (2011): 1167.

Starnes and colleagues also evaluated the potential facilitators and barriers to trail use by participants based on 31 reviewed studies; their results are shown in Table 10.7.[25] As you review Table 10.7, which items do you think would enhance or facilitate trail use? Which items do you perceive as being barriers to trail use? Some obvious facilitators supporting trail use as listed would include a person seeking opportunities for personal fitness and health who can exercise on a trail with a friendly atmosphere where he or she could meet new people, in a safe, well-maintained setting with numerous amenities. An example of barriers related to trail use might include an older adult who has limited time for physical activity who tries to use a trial that is not well maintained, that presents challenges to personal safety, has poor aesthetics, and has poor trail design (uneven surfaces and trail segments that are not effectively connected with clear signage). As you probably have noticed (similar to Table 10.6), each item listed in Table 10.7 could be rated as a facilitator or a barrier depending upon individual/population opinions, judgments, and perceptions.

Godbey and Mowen concluded that not only are the physical activity benefits of parks and recreation substantial and economically a bargain for users, communities, and city policy makers, but the levels of benefits can still be increased significantly at a low cost.[26] They provided seven recommendations through which parks and recreation programs can increase the health and physical activity benefits for consumers:

1. Make park and recreation services closer and more accessible—"creating parks and new park connectors from former industrial and commercial sites is an emerging tool being used to build urban park capacity."

2. Enhance travel connections (e.g., access to all parts of a park, trail, or playground) to new and existing park and recreation facilities—"the presence of active features at parks (e.g., trails, sports fields, playgrounds) enhances park use and physical activity levels."

3. Design and renovate parks to enhance active options across the lifespan—"today's park renovations and redesigns could be made with an eye toward active participation from all visitors by providing a wide range of active features."

4. Promote park and recreation services as an essential component of the health care system—"large scale advertising or promotion of parks and recreation can be used to position them as a fun and alternative place for enjoyable physical activity."

**Table 10.7** | Potential Facilitators and Barriers That Affect Trail Use

| INTRAPERSONAL |
| --- |
| Appreciation of nature or the outdoors |
| Personal fitness or health |
| Relaxation, solitude, or physical/psychosocial escape |
| Perception of a challenge, personal control, autonomy |
| Fun and enjoyment |
| Information about or awareness of the trail |
| Attachment to the trail |
| Desire to learn about the history of the area |
| Lack of time |
| Lack of money |
| Age |
| Education |

| INTERPERSONAL |
| --- |
| Negative interactions among users |
| Friends or family member to use trail with |
| Community pride and community identity |
| Friendly atmosphere and opportunity to meet new people |

| ENVIRONMENTAL |
| --- |
| **Trail** |
| Trail availability or convenience to home |
| Trail design (e.g., surface, street crossings, width, length, access points, terrain level, accessible for disabled) |
| Aesthetics or scenic features |
| Amenities (e.g., restrooms, water fountains, trash cans, recycling cans, parking for vehicles, signage, mile markers, lighting, etc.) |
| Safety |
| Maintenance or cleanliness |
| Freedom from motorized transportation |
| Active transportation or commuting opportunity |
| Cultural history of the area |
| Lack of services (e.g., food and bike repair) |
| **Policy** |
| Preservation of open space |
| Land-use patterns that support multiple uses |
| Development of trails |
| Funding for trails |

*Source:* From H. A. Starnes et al., "Trails and Physical Activity: A Review," *Journal of Physical Activity and Health* 8 (2011): 1171.

5. Create more recreation programs that provide physical activity.

6. Increase physical activity opportunities within existing programs—"a wide range of park and recreation programs could be modified or adapted to include bouts of moderate-to-vigorous physical activity."

7. Partner with and promote recreation programs to entire organizations—"participation in physically active recreation programs could be enhanced by promoting them to entire organizations rather than individuals."

Kinesiology professionals interested in pursuing a career in recreation-related areas should use the seven recommendations made by Godbey and Mowen to help them prepare and integrate their skills for success.[27]

## Physical Activity in Career Personal Training Settings: Basic Terms, Common Components, and the Physical Activity Continuum

**Personal training** is an occupation in which fitness professionals, usually with an academic training background in kinesiology and national professional certification, teach and coach individuals and groups how to achieve functional health, improved levels of physical fitness, high levels of performance fitness, wellness, and adopt other healthy behaviors. Personal trainers help clients set goals, provide feedback, and help monitor progress over time. Personal trainers are often called *wellness coaches* or *life coaches*, although there are distinctions among the three professional roles. Wellness and life coaches usually focus more on behavioral changes for individuals and groups, and physical activity may not be their primary focus.

### What Options Do Personal Trainers Have?

Conduct an Internet search to determine the differences among the terms *personal trainer*, *wellness coach*, and *life coach*.

According to the Bureau of Labor Statistics of the U.S. Department of Labor, there were at least 279,100 personal fitness trainers and instructors in 2014, and by 2024 the field is expected to grow by 8%.[28] Important personal trainer skills for entering the field are outlined in Table 10.8.

Many personal trainers in entry level positions at large commercial fitness centers often only have a high school education and usually are not nationally certified. In order to achieve higher-paying professional positions, most personal trainers obtain formal kinesiology academic training (like an associate, bachelor, or master's degree) and professional certification (see Chapter 1 for a discussion of professional development in kinesiology). A variety of professional organizations, associations, and agencies provide personal training certifications. However, certification programs such as those promoted by the American College of Sports Medicine (ACSM), the National Strength and Conditioning Association (NSCA), and a few other organizations (e.g., ACE, NASM, AFAA, Cooper Institute) require more rigorous written and practical examinations and thus are more respected than some lesser known programs.

**Table 10.8** | Common Personal Trainer Skills for Success

1. Customer service skills: the ability to interact with a diversity of individuals and groups and sell one's professional proficiencies through a variety of communication styles.

2. Listening skills: the ability to learn the specific physical activity and physical fitness needs of one's clients and to develop realistic, obtainable goals.

3. Motivational skills: the ability to help clients focus, stay engaged with physical activity programming, and avoid permanent relapses.

4. Physical fitness: the ability to develop and maintain acceptable levels of personal physical activity and physical fitness in order to serve as a role model (not necessarily athletic) for clients.

5. Problem-solving skills: the ability to integrate and use kinesiology subdisciplines to evaluate individual and group barriers and facilitators for success.

6. Speaking skills: the ability to verbally communicate and motivate spontaneously and effectively while working with clients.

7. Effective business skills: the ability to provide basic accounting, sales, marketing, and daily operations management and strategic planning.

*Source:* Adapted from Bureau of Labor Statistics, U.S. Department of Labor, *Occupational Outlook Handbook, 2014–2015, Fitness Trainers and Instructors,* available at www.bls.gov.

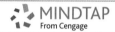

**Personal Fitness Certifications**

**Go to your MindTap course** to learn more about professional development in personal fitness training. Links to many of the programs mentioned above are included.

As you learned earlier in this chapter, it is helpful for kinesiology professionals to understand the population-level leisure time trends in order to forecast future opportunities and strategies for program development and implementation. Professionals interested in personal training can use resources such as the 2016 Annual ACSM Worldwide Survey of Fitness Trends to help them identify the KSAs they currently have that will help to meet their clients' needs, as well as the ones they need to acquire for future success. The ACSM surveys certified exercise professionals worldwide annually to help researchers determine physical activity- and physical fitness-related trends and fads. **Trends** refer to physical activity developments or changes that appear to be sustained over several years, whereas **fads** are activities that produce high levels of individual and group enthusiasm for brief periods of time. It is important for exercise professionals to understand the distinctions between trends and fads if they are to accurately predict future economic and professional changes that will help personal training programming remain effective. Fads come and go quickly, and are commonly observed in the personal fitness industry; however, they are not new to

fields like kinesiology. For example, in *Trends Toward the Future in Physical Education,* Massengale builds a strong case for forecasting future events in the field of physical education when he states:[29]

> The field of physical education has witnessed too many hula hoops, too many parachutes, too many movements, too many behavioral objectives, and most recently too many people from too many fields who proclaim themselves experts in health promotion.

By thinking about the future of the field of kinesiology, you can learn to distinguish between fads and true trends (or sound ideas) that can enhance your physical activity integration abilities and your potential professional career opportunities.

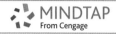

**The Future of Kinesiology**

**Go to your MindTap course** to learn more about future trends and recent or past fads in personal training. You can also track future trends and recent or past fads by following the annual ACSM survey results.

The 2016 ACSM annual survey on fitness trends included 2,833 responses worldwide, and Table 10.9 lists the occupational categories for those participating. As shown in Table 10.9, the number one category was part-time personal trainer, which has become a popular career move for many workers since the U.S. economic downturn in 2007.

**Table 10.9** | Respondents' Occupation (by Percentage of Total)

| OCCUPATION | % OF TOTAL |
|---|---|
| Personal trainer (part-time): | 14.12 |
| Personal trainer (full-time): | 10.30 |
| Health fitness specialist (or equivalent): | 7.71 |
| Health/fitness director: | 6.53 |
| Clinical exercise physiologist: | 6.33 |
| Graduate student: | 4.92 |
| Professor: | 6.25 |
| Medical professional (M.D./D.O., R.N., physical therapist, occupational therapist): | 6.37 |
| Undergraduate student: | 3.78 |
| Program manager: | 4.17 |
| Clinical exercise specialist (or equivalent): | 2.71 |
| Owner/operator: | 3.22 |
| Group exercise leader: | 2.36 |
| Teacher: | 2.01 |
| Other: | 14.94 |

*Source:* W. R. Thompson, "Worldwide Survey of Fitness Trends for 2016," 10th Anniversary Edition, *ACSM's Health and Fitness Journal* 19, no. 6 (2016): 11.

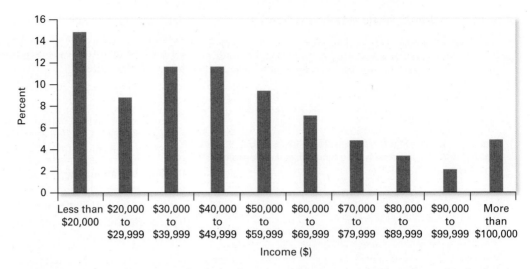

**Figure 10.10** | Sample Range of Salaries for Personal Trainers and Other Fitness Professionals

*Source:* W. R. Thompson, "Worldwide Survey of Fitness Trends for 2016," 10th Anniversary Edition, *ACSM's Health and Fitness Journal* 19, no. 6 (2016): 11.

The distribution of annual salaries reportedly earned by the survey respondents are shown in Figure 10.10. These results closely match job forecasting salary indicators available from the US. Department of Labor.

Trends can change readily. Group fitness activities such as Zumba, Pilates, spinning, stability ball exercises, pregnancy/postnatal classes, water workouts, mixed martial arts kickboxing, power training ropes, exercise at unmonitored fitness facilities, barefoot walking and running, and hula hoop workouts were all included in previous trend lists, but did not appear in 2016. The three trends from the 2015 ACSM survey list, children and exercise for "the treatment/prevention of obesity," "worker incentive programs," and "boot camp" fell out of the 2016 top 20. Many of these physical activities, though effective at promoting moderate and vigorous physical activity levels, may be more fad like, or may have lost popularity. As summarized by Thompson, "the annual survey may help the health and fitness industry make some very important investment decisions for future growth and development. Important business decisions should be based on emerging trends and not the latest exercise innovation peddled by late-night television infomercials or the hottest celebrity endorsing a product."[30]

individual progress is related to physical and mental challenges. Those with higher-order physical activity or health promotion goals must focus on making adjustments using the principles of overload, specificity, and adaptation to achieve higher levels of physical activity performance, health promotion, or disease prevention/management.

Personal trainers must always keep up with current fitness trends. Data from the same survey, presented in Table 10.10, provide a glimpse at 2016 popular fitness trends.

For example, in the leisure, recreation, and personal settings, kinesiology professionals should use health promotion programming to increase the physical activity and fitness of individuals or populations—or at least try to move them from sedentary patterns toward achieving functional health. Kinesiology professionals should recognize opportunities and develop strategies to help individuals/populations use their discretionary time to increase their physical activity and health. For effective implementation in leisure, recreation, and personal settings, we recommend that you integrate the concepts of the physical activity continuum; the principles of overload, specificity, and adaptation; and the strategies listed in Table 10.1.

## The Physical Activity Continuum and Leisure Time, Recreation, and Career Personal Training Settings

As you have learned in Chapters 4 through 9 of the text, the physical activity continuum (see Physical Activity Continuum icon figure) should be used as a model for moving from sedentary behaviors (or nonparticipation in physical activities or other health-promoting activities, for example) to achievement of health by meeting the 2008 U.S. Physical Activity Guidelines across the lifespan, and

## How Do You Know You Are Being Effective? The Evaluation of Leisure Time, Recreation, and Career Personal Training Health Promotion Programs

The development and implementation of physical activity programs (as well as other health-related targeted interventions) for leisure time, recreation, or personal training purposes should be evaluated to determine the

**Table 10.10** | Top 20 Worldwide Fitness Trends

1. *Wearable technology: includes* pedometers, fitness trackers, heart rate monitors, digital watches, and GPS monitors. New to the ACSM survey's top 20, the explosion in manufacturing, sales, and consumer use of wearable technology may reflect a better U.S. economy and more affordable access to physical activity for the masses.

2. *Body weight training:* involves using one's own body weight as the primary form of resistance for movements and exercise. It includes performing traditional physical activities such as push-ups, pull-ups, and other activities involving minimal equipment, which makes it an inexpensive way to train. Body weight training was rated as #3 in the 2013 ACSM survey, #2 in 2014, and has become a defined trend to watch.

3. *High-intensity interval training (HIIT):* includes short bursts of high-intensity activity followed by brief sessions of rest (often for less than 30 seconds); a total workout usually lasts less than 30 minutes. These activities are very popular with clients and can produce quick results, but they present a high risk for injuries, especially for unfit and/or older individuals or groups. HIIT activities were rated as #1 in the 2014 ACSM survey but did not even make the 2013 list, so it will be interesting to see if HIIT continues to be a trend or becomes a fad (see exercise physiology example in Lesson 2 for more).

4. *Strength training:* as you learned in Chapter 6, the strengthening and conditioning of the musculoskeletal system has become recognized as just as important to health and human performance as aerobic activities. Unfortunately, far fewer middle-aged and older adults participate regularly in strength and conditioning physical activities than in aerobic physical activities.

5. *Educated and experienced fitness professionals:* with the expanding opportunities for personal trainers and degreed fitness professionals, the number of certifications has grown exponentially. This growth has made the fitness industry more rigorous and accountable (in terms of safety and positive outcomes); however, because obtaining certification can be relatively expensive, many unscrupulous groups offer certifications that are fairly easy to obtain and lacking in quality.

6. *Personal training:* an expanding career field (full and part time) that provides opportunities in communities, commercial settings, business and corporate settings, and clinical settings. Personal training has appeared in nine of the last top 10 ACSM survey lists.

7. *Functional fitness:* the development and maintenance of day-to-day physical activity levels associated with positive health outcomes, while avoiding the negative outcomes of remaining sedentary.

8. *Fitness programs for older adults:* expanding opportunities to work with the aging population in the United States (as well as globally) to help individuals and groups adjust to specific health-related limitations while becoming and remaining physically active.

9. *Exercise and weight loss:* as you learned in Chapter 7, energy balance is the relationship among energy intake, energy expenditure, and energy storage associated with the maintenance of body homeostasis. It is influenced by caloric intake (eating) and caloric expenditure (physical activity). Weight control (maintenance, loss, or gain) refers to the interaction of participation in regular physical activity with the kinesiology science subdisciplines (exercise physiology, biomechanical, behavioral) and environmental challenges to influence individuals' or populations' ability to achieve and maintain a healthy body composition.

10. *Yoga:* a traditional form of physical activity combined with relaxation techniques that are very popular among health-conscious individuals and groups. Yoga is practiced in many forms and the number of yoga certification opportunities has increased significantly.

11. *Group personal training:* training small groups of individuals provides an economic incentive (savings) for participants and opportunities for personal trainers to provide their own expertise more widely.

12. *Worksite health promotion:* as you learned in Chapter 9, workplace health promotion programs that focus on increasing and maintaining physical activity levels for employees and their families can create a positive culture for business and industry that can translate into healthier communities.

13. *Wellness coaching:* as mentioned at the beginning of this section, wellness coaching is more focused on behavioral changes for individuals and groups than physical activity. This appears to be a growing trend and reinforces the integration of kinesiology subdisciplines for physical activity problem solving.

14. *Outdoor activities:* as you learned earlier in this chapter, new career opportunities are developing as the interest in physical activity, health, physical fitness, and peak performance related to all aspects of recreation, including outdoor activities, increases. Many new career opportunities will involve addressing barriers and facilitators of the built environment (such as development and renovation of parks, greenbelts, and trails).

15. *Sport-specific training:* fitness programming that is used by many personal trainers to prepare individuals and groups for participation in club sports, school sports, and professional sports.

16. *Flexibility and mobility rollers:* these activities are designed to provide massage and reduce muscle tightness that can increase one's mobility. A variety of assessments and treatments have been promoted in the emerging literature, and it will be interesting to evaluate this new top 20 trend in the future.

17. *Smartphone exercise apps:* with the explosion of electronic media, numerous applications are available free or at low cost to monitor health and track fitness progress. Errors of measurement of many of the smartphone apps is a concern, but they are very popular with younger individuals who have grown up using electronics their whole lives.

18. *Circuit training:* a form of resistance training that includes multiple stations (6 to 10) such that an individual or a group can rotate through the stations, exercising and then resting briefly before performing at the next station. Circuit training is similar to HIIT, but conducted at lower intensities.

19. *Core training:* strength and conditioning of the stabilizing muscles of the abdomen, thorax, and back. Core exercises involve the hips, lower back, and abdomen, all of which provide support for the spine and thorax.

20. *Outcome measurements:* a newer trend that refers to accountability as regards the fitness benefit claims promoted by one form of training versus another. This is an important trend that you have learned about throughout this text and that has been presented to you as evidence-based programming and evaluation.

*Source:* Adapted from W. R. Thompson, "Worldwide Survey of Fitness Trends for 2016," 10th Anniversary Edition, *ACSM's Health and Fitness Journal* 19, no. 6 (2016): 11–16.

programs' effectiveness. From measuring and evaluating the progress made by an individual client or athlete to broad changes in a community, understanding effectiveness is crucial. As you learned in Chapter 9, several steps must be completed when developing evaluation outcomes to determine whether worksite health and physical activity programs are effective. Program evaluation is often the critical component that is omitted during program development and implementation for physical activity interventions (and other health/fitness initiatives). This omission creates a major gap for program supporters (internal and external to the program), who are then unable to demonstrate that the program was effective and should continue as initiated.

The CDC proposed framework for evaluating physical activity programming includes the following six steps:

1. Engage stakeholders (all with direct and indirect interests in the program).
2. Describe and plan the program.
3. Define the evaluation.
4. Gather data.
5. Develop conclusions from the evaluation.
6. Communicate findings to ensure use.

Although a full treatment of techniques for evaluation of effectiveness is beyond the scope of this text, physical activity program evaluation can be categorized into four broad areas (Figure 10.11).[31] The four categories are formative, process, outcome, and cost-effectiveness evaluation.

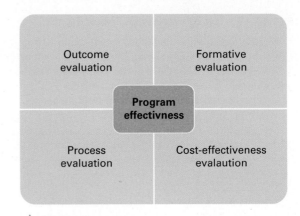

**Figure 10.11** | Four Evaluation Categories for Physical Activity Promotion Programs

*Source:* H. W. Kohl III and T. D. Murray, *Foundations of Physical Activity and Public Health* (Champaign, IL: Human Kinetics, 2012).

**Formative evaluation** involves determining the needs, utility, and design features of the physical activity program. **Process evaluation** focuses on the quality of the program and delivery options. **Outcome evaluation** involves determining the direct impact of the programming on physical activity (e.g., whether it affected behavior or physical fitness levels). Finally, **cost-effectiveness evaluation** involves determining if the program costs and potential income (if applicable) are appropriate or might be improved with alternative approaches. Figure 10.12 shows a sample schematic **logic model** (framework or road map) for physical activity evaluation.

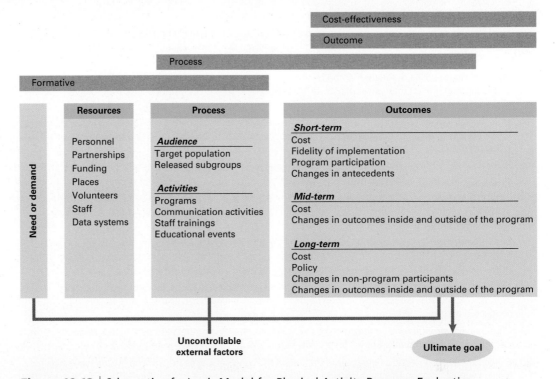

**Figure 10.12** | Schematic of a Logic Model for Physical Activity Program Evaluation

*Source:* H. W. Kohl III and T. D. Murray, *Foundations of Physical Activity and Public Health* (Champaign, IL: Human Kinetics, 2012).

# EXAMPLES OF APPLYING LEISURE TIME, RECREATION, AND PERSONAL TRAINING PRINCIPLES OF PHYSICAL ACTIVITY IN RELATIONSHIP TO THE KINESIOLOGY SUBDISCIPLINES

*In Lesson 1, you learned about the integration of leisure time, recreation, and personal training with the principles of physical activity and kinesiology. You learned about disparities among population subgroups in physical activity and how physical activity can be promoted through recreation and personal training experiences. By understanding leisure time, recreation, and personal training trends, kinesiology professionals can more effectively plan and implement successful physical activity programming. In Lesson 2, you will learn about examples of applying leisure time, recreation, and personal training principles*

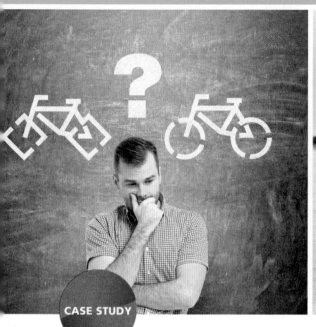

CASE STUDY

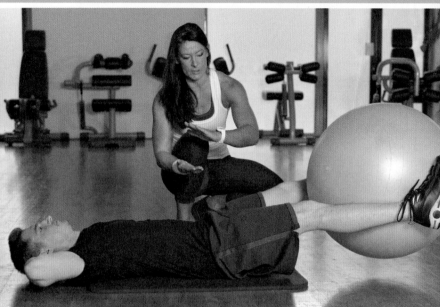

## In the real world . . .

As described earlier in this chapter, Jerald is becoming more physically active by using the Bulldog Trail. He wants to lose weight and become healthier by walking, jogging, and cycling the three-mile trail. Jerald, like many adults, has been inactive during much of his leisure time but now is managing to adjust his daily schedule to devote an hour to active commuting and participation in recreational physical activity. If he can cover two to three miles per day, he should be able to expend 200 to 500 calories more than he has been, which should improve his fitness levels and help him achieve a healthier weight. The Bulldog Trail will most likely increase the physical activity levels of students, faculty, and staff as the trail is very accessible—it is located on campus and is close to many area neighborhoods.

Jerald increased his use of the trail for the first 6 weeks of his 16-week semester, but by weeks 7 through 12, he hardly used the trail because he got too involved with more sedentary activities (videos and gaming) during his discretionary time. His initial time management plan did not work out for the long haul, but he did learn to think about using his discretionary time to get more physically active. He developed a new time management plan for the next semester to get more opportunities to use the Bulldog Trail because he did lose five pounds and felt healthier and more focused after weeks 1 through 6, before he stopped participating.

As a kinesiology professional, and based upon what you learned in Lesson 1, you could discuss with Jerald the factors that might affect his use of Bulldog Trail, including both the potential barriers and facilitators, to help him succeed in achieving his physical activity goals. You might even advise

*to physical activity within the related subdisciplines of kinesiology, and how to integrate them into effective programming strategies. You should also think about how you can use the examples in Lesson 2 to investigate new or optional kinesiology career opportunities for yourself.*

- Exercise Physiology
- Biomechanics
- Public Health
- Sport/Exercise Psychology
- Motor Learning
- The Practice of Kinesiology

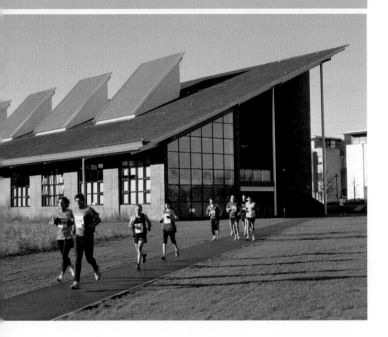

Jerald to hire a personal trainer individually, or encourage him to participate in group personal training in an outdoor physical activity program (e.g., Bulldog Trail Challenge, which consists of high-intensity interval training (HIIT) sessions two to three times per week). By understanding the evolving trends in leisure time physical activity, recreation, and personal training, kinesiology professionals can help individuals like Jerald and groups engage more effectively in traditional and emerging physical activity opportunities.

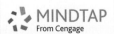

| MINDTAP From Cengage | Go to your MindTap course to complete the Case Study activity for this chapter. |

# Exercise Physiology

High-intensity interval training (HIIT) was the most popular fitness ACSM fitness trend for 2014, number 2 in 2015, and number 3 in 2016, and this has important implications for those interested in personal training careers. You learned about interval training in Chapter 5. Although HIIT is currently very popular, it is often implemented inappropriately; specifically, the rest (or lower-intensity) interval is often too short to allow recovery prior to the next high-intensity bout of physical activity. Interval training is said to have evolved as early as the 1920s among distance running athletes known as the "Flying Finns," a group of outstanding Olympians from Finland that included Paavo Nurmi, Hannes Koehmainen, and Emil Zatopek. Most highly fit, long-time elite runners engage in interval training only two to three times per week to allow appropriate recovery from exercise. However, some new and popular HIIT programs encourage participants to perform intervals five or more times per week, which is not consistent with modern periodization (alternating training and recovery to minimize overtraining) recommendations.

Interval training can cause quick physiological changes (big gains for a little pain) such as increases in $VO_2$ max, positive changes in oxidative metabolic enzymes, and weight loss with increases in lean muscle mass. Intervals challenge the spectrum of energy demands (anaerobic power, anaerobic capacity, and aerobic power) based on the intensity and duration of each interval, as well as total number of intervals. As early as the 1950s, exercise physiologists such as Per-Olaf Åstrand advocated that those interested in high-performance interval training should pay close attention to the work-to-rest ratios in relation to the time length of the work interval. Rest (recovery) intervals can be passive (e.g., standing) or active (e.g., low- to moderate-intensity walking/jogging). Active recovery has been found to be more effective with intervals lasting longer than 30 seconds.

Short intervals that last less than 10 to 30 seconds (anaerobic power) primarily stress the adenosine triphosphate (ATP) and creatine phosphate (CP) anaerobic energy stores of the body. The body requires a rest period that is three to five times the length of the interval bout to resynthesize ATP and CP, which allows for performance of the next interval (work-to-rest ratio of 1:3–5). For example, if you perform a series of eight 10-second sprints at maximum sprint speed, you should recover for at least 30 seconds (passive or low active recovery) between sprints if you want to maintain the same high intensity. Unfortunately, many currently popular HIIT workouts encourage participants to cut the recovery time to less than what is required (e.g., 10 to 20 seconds), which creates additional fatigue and increases the risk of injury, or at minimum decreases the participants' ability to complete the workout.

Intermediate intervals that last between 30 seconds and 3 minutes (anaerobic capacity) primarily stress the ATP/CP and anaerobic glycogen energy stores of the body and require a work-to-rest ratio of 1 to 2. For example, if you perform a series of eight 400-meter runs at 70 seconds per lap, you should rest (low or moderate active recovery preferred) for 140 seconds between runs early in training, and maybe 105 seconds between runs after 8 to 10 weeks of interval training.

Longer intervals that last three to five minutes (aerobic power) primarily stress the aerobic energy system and require a work-to-rest ratio of 1 to 1. For example, if you perform a series of three one-mile runs at six minutes per mile, you should rest (moderate active recovery preferred) five to six minutes after finishing one mile interval prior to beginning the next mile interval. Remember, reducing the rest interval too much will result in earlier fatigue, compromise completion of the planned number of intervals, and possibly increase injury risk.

## Biomechanics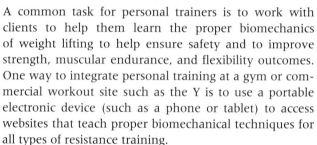

A common task for personal trainers is to work with clients to help them learn the proper biomechanics of weight lifting to help ensure safety and to improve strength, muscular endurance, and flexibility outcomes. One way to integrate personal training at a gym or commercial workout site such as the Y is to use a portable electronic device (such as a phone or tablet) to access websites that teach proper biomechanical techniques for all types of resistance training.

For example, there are commercial exercise prescription websites that provide personal trainers and their clients with detailed information on how to develop weight-training workouts, national recommendations for resistance, practical research findings, fitness performance calculators, sample workouts for specific client needs, and much more. Personal trainers can use the sites to interact with their clients and show them videos that demonstrate specifically how to perform all types of exercises (for all muscle groups). Not only can the personal trainer instruct his or her client more effectively with the videos and specific instructional guides, but the trainer can have clients return to the same website at their leisure to reinforce training concepts and provide feedback.

Incorporating electronic technology from readily available websites into personal training sessions may become a new trend in the industry over time. For now, we encourage practitioners to integrate electronic technology into their instruction and interactions with individuals and population.

## Public Health

An example of the integration of public health policies into school settings and community recreational settings can be found in the 2013 Research Digest under *Policies to Increase Youth Physical Activity in School and Community Settings.*[32] Physical activity levels among youth (children and adolescents) can be increased by alterations in the built environment and through policy changes such as joint land use agreements between a school district and a city/county that lay out the terms and conditions for the shared use of public property. Usually, each entity involved in a joint use agreement helps fund the development, operation, and maintenance of the recreational facilities. In this way, the costs and liabilities associated with the facilities are shared. For example, a school and a swim team might share a pool, or a school might allow a local soccer league to use its fields on weekends. Preliminary research suggests that joint use agreements have the potential to increase levels of physical activity while also providing safer environments in which to be physically active.

Figure 10.13 and Table 10.11 show how the energy expenditure of youth can be increased, not only by changing physical activity policies in schools (see Chapter 11) but also by changing the built environment and community (parks and recreation).

## Sport/Exercise Psychology

Physical activity and exercise are often recommended for cancer survivors to improve their physiologic and psychologic health. Emerging evidence suggests that the major primary benefit of physical activity for those with cancer may be improved quality of life. A significant challenge for cancer survivors is to adjust positively to the physiologic and psychologic changes that result from the disease and the therapeutic treatments encountered. Common cancer treatments such as chemotherapy, radiation, and

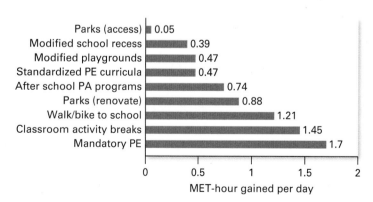

**Figure 10.13** | Impact of School-Based Policies and Changes on Physical Activity Energy Expenditure in Youth

*Source:* D. Bassett et al., "Policies to Increase Youth Physical Activity in School and Community Settings," *Research Digest* 14, no. 1 (March 2013): 2.

**Table 10.11** | Estimated Kilocalorie Expenditures among Youth Associated with School Policies and Built-Environment Changes

|  | KCAL/DAY FOR 50-LB YOUTH | KCAL/DAY FOR 100-LB YOUTH | KCAL/DAY FOR 150-LB YOUTH |
|---|---|---|---|
| Mandatory, Daily PE | 39 | 77 | 116 |
| Classroom Activity Breaks | 33 | 66 | 99 |
| Walk/Bike to School | 27 | 55 | 82 |
| Park Renovations | 20 | 40 | 60 |
| After School PA Programs | 17 | 34 | 50 |
| Standardized PE Curriculs | 11 | 21 | 32 |
| Modified Playgrounds | 10 | 21 | 31 |
| Modified School Recess | 9 | 18 | 27 |
| Parks (Access) | 2 | 4 | 5 |

PE = physical education; PA = physical activity.

*Source:* D. R. Bassett et al., "Policies to Increase Youth Physical Activity in School and Community Settings," *Research Digest* 14, no. 1 (March 2013): 2, 3.

surgery can reduce or eliminate cancerous tissue, but can also negatively affect the body (e.g., lower immune response, increase fatigue). Treatments such as hormone therapy and steroids administered during and after primary cancer treatments can produce a variety of negative physiologic and psychologic consequences including fluid retention, reduced cardiorespiratory fitness, reduced muscular strength and endurance, poorer quality of life, lower self-esteem, and increased vulnerability to adverse events (e.g., falls).

Table 10.12 summarizes psychological effects of physical activity among cancer survivors.

## Motor Learning

Physical activity skills (e.g., jumping, throwing, and hitting inanimate objects) are important predictors of increased levels of physical activity in children, adolescents, and adults.[33] By participating in a variety of leisure and recreation physical activities, individuals/populations can acquire valuable motor skills that can translate into greater physical activity participation during discretionary time.

The Seguin (Texas) Outdoor Learning Center is an example of a partnership between a donated outdoor education park and the Seguin school district (Seguin ISD). The purpose of the SOLC is to promote physical activity experiences for local children and adolescents for nominal fees that support the operation and maintenance of the facilities. The SOLC helps youngsters develop a variety of motor skills that are important now and in the future to encourage appropriate and higher levels of physical activity for health.

The SOLC hosts a variety of programs (e.g., science/cognitive based, arts and crafts, and adventure courses). The adventure course programming focuses on numerous physical activities including:

*Canoeing and kayaking*—students learn to paddle effectively and safely

*Hiking*—students hike numerous mulched trails through the woods and learn to identify local plants and trees

**Table 10.12** | Psychological Effects of Physical Activity Among Cancer Survivors

| PARAMETER | IMPROVEMENT AFTER CANCER TREATMENT | IMPROVEMENT DURING CANCER TREATMENT |
|---|---|---|
| Overall quality of life | Small to moderate | Small to moderate |
| Anxiety | Not enough evidence | Small to moderate |
| Self-esteem | Not enough evidence | Small to moderate |

*Source:* H. W. Kohl and T. Murray, *Foundations of Physical Activity and Public Health* (Champaign, IL: Human Kinetics, 2012). Table based on data from R. M. Speck, et al., "An Update of Controlled Physical Activity Trials in Cancer Survivors: A Detailed Systematic Review and Meta Analysis," *Journal of Cancer Survivorship* 4 (2010): 87–100.

*Geocaching*—students participate (walk/jog) in scavenger hunts using GPS systems

*Biking*—students learn to ride mountain bikes safely and perform basic bicycle maintenance

Field trips to the SOLC are age and developmentally appropriate, as designed initially by Erma Lewis (a long-time Seguin ISD physical educator and outdoor specialist who died in 2013). The SOLC programs offer local youth opportunities to experience outdoor physical activity that many of them would not have otherwise. The physical activity programming at the SOLC (such as mountain biking) allows youth who do not have previous experience or skills to ride a bike for the first time.

## The Practice of Kinesiology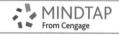

The HEB Foundation Free Camps are an example of physical activity promotion that targets children through a partnership between a large corporation that owns an outdoor education camp in Leakey, Texas, and Texas schools. The HEB Foundation acquired 1,900 acres of land near the headwaters of the Frio River in 1954. The HEB Foundation Free Camps were initiated and have been focused on family-owned beliefs and values that link to the basic integration of philosophical, historical, and sociological kinesiology related concepts that promote good health and quality of life.

Currently the foundation promotes free camping experiences (three days and two nights) in the Frio River Canyon (about 100 miles west of San Antonio, Texas) for a variety of youth groups, including schools. For example, all Seguin fifth graders have visited the HEB camp for each of the past three years. The Seguin district has provided funds for the busing of students, a few staff members for supervision and food service, and verification of insurance coverage for participants so that students from the district can attend and participate in these free, unique, on-site camping and outdoor physical activity experiences.

The HEB Foundation Camp provides outdoor activities in a remote area that many students would not otherwise encounter. The outdoor physical activities at the foundation camps are similar to the ones previously described for the SOLC. The foundation camps provide students and the teachers/staff that accompany them opportunities to be physically active together, cook and eat together, and learn to appreciate outdoor experiences. Kinesiology professionals run the HEB Foundation camps and have integrated the subdisciplines of kinesiology into their current programming.

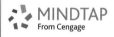
## Chapter Summary

▸ The opportunities and potential to promote physical activity and kinesiology-related subdiscipline concepts for leisure time, recreation, and careers in personal training to large populations are considerable. The career opportunities for kinesiology professionals who wish to work with individuals and populations during leisure time, recreation, and personal training are expanding rapidly and are forecast to continue expanding.

▸ The trends in U.S. adults who reported no leisure time physical activity from 1988 to 2010 indicate that, despite a slight improvement, there are still about 1 in 4 Americans who do not engage in *any* leisure time physical activity.

▸ By monitoring the trends in leisure time physical activity over time, kinesiology professionals can gain a better understanding about how to develop integrated strategies to increase physical activity levels of individuals and populations. Tracking physical activity trends also helps professionals evaluate the progress of specific physical activity interventions such as those delivered in recreation or personal training settings.

▸ Career opportunities in recreation are developing as the interest in physical activity, health, physical fitness, and peak performance is currently increasing rapidly. Many new career opportunities will involve addressing barriers

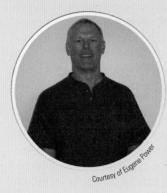

Courtesy of Eugene Power

**Q: Why and how did you get into the field of kinesiology?**

**A:** *Originally I was a marketing major in college but soon realized that I didn't want to wear a suit every day for the rest of my life. I had always been involved in sports and loved the strategies, tactics, and techniques involved, so I became a PE major with a goal of going into coaching. I have since been fortunate in my 40-year career to have taught and coached at every level from junior high to minor league baseball. Living the dream!*

**Q: What was the major influence on you to work in the field?**

**A:** *My college roommate and I both felt the same way about being fit and healthy and of not being chained to a desk all day. Plus I had some really good PE instructors in college who encouraged me to pursue coaching and teaching. I think they saw something in me that maybe I was not aware of at the time and tried to give me direction in my life. I would also say that my parents and both of my older brothers encouraged me to do what I loved and not what other people might have wanted me to do, since the definition of success in life is different for everyone. I am thankful for the input and direction of a great many friends, educators, and mentors who have helped shape my life and career along the way.*

**Q: What are your current research interests, and how do you translate your research results to practitioners?**

**A:** *Over the last five years or so, my colleagues and I have collected a tremendous amount of data regarding movement competency in our students through the various screening instruments that we have employed at the outset of our semester-long fitness classes. By using these movement screens, especially the FMS as developed by Gray Cook, we have been able to sample or profile fundamental movement patterns and identify possible dysfunctions in mobility and motor control to better help us to design a fitness program that will be the most productive over the course of the semester. At the end of each 16-week term we then look for improvement in any particular patterns that the kids may have been deficient or lacking in as a way to appraise whether our exercise programming is actually helping the classes develop better movement qualities. We have since presented our data at numerous conventions and workshops, and have received very positive feedback from our peers as to implementation of movement screening in a wide variety of settings.*

**Q: How do you stay physically active yourself and promote good health to others directly around you?**

**A:** *I have always subscribed to the idea that the human body should be exercised daily. Not*

and facilitators within the built environment (such as development and renovation of parks, greenbelts, and trails).

▸ Family-based approaches that promote physical activity such as park and recreation activities are important strategies that can shape the future physical activity levels of children and adolescents. Parents can significantly influence the physical activity levels of their children in several ways (including leisure time physical activity and recreation).

▸ Personal trainers help clients set goals, and they provide feedback and help monitor progress over time. Personal trainers are often called *wellness coaches* or *life coaches*, although there are distinctions among the three categories. Wellness and life coaches usually focus more on behavioral changes for individuals and groups, and physical activity may not be their primary focus.

▸ Program evaluation is often the critical component missing from program development and implementation for physical activity interventions (and other health/fitness initiatives); this omission creates a major gap for program supporters (internal and external to the program), who are then unable to demonstrate the program was effective and should continue as initiated.

## Remember This

| | | | |
|---|---|---|---|
| cost-effectiveness | formative evaluation | logic model | process evaluation |
| evaluation | leisure time physical | outcome evaluation | recreation |
| fads | activity | personal training | trends |

*necessarily hard every day, but you must do something, even if it is as simple as walking your dog or playing in the park with your kids. In a perfect world we would all train every day! However, I accept that that is not possible for most people. I do firmly believe that movement and physical activity is not a means to an end, but an end in and of itself. My number one rule in my classes and my personal life is to have fun when exercising or moving—find the things you like to do and you will have better compliance, do them more often, and ultimately attain better results. I "preach" this philosophy to my students and hope that my own example of being active on a daily basis sets a standard for them to aspire to.*

**Q:** **How have you had to integrate the subdisciplines of kinesiology in your professional practice?**

**A:** *As a college fitness instructor, I employ the knowledge and ideas of many different areas in my teaching including, but not limited to, anatomy, exercise physiology, biomechanics, nutrition, motor learning, early childhood development, movement screening, and the neurodevelopmental sequence. I also emphasize appropriate program design in terms of resistance training, core stability, cardiorespiratory activities, and metabolic conditioning.*

*Essentially, I will use anything and everything that I think will help my students become happier and healthier individuals through improved competency in their movement patterns and physical activities. I am not afraid to change my mind (or philosophy) about training and exercise and continually seek out new knowledge through seminars, workshops, podcasts, membership in professional organizations, and just plain old networking. I make the promise to my classes at the start of every semester that I will deliver as up-to-date information to them as I can, and I strive to study harder in preparing for my lessons than the students do. A large part of my enjoyment in teaching does come from learning new philosophies, sciences, and techniques, and with the advent of computers and cell phones, the wealth of information about fitness and health is easily accessed and put into practice, which makes it all the more exciting for me and, hopefully, my classes.*

*Eugene Power is a Professor of Kinesiology at Del Mar College in Corpus Christi, Texas. He is a Certified Strength and Conditioning Specialist (NSCA–National Strength and Conditioning Association), as well as being certified in the Functional Movement Screen (FMS). He is also a member of the Texas Chapter of the American College of Sports Medicine (ACSM), Texas High School Coaches Association (THSCA), Texas Association for Health, Physical Education, Recreation and Dance (TAHPERD), and the Association of Professional Ballplayers of America (APBPA).

## For More Information

Access these websites for further study of topics covered in the chapter:

- Find updates and quick links to these and other evidence-based practice related sites in MindTap.
- Search for further information about physical activity measures and programs related to leisure time, recreation, or personal training at activelivingresearch.org.
- Search for information and resources about the objectives for physical activity in leisure time, recreation, and personal training settings by choosing the "Physical Activity" topic on the Healthy People 2020 website at www.healthypeople.gov.

- Search the internet for websites that contain information about leisure time, recreation, and personal training information and ask your instructor which commercial websites they would recommend that integrate electronic technology into practice.
- Search for more information about physical activity in leisure time, recreation, or career personal training settings related to the National Physical Activity Plan at www.physicalactivityplan.org/index.html.
- Search for more information about parks, recreation (indoor and outdoor), and emerging personal training-related activities at www.nrpa.org/.

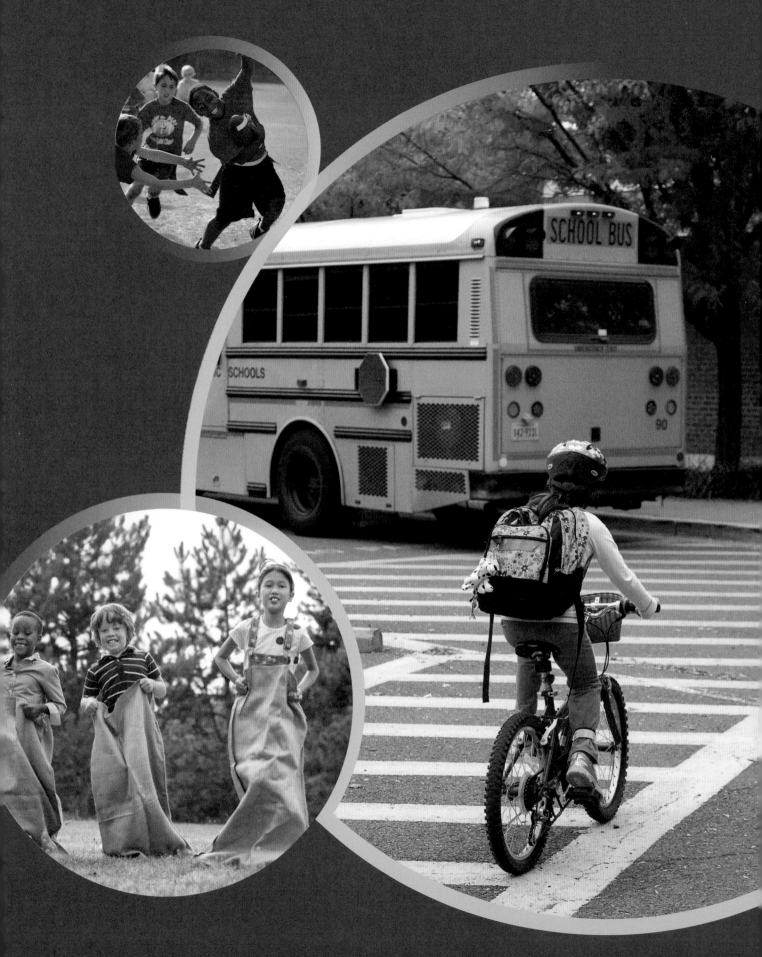

# Integration of Kinesiology and Physical Activity into School Settings

*What knowledge, skills, and abilities do kinesiology majors need to acquire and use for pursuing careers in schools?*

**LESSON 1** PHYSICAL ACTIVITY IN SCHOOL SETTINGS

**LESSON 2** EXAMPLES OF APPLYING KINESIOLOGY SUBDISCIPLINES IN SCHOOL SETTINGS

## Learning Objectives

*After completing this chapter, you will be able to:*

**Explain** common terms associated with physical activity opportunities in school settings.

**Discuss** the importance of promoting participation in physical activities in school settings.

**Explain** how to promote participation in physical activities in school settings by integrating the kinesiology subdisciplines across the physical activity continuum.

**Describe** the specific health benefits of participating in physical activity programs in schools vis-a-vis the physical activity continuum.

**Explain** how the health benefits of participating in physical activity programs in schools can positively influence student health and academic performance.

**Explain** a systematic process for developing school physical activity promotion programs.

**Give** examples of barriers to the development of school physical activity promotion programs.

**Explain** a variety of examples of application of kinesiology subdisciplines in school settings.

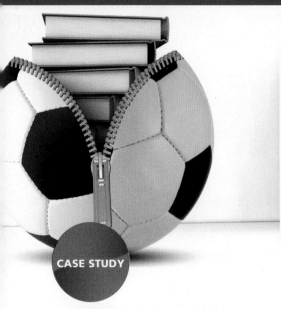

CASE STUDY

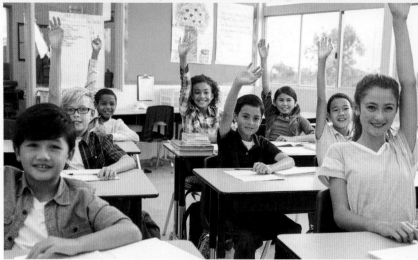

# In the real world . . .

In Chapters 6 and 7 we learned that 10-year-old Eugene Casey is enrolled in a physical education (PE) class at his school. Eugene's parents are excited that he enjoys lifting weights and that he has added muscle and his BMI has dropped. His mother, Maria, was recently at a parent/teachers meeting and heard from the principal that next year PE at Eugene's school will be cut from five days per week to only two days per week. Because of the budget cuts, a PE teacher will also be laid off, resulting in class sizes nearly doubling. Although many of the parents at the meeting did not really react to the announcement, Maria was upset. Eugene had been making really good progress with his weight lifting program. She had also recently heard on one of her favorite daily television talk shows that a recent study

showed that elementary school students who were regularly taking PE (three or more days per week) in school had better grades, were more attentive and recalled information faster than students who did not take PE. The television report listed several benefits:

▸ Physically active and fit children tend to have better academic performance, better school attendance, and fewer disciplinary problems than children who are not active and fit.

▸ Allocating time for daily physical education in schools does not hurt academic performance, and regular exercise may improve students' concentration and cognitive functioning.

▸ More time in physical education is associated with better grades and standardized test scores.

Maria is curious about whether there is any truth to what she heard because most of Eugene's grades improved

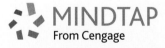
## MINDTAP
### From Cengage

Go to your MindTap course now to answer some questions and discover what you already know about the integration of kinesiology and physical activity into school settings.

## INTERACTIVE ACTIVITIES

### Research Focus

In 1972 a major piece of federal legislation known as Title IX of the Educational Amendments of 1972 was enacted in the United States. Go to your MindTap course to learn more about Title IX and the rise of sports participation among girls.

### Career Focus

Go to your MindTap course to learn more about Directors of Physical Activity (DPA). The idea of a Whole of School approach to physical activity promotion in schools has inspired identifiable programs in schools termed Comprehensive School Physical Activity Programs (CSPAP).

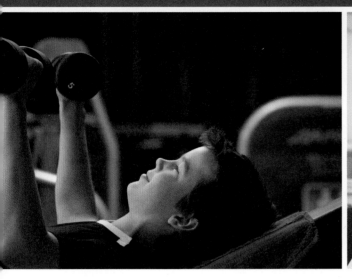

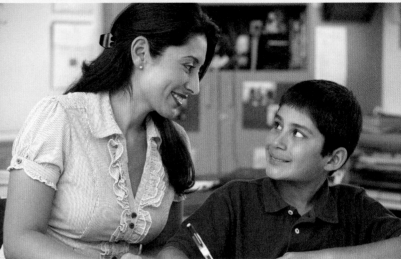

during the most recent six-week grading cycle. She wonders: Did Eugene perform better academically because he became more physically active while taking PE, or was it just a coincidence? If the physical activity was part of Eugene's improved performance in school, it didn't seem to make sense to Maria that the school was cutting back on PE. She made an appointment with the principal to discuss the decision. Obviously, there are other opportunities for physical activity in the school setting. Sports, active transportation, active classroom breaks all contribute and have the potential for increasing physical activity. Maria really wanted answers from the principal. What do you think? Does participating in regular physical activities in school (like PE) improve academic performance? If so, how does it affect cognitive function? What evidence is available that supports the old philosophical adage, "a sound mind in a sound body," which was coined by the ancient Greek philosopher Thales? What are ways that children can reach 60 minutes/day of physical activity each day while at school?

We will follow up with Eugene's case story in Lesson 2 of this chapter, after you have had a chance to learn about the types of opportunities for physical activity in and around school settings.

# Introduction: Physical Activity, Kinesiology, and School Settings

In today's world, children, like adults, are faced with many choices that make adopting sedentary behaviors easy but exercise and physical activity more difficult. We have successfully engineered opportunities out of daily life in situations where youth could automatically be physically active. Computers, televisions, video games, and other sedentary entertainment have dislodged more active pursuits such as pick-up basketball, outdoor play, etc. In many places, it is not safe for children to play outside, further inhibiting opportunities for physical activity. It has been estimated that 80% of youth in the world are not physically active enough to promote their health, which requires 60 minutes of activity each day.[1] This has been an urgent wake-up call for kinesiology and health professionals to make changes to reverse this problem. Schools have been a frequent target of such efforts.

Why schools? Schools are logical settings for promoting physical activity and integrating the principles of kinesiology because of the large number of children and adolescents they serve. Schools usually also have infrastructures for physical activity, such as gyms, fields, and large spaces in which to move. Schools provide kinesiology majors with numerous career opportunities, such as teaching, coaching, and coordinating events that promote physical activities. In the United States, a historical focus on athletics and physical education has begun to shift toward inclusion of physical activity for all students to improve health and promote safety. National legislation and the 2013 Institute of Medicine report, *Educating the Student Body: Taking Physical Activity and Physical Education to School*, promote the integration of physical activity and kinesiology-related concepts into the school environment before, during, and after school.[2] The U.S. National Physical Activity Plan also contains several strategies to promote physical activity in the education sector or schools, outlined in Table 11.1 (specific implementation tactics are also included within the sector).

Physical education has traditionally been the sole source of physical activity in schools. Optimally, children would have a physical education class each day in which physical activity as well as skills development, sportsmanship, and other concepts are taught. In reality, very few children in the United States have the opportunity for daily physical education and, more likely, it is a rare or nonexistent opportunity particularly for high school children. Pressures for increasing academic performance have led to the misguided sacrifice of physical education in favor of more classroom (sedentary) time. The further challenge is that even the most traditional approaches to providing in-school opportunities for physical education will only keep children active for (at most) 10 to 20 minutes each class period—far less than the 60 minutes of physical activity each day required to meet the guideline for children. How are children supposed to achieve the remainder of the recommended physical activity during the school week? Physical education alone is inadequate. Alternate solutions are needed, and kinesiology professionals are well positioned to provide physical activity opportunities beyond traditional physical education.

Schools can be a catalyst for helping children meet daily physical activity guidelines. The Institute of Medicine has proposed a "Whole of School" approach for transforming a school into a hub for children's physical activity, enabling children to be active at least 60 minutes each day they are in or around schools.[3] This is a critical area in which kinesiology integrates into schools and the educational system. The Whole of School approach to physical activity is diagramed in Figure 11.1. Children are typically in school six to

**Table 11.1** | Strategies to Promote Physical Activity in the Educational Sector or Schools

| | |
|---|---|
| STRATEGY 1 | States and school districts should adopt policies that support implementation of the Comprehensive School Physical Activity Program model. |
| STRATEGY 2 | Schools should provide high-quality physical education programs. |
| STRATEGY 3 | Providers of afterschool, holiday, and vacation programs for children and youth should adopt policies and practices that ensure that participants are appropriately physically active. |
| STRATEGY 4 | States should adopt standards for childcare and early childhood education programs to ensure that children ages zero to five years are appropriately physically active. |
| STRATEGY 5 | Colleges and universities should provide students and employees with opportunities and incentives to adopt and maintain physically active lifestyles. |
| STRATEGY 6 | Educational institutions should provide preservice professional training and in-service professional development programs that prepare educators to deliver effective physical activity programs for students of all types. |
| STRATEGY 7 | Professional and scientific organizations should develop and advocate for policies that promote physical activity among all students. |

*Source:* National Physical Activity Plan Alliance (NPAPA), www.physicalactivityplan.org/index.html.

seven hours each day (middle of figure). Physical activity opportunities at school can consist of the traditional PE and recess periods as well as new approaches such as classroom breaks and academic lessons that include physical activity. Additionally, the time windows before and after school provide another one to four hours of physical activity possibilities, including active travel to and from school, after-school programs, and sports. Taken together, these represent 11 hours each school day into which physical activity opportunities for children may be incorporated. Suddenly, 60 minutes each day seems an entirely reasonable goal.

**Figure 11.1** | Whole of School Approach to Physical Activity Promotion in Schools

*Source:* Adapted from Institute of Medicine, *Educating the Student Body: Taking Physical Activity and Physical Education to School* (Washington, DC: The National Academies Press, 2013), S-8, available at books.nap.edu.

## MINDTAP
From Cengage

### Educating the Student Body

In 2013, a major report from the U.S. Institute of Medicine, part of the National Academies of Science, detailed six high-level recommendations for action needed to improve opportunities for physical activity in school children, using the school as the hub for these activities. **Go to your MindTap course** for information on these six recommendations and a video infographic on the report.

The Whole of School approach for physical activity also reinforces the idea of the physical activity continuum. School-based professionals can help move students from sedentary behaviors toward the achievement of better health by meeting or exceeding the amount of physical activity from the U.S. Physical Activity Guidelines. Further, students who desire higher-order physical activity such as sports competitions or health promotion outcomes should be encouraged to focus on making adjustments using the principles of overload, specificity, and adaptation to achieve higher levels of physical activity performance. Kinesiology professionals in schools and their fellow colleagues should combine and integrate the concepts of the physical activity continuum (see the inserted Physical Activity Continuum icon ) into the recommended Whole of School approach model.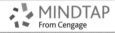

## Physical Education

**Physical education** is a formal, standards-based content area of study in schools that encompasses assessment according to standards and benchmarks. It is defined in Chapter 1 as "a planned sequential kindergarten–grade 12 standards-based program of curricula and instruction designed to develop motor skills, knowledge, and behaviors of healthy active living, physical fitness, sportsmanship, self-efficacy, and emotional intelligence." As a school subject, physical education focuses on teaching the science and methods of physical activity as a part of healthful living.[4] Physical education is a means to engage children in developmentally appropriate physical activities that develop their fitness, gross motor skills, and health.

Physical education has a long history as a prominent discipline of kinesiology. Referred to as "gymnastics" in the early years, it was a subject in schools at the beginning of the nineteenth century.[5] The role of physical education in human health was quickly recognized, and the subject evolved into school-based instruction on personal hygiene and exercise for bodily health. In the early twentieth century, this emphasis on health was perceived by some as too narrow because it ignored the role that physical activity can play in supporting the growth and development of children, particularly through the pubertal years. This realization helped to expand school physical education to include games and developmentally appropriate skill movements by the mid-twentieth century. In recent years, the two schools of thought have merged somewhat to connect physical activity to its consequences (e.g., physical activity and health), teaching children the science of healthful living and skills needed for an active lifestyle.

Physical education, like any other school subject, should be used to teach skills and provide guided experiences; the aim is for youth to learn how to become physically active, have confidence doing so, and to remain active throughout their lives. As such, physical education has evolved as a field with clear learning goals and objectives at all educational levels. A modern definition of physical education is "…education content using a comprehensive but physically active approach that involves teaching social, cognitive, and physical skills, and achieving other goals through movement."[6] Physical education can be viewed as having two overarching goals: (1) to prepare children and youth for a lifetime of physical activity and (2) to engage them in physical activity during physical education sessions.

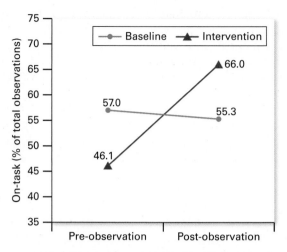

Figure 11.2 | Mean Percentages of On-Task Behavior during Academic Instruction Time among the Least On-Task Students (N = 10)

*Source:* From M. T. Mahar et al., "Effects of a Classroom-Based Program on Physical Activity and On-Task Behavior," *Medicine and Science in Sports and Exercise* 38, no. 12 (2006): 2086–2094.

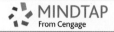

### Physical Activity versus Physical Education

Is physical activity identical to physical education? No. Although schools can offer many opportunities for physical activity, physical education should be viewed as a distinct educational program with distinct learning goals and objectives. Physical activity, in general, is more behavioral in nature and involves movement. Physical activity can (and should) happen during physical education class, but physical education need not occur each time a child is physically active. **Go to your MindTap** course to visit the Shape America website, view the *Shape of the Nation* report, and to learn more about many facets of physical education in the United States, including legislative requirements, teacher training, and certification.

## Classroom Activity Breaks

Another place that kinesiology is relevant in schools is in the academic classroom. Unlike recess, lunchtime, and other physical activity opportunities, structured **classroom-based physical activity breaks** refer to all activity, regardless of intensity, performed in the classroom during normal classroom time. Both physical activity during academic classroom instruction and breaks from instruction that are specifically designed for physical activity fall into this category. Physical education and recess are not considered classroom-based physical activity breaks even if they happen to be conducted in the classroom by the usual classroom teacher. Physical activity breaks during lunchtime are also excluded from this category. Classroom teachers will use such breaks to help refocus students during learning activities.

Can structured physical activity breaks actually be used effectively in schools? A typical break consists of 10 to 15 minutes of activities and emphasizes vigorous or moderate-intensity physical activity. This strategy is effective in significantly increasing physical activity levels

of school-age children. One study reported a nearly 20% increase in steps per day among third and fourth grade students who participated in a classroom physical activity break program, as shown in Figure 11.2.[7] In addition to helping to refocus learning and increasing physical activity, such breaks may be effective for weight control among students when continued over 2 years.[8]

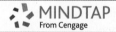

### TAKE 10!™

While in school, children are most sedentary during the time spent in the classroom. Can physical activity be incorporated into traditional classroom lessons? Can mathematics, language arts, or history be taught using physical activity by getting children out of their chairs and moving around? The TAKE 10!™ program is an example of such a creative approach. This program seeks to integrate 10 minutes of physical activity into otherwise sedentary lesson time. Instead of substituting physical activity for academic lessons, TAKE 10! integrates physical activity into the academic lesson. Research supports this approach as yet another way to engineer physical activity back into children's lives. In addition to increasing physical activity, programs like TAKE 10! may improve students' concentration abilities as well as time-on-task to aid learning. They represent another way that kinesiology integrates with schools and the education system. **Go to your MindTap** course to learn more about TAKE 10!.

The main reason children attend school is to learn. Everything schools do centers around teaching children knowledge and skills for the future. Traditionally, children sitting in their seats for extended periods of time, as opposed to being physically active, has been promoted as the best way to learn school lessons. What if we actually are impeding learning by making children sit too long, remaining sedentary for several hours? Do classroom physical activity breaks impede learning? This argument has been used to support more sedentary classroom learning time, artificially positioning physical activity as being unrelated to learning. Emerging research seems to support the idea that physical activity breaks are not only effective at increasing physical activity but also may enhance learning, academic performance, and related classroom behaviors such as focus, and classroom climate.

## Recess

Another way kinesiology is integrated into schools is through physical activity opportunities during recess. Recess is one of the most common forms of physical activity breaks during the school day. Recess may represent up to 40% of daily physical activity time for school children.[9] **Recess** is the time of day set aside for students to take a break from their class work, engage in play with their peers, and take part in independent, unstructured activities. Recess is most common in elementary schools but is rare during the secondary years.

Recess is an important part of the educational experience for elementary-age children and is a key way that more physical activity can be attained during the school day. Like that encountered during physical education, physical activity during recess can be an early, positive experience for children and adolescents. In addition, quality recess activities can also help children develop and practice important life skills including socialization, conflict resolution, problem-solving, and sharing, among others. Recess is also a developmentally appropriate outlet for reducing stress in children.

### Importance of Recess

» Recess is a complement to but not a replacement for physical education. Physical education is an academic discipline.

» Recess can serve to offset sedentary time and contribute to the goal of 60 minutes or more of vigorous or moderate-intensity physical activity each day.

» Peer interactions and socialization during recess complement those occurring in the classroom.

## Sports

Another prominent way that kinesiology is integrated into schools and the educational system is through sports programs. Intramural (within a school) and extramural (outside of schools) sports programs are extremely popular ways for youth to be physically active. Sports can be conceptualized anywhere from unstructured play to very well planned events that are also an occupation. According to Woods, **play** is a "free activity that involves exploration, self-expression, dreaming, and pretending. Play has no firm rules and can take place anywhere."[10] Children's play often involves physical movement. **Games** are forms of play "that have greater structure and are competitive. Games have clear participation goals … [and] are governed by informal or formal rules." Games can be sedentary or physical; involve competition, planning, and strategizing; and result in "prestige or status." **Sports** represent a specialized or higher order of play or games with special characteristics. Sports involve physical movement and skill. They must be "competitive with outcomes that are important to those involved"; in sports, "winning and losing are a critical part of competition." Thus, an important aspect of sports is institutionalized competition under formal rules. Lastly, work is "purposeful activity that may include physical and mental effort to perform a task, overcome an obstacle, or achieve a desired outcome." Sports can be work. A hierarchy of sports is shown in Figure 11.3.

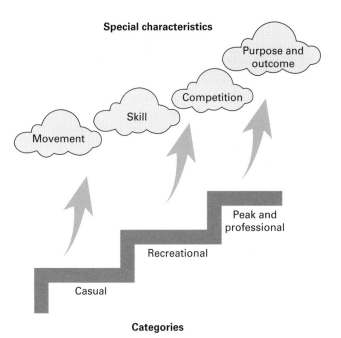

**Figure 11.3** | A Hierarchy of Sports: Levels of Competition and Special Characteristics of Physical Activity Linked to all Categories of Participation

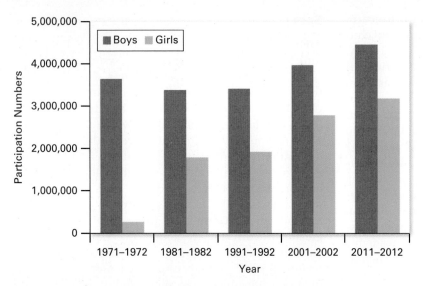

**Figure 11.4** | Overall Participation in High School Sports in the United States from 1971 to 2012

Data from the National Federation of State High School Association, www.nfhs.org/ParticipationStatics/ParticipationStatics.aspx/ and published in H. W. Kohl III, H. D. Cook, and the Institute of Medicine, *Educating the Student Body: Taking Physical Activity and Physical Education to School* (Washington, DC: The National Academies Press, 2013).

approximately 58.3% of 6- to 17-year-olds participated in sports teams or lessons over a 12-month period.[12] Further, the CDC reported that, in 2011, 58% of high school students played on at least one sports team.[13] Intramural sports clubs in middle and high schools also involve large numbers of students. Many students who do not play on school teams may participate in sports programs outside of school. CDC data suggest that an estimated 31 million of the 55 million high-school-aged youth participated in sports outside of school.[14] Participation in sports in and outside of school has increased considerably in the past 20 years. Although boys' participation increased by about 22% during these years, girls' participation increased about 10-fold. Changes in high school sports participation since the early 1970s are shown in Figure 11.4.

Children in schools can take part in sports as either participants or spectators. Although participants theoretically grow into adulthood and can continue participation, that does not happen as much as thought. In fact, it has been suggested that sports participation at a young age results in those participants only becoming loyal spectators in later years. Being a spectator at a young age, although it may be related to a better understanding of the sport being played, probably does not result in actual participation.[11]

Sports programs in schools typically fall into two broad categories based on the nature of the competition: *intramural*, or within a school, and *interscholastic*, or between schools. Intramural sports frequently include leagues for group participation or individual opportunities for a variety of pursuits. Intramural sports can be a major venue for physical activity among youth in schools if the appropriate infrastructure (fields, gymnasiums, coaching/supervision) is in place. Interscholastic sports such as soccer, basketball, and football are designed for athletic competition and most often match schools of similar enrollment and geographic location. The type and scope of each of these categories of sports offered vary by school size and location and the socioeconomic status of students.

Participation in sports has flourished both within and outside of schools. Although young children are not eligible for formal interscholastic competition until they reach secondary schools, children with athletic aspirations (or enthusiastic parents) start preparation for competition at a very young age. Results of the National Survey of Children's Health showed that

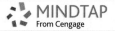
From Cengage

### Title IX and the Reshaping of Sports Opportunities for Females

**Go to your MindTap course** to learn more about Title IX and the rise of sports participation among girls. In 1972 a major piece of federal legislation known as Title IX of the Educational Amendments of 1972 was enacted in the United States. Title IX is a public law designed to forbid discrimination based on gender under any educational program receiving federal financial assistance. Because many universities receive some kind of federal funds, and because intercollegiate sports were dominated by male competition up to that point, Title IX has been widely credited with reshaping sports opportunities for females, not only in college settings but also in high school settings, as high school opportunities and training will often lead to college competition. The law, in 2002 renamed for Patsy Mink, a congressional representative from Hawaii who co-authored the legislation, has allowed for more resources (fields, locker rooms, coaching staff, etc.) to be channeled to women's sports around the country.

Students have many choices of interscholastic sports. Lee and colleagues cite 23 popular sports, grouped in Table 11.2 as team or individual sports. The degree to which sports participation among youth translates to

**Table 11.2** | Interscholastic Sports Choices and Percentage of Middle and High Schools Offering Them

| SPORT | MIDDLE SCHOOLS (PERCENT) | HIGH SCHOOLS (PERCENT) |
|---|---|---|
| **Team Sports** | | |
| Baseball | 35.7 | 79.6 |
| Basketball | 76.4 | 90.9 |
| Cheerleading | 50.9 | 77.3 |
| Softball | 45.2 | 77.9 |
| Field hockey | 7.1 | 10.2 |
| Football | 53.0 | 71.0 |
| Ice hockey | 2.4 | 14.3 |
| Lacrosse | 2.1 | 3.8 |
| Soccer | 32.3 | 60.3 |
| Volleyball | 57.3 | 71.4 |
| Water polo | 0.5 | 2.6 |
| **Individual Sports** | | |
| Badminton | 4.2 | 7.2 |
| Bowling | 3.0 | 17.2 |
| Cross-country | 38.9 | 68.4 |
| Cross-country skiing | 3.2 | 5.9 |
| Golf | 22.1 | 68.4 |
| Gymnastics | 5.2 | 10.1 |
| Riflery | 2.1 | 3.8 |
| Swimming | 6.9 | 37.8 |
| Tennis | 12.6 | 53.0 |
| Track and field | 52.1 | 73.2 |
| Weight lifting | 9.9 | 23.8 |
| Wrestling | 28.7 | 49.6 |

*Source:* Adapted from S. M. Lee et al., "Physical Education and Physical Activity: Results from the School Health Policies and Programs Study 2006," *Journal of School Health* 77 (October 2007): 435–463.

lifelong physical activity, while presumed, is really unknown. The issue is complicated. Do participants in team sports have a different experience than those in individual sports? Does the self-esteem gained from sports participation (as well as the skills) translate to a better chance that former participants will continue to be physically active throughout their lives? Is the experience of working on a team different than that of an individualized sport? What is your experience?

### Barriers to Participation in Sports

Kinesiology offers several potential solutions to challenges faced by students participating in sports through schools. Although the benefits of participating in high school sports—such as increases in physical activity, academic performance, and increased school attendance and self-esteem—are beginning to be understood, there are barriers to implementation. Transportation costs and inadequate facilities and equipment are important

barriers to sports participation. Such disparities differentially affect youth from low-income families. Where facility and land limitations prevail, school districts have resorted to developing partnerships and contractual agreements with local community recreation centers or universities to use their facilities for various sports programs. A lack of funding for sports equipment has further reduced the number of participating students, as the number of uniforms available per sport has caused the selection process to become more stringent. It is clear that the percentage of students participating in interscholastic sports at a school or in a school district depends largely on the type and number of facilities available. (See Figure 11.5.)

The availability of quality coaches as well as fewer overall sports offerings are two additional problems faced by schools. Declining financial incentives and increasing time commitments to other needs have resulted in fewer school personnel able to coach intramural and interscholastic teams. Budget reductions have resulted in fewer sports offerings, with primary sports (and their associated revenue) being retained and the tier-two sports, such as golf and tennis, either being eliminated or requiring that students pay 100% of the cost of participation. Indeed, many school districts across the United States have implemented a pay-to-play policy, in which students (and their families) must pay money in order to participate in the sport. It has been estimated that more than 30% of schools in the United States require students to pay to participate in interscholastic sports. Such a system reduces access to sports participation, particularly among children and adolescents from low-income households. Clearly sports participation, while an avenue for physical activity for some youth, cannot reach all.

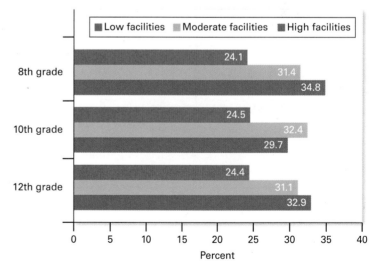

**Figure 11.5** | Participation in Interscholastic Sports among Boys and Girls by Availability of Sports Facilities, 2009–2011

*Source:* From Figure 2 of N. Colabianchi, L. Johnston, and P. M. O'Malley, *Sports Participation in Secondary Schools: Resources Available and Inequalities in Participation—A BTG Research Brief* (Ann Arbor: Bridging the Gap Program, Survey Research Center, Institute for Social Research, University of Michigan, 2012), available at www.bridgingthegapresearch.org.

- Only one-third of lower-income parents reported that their child participated in school sports, compared with more than half of higher-income parents.

- In lower-income households, nearly one in five parents reported a decrease in their child's participation in school sports because of cost.

Socioeconomic status very much influences sports participation in schools, and schools in low socioeconomic areas have fewer facilities and places to be active. Colabianchi and colleagues determined that the percentage of students participating in sports varied almost linearly with availability of facilities.[15] Participation was higher at schools with moderate facilities availability than at those of with few, and even higher at schools of the highest availability. (See Figure 11.6.) Comparing Figure 11.5 with Figure 11.6, which substitutes socioeconomic status instead of facilities availability, the similarity is difficult to ignore.

To provide students with the physical activity and psychosocial benefits of engaging in sports at school, educational systems need to reevaluate their budgets to ensure that equitable sports opportunities are available for youth in all types of school settings and at all levels of socioeconomic status. The same holds true with respect to ensuring that school-based intramural sports opportunities are available before or after school hours to increase participation in physical activity among all students.

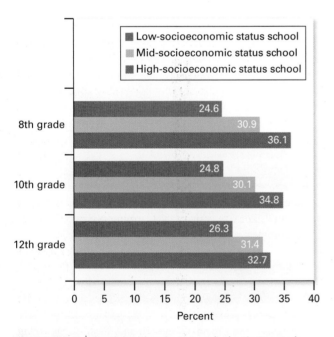

**Figure 11.6** | Participation in Interscholastic Sports by School Socioeconomic Status among Boys and Girls, 2009–2011

Source: From Figure 1 of N. Colabianchi, L. Johnston, and P. M. O'Malley, *Sports Participation in Secondary Schools: Resources Available and Inequalities in Participation – A BTG Research Brief* (Ann Arbor, MI: Bridging the Gap Program, Survey Research Center, Institute for Social Research, University of Michigan, 2012), available at www.bridgingthegapresearch.org.

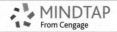

**Programs for Students with Disabilities**

The 2010 Government Accountability Office (GAO) report *Students with Disabilities: More Information and Guidance Could Improve Opportunities in Physical Education and Athletics* notes that students with and without disabilities are provided similar opportunities to participate in physical education in schools, but identifies several challenges to serving students with disabilities. Likewise, opportunities were provided for students to participate in sports, but students with disabilities were much less likely to participate than those without disabilities. Yet the effects of sports programs for students with and without disabilities have been shown to be similar, including not only obesity reduction but also higher self-esteem, better body image, and greater academic success; more confidence and a greater likelihood of graduating from high school and matriculating in college; and greater career success and options.[16]

## Active Transport

Although not traditionally a focus in kinesiology, active transportation to and from school is another opportunity for physical activity. **Active transport**, or active commuting, refers to walking, cycling, or other human-powered methods (e.g., skate boarding) of transportation. It includes using public transportation, using walking school buses, and being driven part of the way to school and allowed to walk the remainder of the way. Active transport equates to moderate-intensity physical activity, which, as discussed in earlier chapters, provides important health benefits.

**Safe Routes to School**

Active transportation to school has declined rapidly since the mid-1970s. This decline is a multidimensional problem that involves perceived safety, the distance children must travel to and from school, and transportation infrastructure. The U.S. National Center for Safe Routes to School was formed to assist states and communities in enabling and encouraging children to safely walk and bicycle to school. The center sponsors a Walk to School Day each year in October and has many resources available to help plan programs.

Do you walk or bicycle to school or between classes? Active commuting has been proposed as an ideal low-cost strategy to increase physical activity within the general population and can account for a substantial portion of recommended daily physical activity.[17] These benefits, together with concern about increased traffic congestion, safety, and vehicle pollution, have contributed to growing interest and enthusiasm for youth using active transport to and from school. In addition to health and environmental benefits, active transport may help to increase social interaction among youth

Five decades ago, children actively commuting to school were a common sight. At that time, nearly 90% of children who lived within a one-mile radius of school either walked or biked to school. Since 1969, however, the prevalence of youth walking or biking to school has steadily declined, paralleling a decline in active commuting among American adults.[18] Figure 11.7, based on data from the U.S. Department of Transportation, shows the decline in active transportation to and from school between 1969 and 2001.

From an international perspective, active transport among children and adolescents is more prevalent in European countries such as the Netherlands and Germany, which have a culture of active transport, than in other regions. Not surprisingly, the health profile among youth in these countries is better than in the United States. There is inverse relationship between the percentage of the population who report using active transport and obesity among residents of the United States, Canada, Australia, and 14 European countries.[19] In this study, the United States ranked the lowest for active transport and the highest for obesity prevalence.

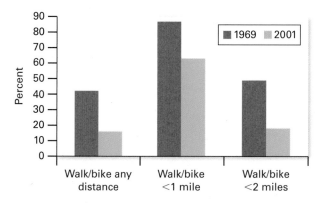

**Figure 11.7** | Decline in Active Transportation to and from School among Youth from 1969 to 2001 in the United States

*Note:* The "walk/bike any distance" category signifies children who walked or biked a distance greater than two miles.

*Source:* S. A. Ham, S. Martin, and H. W. Kohl III, "Changes in the Percentage of Students Who Walk or Bike to School – United States, 1969 and 2001," *J Phys Act Health* 5 (2008): 205–215.

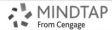

Several factors contribute to the lack of active transport of youth to and from school. The first is accessibility, which depends on the proximity (i.e., within a one-mile radius) of the children's homes to the school. Land and construction costs for new schools has driven such projects away from city centers and existing neighborhoods, often miles away from residential areas. In fact, long distances to school is the most frequently cited reason why active transportation is not used more.[20]

In addition to proximity, a second key determinant of active transportation is infrastructure. For active transport to be effective, not only must schools be in close proximity to the neighborhoods of students, but sidewalks, pedestrian crossings, and traffic lights must be adequate. Boarnet and colleagues found that children's walking and cycling behavior to and from school was substantially higher in urban areas where improvements in sidewalks, traffic lights, pedestrian crossings, and bike paths had occurred.[21] What about your life? Is your choice to walk or cycle influenced by infrastructure that makes active transportation safer and easier?

Related to infrastructure issues are parental concerns about safety, including traffic dangers. Even if the infrastructure exists, does that mean the routes are safe? Even with sidewalks, does the perception of safety from crime or other hazards prevent active transport to school? Safe Routes to School initiatives, specifically designed to bring traffic engineers together with school officials to make school trips safer, including traffic calming techniques such as speed bumps, four-way stop signs, traffic circles, and lowered speed limits, have resulted in dramatic improvements in participation. One study reported a 64% increase in the percentage of students walking to school in urban areas after a Safe Routes to School initiative was implemented.[22] The "walking school bus" (i.e., a group of children who walk to school with an adult escort) has been shown to be an effective method for safely transporting children to and from school.[23]

## Walking School Bus Programs

School-endorsed walking school buses may address several of the barriers tied to active transport to and from schools—in particular, traffic and crime dangers. Walking school buses have been a popular means for walking young children to school securely in Europe and Australia and are beginning to catch on in the United States. A **walking school bus** often entails one or two adult volunteers escorting a group of children from pick-up points (walking school bus stops) or their homes to school along a fixed route, starting with the pick-up point or home that is farthest from the school and stopping at other pick-up points or homes along the way. For increased security for the youngest children, a rope that surrounds

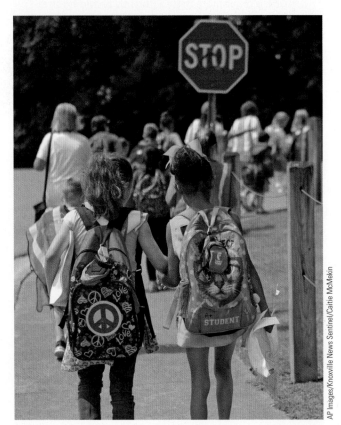

AP Images/Knoxville News Sentinel/Caitie McMekin

the group can be used. On the way back from school, the same system is used in the opposite direction.

Walking school buses are a low-cost initiative communities can undertake to increase physical activity among elementary school children. The prevalence of walking school buses remains low in the United States but is growing; in 2008–2009, about 4.2% of a representative sample of public elementary schools organized walking school buses, with an increase to 6.2% in 2009–2010.[24]

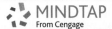
From Cengage

### Examples of Walking School Bus Programs

Many resources are available to schools and communities that are interested in starting a walking school bus program. **Go to your MindTap course** to learn more about the CDC KidsWalk-to-School program. The CDC's Nutrition and Physical Activity Program has developed KidsWalk-to-School, a community-based program that encourages children to walk and bicycle to school. It provides resources and training modules for creating walk-to-school programs. The program increases awareness of the importance of physical activity for children and mobilizes communities to advocate for the creation of safe routes to school.

Parents' engagement in school-based health promotion activities is another significant benefit of walking school buses. In some communities, walking school buses have provided opportunities for parents and other volunteers to remain engaged in the life of the community while increasing their own physical activity.

# EXAMPLES OF APPLYING KINESIOLOGY SUBDISCIPLINES IN SCHOOL SETTINGS

*In Lesson 1, you learned about the integration of physical activity and the principles of kinesiology in schools. You learned about why physical activity and other positive health behaviors are promoted in school settings. Effective physical activity and health promotion in schools can provide cognitive, health,*

*and social benefits for all students. In Lesson 2, you will learn about examples of how physical activity promotion concepts in schools are integrated with the subdisciplines of kinesiology.*

▶ Exercise Physiology
▶ Biomechanics

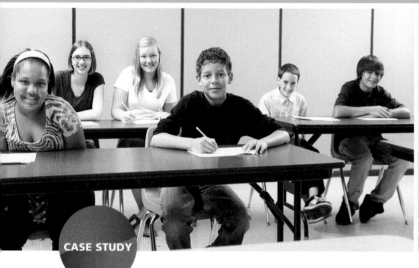

CASE STUDY

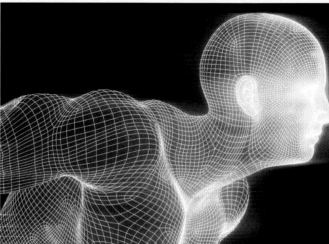

# In the real world . . .

Recall that Eugene's mother, Maria, is interested to know whether recent improvements in his grades in school are linked to his participation in school physical education and whether what she heard on television about this relationship is accurate. The kinesiology research literature supports the hypothesis that participation in school physical activity, including physical education, is correlated with better academic performance.[25] Participation in physical activity improves the cognitive and motor skills of children and adolescents by positively influencing the following physiological factors:

▶ Cerebral capillary growth
▶ Blood flow
▶ Oxygenation
▶ Production of neurotrophins (help in the development and regulation of nerves)
▶ Growth of nerve cells in the hippocampus (center of learning and memory)
▶ Neurotransmitter levels

▶ Development of nerve connections
▶ Density of neural network
▶ Brain tissue volume

The physical activity-related physiological changes may be associated with:

▶ Improved attention
▶ Improved information processing
▶ Enhanced storage and retrieval of information
▶ Enhanced coping abilities
▶ Enhanced positive affect (emotion)

Additionally, physical activity, including organized sports participation, is correlated positively with academic performance and positive behaviors in middle school and high school students—athletes perform better than non-athletes on cognitive performance tests.

Recent data suggests that athletes, as compared with non-athletes, are at lower risk for dropping out of school, perform better academically at the minimal and commendable levels in standardized testing battery, and are subject to fewer disciplinary actions. For example, a recent study of nearly than 35,000 male and female high

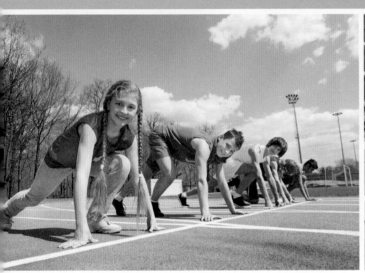
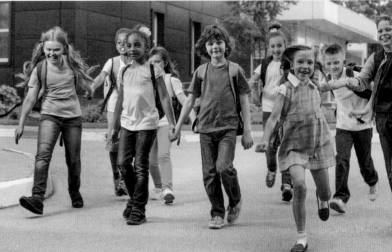

school athletes and non-athletes (grades 7–12) reported that a significantly higher proportion of athletes than non-athletes passed their standardized tests in math, language arts, reading, writing, science, and social studies. Further, athletes in this study were less likely to drop out of school and have disciplinary problems compared to non-athletes.[26] Other research findings have supported associations between children's and adolescents' participation in physical activity and improvements in their lifelong learning capacity and quality of life, as well as the quality of their community. However, further studies are needed to determine whether there are cause-and-effect relationships between academic and behavioral performances when comparing athletes and non-athletes. For example, does the type of sport matter? Is any effect really due to the physical activity in which athletes participate, or could there be other explanations?

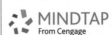

Go to your MindTap course to complete the Case Study activity for this chapter.

## Exercise Physiology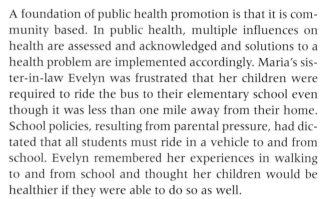

One of the U.S. national goals for school physical education classes is to engage students in vigorous or moderate-intensity physical activity for at least half (50%) of total class period time. For a physical education class that meets for 60 minutes five days a week, students should be engaged in moderate- or vigorous-intensity physical activity for at least 30 minutes. However, most students do not even obtain 30 minutes of physical activity before, during, or after school.[27] Eugene's PE teacher Mr. Daniels has been trying to learn new instructional techniques to increase the amount of physical activity time in his classes. He was able to purchase 30 new heart rate monitors to use with students by getting a small grant through the school foundation. He also attended a recent state conference workshop that focused on how to use heart rate monitoring to facilitate increased student physical activity in PE time. Mr. Daniels learned about evidenced-based techniques that were effective at getting students more physically active for 50% of PE class time.

For example, Jago and colleagues designed studies that modified physical education curricula to increase student vigorous and moderate-intensity physical activity using cutoff points based on heart rate: >130 to 140 beats per minute was defined as moderate physical activity and >140 beats per minute as vigorous physical activity.[28] Measures of randomized heart rate monitoring for over 2,000 students in school physical education classes indicated that physical education lessons can be modified to yield increased physical activity. The authors' modifications of physical education lessons included instant activities (moving immediately upon arriving at class), a "health related physical activity" lasting five to six minutes, a portion focused on the acquisition of skills and knowledge, and practice time related to the day's lesson. The interventions allowed students to spend more than 50% of the time available in the class engaged in health-enhancing moderate- to vigorous-intensity physical activity.

## Biomechanics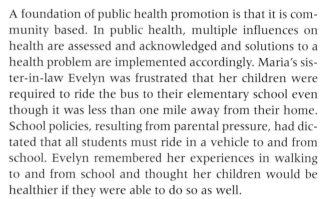

In addition to learning about heart rate monitoring at his state conference meeting, Mr. Daniels attended a couple of sessions focused on the biomechanics of movement for children and adolescents. The speakers reminded him that physical activity promotion in youth, particularly in schools and in sports programs, must account for the fact that children and adolescents are still growing and developing. In fact, peak bone mass is not normally achieved until we reach our mid-20s. Moreover, all youth develop on differing trajectories. Some mature faster and have better biomechanical control of their musculoskeletal system (and may be better athletes), while other students develop more slowly. Coaches and physical educators must realize these differences and plan accordingly. As discussed in Chapter 2 (Figure 2.1), running economy (lower $O_2$ cost at a given speed) is influenced by psychomotor factors, physiological factors, biomechanical factors, biochemical factors, and other factors. Growth and developmental trajectories affect primarily the biomechanics of running economy in children and adolescents as compared to adults. Researchers collected yearly physiological data (including $VO_2$ max and $O_2$ uptake at various submaximal running speeds on a treadmill) on runners from the age of 10 to adulthood.[29] In these studies, $VO_2$ max did not change significantly over time. The authors concluded that biomechanical factors related to growth and development—such as increased limb length, motor unit recruitment, and natural stride length changes—helped explain common differences between trained adolescents and trained adults in running economy (adults are more economical). Clearly this is one reason why young runners compete against peers of a similar age and older runners (with more advanced biomechanics) similarly are matched.

## Public Health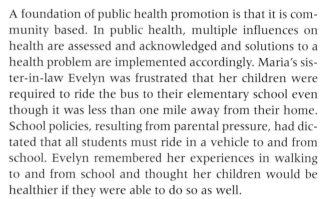

A foundation of public health promotion is that it is community based. In public health, multiple influences on health are assessed and acknowledged and solutions to a health problem are implemented accordingly. Maria's sister-in-law Evelyn was frustrated that her children were required to ride the bus to their elementary school even though it was less than one mile away from their home. School policies, resulting from parental pressure, had dictated that all students must ride in a vehicle to and from school. Evelyn remembered her experiences in walking to and from school and thought her children would be healthier if they were able to do so as well.

Evelyn met with the principal and the school parent-teacher association. Each offered various explanations as to why active transportation to school was not allowed: the crosswalks at a major intersection were not painted clearly; traffic moved too quickly; there were stray dogs in the neighborhood that frightened some children; parents perceived that walking to school was not safe; and students were always late if they walked to school. Evelyn was frustrated because these reasons seemed like excuses to her.

Evelyn contacted her state Safe Routes to School coordinator for suggestions on how to overcome the barriers she heard about from the principal and the parent-teacher association. With other parent volunteers in the neighborhood, Evelyn organized a walking school bus for the younger children and a "Bicycle Posse" for the older ones. Each group was supervised by a responsible adult(s) and devised pathways to get to school safely either on foot or by bicycle. Evelyn contacted the city roads department and had the crosswalks around the school repainted so they were clearly marked. A schedule of parent volunteer crossing guards was developed to help the walking school bus cross the road safely. Animal control was contacted to collect the stray dogs. At the beginning of the next school year, Evelyn contacted the principal and parent-teacher association again and convinced them to support a pilot program to determine interest. She passed out flyers for students to take to their parents. On National Walk-to-School Day, the program was launched. Through hard work and a dedication to public health, Evelyn was able to overcome barriers and change the culture in her children's school to encourage active transport to school. Now, children who participate accrue nearly 25 minutes of physical activity per school day that they didn't get when they were riding in the bus or in cars to school.

## Sport/Exercise Psychology

There are clearly mental aspects to physical activity participation all along the continuum, for those just beginning an exercise program all the way to elite athletes in competition. Concepts such as motivation, goal setting, confidence, communication, and performance anxiety can affect even the youngest children interested in being physically active and playing sports. Eugene's cousin Marion plays interscholastic softball for a large high school. She enjoys the physical activity and being with her friends on the team. She is an infielder who plays great defense, but she freezes when she is in the batter's box. Her season batting average is only 0.160. The coach has benched her for a pinch-hitter several times, but the team needs her on the field because of her defense. The team is counting on her, and each time she is at bat she feels less confident that she can hit the ball. Marion feels like she is letting her team down and has seriously considered quitting.

Marion's coach noticed that Marion's father attended all the games and cheered the loudest when Marion was in the batter's box. That seemed to make Marion even more nervous and distracted, not allowing her to focus on the moment the pitch was released from the pitcher's hand. After sitting with Marion after the game, her coach realized that Marion felt she was letting her father down each time she did not hit an extra-base hit or a home run. Although Marion's father was very supportive, Marion was not managing the expectations as well as she could. Not even the best hitters can hit an extra-base hit every at-bat. Through some individual meetings and one-on-one coaching sessions, Marion's coach was able to help to learn how to manage her expectations in the batter's box. She was able

to help Marion focus on the process of hitting a softball instead of only on the outcome. She also helped Marion develop skills to let go of any mistakes she made in the batter's box and focus on her successes. Through the season, Marion's confidence improved along with her batting average, and she became a well-rounded confident player by the time the playoffs arrived.

## Motor Learning and Motor Skills Development

After attending conference sessions about heart rate monitoring and biomechanical factors, Mr. Daniels chose to attend a session to update his knowledge and skills related to motor skill development research and the use of motor learning concepts/strategies to promote increased youth physical activity. The research findings for youngsters that was shared at his conference reinforced concepts that he was familiar with but also helped expand his knowledge of evidenced-based strategies to increase vigorous and moderate-intensity physical activity within his own classes.

Growth, development, and maturation factors influence the physical activity participation and physical fitness levels of children and adolescents. Both teachers and coaches should take individual differences such as age, sex, and developmental stage into consideration when they plan physical activities for children and adolescents. Malina and colleagues have suggested a paradigm for physical education and physical activity programs designed for youth based on growth and developmental considerations.[30] Figure 11.8 shows their recommendations for changing the emphasis of physical activities to complement growth and development during childhood and adolescence.

Figure 11.8 indicates that during preschool and elementary school, physical education and physical activity programs should focus on improving motor skills such as moving, fleeing, dodging, jumping, landing, balancing, kicking, throwing, and catching. Physical activities for this age range (2 to 10) should help students develop physical competence, optimize fun and enjoyment, and minimize anxiety and stress.

As students reach ages 10 to 18 years, the focus for physical activities should shift toward individual and group activities including in-school and out-of-school sports. For older students, it is important for physical educators and coaches to emphasize health and fitness concepts that can be carried over into adulthood.

It is important for children and adolescents to develop motor skills in physical education and sports because they contribute to increased levels of participation in physical activity. It has been estimated that competence in motor skill activities such as basketball, golf, and bicycling contributes significantly to an adult's choice to be physically active (meeting U.S. guidelines) or inactive.

McNamee and colleagues developed a games-skills teaching strategy that focuses on small group skills instruction while maintaining at least moderate-intensity physical activity (heart rates between 130 and 140 beats per minute) called high activity skills progression (HASP).[31] The HASP format promotes the process of developing motor skills (like proper throwing form) versus products outcomes (like throwing five times). The implementation of HASP activities by physical educators can facilitate student skill demonstrations, practice opportunities, teacher feedback, and immediate feedback during transitions. Table 11.3 contains a HASP

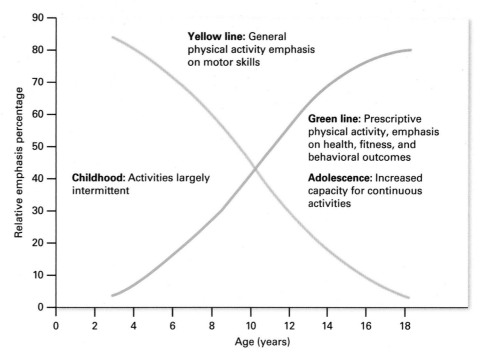

**Figure 11.8** | Changes in Physical Activity Needs with Increasing Age of Children and Adolescents

*Source:* From R. M. Malina, "Fitness and Performance: Adult Health and the Culture of Youth," in *New Possibilities, New Paradigms?*, edited by R. J. Park and H. M. Eckert (Champaign, IL: Human Kinetics Publishers, 1991), 30–38.

**Table 11.3** | HASP Lesson

| LESSON OUTCOMES |
| --- |
| ▸ Demonstrate a chest pass. |
| ▸ Execute a fake chest pass. |
| ▸ Move to an open area without the ball. |

| BEFORE-CLASS SET-UP |
| --- |
| ▸ Set up grid area for every six students, about the size of one-fourth of a basketball court. |

| SKILL PRACTICE (3 MIN.) |
| --- |
| ▸ Teacher demonstrates a chest pass. |
| ▸ Students shadow-practice chest pass without a ball. |
| ▸ Teacher demonstrates faking a chest pass. |
| ▸ Students shadow-practice faking a pass both to the left and right. |

| SKILL DRILL (6 MIN.) |
| --- |
| ▸ Teacher uses a partner strategy and students perform chest passes with one ball. |
| ▸ HASP set-up—separate class into two lines facing each other. One student at a cone passes to a partner whose back is to the wall. |
| ▸ Students include faking a pass either left or right. |
| ▸ Challenges: |
|   • How many passes can you catch in 20 seconds? |
|   • Can you improve your score? |
|   • Every two catches the outside student moves a step back. |
|   • Every two catches you and your partner move to a lower position. |
| ▸ After a few minutes of chest passes, move to bounce chest passes and repeat the challenge. |
| *Transition to next activity* |

lesson that promotes vigorous and moderate-intensity physical activity and skill development.

# The Practice of Kinesiology 🛑

The Seguin Independent School District (SISD, USA) serves as an excellent example of school physical activity promotion and integration within a local community. The SISD was recognized in 2013 as having the best Student Health Advisory Committee (SHAC) in Texas. One of the goals of SHACs is to promote a culture of physical activity and health within schools. The SISD SHAC was designed after the CDC Coordinated School Health model with a primary emphasis on promoting physical activity to students, faculty/staff, and the community. The purpose of this section is to share the documented outcomes of the SISD SHAC Physical Activity Initiative.

## Outcomes of the SISD SHAC Physical Activity Initiative

### Demographics

Seguin, Texas, has a total population of 25,000. The SISD has 7,440 students; 66.13% of students are considered economically disadvantaged (or low socioeconomic status, SES); 65.9% are classified as Hispanic, 26.7% as white, and 5.7% as African-American.

### History

The SISD Student Health Advisory Committee (SHAC) was formed in 2007 as mandated by 2005 Texas legislation using an evidence-based model of physical activity (PA) promotion for health (consistent with the U.S. National Physical Activity Plan).

Partners included the Seguin ISD school physical education and faculty/staff wellness departments, the Seguin Outdoor Learning Center, the Guadalupe Regional Medical Center, Seguin local community and business leaders, local universities Texas Lutheran and Texas State, and the HEB Foundations Free Camp (Leakey, Texas). Physical activity and health promotion programming included the following activities, amenities, and services for students, shown in Table 11.4.

### Results

Several key findings from the SISD physical activity initiative show the potential for such school-based programming:

▶ Campus walking trails for nine schools constructed with improved connectivity/assess to city parks.
▶ Increased student, faculty, and staff physical activity opportunities.

**Table 11.4** | Physical Activity and Health Promotion Programming of the SISD SHAC Physical Activity Initiative

| PROGRAMMING CATEGORY | ACTIVITIES |
|---|---|
| On-Campus Physical Education, Concept, and Skill Instruction | ▶ Basketball<br>▶ Volleyball<br>▶ Soccer<br>▶ Flag football<br>▶ Tennis<br>▶ Badminton<br>▶ Frisbee golf<br>▶ Ultimate Frisbee |
| Health Promotion Educational Topics | ▶ Mental and emotional health<br>▶ Growth and development<br>▶ Body systems<br>▶ Personal health and physical activity<br>▶ Violence and injury prevention<br>▶ Alcohol, tobacco, and drugs<br>▶ Chronic disease<br>▶ Communicable disease |
| Off-Campus Outdoor Education and Community-Based Recreation | ▶ Swimming<br>▶ Golf<br>▶ Fishing<br>▶ Ropes course<br>▶ Canoeing<br>▶ Rock climbing<br>▶ Archery<br>▶ Mountain biking<br>▶ Geocaching |
| Fitness | ▶ Jogging and walking trail<br>▶ Wellness center |
| Cardiovascular Development | ▶ Treadmills<br>▶ Rowing machines<br>▶ Stationary bikes<br>▶ Elliptical machines<br>▶ Stair climbers |
| Resistance Training | ▶ Dumbbells<br>▶ Weight machines |

▶ Several state and local presentations along with a publication of an implemented plan that improved FITNESSGRAM scores.
▶ 6,500+ students who participated in the Seguin Outdoor Learning Center and HEB Foundation camping/outdoor PA experiences.
▶ Named best District SHAC in Texas, 2013.

# People Matter  Michelle Hairston, Physical Education Instructor*

**Q:** Why and how did you get into the field of kinesiology?

**A:** *From as far back as I can remember, I was always a very active kid. I loved being outside running and playing with my friends! When I was in elementary school, my school didn't provide physical education for grades 1–4. We only had recess, which I loved because it was my time to be free. It was my time to play kick ball, jump rope, and tag.*

*When I turned eight, my friends Phillip, Carlos, and Willie were all going to play little league baseball. If you notice, the names I listed above are all boys. Yes, I was a huge tomboy and I had always played football, baseball, wrestled, and did whatever Phillip, Carlos, and Willie did, so when they said they were signing up for Little League, I was trying to figure out how I was going to convince my mother to let me sign up on this all-boys' baseball team. So, I got my permission slip and took it home to my mom, she read the information and to my surprise, she signed it and that's where it all began! I played Little League with the boys, being the only girl on the team until my little sister Jimmie (yes, her name is Jimmie) was old enough to join the team. I played sports throughout middle school and high school, excelling in basketball and track. Some of my favorite teachers were my physical education teachers. I knew I loved sports and I knew I loved kids, so majoring in Physical Education and Health was my ticket to be involved with both!*

**Q:** What was the major influence on you to work in the field?

**A:** *Being an athlete helped tremendously, but I had some pretty awesome teachers who inspired me to want to become a teacher. I love showing young people that being physically active can be fun and at the same time help them maintain a healthy lifestyle. I love working with young people and watching them develop and mature into healthy, happy adults.*

**Q:** What are your current research interests, and how do you translate your research results to practitioners?

**A:** *Since I am a practitioner, I rely on physical education and physical activity researchers to inform me on proven practices that will help me continue to best lead my students in becoming active for a lifetime. I am also interested in research on ways of expanding my role as the physical activity leader in the school and incorporating the components of Comprehensive School Physical Activity Programming (CSPAP) using physical activity as the core.*

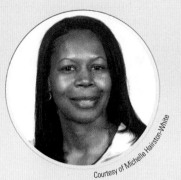

Courtesy of Michelle Hairston-White

**Q:** How do you stay physically active yourself and promote good health to others directly around you?

**A:** *I'm not as physically active as I once was, but I do manage to participate during my PE classes when my classes are taking part in team sports. Occasionally, my husband and I enjoy hiking while four-wheeling in the mountains. As far as promoting good health to those around me, activities such as karate, after-school open gym, gymnastics, and Zumba have been offered to our students, families, and community. I also sponsor an annual Breast Cancer Awareness Walk for our students, families, and community. Our classroom teachers also provide physical activity breaks throughout the school day. And by promoting the National PE Standards, it helps with maintaining a well-rounded curriculum.*

**Q:** How have you had to integrate the subdisciplines of kinesiology in your professional practice?

**A:** *I utilize motor learning and motor skill development a great deal in my PE classes. Students in grades K–2 are taught basic locomotive movements to teach them how we move through space. (Examples: walking, running, skipping, hopping, jumping, leaping, and galloping) Students in grades 3–5 are taught fundamental skills when learning a new team sport. (Examples: ball-handling skills, shooting skills, and passing skills for basketball)*

*I introduced my students to the Minds-In-Motion-Maze this school year. It's a 15-station program designed to stimulate a child's visual processing and auditory processing, as well as their motor skills.*

*Michelle Hairston-White is currently the physical education instructor at Welch Elementary School in Welch, WV. She is chairperson of her school Wellness Committee and a member of the McDowell County Schools Wellness Committee. She is a 1987 graduate of Concord University in Athens, WV.

- 2013 SISD bond election that resulted in $88.3 million of funding for new school and community improvements based on several SHAC integrated physical activity policy recommendations.

- 2014 Award of Excellence in Texas School Health and Reaching for Excellence Grant Winner—Texas Department of State Health Services

- 2015 Partner Project with hospital partners—Greenhouse and Gardens

## Discussion/Conclusion

The SISD SHAC Physical Activity Initiative provides an effective community-wide, school-based physical activity model for others interested in promoting school health through physical activity promotion and effective physical activity policy advocacy. The ongoing success of the SISD SHAC Physical Activity Initiative is also based upon the effectiveness of the program's leadership to integrate the kinesiology subdiscipline of philosophy, history, and sociology into planning and implementation.

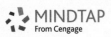

**MINDTAP** From Cengage

Now that you have completed this chapter, go to your MindTap course to complete all assigned activities. Check out the additional resources developed to help you apply the material in this chapter to your course and career goals.

## Chapter Summary

- Schools are logical settings for promoting physical activity and the principles of kinesiology because of the large number of children and adolescents they serve.

- Physical education is a planned sequential K–12 standards-based program of curricula and instruction designed to develop motor skills, knowledge, and behaviors of healthy active living, physical fitness, sportsmanship, self-efficacy, and emotional intelligence.

- A classroom physical activity break typically consists of 10–15 minutes of activities focused on vigorous or moderate-intensity physical activity. This strategy has been found to be effective in significantly increasing physical activity levels of school-age children.

- One of the most common opportunities for physical activity during the school day is recess. Recess is most common in elementary schools and is rare during the secondary years.

- In-school sports programs typically fall into two categories based on the nature of the competition: *intramural*, or within a school, and *interscholastic*, or between

schools. In the past 40 years, participation in sports has flourished both within and outside of schools.

- Active transport or active commuting refers to walking, cycling, or other human-powered methods (e.g., skate boarding) of transportation. It includes using public transportation, using walking school buses, and being driven part of the way to school and allowed to walk the remainder of the way. Active transport equates to moderate-intensity physical activity, which, as discussed in earlier chapters, provides crucial health benefits.

- Scientific evidence indicates that participation in physical activity improves cognitive and motor skills in children and adolescents by positively influencing numerous physiological factors. Additional emerging research evidence suggests that physical activity including organized sports participation is correlated positively with academic success and positive behaviors in middle school and high school students and that athletes perform better than non-athletes on cognitive performance tests.

## Remember This

| | | |
|---|---|---|
| active transport | games | recess |
| classroom-based physical activity breaks | physical education | sports |
| | play | walking school bus |

# For More Information

Access these websites for further study of topics covered in the chapter:

- Find updates and quick links to these and other evidence-based practice-related sites in MindTap.
- Search for information about the Institute of Medicine's *Educating the Student Body* at http://www .nationalacademies.org/hmd/Reports/2013/Edu- cating-the-Student-Body-Taking-Physical-Activity -and-Physical-Education-to-School.aspx.
- Search for more information about the U.S. National Physical Activity Plan at www.physicalactivityplan.org.
- To learn more about the Whole School, Whole Child, Whole Community model, see https://www.cdc.gov /healthyyouth/wscc/.
- Learn more about promoting physical activity in school physical education and sports for those with disabilities, see http://www.gao.gov/products/GAO-10-519.
- Find more about career options involving kinesiology and school careers at the American Kinesiology Association website: www.americankinesiology.org.

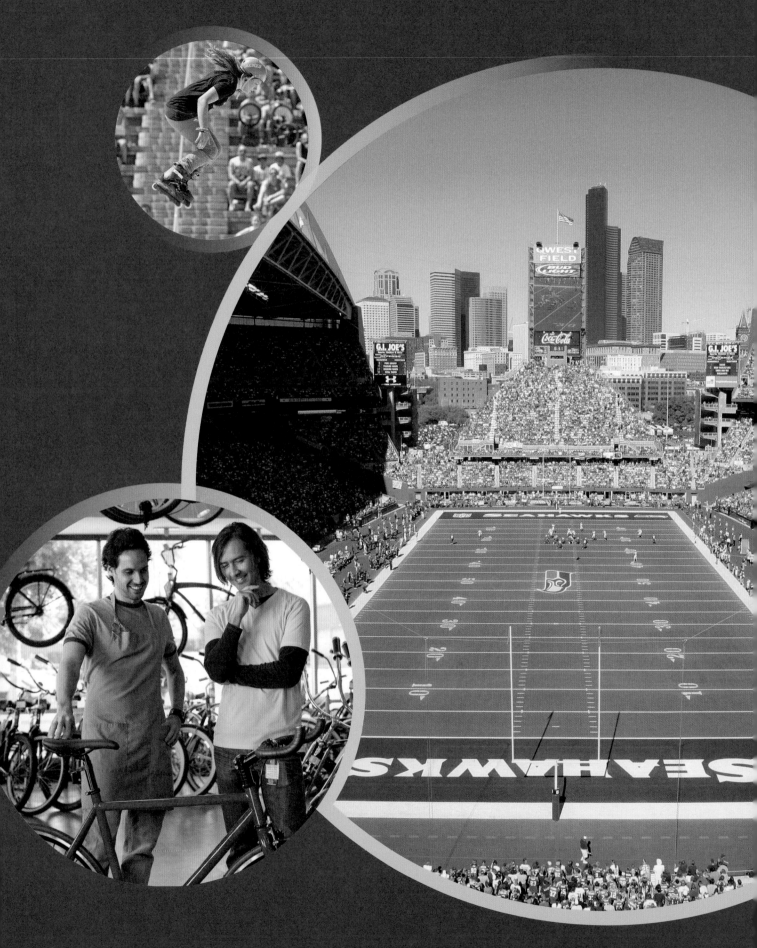

# Integration of Kinesiology with Careers in Sports

*What knowledge, skills, and abilities do kinesiology majors need to acquire and use for pursuing careers in sports settings?*

**LESSON 1** INTEGRATION OF CAREERS IN SPORTS WITH THE PRINCIPLES OF PHYSICAL ACTIVITY AND KINESIOLOGY

**LESSON 2** EXAMPLES OF APPLYING SPORTS MEDICINE, SPORT MANAGEMENT, AND COACHING PRINCIPLES OF PHYSICAL ACTIVITY IN RELATIONSHIP TO THE KINESIOLOGY SUBDISCIPLINES

## Learning Objectives

*After completing this chapter, you will be able to:*

**Define** common terms associated with the sports principles that promote health, physical fitness, and optimal human performance.

**Justify** the importance of understanding sports and participation in physical activities in the context of the various subdisciplines of kinesiology.

**Explain** why participating in sports is an effective way of achieving physical activity across the physical activity continuum.

**Describe** the essential elements of effective sport management and coaching programs.

**Explain** how effective sport management and coaching programs integrate with kinesiology careers.

**Give** examples of the trends of participation in sports.

**Understand** how the trends of participation in sports relate to career planning for kinesiology professionals.

**Describe** common adverse events related to sports participation.

**Explain** how the application of integrated kinesiology-related principles in sports programming can improve the management of adverse events related to sports participation and help reduce their prevalence and severity.

**Give** examples of application of sport management and sport coaching concepts on participation in physical activity.

**Explain** how the application of sports medicine, sport management, and sport coaching concepts on participation in physical activity is related to the kinesiology subdisciplines.

**Explain** the examples of application of sport management and sport coaching concepts on participation in physical activity.

# INTEGRATION OF CAREERS IN SPORTS WITH THE PRINCIPLES OF PHYSICAL ACTIVITY AND KINESIOLOGY

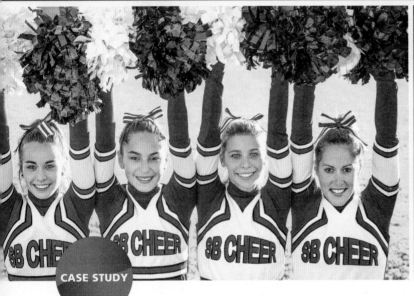

**CASE STUDY**

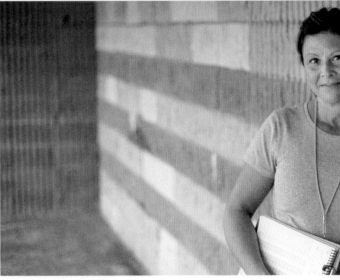

## In the real world...

As you may recall from Chapter 8, Cara Casey, a high school freshman, was considering trying out to be a cheerleader or a dancer, but her friend Amy was attempting to talk her into trying out for the cross-country team instead. Cara decided to run cross-country after all, and she is very happy that she chose not to try out for cheerleading because some of her other friends do not like being on the team. For example, Cara's friend Katy made the freshman cheerleading team, but she is frustrated with the cheer sponsor/coach, Ms. Reeves. Ms. Reeves was a cheerleader herself 15 years ago and has been coaching cheerleaders for 10 years with minimal administrative supervision until this year. She has often failed to balance her cheer budget effectively in years past, and she has had numerous complaints about how she manages her program. However, no one from her school campus has held her accountable on these measures because she has won many local and regional championships. Her college degree is in English, and she has little knowledge or skills (except through her own personal experiences) that apply to proper conditioning, injury prevention, or the importance of applying kinesiology subdiscipline concepts to improve performance. Ms. Reeves also has no formal training related to sport management issues such as ethics, leadership, business, or economics. Therefore, she coaches much like she was coached many years ago, without regard to available science-based training and safety methods.

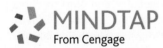
**From Cengage**

Go to your MindTap course now to answer some questions and discover what you already know about the integration of kinesiology with careers in sports.

## INTERACTIVE ACTIVITIES

### Research Focus

Go to your MindTap course to learn more about participation trends in selected sports activities using information from the Physical Activity Council and the U.S. Census.

### Career Focus

Go to your MindTap course to learn more about the Global Physical Activity Network. Activities include searches for articles related to sports and physical activity that affect societal issues such as politics, business, culture, and technology.

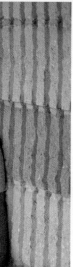
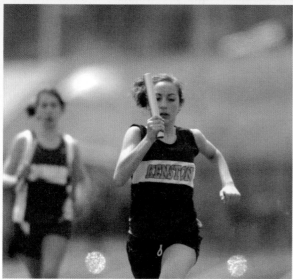

Katy likes Ms. Reeves as a person but has begun to lose respect for her as a coach. Ms. Reeves berates girls on the team (calls them unflattering names) when they make errors while performing stunts, and she uses exercise as a punishment (a girl who makes an error must run laps around the gym or do 20 push-ups before continuing practice). Katy is also upset with Ms. Reeves for encouraging the girls' parents to attend practice and watch them from an enclosed upstairs observation room in the gym, which Katy thinks creates a climate of favoritism. Katy's mom has told her that the interactions among many of the cheer team parents create an atmosphere that reinforces criticism of and sarcasm toward the cheer team girls who have less experience than others, and that these attitudes are endorsed by Coach Reeves. Katy's mom said she would rather walk around the gym on the school grounds trail for exercise during cheer practice than listen to the constant bickering of the cheer parents. Finally, Ms. Reeves coaches a cheer club team (the All Stars) off campus and often appears to be far more interested in the All Stars than the school team.

Although Katy enjoys many aspects of being on the cheer team, she is considering quitting because she has struggled to perform well since sustaining an early-season hamstring injury. Coach Reeves determined Katy's injury was minor, but offered no effective strategies for evaluation or treatment. She told Katy it would get better in a few days if she stretched her hamstring a couple times per day for five minutes each time, but the injury still hurts three weeks later. Cheer just isn't much fun for Katy anymore.

Have you or someone you know been on a sports team like Katy's? What do you think coaches (or their assistants) at any level (youth, high school, college, professional) should know about evaluating and developing sports skills, competing and practicing safely, and building a culture of positive sportsmanship that promotes appropriate sport psychology concepts? How might a degree in kinesiology prepare sports coaches effectively? Do you think coaches who do not have degrees in kinesiology need certification training to coach more effectively?

What skills, if any, might a sport management trained professional use to help Coach Reeves improve her cheerleading team? Even though sports coaching and sport management are two distinct and separate professions, Coach Reeves's new supervisor (the school athletic director) has a sport management degree and extensive experience applying ethics, leadership, business, and economic principles that could enhance the effectiveness of her cheer team. He is planning on visiting with Ms. Reeves following the cheer season to conduct a complete employee performance and program evaluation. We will follow up with Katy in Lesson 2 to see how her cheerleading experience might be improved or restructured through the application of kinesiology subdisciplines to coaching strategies and the application of appropriate sport management techniques.

# Introduction: Sports and Kinesiology

As you learned in Chapter 11, **sports** refers to a specialized or higher order of play or games with particular characteristics. It must involve physical movement and motor skills. It must be "competitive with outcomes that are important to those involved," and "winning and losing are a critical part of competition." Sports participation allows many individuals to refine their skills (e.g., golf, skeet shooting), enjoy psychological and cognitive challenges, and achieve peak performance at their own levels.

Historically, kinesiology and sports have been closely intertwined with programs designed for the professional preparation of teachers and coaches for in-school and out-of-school sports as part of major curricular plans in many collegiate kinesiology departments. Since the 1970s, sports and sports preparation programs in universities have been primarily managed by athletic departments, student affairs departments, and recreational sports programs. Within kinesiology departments, specializations in sports (where they exist) are now usually part of sports medicine (such as athletic training or pre-physical therapy; review Chapters 1 and 2 for more on these topics), sport management, or coaching degree programming. Today, many sport management programs have also become more aligned with university business schools that supervise or are more closely linked to curricular programming with kinesiology departments. Sports programs (outside of school) are managed by local, regional, national, and international sports organizations or governing bodies.

Since ancient times, sports and sports participation have been tied to politics, culture, business, cheating, violence, technology, and other aspects of society that influence nationalism (e.g., World Cup soccer), global power, and recognition. Ideally, participation in sports is associated with positive outcomes such as peak performance, good sportsmanship, traditional rivalries, respectful competition, and other attributes usually associated with being a champion or part of a championship team. However, as may readily be observed and regularly experienced through various media resources, sports and sports participation can also sometimes be associated with negative outcomes such as drug use, illegal gambling, excessive violence, injuries, abuse of power, racism, and inappropriate stereotyping (see Chapters 14 and 15 for more about negative outcomes associated with poor physical activity leadership, ethics, and/or management). It takes little time to either think of, or search the Internet for, a list of sports champions, teams, and organizations that were once revered as heroic only to fall from grace due to faults or misdeeds that have been judged to be disgraceful, illegal, or both. Perhaps it should not surprise us as kinesiology professionals that, although we expertly promote a variety of subdisciplines that enhance sports and sports participation (e.g., exercise physiology, biomechanics, and sport psychology), we are often only peripherally involved in providing quality sports participation programming at various levels (youth, high school, collegiate, and professional). In any case, as you learned in Chapter 11, the U.S. National Physical Activity Plan (NPAP) and the 2008 Physical Activity Guidelines for Americans recommend sports as an important sector in which to promote physical activity to various ages across the lifespan, using integrated kinesiology subdisciplines. The specific strategies of the NPAP are shown in Table 12.1.

Participation in sports across the lifespan and across the physical activity continuum (low, functional health, physical fitness, and peak) can promote positive health outcomes for a lifetime. As you recall, understanding the physical activity continuum can help kinesiology professionals apply the major principles of training such as overload, specificity, and adaption for achieving specific

**Table 12.1 | Strategies to Increase Physical Activity in the Sport Sector**

| | |
|---|---|
| STRATEGY 1: | Sports organizations should collaborate to establish a national policy that emphasizes the importance of sports as a vehicle for promoting and sustaining a physically active population. |
| STRATEGY 2: | Sports organizations should establish an entity that can serve as a central resource to unify and strengthen stakeholders in the sports sector. |
| STRATEGY 3: | Leaders in multiple sectors should expand access to recreational spaces and quality sports programming while focusing on eliminating disparities in access based on race, ethnicity, gender, disability, socioeconomic status, geography, age, and sexual orientation. |
| STRATEGY 4: | Sports organizations should adopt policies and practices that promote physical activity, health, participant growth, and development of physical literacy. |
| STRATEGY 5: | Sports organizations should ensure that sports programs are conducted in a manner that minimizes risk of sports-related injuries and illnesses. |
| STRATEGY 6: | Public health agencies, in collaboration with sports organizations, should develop and implement a comprehensive surveillance system for monitoring sports participation in all segments of the population. |
| STRATEGY 7: | Coaches, game officials, parents, and caregivers should create safe and inclusive environments for sports participation that promote physical activity and health for youth and adult participants. |
| STRATEGY 8: | Sports organizations should use advances in technology to enhance the quality of the sport experience for participants. |

*Source:* National Physical Activity Plan Alliance (NPAPA), http://www.physicalactivityplan.org/index.html.

desired outcomes. Students who are interested in careers such as sports medicine, sport management, or coaching can improve the effectiveness of their programs by understanding and applying the upper end of the physical activity continuum; making sound leadership, management, and ethical decisions; and by developing quality training plans. By combining and integrating the concepts of the physical activity continuum (see the inserted physical activity continuum icon) into the process of sports medicine, sport management, or sports coaching strategic planning sessions, positive outcomes for achieving peak performance are far more likely to occur.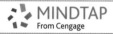

The purposes of this chapter are to (1) highlight the importance of understanding sports and participation in physical activities, integrating the various subdisciplines of kinesiology; (2) describe and explain the essential elements of effective sports training programs and explain how they integrate with careers such as sports medicine, sport management, and coaching (building off the concepts first introduced in Chapters 1 and 2); and (3) describe common adverse events related to sports participation and how the application of integrated kinesiology-related principles in sports programming can improve the management of such events and help reduce their prevalence and severity.

A complete review of the sports participation topics related to politics, culture, business, cheating, violence, technology, and other aspects of society that influence nationalism, global power, and recognition is beyond the scope of this text. However, students pursuing careers in sports medicine, sport management, or coaching should take course work as described in the career preparation sections covered in Chapter 2 or later in this chapter. This chapter is focused more on sport management or coaching careers than sports medicine careers except in the section on prevention and management of adverse events. Those students interested in sports medicine careers such as athletic training, physical therapy, and occupational therapy will need to complete detailed specific degree programming based upon national organization certifications (such as the National Athletic Trainers' Association [NATA] and others; please see Chapter 2, Lesson 1 for more specifics).

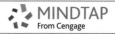
# Physical Activity in Sports Settings: Components of Sports and Kinesiology

When asked to think about sports and various sports participation opportunities, most people traditionally think of sports such as baseball, basketball, football, softball, and soccer. In today's society, however, it seems that a newly developed sport with individual and group participants emerges every six months or so. For example, Moms Team (www.momsteam.com) provides a current listing of a variety of sports and related physical activities with descriptions. The sample list of sports and related physical activities organized by category in Table 12.2 illustrates the

**Table 12.2 | Common Sports and Related Physical Activities**

| |
|---|
| *Extreme Sports*—bike (stunt), motocross, skiing and snowboarding, and sky surfing |
| *Fishing*—fly, freshwater, and saltwater |
| *Fitness Sports Activities*—step aerobics, cardio kickboxing, fitness cycling, fitness swimming, fitness walking, Pilates, running, and yoga/Tai Chi |
| *Indoor Sports*—billiards, bowling, darts, and gymnastics |
| *Outdoor Sports/Activities*—camping, equestrian activities, golf, hiking, rock climbing, cross-country running, and track and field |
| *Personal Contact Sports*—boxing, martial arts, and wrestling |
| *Racquet Sports*—badminton, racquetball, squash, table tennis, and tennis |
| *Shooting Sports*—archery, bow hunting, gun hunting, shooting clays/trap/skeet, and target shooting |
| *Team Sports*—baseball, basketball, cheer and spirit, dance, football, ice hockey, in-line hockey, lacrosse, rugby, soccer, softball, and volleyball |
| *Water Sports*—canoeing, diving, jet skiing, kayaking, rafting, sailing, scuba diving, snorkeling, swimming, wake boarding, water polo, water skiing, kite surfing, and wind surfing |
| *Wheel Sports*—BMX biking, road cycling, in-line skating, mountain biking, roller hockey, and skateboarding |
| *Winter Sports*—cross-country skiing, downhill skiing, figure skating, freestyle skating, luge, snowboarding, snowmobiling, and speed skating |

*Source*: Adapted from www.momsteam.com.

wide variety of opportunities for participation in sports, as well as potential kinesiology-related career opportunities for instructing, coaching, or the management of sports.

In *Trends Toward the Future in Physical Education*, Van der Smissen describes a variety of roles that sports play in relationship to kinesiology subdiscipline knowledge, skills, and abilities (KSAs) and sport management.[1] **Sport management** can be defined as the organization of educational and business aspects of sports and sports-related physical activities. Sport management incorporates an array of perspectives such as those of participants, spectators, the media, team owners, and the sporting goods industry.[2]

Van der Smissen discusses how sports may be approached as (1) a physical activity, (2) a modality, (3) a service, (4) a tenant, and (5) a sales product.[3] These various perspectives of sports can all be linked to the integration of kinesiology subdisciplines with the business principles of sport management (such as accounting, business law, marketing, management, and so on).

It is easy to understand how sports serve as physical activity since many of us have participated in sports at school, in recreation programs, in programs like the Y, in church leagues, or in community-sponsored events. Sports as an important source of physical activity is commonly promoted by kinesiology-trained individuals who instruct and/or organize events to promote positive socialization and improved health.

Sports provide a means through which participants and spectators experience pleasure. As noted by Smissen, participation in sports can help reduce stress, improve fitness, manage obesity and diabetes, and provide spectator entertainment and rehabilitation therapy.[4] Professional athletes and performers (e.g., ice skaters or Harlem Globetrotters) have fun competing but also make a living through sports. Kinesiology professionals are often actively involved in managing programs that use sports as a modality. Many kinesiology students are also interested in the prevention and rehabilitation of injuries and are pursuing careers as athletic trainers, physical therapists, and sports physicians.

Sports are considered a service in business enterprises such as fitness centers, golf courses, ski resorts, aquatic centers, hospital-based wellness centers, and the like. A primary goal in providing sports as a service is for a facility owner/manager to generate a profit based upon services delivered. Obviously, sports services will likely require much more than just the basic instruction and organizational skills of many kinesiology-trained professionals. For example, successful owners/managers use sports services and management skills to rent/purchase equipment, develop variable payment plans related to memberships, and coordinate amenities such as hot tubs/spas, massage therapy, physical therapy, and athletic training. Mastery of these skills requires additional business-based experiences.

Sports can be viewed as a tenant of facilities such as a city park composed of athletic fields (sports complex), a sports stadium, or a convention center. Successful management of tenant facilities requires owners/managers to ensure that the facilities are used regularly—often not only for sports but also for other community or city events. For example, many local community recreation facilities are used at different times for a variety of events such as baseball/softball leagues, car exhibits, rodeos, concerts, fairs, and special events. A traditionally trained kinesiology professional who seeks a career in tenant sport management needs to develop strong marketing, advertising, and promotional skills to be successful in keeping his or her facility fully utilized.

Sports as a sales product includes a wide spectrum of goods that can be purchased by consumers for participating in sports, experiencing sports as a spectator, or participating as a virtual player (via computer-based gaming). Sports sales include retail and wholesale clothing lines, equipment sales (e.g., shoes, basketballs, soccer equipment), technology items (e.g., heart rate monitors, cell phone applications, commercial GPS-based mapping and logging programs), coaching educational programs (e.g., USA soccer certification programming for coaches and referees, video instruction and evaluation websites), wellness and personal trainer coaching applications for electronic devices, marketing and advertising programming (e.g., minor league baseball ticket sales and game day promotions), and instructional media and public broadcasting opportunities (e.g., sports freelance feature writer/blogger, journalist, or sports information director).

Prior to exploring the details of preparing for kinesiology-based careers in sport management or coaching, it is important to learn how to monitor and follow trends in sports participation over time (for example as discussed in Chapter 10 for leisure-time physical activity and personal training). By tracking sports participation and population trends (surveillance), kinesiology professionals can gain a better understanding about how to develop integrated strategies to increase physical activity levels through sports. They can also develop career paths and learn to modify them for new job opportunities as trends change. The process also helps them evaluate the progress of specific sports participation/promotion programming and possible career paths in recreation and personal training settings as discussed in Chapter 10.

## Sports Trends, Tracking, and Surveillance

One of the easiest methods to follow sports trends and develop surveillance for factors that influence careers like sports medicine, sport management, and coaching is to refer to the annual Physical Activity Council (PAC) Report.[5] The PAC is made up of eight leading

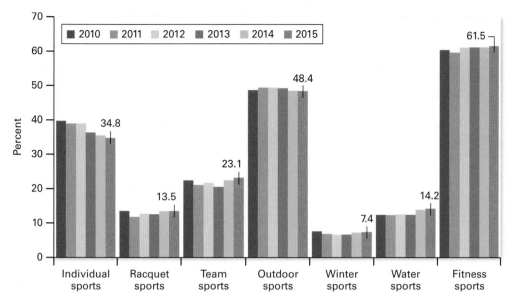

**Figure 12.1** | Sports Participation Trends 2010–2015 (% of Individuals Ages 6+ Participation by Sport)

*Source:* Physical Activity Council, "2016 Participation Report," p. 7, available from www.physicalactivitycouncil.com.

sports and manufacturer associations that survey sports participation trends within the United States. The 2016 PAC Participation Report represented 32,658 online interviews nationwide and was representative of the U.S. population ages 6 and older. The results were adjusted through statistical weighing techniques to reflect the total 2016 U.S. population, 294,141,894 people. The following section provides you with an overview of the 2016 PAC report as it relates to integrating sports with kinesiology.

Participation percentages by sports categories for individuals from 2010 to 2015 are shown in Figure 12.1. Individual sports participation has dropped slightly since 2010, while other participation proportions remained stable.

The prevalence of physical inactivity by age from 2010 to 2015 are displayed in Figure 12.2. These data reinforce the population trends for engaging in no leisure-time physical activity you learned about in Chapter 10. The data from PAC show some small changes year to year, but generally younger individuals are more active than those aged 45 and older.

Surveillance and trend data can also reveal age-differences and possibly preferences related to sports participation. A breakdown of sports participation percentages by birth cohort is shown in Figure 12.3. The birth cohorts shown are: Baby Boomers-born between 1945 and 1965; Generation X-born between 1965 and 1979; Generation

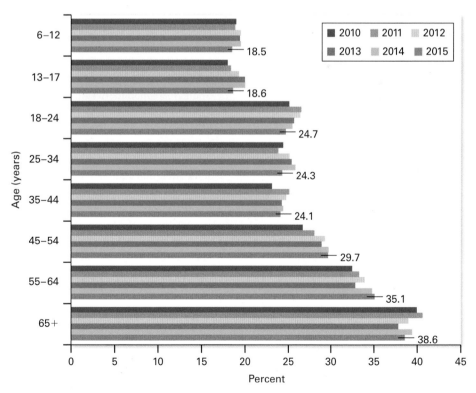

**Figure 12.2** | Physical Inactivity Percentages in the United States by Age Group, 2010–2015

*Source:* Physical Activity Council, "2016 Participation Report," p. 12, available from www.physicalactivitycouncil.com.

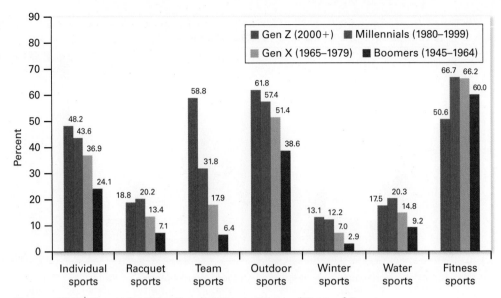

**Figure 12.3** | Sports Participation by Generation and Type of Sport

*Source:* Physical Activity Council, "2016 Participation Report," p. 9, available from www.physicalactivitycouncil.com.

Y/Millenials-born between 1980 and 1999; and Generation Z-born in 2000 or later. As evidenced in the figure, fitness sports are reportedly more popular with older participants while team and other outdoor sports are most popular with Generation Z. What other patterns can you spot?

Economic trends for sports-related spending from 2013 to 2015 are shown in Figure 12.4. The data show that spending increased over time on sports/recreation footwear and clothing, while other categories show slow growth or minimal changes.

The PAC survey results regarding interest in future participation in a sport or sports activity among current non-participants by age group are shown in Table 12.3. The data in the table highlight the potential for future participation in the various sports and activities (top 10 ranked) in which these age groups expressed interest. According to the PAC report, camping and swimming for fitness are popular for all age groups, and hiking, bicycling, and working out with weights are of growing interest for most age groups as well.

By using sports data like that from the 2016 PAC Participation Report, kinesiology professionals can gain a better understanding of trends in

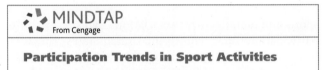

**Participation Trends in Sport Activities**

**Go to your MindTap course** to learn more about participation trends in selected sports activities using information from the Physical Activity Council and the U.S. Census.

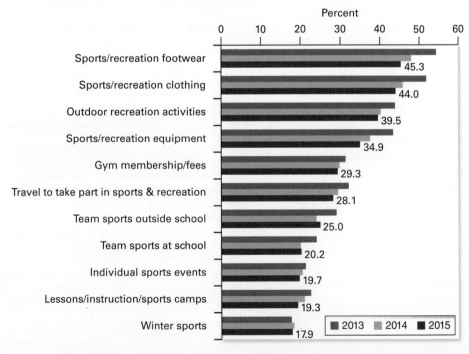

**Figure 12.4** | Spending Trends: Fitness and Activity Related Spending 2013–2015

*Source:* Physical Activity Council, "2016 Participation Report," p. 15, available from www.physicalactivitycouncil.com.

**Table 12.3** | Nonparticipant Interest in Future Sports Participation (Top Ten for Each Age Group)

| AGES 6–12 | AGES 13–17 | AGES 18–24 | AGES 25–34 |
|---|---|---|---|
| Camping | Camping | Camping | Swimming for fitness |
| Swimming for fitness | Swimming for fitness | Bicycling | Camping |
| Bicycling | Bicycling | Swimming for fitness | Bicycling |
| Basketball | Working out w/machines | Hiking | Hiking |
| Running/jogging | Running/jogging | Backpacking | Running/jogging |
| Soccer | Hiking | Working out w/weights | Canoeing |
| Fishing | Fishing | Running/jogging | Backpacking |
| Football | Working out w/weights | Martial Arts | Working out w/machines |
| Swimming on a team | Shooting | Working out w/machines | Working out w/weights |
| Hiking | Martial arts | Climbing | Kayaking |

| AGES 35–44 | AGES 45–54 | AGES 55–64 | AGES 65+ |
|---|---|---|---|
| Camping | Camping | Bicycling | Birdwatch/wildlife viewing |
| Swimming for fitness | Swimming for fitness | Swimming for fitness | Swimming for fitness |
| Bicycling | Bicycling | Camping | Working out w/machines |
| Hiking | Hiking | Birdwatch/wildlife viewing | Fishing |
| Working out w/weights | Working out w/machines | Hiking | Hiking |
| Working out w/machines | Fishing | Fishing | Bicycling |
| Running/jogging | Birdwatch/wildlife viewing | Working out w/machines | Fitness classes |
| Fishing | Canoeing | Working out w/weights | Working out w/weights |
| Canoeing | Working out w/weights | Canoeing | Camping |
| Backpacking | Backpacking | Fitness classes | Canoeing |

*Source:* Physical Activity Council, "2016 Participation Report," p. 19, available from www.physicalactivitycouncil.com.

sports as physical activity, as a modality, as a service, as a tenant, and as a sales product. The tracking and surveillance of sports data over time can help kinesiology professionals plan, implement, and evaluate current and future sports programming to make them more effective.

# Preparation for Sport Management Careers

Sport management undergraduate and graduate programs can be found at numerous universities in the United States. Though one can obtain a degree in sport management by completing a curriculum in either kinesiology departments or business schools, this section will focus on the integration of sport management with undergraduate kinesiology training. To prepare for a successful career in sport management, students need to acquire a variety of KSAs from courses in the following categories (or grouped similarly):

▸ General education courses (e.g., English, literature, history, and science)

▸ Core courses in sports management; options will *vary greatly* but may include:

• Scientific bases of physical activity and sports (e.g., exercise physiology, biomechanics, sport psychology, and care and prevention of athletic injuries)

• Specific sports-related courses in kinesiology (e.g., introduction to sport management, sports in society, cross-cultural influences of sports, politics of sports, sports ethics, and the economics of sports)

- Business management-related course work (e.g., introduction to management, marketing and advertising, computer applications, effective leadership, effective communications, and legal aspects [business law])
- Business economics-related course work (e.g., accounting, budgeting, finance, and basic business statistics)
- Leadership skills-related course work (usually contained in kinesiology or business core courses; see Chapter 14 and 15 for more information about leadership and ethics)
- Specialization tracks or course work for specific career interests (sports as related to physical activity, modalities, services, tenants, or sales)
- Practicum or internship (e.g., one semester spent working in a sports management environment that is specifically career related)
- Electives (usually limited)

If opportunities are available, we suggest acquiring unique sport management specialization skills such as social networking, digital video production, and electronics or computer-related application.

---

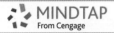

**The Benefits of Membership**

As part of professional sport management undergraduate preparation, you should consider joining a professional organization like the North American Society for Sport Management or others; see www.nassm.com.

By joining a professional sport management organization, you will make important professional contacts and expand you career KSAs. Membership can help you practice the business of sports with integrity and professionalism as promoted through ethical sport management policies. **Go to your MindTap course** to read the Ethical Creed of the North American Society for Sport Management, and see Chapters 14 and 15 for more about leadership and ethics.

---

## Preparation for Coaching Careers

**Coaching** in relationship to sports is defined as "the consistent application of integrated professional, interpersonal, and intrapersonal knowledge to improve athletes' competence, confidence, connection, and character in specific coaching contexts."[6] A less formal definition by Pate and colleagues suggests that a coach is "a professional whose occupation is to assist athletes and athletics teams in the enhancement of sports performances."[7] Pate and colleagues also note that good coaches should possess science knowledge (e.g., exercise physiology, biomechanics, and sport psychology) related to sports and regularly seek out new KSAs to improve their coaching skills.[8]

Many people (including kinesiology majors) are drawn to the coaching profession because it can be glamorous and financially rewarding for top collegiate and professional coaches of popular sports (e.g., football, basketball, baseball, and soccer). However, collegiate and professional coaches are often ex-athletes themselves and many have at least a master's degree in kinesiology or business. The chances of a high school athlete becoming an NCAA athlete are less than 6 to 7% (depending on the sport), and the percentage of collegiate athletes who go on to be a professional athlete is variable but well below 2% for football, men's and women's basketball, and men's soccer.[9] Because most coaches are former athletes, the probability of becoming a collegiate or professional coach is linked to the odds of having been a college or professional athlete, and is also limited further due to fewer career opportunities (smaller number of collegiate and professional teams) as compared to adaptive, community, youth, school, club, and private coaching positions.

A majority of career coaches move about often in order to improve their future opportunities and earn only modest amounts of money based upon their win/loss records. Most coaches at all levels (adaptive, community, youth, school, club, private, college, and professional) truly love sports and coaching because they are respected and admired by those they coach. Obviously, however, there are coaches (and you may have had one or more) who abuse their leadership roles and perhaps do more harm than good in working with individual athletes or teams. Fortunately, our currently strong societal emphasis on sports, sports participation, and increased leadership expectations for coaches beyond just win/loss records (e.g., improving athletics skills for all populations, promoting health and safety for athletes, acquiring and maintaining coaching certification, and ethical decision making) has significantly improved the quality of the coaching profession.

Good coaches are good leaders (see Chapters 14 and 15 for more on leadership and ethics) and they are coachable (personality that is receptive to continued personal and professional self-improvement) themselves, which means they are able to observe, listen, learn, develop effective practices, teach athletes to perform, and do

**Table 12.4** Are You Coachable?

- Who is your current coach/mentor or who are your coach/mentor role models?
- Do you have a good working relationship with your current coach or mentor?
- Do you receive and follow directions easily?
- Are you ready to learn new concepts that will enhance your role as a leader?
- Are you working with the rest of your coaching staff as part of the team to perform (effective communication and the sharing of new ideas and strategies)?
- Are you becoming or staying engaged in the coaching and continuing education culture? In other words, are you gaining knowledge about your sport and teaching that will help you perform better (e.g., about health and fitness, nutrition, safety, injury prevention and rehabilitation, etc.)?
- Are you currently engaging in regular physical activity, eating a healthy diet, and avoiding risky behaviors?

*Source:* Adapted from E. B. Power and T. D. Murray, *101 Healthy Lifestyle Tips for Coaches* (Monterey, CA: Coaches Choice, 2013).

their part as the leader of a team.[10] Table 12.4 contains questions that any coach should ask him- or herself if interested in career coaching (also review Chapter 2 on coaching as a career).

If you answered "no" to more than two of the questions in Table 12.4, you probably are not very coachable. You should probably think about ways in which you can become more coachable for your future success as a coach, as well as in other areas of your professional and personal life. How can you become more coachable or remain coachable? One good way is to arrange to attend and participate in regular continuing education activities such as those provided by the USA Track and Field Coaching Schools (levels 1, 2, and 3).

The Society of Health and Physical Educators (SHAPE America) has produced national standards for sports coaching.[11] The standards, listed in Table 12.5, address eight domains for effective coaching. Although a single coach would be challenged to fulfill all of the standards, most sports teams have multiple coaches who could work together to achieve compliance with the eight domains.

Some helpful behavioral guidelines for future coaches are shown in Table 12.6 and Table 12.7, offering strategies for developing an ethical and supportive coaching environment for participants.

To prepare for a successful career in coaching through undergraduate studies with a kinesiology focus, students need to acquire a variety of KSAs from courses in the following categories (or grouped similarly):

- General education courses (e.g., English, literature, history, and science)
- Core courses in coaching—options will *vary greatly* but may include those below:

  - Scientific bases of physical activity and sports (e.g., exercise physiology biomechanics, sport psychology, and care and prevention of athletic injures)
  - Specific sports-related courses in kinesiology (e.g., introduction to coaching, sports in society, and the business of sports)
  - Coaching leadership-related course work (e.g., computer applications, effective leadership, effective communications, and legal aspects of coaching; also see Chapter 15 for more on leadership)
  - Specialization course work for the sport(s) one is interested in coaching (e.g., baseball, football, and tennis)
  - Practicum or internship (e.g., one semester spent working in a sports program environment that is specifically related to one's career interest at the target level [community, youth, school, club, private, college, or professional])
  - Electives (usually limited)

If opportunities are available, we suggest acquiring unique coaching specialization skills such as social networking, digital video developing and editing, and electronics or computer-related application.

For many students interested in school coaching (seventh through twelfth grades in many states), you will need to become a certified teacher in a specific area (e.g. English, math, or science) in addition to having academic skills and preferred experience as a coach at least at the volunteer level. The primary portion of a school coach's salary is paid for their teaching duties, and a stipend is usually added for coaching a single or multiple sports.

As part of undergraduate coaching preparation, you should consider acquiring a coaching certification at the appropriate level along with your degree because this is required or preferred for many entry-level jobs. Many states require coaches to obtain and maintain coaching certification as part of their professional standards. You can learn more about coaching education and continuing education opportunities through your state coaching association (e.g., for Texas High Schools) or groups like the National Alliance for Youth Sports. Future coaches should also become familiar with the specifics of national, regional, state, and local legislative bills/acts and policies such as the 1991 Controlled Substance Act (CSA), Title IX of the Civil Rights Act of 1964 and amendments, the Americans with Disabilities Act of 1990, and the USA Paralympics

**Table 12.5** | National Standards for Sports Coaching

**Domain 1: Philosophy and Ethics**

Standard 1—Develop and implement an athlete-centered philosophy

Standard 2—Identify, model, and teach positive values learned through sport participation

Standard 3—Teach and reinforce responsible personal, social, and ethical behavior for all people involved in the sport program

Standard 4—Demonstrate ethical conduct in all facets of the sport program

**Domain 2: Safety and Injury Prevention**

Standard 5—Prevent injuries by providing safe facilities

Standard 6—Ensure that all necessary protective equipment is available, properly fitted, and used appropriately

Standard 7—Monitor environmental conditions and modify participation as needed to ensure the health and safety of participants

Standard 8—Identify physical conditions that predispose athletes to injuries

Standard 9—Recognize injuries and provide immediate and appropriate care

Standard 10—Facilitate a coordinated sports health care program that includes prevention, care, and management of injuries

Standard 11—Identify and address the psychological implications of injury

**Domain 3: Physical Conditioning**

Standard 12—Design programs of training, conditioning, and recovery that properly utilize exercise physiology and biomechanics principles

Standard 13—Teach and encourage proper nutrition for optimal physical and mental performance and overall good health

Standard 14—Be an advocate for drug-free sport participation and provide accurate information about drugs and supplements

Standard 15—Plan conditioning programs to help athletes return to full participation following injury

**Domain 4: Growth and Development**

Standard 16— Apply knowledge of how developmental change influences the learning and performance of sport skills

Standard 17—Facilitate the social and emotional growth of athletes by supporting a positive sport experience and lifelong participation in physical activity

Standard 18— Provide athletes with responsibility and leadership opportunities as they mature

**Domain 5: Teaching and Communication**

Standard 19—Provide a positive learning environment that is appropriate to the characteristics of the athletes and goals of the program

Standard 20—Develop and monitor goals for the athlete and program

Standard 21—Organize practice based on a seasonal or annual practice plan to maintain motivation, manage fatigue, and allow for peak performance at the appropriate time

Standard 22—Plan and implement daily practice activities that maximize time on task and available resources

Standard 23—Utilize appropriate instructional strategies to facilitate athlete development and performance

Standard 24—Teach and incorporate mental skills to enhance performance and reduce sport anxiety

Standard 25—Use effective communication skills to enhance individual learning, group success, and enjoyment in the sport experience

Standard 26—Demonstrate and utilize appropriate and effective motivational techniques to enhance athlete performance and satisfaction

**Domain 6: Sport Skills and Tactics**

Standard 27—Know the skills, elements of skill combinations, and techniques associated with the sport being coached

Standard 28—Identify, develop, and apply competitive sport strategies and specific tactics appropriate for the age and skill levels of participating athletes

Standard 29—Use scouting methods for planning practices, game preparation, and game analysis

**Domain 7: Organization and Administration**

Standard 30—Demonstrate efficiency in contest management

Standard 31—Be involved in public relations activities for the sport program

Standard 32—Manage human resources for the program

Standard 33—Manage fiscal resources for the program

Standard 34—Facilitate planning, implementation, and documentation of the emergency action plan

Standard 35—Manage all information, documents, and records for the program

Standard 36—Fulfill all legal responsibilities and risk management procedures associated with coaching

**Domain 8: Evaluation**

Standard 37—Implement effective evaluation techniques for team performance in relation to established goals

Standard 38—Use a variety of strategies to evaluate athlete motivation and individual performance as they relate to season objectives and goals

Standard 39—Utilize an effective and objective process for evaluation of athletes in order to assign roles on positions and establish individual goals

Standard 40—Utilize an objective and effective process for evaluation of self and staff

*Source:* Gould et al., "Effective Education and Development of Youth Coaches," *Research Digest Series* 14, no. 940 (December 2013), President's Council on Fitness, Sports & Nutrition, www.fitness.gov/resource-center/research-and-reports/.

**Table 12.6** | Behavioral Guidelines for Youth Sport and Coaches

- Focus on praise and encouragement by looking for and rewarding what young athletes do correctly; give praise sincerely by making sure it is earned
- Minimize punishment and hostile and controlling behaviors
- Reward effort as much as outcome
- Develop realistic expectations based on the young athletes' age and developmental level
- Give a high frequency of affirmative, instructive, and supportive behavior
- Focus on instruction—teaching and practicing skills
- Modify skills and activities so that they are developmentally appropriate
- Focus more on self-improvement goals versus competitive outcomes
- Use the sandwich approach to error correction (a sincere positive statement, corrective feedback, encouraging statement)
- Modify rules to maximize activity
- Reward correct performance technique, not just the outcome of a skill (e.g., how a shot was executed, not just whether it went in)
- Create environments that reduce fear of failure
- Be enthusiastic!

*Source:* Gould et al., "Effective Education and Development of Youth Coaches," *Research Digest Series* 14, no. 940 (December 2013), President's Council on Fitness, Sports & Nutrition, www.fitness.gov/resource-center/research-and-reports/.

**Table 12.7** | Strategies for Providing an Autonomy Supportive Coaching Environment

- Give young athletes choices within rules and safety limits (e.g., let the players call some plays in football)
- Be sure to provide rationales for rules, limits, and tasks (e.g., we should not yell at officials, because they are human and make errors just like we do)
- Strive to understand others' feelings (e.g., a coach carefully observes how her players respond to failure)
- Allow young athletes opportunities to work independently and to take initiative (e.g., allow the athletes a few minutes each practice to coach one another)
- Provide feedback about competence in a noncontrolling manner (e.g., "Sarah, you did a nice job on that play," versus, "Sarah, if you don't get it right I will bench you")
- Do not use guilt. controlling statements, or tangible rewards to control young athletes' behaviors (eg., a coach stops giving every player a trophy)
- Keep winning in perspective by not becoming ego-involved in competition (e.g., a coach does not get overly competitive when an opposing coach uses dirty tricks against his team)

*Source:* Gould et al., "Effective Education and Development of Youth Coaches," *Research Digest Series* 14, no. 940 (December 2013), President's Council on Fitness, Sports & Nutrition, www.fitness.gov/resource-center/research-and-reports/.

and Special Olympics Programs. By promoting physical activity opportunities for their communities, coaches produce a win-win situation for their own programs while helping community members improve their health.

# Preparation to Prevent and Manage Adverse Events

Any discussion about sports participation, and one inherent to sport management and coaching, that is integrated with kinesiology should include the recognition of the benefits of physical activity participation, but also the risks of experiencing **adverse events** (defined as undesired health events like musculoskeletal injuries or heat-related illness). Chapter 10 of the Physical Activity Guidelines Advisory Committee Report (PAGACR) is devoted to adverse events associated with participation in physical activities (not necessarily sports) from a public health perspective.[12]

In this section, we use a public health approach to discuss common adverse events as they relate to sports participation and the professions of sports medicine, sport management, and coaching because most research evidence on adverse events involves competitive athletics or sports. The information covered in this section is developed to encourage you to prepare yourself professionally to help prevent and manage adverse events. Today, kinesiology professionals at all levels are regularly (e.g., daily or weekly) facing the realities and pressures of strong public scrutiny regarding their role in promoting the health and safety of sport for participants.

Sports medicine professionals will become well versed at dealing with adverse events based on the specific certification and/or registration requirements of their professions such as athletic training, physical therapy, sports physician, and others. Future career opportunities for sports medicine students require the integration of many KSAs from the various subdisciplines of kinesiology.

Future sport management professionals will need to prepare themselves to understand how to develop sound policies and regulations that deal with adverse events in order to effectively manage, administrate, and maintain positive public relations for their programs. As you learned in the Chapter 2 sport management career example, adverse events can affect the health, safety, and number of total participants that might be attracted to participate in an event like a large marathon. Although not all sport management-related careers require event development, promotion, and implementation of job duties, most will, and a basic understanding of common adverse events is necessary to provide a reasonable standard of care to deal with a wide variety of potential health and safety issues (also see Chapter 16 and legal issues).

Future coaches will also need to prepare themselves by acquiring an understanding of adverse events because they are part of the athletic management team that works with physicians, athletic trainers, physical therapists, occupational therapists, and other health care personnel to maintain the health and safety of their athletes (see Chapter 2 coaching example). In fact, if today's coaches have not learned to integrate kinesiology and adverse event management as part of their coaching strategies, they may find themselves negligent or facing constant criticism for not having an adverse management plan.

**Table 12.8** | Factors Associated with the Risk of Activity-Associated Adverse Events

| |
|---|
| 1. Type of activity* |
| 2. Dose of activity* |
| 3. Personal characteristics |
|    a. Demographics |
|    b. Behavioral factors* |
|    c. Health status |
| 4. Protective gear and equipment |
| 5. Environmental conditions |

*Key factors under individual control.

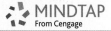

**MINDTAP**
From Cengage

**Adverse Events as Described in the Physical Activity Guidelines for Americans**

Go to your **MindTap course** to learn more about adverse events, physical activity, and sports participation as developed in the Physical Activity Guidelines for Americans.

Adverse events related to sports participation or of importance to sports medicine, sport management professionals, and coaches include mild, severe, and life-threatening situations. Sports participation (as compared to nonparticipation) is automatically associated with a greater risk for common injuries such as muscle sprains, strains, and blisters. However, the risks for other adverse events including cardiac events and sudden death, musculoskeletal or spinal cord injuries, and traumatic brain injuries (e.g., concussions) may also be increased for some sport participants. By adopting and applying a public health approach to common sport injuries and other adverse events, kinesiology professionals can play a public, proactive role instead of a reactive, defensive one. Section G of the PAGACR reports that certain factors affect an individual's susceptibility to adverse events. These factors (see Table 12.8) include the type of activity being performed (e.g., walking versus rugby), dose of activity (the total volume, as determined by the frequency, duration, and intensity), personal characteristics of the individual (e.g., age, physical activity habits), equipment or protective gear used (e.g., bike helmets), and environmental conditions (e.g., proximity to traffic, weather).[13]

The severity of adverse events can also be influenced by the safety of sports testing or sports facilities. The availability of athletic trainers and physicians onsite as well as emergency transportation availability at sporting events can help reduce the severity of adverse events. To prepare for adverse events, sport management and coaching professionals should develop emergency plans for a diversity of sporting events from leadership and administrative perspectives. Many sport management and coaching professionals are now considered part of new models pertaining to athletic program administration that include the involvement of research coordinators and all sports staff (e.g. sports medicine personnel, coaches, administrators, and so forth) as part of an integrated team to promote the health, safety, and welfare of athletes. For example, the University of Nebraska Athletic Performance Laboratory is the first in-stadium, on-campus facility devoted to understanding of performance, safety, brain function, health, and long-term well-being that benefits student athletes, the military, and society.

Once developed, emergency plans should be practiced regularly and implemented to optimize emergency response time and initial clinical care. Finally, it is important to ensure the safety of nonparticipants (e.g., spectators) at sporting events by having emergency equipment (e.g., automatic defibrillators [AEDs]) and additional emergency plans in place.

Specific data regarding adverse events are often lacking or difficult to interpret because only the number of cases of injury are recorded, without reference to the total population at risk or number of participants. To determine the prevalence of a specific adverse event, the total number of events that occur must be compared to the total possible events in a population (number of participants at risk).

Three of the most common adverse events (besides heat illness) that specifically confront sports medicine, sport management, and coaching professionals today are cardiac (heart-related) events associated with cardiac arrest or cardiac death, musculoskeletal injuries, and concussions (or **traumatic brain injury [TBI]**). In the following sections, we will provide brief overviews of these three adverse events and a rationale for the strategies by which sport management and coaching professionals can help prevent them or reduce their severity. The examples chosen are common adverse event challenges of interest to coaches, sports medicine professionals, sport program managers, administrators, media, and other sports professionals. The examples impact and affect professionals at the "hands-on level" (coach instruction) along a continuum that includes traditional sports medicine care and management, plus leadership personnel who develop policies and regulations to optimize the management of adverse events. Adverse events can obviously occur in other settings than just sports, such as community recreational settings, the workplace, in schools, and so forth. Thus, standard training of kinesiology majors in first aid, cardiopulmonary resuscitation (CPR), and automatic external defibrillator (AED) are common skills and essential to careers in sports.

## Cardiac Events

Participating in vigorous-intensity physical activity and/or sports (as compared to participating in moderate-intensity physical activity or inactivity) increases the risks for sudden cardiac death for those who already have heart disease (e.g., atherosclerosis—significant plaque buildup in the coronary arteries) or underlying heart dysfunction (e.g., hypertrophic cardiomyopathy [HCM]—enlarged heart due to a genetic disorder). Vigorous physical activity can trigger sudden cardiac death by initiating a sequence of events that reduces blood flow to the heart, which in turn results in dangerous arrhythmias (skipped beats). However, most nonsport participants, especially if they are physically active and under the age of 30, are at a lower risk for cardiac events than older participants.

The risk for sudden cardiac death for those individuals under about age 35 is usually not related to atherosclerosis but to genetic/congenital disorders such as HCM, abnormal coronary arteries, abnormal heart valve function, or Marfan's syndrome (weakened tissue of the aorta, a major artery exiting left ventricle of the heart). Genetic/congenital disorders often can be detected by clinicians when they obtain a good family history and perform a physical examination; however, sometimes cardiac adverse events occur without warning, and emergency measures need to be

available and initiated immediately. The risk for sudden cardiac death for those individuals over the age of 35 years is usually associated with atherosclerosis and developing coronary artery disease or other heart-related diseases.

Sport management and coaching professionals should ensure that sports participants they interact with or are responsible for are screened appropriately for risks related to vigorous exercise prior to sports participation. The completion of a signed waiver for participating in sports-related events, while helpful, may not be adequate to protect the professional against a lawsuit for negligence if someone experiences a cardiac event. In most cases, completion of a simple physical activity readiness questionnaire (see Chapter 5) by participants, at a minimum, can help categorize individuals as low, moderate, or high risk for cardiac problems. In other cases (e.g., school-based sports), participants should undergo a **preparticipation physical exam**, a brief physical exam, often required by state law and administered, at least in part, by a physician. If an individual has a strong family history of deadly cardiac events such as HCM, or has been previously diagnosed with heart disease, he or she needs physician clearance to participate in a sport or other physical activity programs.

The period of highest risk for adverse cardiac events is within one hour following vigorous exercise, and therefore sport management and coaching professionals should be aware of the importance of observing participants immediately following exercise—not just during the sporting activity.[14] Fortunately, the overall risk for sudden cardiac death is lower for those who are habitually physically active than for inactive people. As Figure 12.5 shows, the average risk of cardiac arrest for sedentary people is far higher than that for habitually active people. While the risk for active people increases during and immediately after exercise, their overall cardiac risk remains much lower than that of inactive people.

## Musculoskeletal Injuries

The underlying integrated training principles of overload, specificity, and adaptation that you have learned about throughout this text are particularly relevant to understanding musculoskeletal injuries in relationship to physical activity and exercise. Training adaptations based on overloading bones, muscles, joints, and connective tissues allow them to adjust and improve over time. However, bodily systems (e.g., cardiovascular vs. musculoskeletal) do not all adapt at the same rate, and too much overload too soon leads to an increased risk

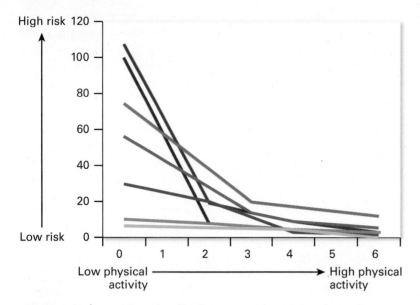

**Figure 12.5** | Risk of Sudden Adverse Cardiac Event by Level of Activity

*Note:* Based on several large population studies. The average risk of cardiac arrest for sedentary people is far higher than that for habitually active people.
*Source:* Physical Activity Guidelines Advisory Committee, *Physical Activity Guidelines Advisory Committee Report* (Washington, DC: U.S. Department of Health and Human Services, 2008), Figure G10.4, p. G10–20.

for injury or to an actual adverse event (e.g., overuse injury like a stress fracture of the lower leg). As discussed previously, few well-designed studies on determining the risks of musculoskeletal injuries have been published due to the inability to compare the number of injuries by type to the total number of participants at risk. Many of the better studies available in the research literature that evaluate adverse events are conducted in research institutes or through branches of the military.

One example of a study on the prevalence of running injuries was conducted by Blair and colleagues.[15] The authors considered the risk factors related to running-associated injuries such as age, height and weight (BMI), health status, motivation, fitness level, previous injury history, and training volume in order to develop a research questionnaire. Data on running practices and history of orthopedic injury (injury requiring the participant to stop running for at least seven days during the 12 months prior to the study) were collected via a survey mailed to 720 men and women who were members of the Cooper Aerobics Activity Center. The researchers received 438 questionnaires back with the following subject demographics: 76% men; mean age = 43.8 years; average weekly mileage = 24.5 miles. Figure 12.6 shows the percentage of runners who responded to the survey who reported a running-related injury during the

previous year. As you can see, injuries increased significantly as weekly mileage increased, which is consistent with musculoskeletal training overload, specificity, and adaptation. Blair and colleagues concluded that there was no association between risk of injury and time or place of running, frequency of stretching, age, or BMI.[16]

In another study, Jones and colleagues investigated physical training injuries among young men in the U.S. Army.[17] Three hundred and three males were evaluated using a questionnaire and fitness assessment at baseline (prior to) and after 12 weeks of physical training consistent with basic training and monitored using Army company logs. Musculoskeletal injury was defined as a case having received treatment for one or more lower extremities (cumulative incidence was 45.9%). Army health care personnel diagnosed all injuries, which were also reviewed by physicians.

The most common injuries following 12 weeks were muscle strains, sprains, and overuse knee conditions. The researchers also found the following risk factors were associated with lower-extremity musculoskeletal injuries: older age, smoking, previous injury (sprained ankles), low levels of physical fitness prior to

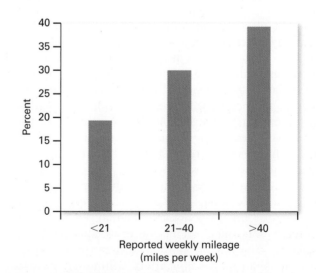

**Figure 12.6** | Relationship between Running Mileage and Running-Related Injury

*Source:* S. N. Blair, H. W. Kohl, and N. N. Goodyear, "Rates and Risks for Running and Exercise Injuries: Studies in Three Populations," *Research Quarterly for Exercise and Sport* 58, no. 3 (1987): 221–228.

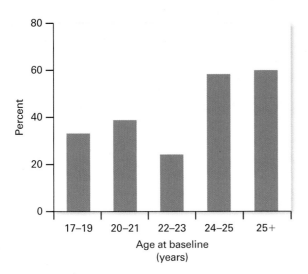

**Figure 12.7** | Musculoskeletal Injury Incidence Rates in U.S. Army Infantry Soldiers by Age

*Source:* B. H. Jones et al., "Epidemiology of Injuries Associated with Physical Training among Young Men in the Army," *Medicine and Science in Sports and Exercise* 25 (1993): 197–203.

entry into the Army, and high running mileage by training unit (see Figure 12.7).[18]

## Concussions

Traumatic brain injury (TBI) is a major cause of death and disability in the United States. TBI is often associated with a head injury that causes at least temporary unconsciousness (about a minute or more). A **concussion** is a type of TBI caused by a bump, blow, or jolt to the head, with or without loss of consciousness, that can change the way the brain normally works. Concussions can also result from a fall or a blow to the body that causes the head—and thus the brain encased within the skull—to move quickly back and forth.[19] Military concussions usually include blunt trauma from an explosive blast and a collision of the head with the helmet. The U.S. military and various sports organizations want to learn and understand more about the potential causes and long-term effects of concussions. Currently, numerous grant sponsors and researchers are engaged in intensive research to determine how soldiers and athletes react to TBI events.

Most concussions associated with participation in sports or other physical activities resolve in 7 to 10 days, although the recovery period may last longer for children and adolescents.[20] Concussions resulting from high school sports are usually associated with full-contact sports such as football and hockey. However, concussions commonly occur in a variety of other sports including

**Table 12.9** | Graduated Return to Play Protocol

| CONSENSUS STATEMENT | | |
| --- | --- | --- |
| REHABILITATION STAGE | FUNCTIONAL EXERCISE OF EACH STAGE OF REHABILITATION | OBJECTIVE OF EACH STAGE |
| 1. No activity | Symptom limited physical and cognitive rest | Recovery |
| 2. Light aerobic exercise | Walking, swimming or stationary cycling keeping intensity <70% maximum permitted heart rate. No resistance training | Increase HR |
| 3. Sport-specific exercise | Skating drills in ice hockey, running drills in soccer. No head impact activites | Add movement |
| 4. Non-contract training drills | Progression to more complex training drills, e.g., passing drills in football and ice hockey. May start progressive resistance training | Exercise, coordination, and cognitive load |
| 5. Full-contact practice | Following medical clearance participate in normal training activities | Restore confidence and assess functional skills by coaching staff |
| 6. Return to play | Normal game play | |

*Source:* P. McCrory et al., "Consensus Statement on Concussion in Sport—the 4th International Conference on Concussion in Sport held in Zurich, November 2008," *British Journal of Sports Medicine* 47 (2012): 250–258.

lacrosse, soccer, basketball, wrestling, gymnastics, cheerleading, and dance. Kinesiology-trained professionals can help reduce the risk of concussions by understanding concussion rates, patterns of injury, and associated risk factors.[21] A step-wise list of factors that should be considered prior to the participant's return to play is shown in Table 12.9 and a list of modifying factors that can and should regulate concussion management and the timeline for the participant's return to play is shown in Table 12.10.

It is especially important that kinesiology majors preparing for sport management and coaching be aware of and understand the latest national and state policies and regulations regarding concussions management due to participant health, safety, and legal implications. The CDC website provides an overview about TBIs and specific information for kinesiology professionals and the public. Laws regarding

**Table 12.10** | Concussion Modifiers

| FACTORS | MODIFIER |
|---|---|
| Symptoms | Number |
| | Duration (>10 days) |
| | Severity |
| Signs | Prolonged less of consciousness (LOC) (>1 min) |
| | Amnesia |
| Sequelae | Concussive concussions |
| Temporal | Frequency—repeated concussions over time |
| | Timing—injuries close together in time 'Recency'—recent concussion or traumatic brain injury (TBI) |
| Threshold | Repeated concussions occurring with progressively less impact force or slower recovery after each successive concussion |
| Age | Child and adolescent (<18 years old) |
| Comorbidities and premorbidities | Migraine, depression or other mental health disorders, attention deficit, hyperactivity disorder (ADHD), learning disabilities (LD). sleep disorders |
| Medication | Psychoactive drugs, anticoagulants |
| Behaviour | Dangerous style of play |
| Sport | High-risk activity, contact and collision sport, high sporting level |

*Source:* P. McCrory et al., "Consensus Statement on Concussion in Sport—the 4th International Conference on Concussion in Sport held in Zurich, November 2008," *British Journal of Sports Medicine* 47 (2012): 250–258.

concussions that occur in sports are currently in force in all states and usually include the following three action steps:

1. Educate coaches, parents, and athletes.
2. Remove the athlete from play.
3. Obtain permission for the athlete to return to play.

The CDC and other professional groups like the ACSM and the National Athletic Trainer's Association (NATA) provide educational materials about concussions for professionals (including those in the kinesiology sub-disciplines: sport management and coaching), parents, and participants. One example is the CDC *Heads Up* online training course about concussions in youth sports. Another example is the CDC *Heads Up Concussion* guide.

---

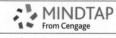
MINDTAP
From Cengage

**Resources to Learn about Concussions in Sports**

**Go to your MindTap course** to read more about concussions in sports and recommended protocols for management. Resources from the CDC, ACSM, and the National Athletic Trainer's Association (NATA) are presented.

---

# EXAMPLES OF APPLYING SPORTS MEDICINE, SPORT MANAGEMENT, AND COACHING PRINCIPLES OF PHYSICAL ACTIVITY IN RELATIONSHIP TO THE KINESIOLOGY SUBDISCIPLINES

*In Lesson 1, you learned about the integration of professions of sports medicine, sport management, and coaching principles with kinesiology. You learned about recent physical activity trends in sports participation and sports promotion at many*

*levels. You also learned how preparation for a kinesiology-related career in sports medicine, sport management, or coaching is integrated with kinesiology subdisciplines. By understanding more about trends in sports participation, sports*

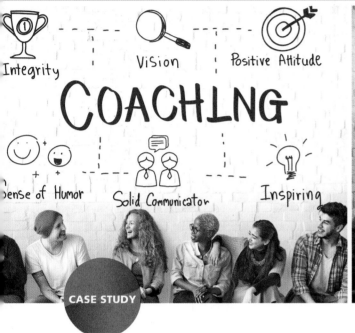

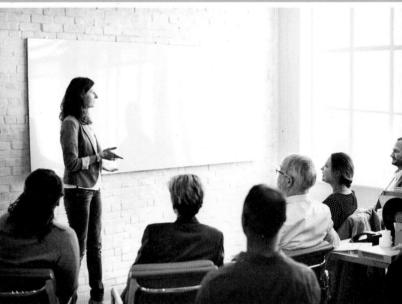

**CASE STUDY**

## In the real world . . .

Recall that Cara Casey is glad that she did not try out for her school cheerleading team because her friend Katy, who did, is very unhappy with the cheer coach and her participation experiences. Katy's cheer coach, Ms. Reeves, coaches a lot. She first became a coach many years ago but lacks the kinesiology background that would help her more effectively evaluate and develop the squad members' cheer skills, teach them to compete and practice safely, and build a positive team culture and experience. She also has managed her program without much outside supervision by school administrators until now. Coach Reeves would benefit from acquiring cheerleading coach certification, which she does not have because her school does not require it for her position. Recently the state passed legislation for all coaches of school sports and activities to obtain two hours of concussion prevention and safety training, but the law has not yet gone into effect.

Several organizations such as the American Association of Cheerleading Coaches and Administrators, National Youth Cheerleading Certification, and U.S. All Star Federation, among others, provide cheerleading coach instruction that focuses on promoting health and safety.[22] It would help Mrs. Reeves and her team members (school and club) to have better practices and competition experiences if she learned more about the following:

1. How to make her coaching a bit more scientific by basing her practices on sound evidence regarding which methods are associated with improving performance skills safely. Cheerleading can be a very dangerous sport if participants do not know how to spot properly or lack the proper physical skills and abilities. Coach Reeves also needs to learn more about common cheer injuries and how to treat them acutely until they can be evaluated by a physician or an athletic trainer.

2. How to deal effectively with parents. Dealing with parents and fans is a common part of coaching.

*products, sports sales, and sports services, kinesiology professionals can more effectively plan and implement successful physical activity programming. In Lesson 2, you will learn about examples of applying sports medicine, sport management, and coaching principles to physical activity in conjunction with the subdisciplines of kinesiology, and how to integrate them into effective programming strategies.*

▶ Exercise Physiology
▶ Biomechanics
▶ Public Health
▶ Sport/Exercise Psychology
▶ Motor Learning and Development
▶ The Practice of Kinesiology

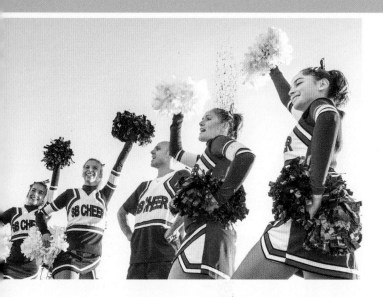

Unfortunately, if not handled effectively, parents can undermine the coach and create a negative atmosphere for participants and supporters of the team. It is helpful for coaches to adopt or develop a policy manual that addresses parent involvement and acceptable expectations. Coach Reeves might also learn to encourage parents to be physically active (e.g., by participating in a walking program) while their children are practicing, as ex-athletes (in this case cheerleaders) often become inactive after their competition days and turn into critical spectators.

3. How to manage her teams more effectively by becoming more organized. This includes learning how to be a good leader (see Chapters 14–16 for more), developing a team policy manual, learning to communicate more effectively, developing a shared yearly calendar vision for planning of practices and competitions, developing fund-raising policies and programs, and planning and coordinating competition opportunities that maximize school and club experiences.[23]

4. Annual evaluations by a school administrator such as her new supervisor, the athletic director (AD), who reviews her program performance annually based upon mutual predetermined goals made by herself and the AD with input from parents and the community.

Like many sports, cheerleading has become very popular in the last decade and the performance and safety expectations of participants and spectators have increased. Cheer coach expectations are also increasing such that coaches are more often expected to acquire and apply kinesiology-related subdiscipline skills promoting principles from exercise physiology, biomechanics, motor learning, and sports psychology.

Sport management professionals may find that they are challenged to develop new strategies to annually review personnel administratively if they do not understand emerging/developing programs like cheerleading. If individuals like Mrs. Reeves have not been part of their administrative chain of command responsibilities in the past, there will be a need for those in sport management to provide program leadership and, as necessary, growth (improvement) plans for subpar evaluations.

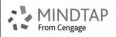

Go to your MindTap course to complete the Case Study activity for this chapter.

# Exercise Physiology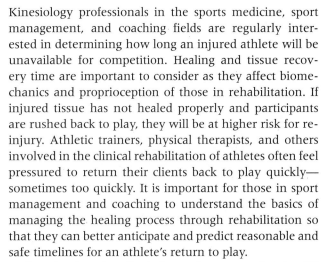

Oftentimes, coaches think that sports science testing such as that done in exercise physiology laboratories provides magical tools for optimizing sports performance and predicting future champions. Laboratory testing can assist coaches and athletes by serving as a training aid that can help to guide training and maintain a positive health status for athletes. MacDougall and colleagues have described the benefits of the regular exercise testing of athletes and the characteristics of an effective testing program.[24]

Physiological testing programs can help coaches and athletes achieve the following:

1. Identify strengths and weaknesses of the athletes and collect baseline data, which is helpful for monitoring progress and returning to baseline fitness levels following an injury.

2. Provide feedback about progress and whether a specific training element is effective.

3. Provide important health status information about the athlete and help coaches verify appropriate adaptations to training, while avoiding overtraining and burnout.

4. Provide an educational process through which the coach and athlete learn how to better manage health and injury challenges. Athletes learn more about their own bodies and the specific demands of their participation.

   - Coaches who are interested in setting up effective physiological testing programs should consider the following factors: Variables tested are relevant or specific to the sport; sometimes general physical fitness assessments administered to athletes, for example, do not provide much sport-specific training help.

   - Tests selected should be valid (test what they should) and reliable (yield consistent results from day to day). Tests should not be considered if no validity or reliability data based on previous studies are available in the sports performance literature.

   - Test protocols should be standardized and specific to sports performance. For example, swimmers should not be treadmill tested to determine their VO$_2$ max.

   - Test administration should be controlled and standardized to minimize errors in measures and variations between test periods.

   - The athletes' human rights must be respected. In Chapter 14 you will learn about ethics and the importance of obtaining informed consent from participants prior to exercise testing.

   - Tests should be repeated at regular intervals based on changes coaches are expecting or hoping to see. Regular testing helps coaches and athletes monitor progress.

   - Results should be shared with coaches and athletes promptly and interpreted effectively so that they understand the results and can apply them to future training. If this last step is ineffective or poorly handled, the testing program probably will be more harmful than helpful to all involved.

# Biomechanics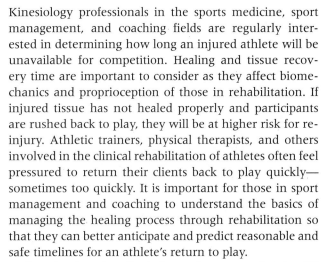

Kinesiology professionals in the sports medicine, sport management, and coaching fields are regularly interested in determining how long an injured athlete will be unavailable for competition. Healing and tissue recovery time are important to consider as they affect biomechanics and proprioception of those in rehabilitation. If injured tissue has not healed properly and participants are rushed back to play, they will be at higher risk for re-injury. Athletic trainers, physical therapists, and others involved in the clinical rehabilitation of athletes often feel pressured to return their clients back to play quickly—sometimes too quickly. It is important for those in sport management and coaching to understand the basics of managing the healing process through rehabilitation so that they can better anticipate and predict reasonable and safe timelines for an athlete's return to play.

Prentice has described three phases associated with tissue healing: the inflammatory stage or response stage, the fibroblastic–repair stage, and the maturation–remodeling stage.[25] He describes the healing process as "a continuum" in which "phases overlap one another with no definitive beginning or end points."

The inflammatory stage or response stage usually lasts two to four days. The fibroblastic–repair stage can last as long as four to six weeks and includes scar development and the healing of connective tissues. The maturation–remodeling stage can take months to years depending upon the severity and extent of the injury. Various tissues (e.g., cartilage, tendons, and bones) heal at different rates and vary in time required to rehabilitate. Prentice encourages sports practitioners to adopt a philosophy of athletic rehabilitation that promotes therapeutic exercise and modalities that:[26]

▸ Stimulate structural function and integrity of the injured part.

▸ Provide positive influences on inflammation and the repair process.

▸ Minimize factors that impede healing.

▸ Focus on preventing reoccurrence by developing structural stability of injured tissue.

## Public Health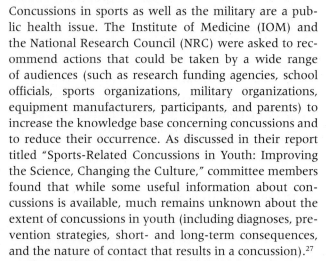

Concussions in sports as well as the military are a public health issue. The Institute of Medicine (IOM) and the National Research Council (NRC) were asked to recommend actions that could be taken by a wide range of audiences (such as research funding agencies, school officials, sports organizations, military organizations, equipment manufacturers, participants, and parents) to increase the knowledge base concerning concussions and to reduce their occurrence. As discussed in their report titled "Sports-Related Concussions in Youth: Improving the Science, Changing the Culture," committee members found that while some useful information about concussions is available, much remains unknown about the extent of concussions in youth (including diagnoses, prevention strategies, short- and long-term consequences, and the nature of contact that results in a concussion).[27]

The IOM/NRC report concluded that more data is needed to achieve the following:

▸ Close the research gaps (regarding specific demographics of participants, history related to the nature and extent of injures, level of competition, and so on).

▸ Gain a better understanding about the diagnosis process, recovery, and resulting health effects.

▸ Improve safety standards and equipment design.

▸ Change the culture surrounding recognizing concussions, reporting them, and determining effective return-to-play criteria.

## Sport/Exercise Psychology

Whereas this chapter has explored the positive aspects of participation in sports in relationship to promoting physical activity and other positive health and socialization factors, critics have posed questions about the negative psychosocial effects of the popularity of participation in high school sports in the United States. Ripley, for example, has argued that in the United States (as compared to other countries), the school day has become too focused on high school sports participation instead of academic pursuits.[28] Although Ripley's article focuses on the sociology and ethics effects of high school sports, her observations also have significant psychological impact for individuals who had their athletic programs cancelled or who participated in sports programs that overemphasize sport participation at the expense of academics.

Ripley builds her case against high school sport participation by noting that a lot of the school culture currently revolves around building numerous high-quality athletic facilities with cases filled with winning athletic trophies, which are often seen as much more prestigious than academic awards. Ripley reports on a school in Texas that had to suspend athletics for a year due to local funding issues

and afterward significantly improved academic scores without sports participation being an option for students. She also argues that sports in high school cost too much (football is the most expensive, yet brings in the most revenue), are a drain on the overall academic budget, and thus disrupt the primary mission of high schools.

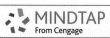

### Is High School Too Focused on Sports?

**Go to your MindTap course** to read Ripley's article. What do you think about the article? You will have the chance to voice your opinions. Based on what you already know, is this author painting an accurate picture of participation in high school sports? Why or why not? What negative psychological effects would you expect for the individuals impacted as examples in the article? Why should sport management professionals and coaches pay attention to articles like this? How should they learn to counter criticisms directed toward their professions at the high school level?

## Motor Learning and Development

What are some of the emerging trends that are driving the business of sports and their integration with sport management in relationship to motor learning/behavior (cues for athletes and active fan engagement) and sports fan behaviors? The Stanford Graduate School of Business reported the following five key trends that are driving the business of sports:[29]

1. During basketball games, data are collected from multiple video cameras that measure the movements and performances of all players on the court. Using analysis of these data, the players' success can be evaluated—based not necessarily on the number of points scored or rebounds pulled down but on their efficiency, or how productive they are per touch of the ball. The data analyses associated with this new technological system are likely to reshape the focus of research into the motor skills involved in basketball and may affect the practical biomechanical teaching aspects as well.

2. The development of smart arenas where mobile technology can help fans experience "ultimate" interactive media experiences at the game or at home by upgrading their seating, adding Wi-Fi connections, acquiring concessions items, reserving parking, and so on.

3. Development of athlete social media engagement through social markets such as YouTube using short

promotional videos to engage fans beyond the competitive experiences.

4. The use of technology to promote additional sponsorships and marketing to more closely tie fans to a team or athlete.

5. The globalization of local or hometown teams to new markets to promote sales.

## The Practice of Kinesiology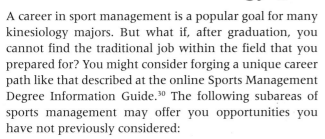

A career in sport management is a popular goal for many kinesiology majors. But what if, after graduation, you cannot find the traditional job within the field that you prepared for? You might consider forging a unique career path like that described at the online Sports Management Degree Information Guide.[30] The following subareas of sports management may offer you opportunities you have not previously considered:

1. Sports blogger
2. Sports philanthropy
3. Player appearances
4. Season ticket management
5. Web master
6. Market research
7. Sports camp director
8. Professor
9. Brand management
10. Social networking/community management
11. Sports event planning
12. Compliance professional
13. Public relations
14. Sports equipment and supply
15. Youth sports organizations
16. Legal services
17. Parks and recreation
18. Resort/club management
19. Digital video editor
20. Olympic involvement
21. Race management
22. Internet production
23. Sports promotions
24. Sponsorship
25. Tournament planner
26. Hospitality specialist
27. Fan development/fan club management
28. Sales
29. Sports mediator/arbitrator
30. Concessions management

The examples provided in Lesson 2 are a few of the ways in which you will find the subdisciplines of kinesiology integrated with real-life issues in sport management and coaching careers. What other examples can you think of where you as a sport management or coaching professional would need to integrate a variety of kinesiology concepts to problem solve in your daily job duties?

---

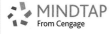

Now that you have completed this chapter, go to your MindTap course to complete all assigned activities. Check out the additional resources developed to help you apply the material in this chapter to your course and career goals.

---

## Chapter Summary

▸ Historically, kinesiology and sports have been closely intertwined with programs designed for the professional preparation of teachers and coaches for in-school and out-of-school sports as part of major curricular plans in many collegiate kinesiology departments. Since the 1970s, sports and sports preparation programs in universities have been primarily managed by athletic departments, student affairs departments, and recreational sports programs. Within kinesiology departments, sports topics (where they exist) are now usually part of sports medicine, sport management, or coaching degree programming. Sports (outside of schools) are currently managed by local, regional, national, and international sports organizations or governing bodies.

▸ Sport management can be defined as the organization of educational and business aspects of sports and sports-related physical activities. Sport management incorporates an array of perspectives such as those of participants, spectators, the media, team owners, and the sporting goods industry.

▸ By using sports participation data like that from the 2016 PAC Participation Report, kinesiology professionals can gain better understanding of trends in sports as physical activity, as a modality, as a service, as a tenant,

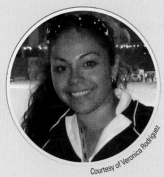

Courtesy of Veronica Rodriguez

**Q:** **Why and how did you get into the field of kinesiology?**

**A:** *As I became more dedicated toward running the last two years of my high school career, my interest grew in how the body functioned and moved. I wanted to learn about nutrition and techniques on staying injury-free; little did I know that kinesiology would also teach me about the importance of communication and leadership development.*

**Q:** **What was the major influence on you to work in the field?**

**A:** *The biggest influence for me was wanting to share my passion and knowledge for movement of the body to people of all ages and interest levels. My love for sports, like many who choose to work in this career field, transformed into a desire of wanting to help others embrace the true importance of being active.*

**Q:** **What are your current research interests, and how do you translate your research results to practitioners?**

**A:** *Currently I am doing research on active recreation and community health for my Master's degree in Park, Recreation, Tourism and Sport Management. This research ranges from the foundations and assessments of physical activity, social ecological frameworks, organization/employee wellness, community resources, youth participation in today's sports, and the relationship of religion, spirituality, and health. Based on the data, logical models for physical activity are then developed and utilized to fit the needs of those in our field.*

**Q:** **How do you stay physically active yourself and promote good health to others directly around you?**

**A:** *Staying physically active has always played a major role in my life, but as my career advances time is not always my friend. Daily reminders to take at least 30 minutes for myself and being creative have been two key elements in staying fit. I play on various intramural sports teams with coworkers, participate in charity fun runs and hikes, and train with friends in the gym throughout the week. Having options to work out in diverse ways and with different people keeps everyone accountable.*

**Q:** **How have you had to integrate the subdisciplines of kinesiology in your professional practice?**

**A:** *When someone hears kinesiology, budgeting and marketing do not immediately come to mind. Yet, they are two of the main elements of our profession. I have found that a sports/physical fitness/health budget is one of the first to be cut or reduced, and you must find ways to improvise. Grant writing will become your best friend. The marketing aspect has taken off because of social media, and you must find ways to reach your clients in this technological takeover. Typically, in this profession having a marketing person is not priority, making you the go-to.*

*Veronica Liz Rodriguez is a facility manager at JDL Fast Track, as well as a track and field coach at Salem Academy High School, in Winston Salem, North Carolina. She also works with TrackTown USA as a sport event manager consultant in Eugene, Oregon, which included working on the 2016 IAAF World Indoor Track & Field Championships and the 2016 U.S. Olympic Team Trials, Track & Field. Prior to JDL, she was an events and high performance manager for USA Track & Field and an assistant coach for the University of Miami (Florida) Track & Field Team, in Miami.

and as a sales product. The tracking and surveillance of sports data over time can help kinesiology professionals plan, implement, and evaluate current and future sports interventions to make them more effective.

▸ Professionals have formally defined coaching in relationship to sports as "the consistent application of integrated professional, interpersonal, and intrapersonal knowledge to improve athletes' competence, confidence, connection, and character in specific coaching contexts." A less formal definition suggests that coaching refers to "a professional whose occupation is to

assist athletes and athletics teams in the enhancement of sports performances."

▸ Any discussion about sports participation that is integrated with kinesiology should include the recognition of the benefits of physical activity participation but also the risks of experiencing adverse events (or undesired health events, e.g., musculoskeletal injuries or heat-related illness).

▸ The severity of adverse events can be influenced by the safety of sports testing or sports participation facilities. The availability of athletic trainers and physicians onsite, as well as emergency transportation availability at sporting events, can also help reduce the severity of adverse events. To prepare for adverse events, sports medicine, sport management, and coaching professionals should develop emergency plans for a diversity of sporting events and ensure they are practiced regularly.

▸ Three of the most common adverse events (besides heat illness) that confront sport management and coaching professionals today are cardiac events associated with cardiac arrest or cardiac death, musculoskeletal injuries, and concussions (or traumatic brain injury [TBI]).

## Remember This

| | | |
|---|---|---|
| adverse events | preparticipation physical exam | traumatic brain |
| coaching | sport management | injury (TBI) |
| concussion | sports | |

## For More Information

▸ Find updates and quick links to these and other evidence-based practice-related sites in your MindTap course.

▸ Search for further information about sports and sports programming for youth at Moms Team, www.momsteam.com.

▸ Search for information about tracking of U.S. participation in sports at the Physical Activity Council website, www.physicalactivitycouncil.com.

▸ Search for educational information about promoting the involvement of girls and women in sports at the Women's Sports Foundation website at www.womenssportsfoundation.org.

▸ Search for information about adaptive sports programming for schools at http://adaptedsports.org/download-resources/.

▸ Search for more information about effective education and the development of youth sports coaches at the President's Council on Fitness, Sports & Nutrition, www.fitness.gov.

▸ Search for more information about sports and adverse events in the 2008 U.S. Physical Activity Guidelines Advisory Committee Report, Part G, Section 10 at www.health.gov/paguidelines/report/g10_adverse.aspx.

▸ Learn more about coaching education and continuing education opportunities through your state coaching association (e.g., for Texas High Schools: www.thsca.com) or groups like the National Alliance for Youth Sports (www.nays.org/coaches). Organizations such as the American Association of Cheerleading Coaches (https://nfhslearn.com/courses/10000/aacca-spirit-safety-certification) and Administrators, National Youth Cheerleading Certification (www.cheercertification.com), and U.S. All Star Federation (www.usasf.net), among others, provide cheerleading coach instruction that focuses on promoting health and safety.

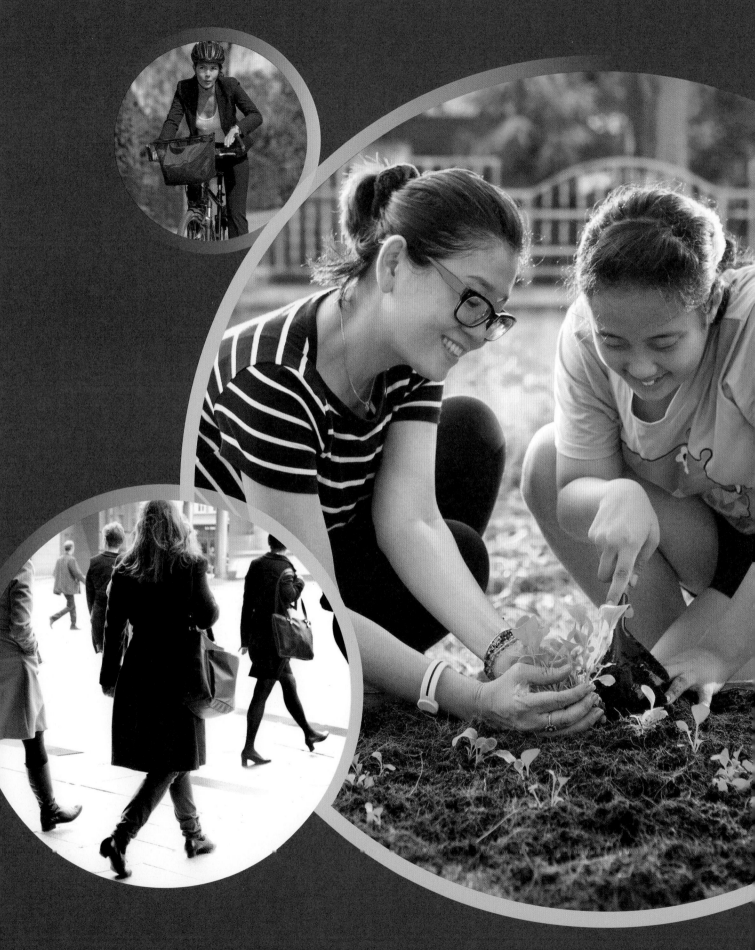

# Integration of Kinesiology in Transportation and Home Environments

*What knowledge, skills, and abilities do kinesiology majors need to acquire and use to understand how physical activity is a part of our home and transportation environment?*

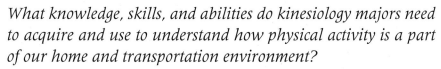

**LESSON 1** INTEGRATING TRANSPORTATION, HOME, PHYSICAL ACTIVITY, AND KINESIOLOGY

**LESSON 2** EXAMPLES OF APPLYING TRANSPORTATION AND HOME ENVIRONMENT PRINCIPLES OF PHYSICAL ACTIVITY BASICS IN RELATIONSHIP TO THE KINESIOLOGY SUBDISCIPLINES

## Learning Objectives

*After completing this chapter, you will be able to:*

**Explain** the common terms associated with the integration of transportation, home, physical activity, and kinesiology.

**Justify** the importance of understanding transportation and home opportunities in relation to participation in physical activities.

**Explain** how transportation and home opportunities of participation in physical activities can be integrated with the various subdisciplines of kinesiology.

**Explain** how active travel and physical activities at home are effective ways of achieving physical activity across the physical activity continuum.

**Describe** the essential elements of the strategies used to promote physical activity through transportation options and home environments.

**Explain** how the promotion of physical activity through transportation options and home environments can be integrated with kinesiology careers.

**Give** examples of application of transportation and home environment principles of physical activity in relation to the kinesiology subdisciplines.

# INTEGRATING TRANSPORTATION, HOME, PHYSICAL ACTIVITY, AND KINESIOLOGY

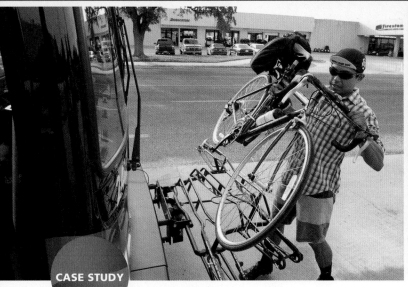

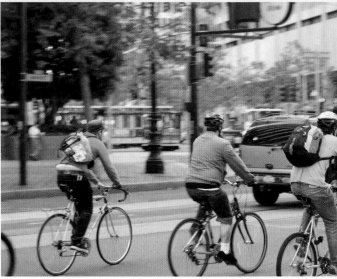

**CASE STUDY**

## In the real world . . .

William Casey, who works at a computer manufacturing company, just received a big promotion. He will now be a team leader for an elite group of engineers working on the company's next big product. The only drawback to this promotion is that he will have to travel to the corporate offices each day rather than to the manufacturing facility where he has worked for over 10 years. The Caseys chose their current home because it was only 8 miles from where William was working. Now he must travel 19 miles in the opposite direction to his new worksite. Although his employer allows flex time and telecommuting arrangements, as a team leader he has supervisory responsibilities

that require him to be in the office most days. William is not looking forward to the longer commute—traffic in his town has been steadily increasing, the price of fuel always seems to be rising, and he is concerned that the extra time in the car will take away from his exercise routine.

At dinner one night, Maria mentions that she heard that the local transportation authority has reworked some bus routes in the city and one of the new routes will pass within a quarter of a mile of their home. The city also purchased new buses that were equipped with bicycle racks, comfortable seats, and even Wi-Fi connections. Maria suggests that using the bus might be an option—it would save on fuel and avoid the stress that would result from driving in traffic each day. William looks into it and learns that the new bus route

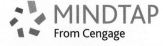

**From Cengage**

Go to your MindTap course now to answer some questions and discover what you already know about the integration of kinesiology and physical activity into transportation and home environments.

## INTERACTIVE ACTIVITIES

### Research Focus

Go to your MindTap course to learn more about details of promoting active travel and physical activity in parks and the National Park Service Parks, Trails, and Health Workbook.

### Career Focus

Go to your MindTap course to learn more about the five strategies and specific tactics that the National Physical Activity Plan recommends to increase physical activity opportunities.

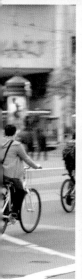
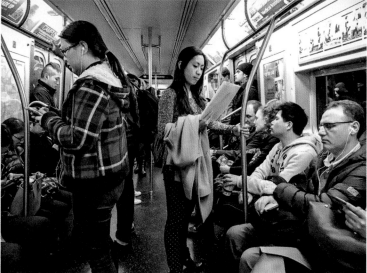
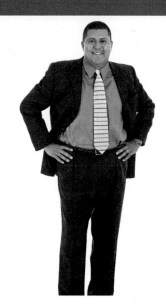

near their home has normal and express bus routes. The line begins near William's home and ends about 0.5 mile from his new workplace. William begins to plan his day around a new commuting schedule, which includes walking 1.5 miles each day as part of commuting to work (0.25 miles in the morning to the bus stop and 0.25 miles home in the afternoon, plus 0.5 mile from the bus to work and another 0.5 mile from work back to the bus). His current exercise plan, walking 4 miles every other day, has been working well; it has helped William lower his blood pressure and lose weight. The new commute offers a chance to increase his weekly walking habit. His children already ride a school bus each day, but taking the bus will be a new experience for William. How do you think William will adjust to his new schedule and transportation challenges? What specific adjustments would you plan in response to a transportation challenge like William's? We'll follow up with William later in Lesson 2.

# Introduction: Transportation, Home, Physical Activity, and Kinesiology

Because all movement is physical activity (Chapter 1), and because kinesiology is the study of movement, settings that involve movement other than exercise training and human performance are also relevant to kinesiology. Although understanding the limits of human performance and seeking ways to maximize it are important, most of the world's population has opportunities to move in two distinctly different areas of life: during transportation and within the home environment. The research literature related to studying physical activity outcomes (e.g., health and fitness) associated with variables in these areas is limited, but they have become areas of emerging interest. In this chapter, we summarize current concepts integrating transportation, home, physical activity, and kinesiology.

## Transportation

Broadly speaking, **active travel** refers to physical activity that helps a person to reach a destination. Active travel is generally taken to mean either walking or biking but can also refer to roller-skating, skateboarding, jogging, or any other form of physical activity involving movement across space to reach a destination. Although the possible destinations are virtually limitless, it helps to classify the major types of destinations for which active travel can be undertaken into five general categories: school, work, shopping, transit, and social or recreation. Categorization by destination is important because it is reasonable to expect the prevalence and determinants of active travel will vary, perhaps considerably, as a function of the destination type. For example, what may predict a person's active travel for a recreation destination such as a neighborhood park may be very different than the reasons for active (or inactive) travel to work or to school, such as access to an automobile.

Research has shown that it is not just enough to suggest to people that they adopt active travel behaviors. There are many barriers to making the active choice the easy choice. If there is no protected bicycle lane on your route home are you more or less likely to ride a bicycle to work? If bus stops (which usually require some active travel to reach) are not convenient or make you feel unsafe, are you more or less likely to use the bus system in your town? The CDC recommends that, to effectively promote active travel, communities must make changes in transportation systems and in the built environment such that the active choice can become the easy choice.[1] Can you think of examples in your own community that would make active travel easier for you?

Active travel to school typically refers to travel by children at the primary or secondary school levels. It could also refer to school-related travel by college or university students, but the bulk of the literature focuses on children under age 18. The prevalence of active travel to school in the United States has changed dramatically over the last several decades. In 1969, approximately 42% of children walked or biked to school. By 2001, that number was reduced to 16.2%.[2] Virtually all the active travel to school was replaced by automobile travel regardless of the distance needed to reach the school (less than 1.0 mile to = >3.0 miles). See Figure 13.1. This steep decrease has been cited as an important contributor to the rising prevalence of childhood obesity, and efforts are currently under way to promote active travel to school as a form of physical activity in children.

Active travel to work is, in a sense, the adult equivalent of active travel to school. Like school, work generally requires a regularly scheduled trip with a well-known end point. However, unlike the substance of primary and secondary education, the substance of jobs can vary greatly from person to person; this in turn may affect the person's ability to actively travel. In the United States, less than 3% of adults walk to work and less than 1% bike to work. The situation in other countries is different; data from England and Wales, for instance, suggest much higher percentages: 10.9% walking and 3.1% cycling.[3] These figures vary by personal and geographic characteristics but collectively suggest that there are important population level differences that must be studied and understood.

Active travel to shopping destinations and active travel to social or recreational activities are similar in that both

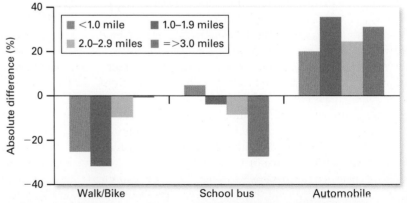

**Figure 13.1** | Absolute Differences between the Percentage of U.S. Students Who Traveled to School by Selected Means (Walk/Bike, School Bus, or Automobile) by Distance (in Miles), 1969 and 2001

*Source:* S. A. Ham, S. Martin, H. W. Kohl III, "Changes in the Percentage of Students Who Walk or Bike to School—United States, 1969 and 2001," *Journal of Physical Activity and Health* 5 (2008): 205–215.

are to some degree discretionary and irregular. This may hinder the ability to understand the causes of active travel to these destinations. Nonetheless, individuals may be more likely to walk or bike to stores or recreational activities than to their workplaces because they have greater freedom to choose destinations that are within reasonable walking or biking distance, as well as the time of travel. No trend data exist for the United States or other countries to indicate the proportion of people who actively travel to shopping, social, or recreational destinations.

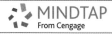

**The Park, Trails, and Health Workbook**

**Go to your MindTap course** to learn more about details of promoting active travel and physical activity in parks and the National Park Service Parks, Trails, and Health Workbook.

Finally, active travel to transit terminals (e.g., bus, light rail, subway, etc.) is unique among travel types because it is an intermediate end point. That is, an individual may walk or bike to a bus stop, but this is not the person's ultimate destination; rather, he or she is headed elsewhere by bus on the next part of the journey. The trip may end with another bout of active travel between the last bus stop and the final destination. This means active travel to transit is actually a subset of active travel to school, work, retail, or social or recreational activities because transit could be used as part of the trip for any of these four destination types. Approximately 3% of the U.S. adult population walks to and from some form of transit, though it is not clear whether this active travel represents part of trips to school, work, shopping, or social or recreational destinations.[4] However, research does indicate that walking is the most prevalent type of physical activity reported by adults.

The U.S. National Physical Activity Plan, as you have learned in other chapters, promotes physical activity in the sectors of business and industry; community, recreation, fitness, and parks; education; faith-based settings; health care; mass media; public health; sports; and transportation, land use, and community design. The sectors of transportation, land use, and community design include the five strategies designed to increase physical activity opportunities shown in Table 13.1.

As you learned in Chapters 9 through 12 and will in this chapter, the U.S. National Physical Activity Plan provides kinesiology practitioners with effective strategies and tactics to promote physical activity for individuals and populations. You should also recognize that the nine sectors contained in the plan are related to potential future job opportunities and career paths for kinesiology professionals.

**Table 13.1** | Strategies to Increase Physical Activity through Transportation, Land Use, and Community Design

| STRATEGY 1 | Community planners should integrate active design principles into land use, transportation, community, and economic development planning processes. |
| --- | --- |
| STRATEGY 2 | Communities should change zoning laws to require or favor mixed-use developments that place common destinations within walking and bicycling distance of most residents and incorporate designated open space suitable for physical activity. |
| STRATEGY 3 | Physical activity and public health organizations should advocate for funding and policies that increase active transportation and physical activity through greater investment in bicycle and pedestrian infrastructure and transit. |
| STRATEGY 4 | Transportation and public health agencies should invest in and institutionalize the collection of data to inform policy and to measure the impacts of active transportation on physical activity, population health, and health equity. |
| STRATEGY 5 | Transportation and public health agencies should implement initiatives to encourage, reward and require more walking, bicycling, and transit use for routine transportation. |

*Source:* National Physical Activity Plan Alliance (NAPA) www.physicalactivityplan.org

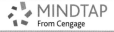

**The U.S. National Physical Activity Plan**

**Go to your MindTap course** to learn more about the five strategies and specific tactics that the U.S. National Physical Activity Plan recommends to increase physical activity opportunities.

### Active Travel to School

As discussed above, there have been major changes in the United States in how children get to and from school. Did you walk or bicycle to elementary, middle, or high school? Did you travel in a car or school bus? In terms of active travel to school, shifts in policy decisions related to school locations have affected the ability of children to use nonmotorized forms of travel. Traditionally, schools in the United States were built within residential communities and were designed to serve the needs of children who lived close to the campus. This minimized the distance between home and school and made walking or biking to school a common behavior. With time, the neighborhood school model evolved such that larger schools were built to serve many neighborhoods, allowing administrators to take advantage of economies of scale with fewer but larger schools. The need for large parcels of land for this newer model often means that newer schools are located farther from any one neighborhood and are sometimes located near major arterial roadways or highways. Not surprisingly, the shift from a neighborhood to a regional school model temporally coincides with the decrease in the prevalence of active travel to school noted previously.

On the other hand, even if a school is located close to a child's home, active travel may not be an automatic behavior. For instance, if the built environment along the path from home to school is inhospitable (litter, traffic, poor lighting, abandoned buildings), active travel may not occur. Recent research has shown that several structural features of the built environment are consistently correlated with active travel. For example, a 2008 systematic review of previous primary studies found that several specific environmental features are associated with active travel to school.[5] First, overall **walkability**—a term that encompasses specific features such as directness of the route to school, sidewalk infrastructure, and greater intersection and residential density—may be an important predictor. Based on this review, living in an urban area, as compared to living in a rural area, was positively associated with active travel to school, but this may be confounded with availability of walking infrastructure. Intuitively it would seem that parental concerns about traffic hazards and crime would be significant predictors of active travel to school; however, this review found no evidence of that.

## Safe Routes to School

As mentioned in Chapter 11, an important effort in the United States to promote active travel to schools is the Safe Routes to School (SRTS) program, which aims to provide support for communities to make improvements to the path between home and school. Funding from SRTS can be used to make structural changes, such as improving sidewalks and crosswalks and installing bike lanes and traffic calming devices. It can also be used for efforts to educate parents and children about how to safely walk or bike to school, and to increase enforcement of existing traffic laws designed to protect active travelers, such as reduced speed limits near schools. Limited evaluation evidence suggests that changes stemming from structural changes to the path to school are effective at increasing walking and biking as a form of active travel to school.

Interestingly, then, sidewalk infrastructure is correlated with active travel to school, whereas parental concerns about traffic and crime are not. Further, distance to school has a significant inverse association with active commuting, whereas the presence of attractive parks and recreational areas in the neighborhood potentially has a positive association, meaning the more attractive parks and open spaces a neighborhood has, the higher physical activity is observed.[6] Much research is being conducted on many factors of the built environment that may impede or promote active travel to school.

### Active Travel to Transit

Although active travel to school represents a trip to a final destination that is well known and predictable, active travel to transit is much more complicated as it involves one part of a trip to a variable final destination. The target destination may vary greatly from person to person walking or biking a route to transit, or even for a single person on different days. William Casey, for example, might get off the bus (if not on the express route) at an earlier stop to shop for some groceries on the way home. The one constant for this form of travel is that it involves an intermediate stop to get on public transit, such as a bus, subway, or train. This variability complicates efforts to understand the reasons why someone would or would not be physically active (e.g., walking or biking) to public transit. Further complicating matters is that active travel to transit usually involves a two-part decision-making process on the part of the commuter. Think about this in your personal context. What decisions are involved in your commute? Researchers must ask two questions: First, what causes an individual to use public transit over other available options? Second, assuming an individual has decided to use transit, what causes her or him to choose walking or biking to the transit stop over other available options, such as driving and parking near the stop or being dropped off? Only with an understanding of both aspects will it be possible to increase population-wide levels of active travel to transit.

Of these two questions, there is relatively more research in the literature on the first. In particular, there is substantial research on understanding an individual's mode choice decisions in the transportation field, especially given the continual increase in the use of motorized vehicles and their adverse impacts such as traffic congestion, increased accidents, and environmental pollution. In the last couple of decades, the efforts of transportation researchers have been even more focused on identifying the behavioral differences in choosing active travel modes or public transit to mitigate these adverse impacts of motorized modes.

It is clear that choice of travel mode is not simple, but influenced by a variety of demographic, socioeconomic, and environmental factors and transportation system characteristics, as well as perceptions and attitudes. For instance, many studies have shown that service reliability (how predictable it is) is one of the most important factors in users' decision to choose public transit. Service quality (new equipment for example) is a key element for making public transit more attractive.[7] Although reliability and quality have been shown to be important, it is likely that other, individualized behavioral factors such as motivation and perceptions of the individual user are central to a decision to switch to and maintain use of public transit. Such individual characteristics can be influenced and even changed by promotional tactics and incentives.

### Fitness Changes

Active travel by definition provides more physical activity to the participant than does sedentary travel and links to the physical activity continuum that you have learned about throughout the last several chapters. The kinesiologist should also ask: Are there health and fitness benefits? Does the physical activity that makes up active travel provide sufficient stimuli for overload, specificity, and adaptation—the three unifying principles of exercise science? Another related question refers to the relative benefits of specific modes of travel. For example, if there are health and fitness benefits to active travel, is there a mode that may yield higher fitness? Bicycling could be hypothesized to result in higher fitness levels than walking does because of its higher intensity. 🏃

Østergaard and colleagues studied children and adolescents from 40 elementary schools and 23 high schools in Norway.[8] These investigators were interested in any associations between the way the youth traveled to school and various fitness and body composition parameters (sum of four skinfolds as a measure of percentage of body fat; review Chapter 7 for more). The study involved taking cardiorespiratory and muscular fitness measures of almost 1,700 youth using standardized testing procedures. Study participants were also asked to complete a questionnaire to determine their usual mode of transportation to and from school: passive (automobile or bus) or active (cycling or walking).

The results of this study pertaining to body fat for adolescent boys and girls are shown in Figure 13.2. Boys and girls who traveled "passively" to school had the highest levels of body fat. Those who walked to school had somewhat lower levels of body fat and those who cycled regularly to school had the least fat. Similar results were generally seen for measures of muscular fitness and for cardiorespiratory fitness—that is, the highest levels of fitness were associated with the most active forms of transport. The authors concluded that active travel to school was associated with better fitness profiles in children and adolescents and that cycling was associated with a better fitness profile than walking.

## The Home Environment

Numerous organizations such as the CDC, the National Institutes of Health (NIH), and the American Heart Association and ACSM advocate the health benefits of participating in physical activities and exercise in home settings. Estimates are available of the numbers of U.S. adults and children who meet national physical activity goals like 150 minutes per week or 60 minutes per day (see Chapter 12). Though the explosion of available

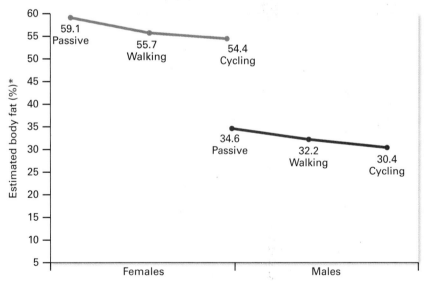

*Percentage of body fat is shown as a function of the sum of 4 skin folds—see source

**Figure 13.2** | Sum of Skinfolds (a Measure of Percent of Body Fat) in Adolescent Girls and Boys Who Traveled to School Passively, by Walking, or by Cycling. Cycling to school was associated with lower levels of body fat for the study population. Østergaard and colleagues concluded that active travel to school was associated with better fitness profiles in children and adolescents and that cycling was associated with a better fitness profile than walking.

*Source:* Based on data from L. Østergaard et al., "Cross Sectional Analysis of the Association between Mode of School Transportation and Physical Fitness in Children and Adolescents," *International Journal of Behavioral Nutrition and Physical Activity* 10 (2014): 91.

consumer wearable devices to track steps, heart rate, etc. would seem to make it easier than ever to be physically active at home, little research has been conducted on the number of Americans who are physically active or exercise at home on a regular basis. The number of consumer products for physical activity and fitness technology continues to increase at rapid rates, while the research about the accuracy and effectiveness for promoting increased physical activity levels of users, for most of the new devices, has lagged. Research supports the fact that wearable devices can help people log and track their physical activity very effectively and then electronically transfer their data to multiple other electronic devices for reflection and further goal setting (remember in Chapter 10 you learned that wearable fitness technology was the number one item in the top 20 of 2016 ACSM Worldwide Survey of Fitness Trends).

Obviously, for many the home setting provides opportunities for physical activity as part of home maintenance and repair. Anecdotally, people who seem to be constantly working on their homes or out in their yards engaging in physical activities such as gardening or mowing probably

reach or exceed the minimum U.S. Physical Activity Guidelines (at least 150 minutes per week of moderate-intensity physical activity) just being physically active in and around their home. However, it is unknown how many Americans actually achieve the standard in this specific manner. Examples of the number of calories expended per hour (based on a weight of 150 pounds) for common home maintenance and repair physical activities that Americans participate in regularly are shown in Table 13.2.

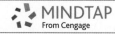
**MINDTAP**
From Cengage

### Physical Activity Guidelines and Home Activities

**Go to your MindTap course** to review the 2008 Physical Activity Guidelines to determine how you could encourage individuals or populations to meet the recommended guidelines by being physically active at their homes and neighborhoods as well as how to determine the caloric costs of home physical activities like mowing the grass or weeding a garden.

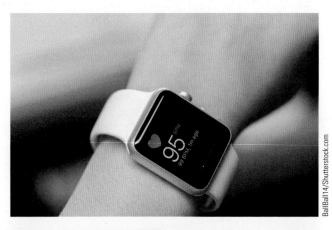

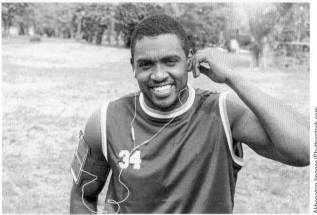

Shown are examples of wearable technology that consumers can use to measure physiological markers (e.g. heart rate, calories, force) of physical activity and that can provide logging/tracking of data for individuals and populations.

**Table 13.2** | Calories Expended per Hour for Common Home Maintenance Activities

| ACTIVITY | CALORIES PER HOUR* |
|---|---|
| Mopping | 170 |
| Heavy cleaning (washing car, washing windows, cleaning garage) | 136 |
| Vacuuming | 170 |
| Carrying groceries upstairs | 442 |
| Walk/run with children vigorously | 200 to 272 |
| Walk/run with pets | 200 to 272 |
| General gardening | 256 |
| Shoveling snow | 576 |
| Installing carpet | 238 |
| Roof repair | 340 |
| Pressure wash fence | 238 |
| Push mowing lawn | 400 |
| Weed whacking | 250 to 300 |
| Painting house | 272 |
| Raking leaves | 384 |
| Cleaning gutter | 272 |

*Data based on 150-pound person. Visit calorielab.com/burned to enter different body weights and recalculate the calories per hour.

*Source:* CalorieLab (www.calorielab.com).

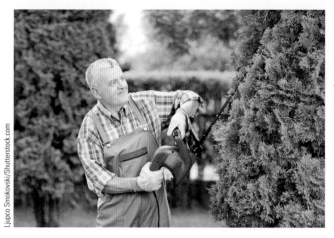

Household chores as pictured can provide physical activity opportunities to expend calories as part of regular (e.g., daily, weekly) leisure time.

Many people probably also participate regularly in physical activities or exercise within their homes, or as part of physically transporting themselves (e.g., walking, jogging, cycling) from their homes to a local park or trail to participate in leisure or recreation (see Chapter 10 for more). Again, however, little is known about how many do so on a regular basis at moderate to vigorous intensities.

Numerous market research groups have reported an emerging trend: Americans are buying home exercise equipment and creating more at-home personal gyms. Home equipment manufacturers have reported that designing home gyms and exercising in the home are becoming more popular for several reasons including:

▶ Baby boomers are aging and health clubs are perceived as places for the young.

▶ Former health club members are familiar with the types of exercise equipment that they like and can afford to buy for use at home.

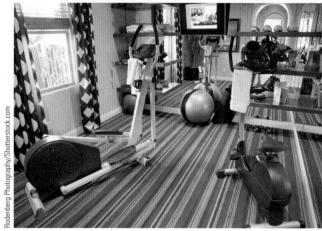

Home gyms have become very popular additions to U.S. households, and market research groups have reported that various equipment items such as treadmills, free weights, exercise balls, machine weights, and floor mats are commonly purchased by consumers.

▶ New equipment includes digital components that complement current home entertainment systems.

▶ Home gyms can be tailored to individual needs economically.

Kinesiology professionals (especially those in personal training; see Chapter 10 for more) can assist individuals and populations in making appropriate home exercise equipment purchases and designing home fitness centers. Several websites found in general Internet searches can help consumers and personal trainers make wise home exercise equipment purchasing decisions (e.g., Harvard Health Publications, tips for choosing the right exercise equipment at www.health.harvard.edu) as well as design home gyms and even learn to exercise at home with minimal equipment.

# EXAMPLES OF APPLYING TRANSPORTATION AND HOME ENVIRONMENT PRINCIPLES OF PHYSICAL ACTIVITY BASICS IN RELATIONSHIP TO THE KINESIOLOGY SUBDISCIPLINES

*In Lesson 1, you learned about the integration of physical activity and the principles of kinesiology in transportation and home environments. You learned about physical activity and active travel to work, school, shopping, and transit. You also learned that there is limited information about the amount of physical activity people perform at home. However, participating in physical activity and exercise in transportation and home settings increases caloric expenditure and both are promoted*

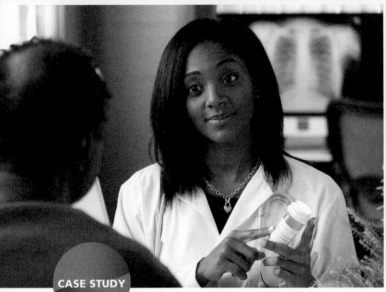

CASE STUDY

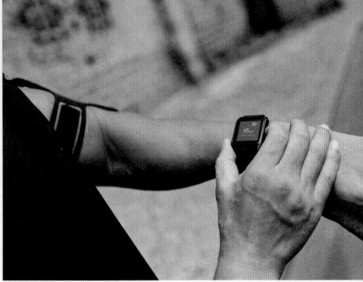

## In the real world . . .

You will recall that William Casey decided to change the way he commuted to work once he received his promotion and had to work in an office much farther from home. He began walking a quarter of a mile each way to and from the bus stop in the morning and afternoon and then a half mile each way to and from his office at the other end of the line. After three months, his routine has been established. He is walking much more each week than when he drove to work and took a walk after dinner in the neighborhood.

What's more, he avoids the stress of sitting in traffic and can relax or work on emails while on the bus each morning and afternoon. He has continued to lose weight and with his physician's approval has been able to discontinue the medicine he was taking for his high blood pressure. Moreover, he has convinced some of his neighbors to do the same thing, at least a few times each week. He also has been working with the human resources department at his job to establish an incentive system (a discounted fare structure) to encourage company employees to take public transportation more frequently.

*as effective ways to achieve the health and fitness goals for individuals and populations. In Lesson 2, you will learn about how physical activity in transportation and home environments is integrated with the subdisciplines of kinesiology.*

- ‣ Exercise Physiology
- ‣ Biomechanics
- ‣ Public Health
- ‣ Sport/Exercise Psychology
- ‣ Motor Learning and Development
- ‣ The Practice of Kinesiology

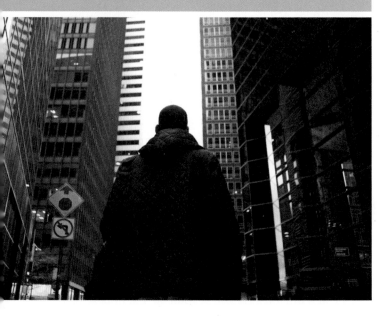

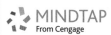
Go to your MindTap course to complete the Case Study activity for this chapter.

## Exercise Physiology

Five days a week, Larry, an attorney, commutes 20 miles from his home to the large city where he works. The commute requires only 30 minutes in light traffic but as much as an hour each way on days when traffic is heavy. Larry is 40 years old, overweight (190 pounds; BMI = 29), and physically inactive and has been diagnosed by his physician as pre-diabetic (blood glucose = 120 mg/dL). Larry has also been feeling increasingly stressed out about commuting in traffic in his car. He has decided to try and make some changes in his commuting lifestyle to improve his physical and mental health. He wants to incorporate as much physical activity as possible into his daily commute.

Larry did some research and found out that he could ride an express city bus for the first 10 miles from his home to a community park walk/cycle trail that connects to his workplace. Additionally, he found out that the express bus has bicycle racks that can accommodate five bicycles, allowing him to bring along his bike and cycle the last 10 miles of his commute. On the days he did not (or could not) use his bus/cycle plan, he could walk two blocks from his office and catch the express bus home to within a block of where he lived. He knew he could always drive to work as a backup plan.

Larry has a quality hybrid mountain bike that he has used only sparingly. Fortunately, he also has a fairly flexible work schedule and a shower facility that he can use for changing as needed.

Once Larry decided to try active travel to work, he figured he should do a trial to determine how long the trip would take him and whether he was fit enough to complete his cycle trip without feeling exhausted for the rest of the day. On his first attempt Larry found that the bus trip took about 20 minutes and his steady, low-level cycle effort took him one hour (about 10 miles per hour). He felt comfortable (not too tired for his low fitness level), and he was happy that his commute only took 1:20, which allowed him 20 minutes to shower and change clothes for work. He decided based on his first effort that he would initially try to actively travel to work two times per week and then add more days as his fitness level improved. Larry wondered whether his active commute would help him lose weight, and he was excited to find out through his Internet search that cycling at 10 miles in one hour expended 340 calories.

If Larry can increase his active commuting to five times per week by adjusting his overload and cycling specificity while adapting to cycling at 12 to 14 miles per hour or 14 to 16 miles per hour, how many calories will he expend through cycling? (Clue: search the Internet to find out how many calories one expends, by weight, for one hour of cycling at various speeds.) Will it be enough to provide significant weight loss?*

---

*The answers are: 12–14 miles/hour = moderate intensity and 518 calories per hour; 14–16 miles/hour = vigorous intensity and 863 calories per hour; and yes, most likely as the cycling portion of his commute increases, it can translate into significant weight loss if he controls his caloric intake, even as he increases his intensity levels and reduces his commute time.

# Biomechanics

Functional movement screening (FMS) is a series of movements designed to assess the quality of fundamental movement patterns and presumably identify an individual's functional limitations or asymmetries.[9] Functional movement screening has been advocated primarily by personal trainers and strength coaches as a tool that integrates biomechanical movements for assessment that can help determine musculoskeletal weaknesses. The weaknesses then can be improved by performing physical activities and exercises (e.g., range of motion stretching, kettle bell movements, and foam rolling), which should theoretically reduce future injury risk.

There is emerging research that supports FMS programming in athletes and military personnel,[10] but it is not clear if FMS programming is effective for children, adolescents, or adults who are not interested or are incapable of performing at peak performance levels. An individual's FMS can be assessed with seven tests that are scored on a scale of 0 to 3. The seven tests are the squat, hurdle step, lunge, shoulder mobility, active straight leg raise, push-up, and rotary stability.[11] A zero score means the person cannot perform a movement free of pain; a 1 indicates the movement cannot be completed as instructed, but there is no pain; a 2 indicates the person can complete the movement pain free, but has some level of compensation (e.g., reaching out an arm for balance); a 3 indicates that the person can complete the movement without compensation. Previous small studies have shown that low FMS scores (<14) are correlated with serious injury in American football players and that FMS scores can be improved following exercise interventions.

As you learned in Chapter 10, personal trainers and strength specialists need a variety of skills to be successful in their careers, and FMS, which is directly related to functional fitness, was listed as number seven on the Worldwide Survey of Fitness Trends for 2016. Although FMS has not been formally studied for home environment physical activity use, a personal training professor at Del Mar College in Corpus Christi, Texas, has recently modified the original seven FMS tests for simple movement evaluations of adults ages 18 to 65 interested in home physical activity, health, and physical fitness. The modified movement screening (MS) tests include shoulder range of motion, toe touch, single leg stance, ankle mobility, squat, leg raise, rotary stability, and a lunge. The new MS programming is currently under study and may provide a new trend for personal trainers and other kinesiology professionals to service their traditional clients, as well as potential new in-home clients seeking improvements in their functional health.

## Movement screen examples

Squat    Lunge    Reach    Push-up

Squatting, lunging, reaching, and push-ups are all part of common movement screen assessments.

# Public Health

One of the most often-cited reasons why people aren't physically active in their neighborhood is a concern for safety. Traffic, crime, lack of sidewalks or cross-walks, stray animals, and other influences can contribute to a perception that walking in your neighborhood is unsafe. Think about where you live. Have you ever felt this way?

Clearly, children's safety is important. How do we encourage active travel to school if safety is not ensured first? One way this concern for safety is being overcome in many communities is with a walking school bus program (see Chapter 11). A walking school bus program removes many of the safety barriers to promoting active travel to school, particularly for younger children. Such programs can take a variety of shapes, but in its simplest form, a walking school bus is a group of children who walk to and from school with guidance and supervision from one or more adults. Walking school buses can include children from only two or three families being walked by one or more of the parents or guardians. They can also be somewhat more elaborate, with time-tables, scheduled "drivers" and conductors, and greater structure on a consistent route to and from school. Some programs have been adapted to include children who ride bicycles to school. In general, the key is to promote active, safe travel to and from school. These programs have flourished recently because they not only provide great opportunities for physical activity but also keep private cars off the street, particularly those that may be idling while the driver waits to pick up a child after school. Naturally, these measures improve ambient air quality as well.

# Sport/Exercise Psychology

You have learned about the physiological benefits of active commuting, but there are obvious psychological benefits as well. However, few studies conducted thus far have evaluated the mental health aspects of active commuting.

Commuting by automobile or public transport alone has been shown to be associated with negative mental health effects such as stress and fatigue, whereas active commuting has been shown to be more relaxing and exciting. The perceived stressors of inactive commuting depend upon the duration of the commute (>60 minutes is worse), lack of predictability, lack of control, and crowding.[12]

Merom and colleagues studied predictors of active commuting in Australia. In their study of 794 workers (ages 18 to 65), they found that individuals who were already physically active were more likely to be active commuters.[13] Subjects responded positively to the prospect of engaging in more active commuting when this allowed them to avoid parking hassles, improve their health, reduce costs, and avoid the stress of driving. The most important finding of the study was that active commuting was much less likely among employees who were sedentary. Have you, or has someone you know, ever commuted regularly by bus or other public transport to school or work? If so, did the experience cause stress that might be avoided by choosing to be make the commute more physically active (by including walking or cycling as part of the commute)? The authors of this text have observed that several of their students have chosen to drive (with their bikes on bike racks) 10 to 15 miles to campus, park in a large parking area on the edge of campus, and then cycle to their classes throughout the day. What kind of active commuting strategies can you think of that would enhance the psychological effects of your (or a fellow student's) daily commute?

## Motor Learning and Development

One form of active transportation is bicycle riding. Most individuals learn to ride a bicycle between the ages of 5 and 8 years old and continue to improve their bike-riding skills until they reach the age of 15 or 16, at which time they may migrate to the passive transportation of the automobile. After the age of 16, many individuals rely so much on the automobile that they rarely if ever ride a bike again. Yet, you have heard of the adage "It is like riding a bike" when describing a skill that, once learned, can be called upon no matter how long the time lapse between situations where you use the skill.

Learning to ride a bicycle is a classic example of motor learning in the development of active transportation. Many individuals started with training wheels, learning to pedal and developing an assemblage of techniques to keep the bike in an upright position while relying heavily on the training wheels. Do you remember the first time you rode a bike without training wheels? At first the bike wobbled from side to side because training wheels were not available to limit the side-to-side motion. You might get a few feet and then crash. An adult may have been behind you, gently pushing, as the increased inertia helped stabilize the bike and your body became more comfortable and at ease in keeping the bike stable during forward motion. And finally, without your realizing it, the adult would let go and you would be bicycling on your own. Remember how proud you felt when you realized that you could ride the bike without help? What you did not realize at the time was that the complexity of the outward performance of bike riding was nothing compared to its complexity within the body. Your brain was detecting and processing hundreds of signals from your eyes,

muscles, joints, and the inner ear each second in an attempt to keep the bike moving forward and upright. All of the signal processing completed by your brain was accomplished without your cognitive awareness that it was taking place. Over time as you continued to ride the bike, you became better because your brain became more efficient at processing these kinesthetic signals, allowing you to gain speed and sometimes do tricks with the bike. The other amazing part of this phenomenon we call motor learning is that the movement data are stored within the brain so that it can be recalled even years after a performance. So, most skill building in kinesiology is like riding a bike: once the brain learns to interpret and process the physical signals, a skill will always be there to use.

## The Practice of Kinesiology

Kinesiology professionals may find future opportunities to work as in-home, mobile personal trainers or functional health specialists setting up physical activity programs or home fitness gyms. As you learned earlier in the chapter, many Americans are buying home exercise equipment and are interested in home personal gyms.[14]

For those thinking about helping others set up their personal home gym, it will be important for them to integrate their own fitness personal training expertise with home design factors and fitness equipment needs based on client budgetary limitations. For example, Jessica Smith, writing for *Shape Magazine*[15] suggests general five steps for your consideration:

1. Find a dedicated space in the house that can be used for working out.

2. Make the home space as attractive as possible; spaces or rooms that are well lighted and not cluttered are more ideal. Based upon the client's budget, you may suggest they add items like Footnote plants, a mirror, music, and video systems to add ambience of the gym.

3. Help the client select physical activity and exercise equipment based on their needs and budget limitations. Adding equipment over time as the client group improves their fitness levels along the exercise continuum is an effective way to save money and meet changing needs and goals.

4. It is important to think about storing fitness equipment when it is not in use, especially if the space/room is used for other functions (e.g., living room or garage). Making sure there are storage bins or a closet can help keep the gym safe and uncluttered.

5. Help the client set up regular times to use the gym and ways to maintain their motivation.

By staying updated through performing regular Internet searches on key words like, "keys to setting up your home gym," and "in home personal fitness training," kinesiology professionals can stay aware of trends in physical activity in the home environment.

## People Matter Tammy Calise, Director of Healthy Communities*

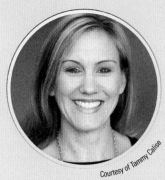

**Q: Why and how did you get into the field of kinesiology?**

**A:** *As a granddaughter and daughter of athletes, I saw the value of fitness, competition, and the positive aspects of team sports. As a mediocre athlete, I also experienced the frustration of wanting to play but not being quite good enough for real competition. While I continued to love sports, and valued fitness, I began to explore group exercise and became very excited about physical activity and chose to major in nutrition and fitness. I went on to get a Master's in health education and obtained my doctorate in public health.*

**Q: What was the major influence on you to work in the field?**

**A:** *At one of my first jobs, I worked with Dr. Robert Pangrazi, a professor at Arizona State University who specialized in youth physical activity. He opened my eyes to a whole new way of thinking about being active and how to engage kids with all athletic abilities, not just the athletes. I learned tips on how to ensure kids stayed active during any given time, were challenged, and most importantly had fun. It became more about the movement and less about the skill. In subsequent work, I also began to see how important the environment was in influencing behaviors. I saw communities, schools, and other places that were not only visually appealing but also provided*

*access to physical activity through well-maintained playground equipment, safe sidewalks and bike lanes, and trails. I also saw places where these things were not available. I began to realize that no matter how much a person was educated and aware of the importance of being physically active, if their environment didn't support these healthy behaviors, it was so difficult for even the most well-intentioned person to be active. This has led me to a career of working across professions (e.g., health and planning) with many diverse stakeholders to make communities and other places where people live, work, go to school, and play more supportive of healthy behaviors.*

**Q: What are your current research interests, and how do you translate your research results to practitioners?**

**A:** *I am the director of Healthy Communities at John Snow Inc., a public health research and consulting firm. In this role, I am responsible for advancing the organization's commitment to place-based efforts where communities flourish and people thrive. My experience includes conducting research and mixed-method evaluations to track the reach, effectiveness, adoption, implementation, and maintenance of complex interventions. I have also used my evaluation experience to enhance implementation, both personally and in providing training and technical assistance to*

---

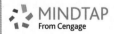
**MINDTAP** From Cengage

Now that you have completed this chapter, go to your MindTap course to complete all assigned activities. Check out the additional resources developed to help you apply the material in this chapter to your course and career goals.

---

## Chapter Summary

▸ Broadly speaking, active travel refers to physical activity undertaken to reach a destination. Active travel is generally taken to mean either walking or biking but can also refer to roller-skating, skateboarding, jogging, or any other form of physical activity involving movement across space.

▸ Virtually all the active travel to school has been replaced by automobile travel, and the steep decrease in active travel has been cited as a possible cause in the rising prevalence of childhood obesity. Efforts are currently under way to promote active travel to school as a form of physical activity in children.

▸ In the United States, fewer than 3% of adults walk to work and less than 1% bike to work. In England and Wales, it has been reported that 10.9% of adults walk and 3.1% bike to work.

▸ Approximately 3% of the U.S. adult population walks to and from some form of transit, though it is not clear whether these were part of trips to school, work, shopping, social, or recreational destinations.

▸ Numerous U.S. agencies and professional organizations advocate the health benefits of participating in physical activities and exercise in home settings. However, little research has been conducted about the number of Americans who are physically active or exercise at home on a regular basis.

*folks at the local and state levels. I have learned firsthand the value and complexity of partnerships in implementing healthy communities efforts and have become increasingly involved in enhancing online knowledge management so partners can share information, document activities, leverage resources, and engage the public and decision-makers in their efforts.*

**Q:** **How do you stay physically active yourself and promote good health to others directly around you?**

**A:** *I try to exercise five to six days a week, but because I have two kids it's hard to get to the gym. I've learned to be flexible with my workouts like going for a run while my 6-year-old bikes next to me or running during nap time so my 3-year-old can nap in the stroller while I get my exercise. I also do a lot of videos at home (e.g., Insanity, T25), and I have done this since my kids were infants. They have seen me work out and think it is what you do. When they were smaller, they would run around me, join me in a "push up," and then go back to playing. I am proud to be a good role model for my girls. If you ask either of them why you need to exercise they will tell you, "to be healthy." I have also recruited a few co-workers to join me in some workouts after work. We usually meet in a large conference room and do some drills using apps on our phone.*

**Q:** **How have you had to integrate the subdisciplines of kinesiology in your professional practice?**

**A:** *Ensuring environments are supportive of health is complex. Healthy community advocates need a network of partners to adopt a shared responsibility to implement policy and environmental changes that support health. Behaviors such as physical activity, and their associated health impacts, need to be viewed as a place-based challenge, not just a personal shortcoming. In this relatively new space, where health is incorporated into all policies, it is not uncommon for there to be a misunderstanding in terms of roles and responsibilities and how entities can work toward a common goal and/or support one another. I integrate the principals of public health, planning, and other disciplines to increase awareness of the value of place-based strategies, the roles of nontraditional organizations in implementing these strategies, and how everyone in a community can benefit.*

*Dr. Calise is the director of JSI Healthy Communities. With almost 20 years of experience at the local, state, and federal government levels, as well as in academia, she is responsible for advancing JSI's commitment to place-based efforts where communities flourish and people thrive. Dr. Calise's interests include the contributions of the physical, social, and cultural environments to health status, particularly in disadvantaged areas. She has a strong background in community-based research, social determinants of health, public policy, and developmental evaluation.

▸ One of the most often-cited reasons why people aren't physically active in their neighborhood is a concern for safety. Traffic, crime, lack of sidewalks or cross-walks, stray animals, and other influences can contribute to a perception that walking in your neighborhood is unsafe.

## Remember This

active travel                    bike share                    walkability

## For More Information

Access these websites for further study of topics covered in the chapter:

▸ To learn more about transportation and home opportunities to increase physical activity related to kinesiology, see the CDC "Take Action for My Community" page at www.cdc.gov/physicalactivity/community -strategies/index.htm.

▸ Search for information and resources about objectives related to physical activity through active transportation and at home at the Healthy People 2020 website: www.healthypeople.gov.

▸ Search for more information about physical activity through active transportation and at home in the "Knowledge Base" of the Global Physical Activity Network at www.globalpanet.com/.

▸ Search for more information about physical activity through active transportation and at home at the U.S. National Physical Activity Plan website at www.physicalactivityplan.org/.

▸ Search for more information about physical activity through active transportation and at home at the President's Council on Fitness, Sports, and Nutrition at www.fitness.gov/.

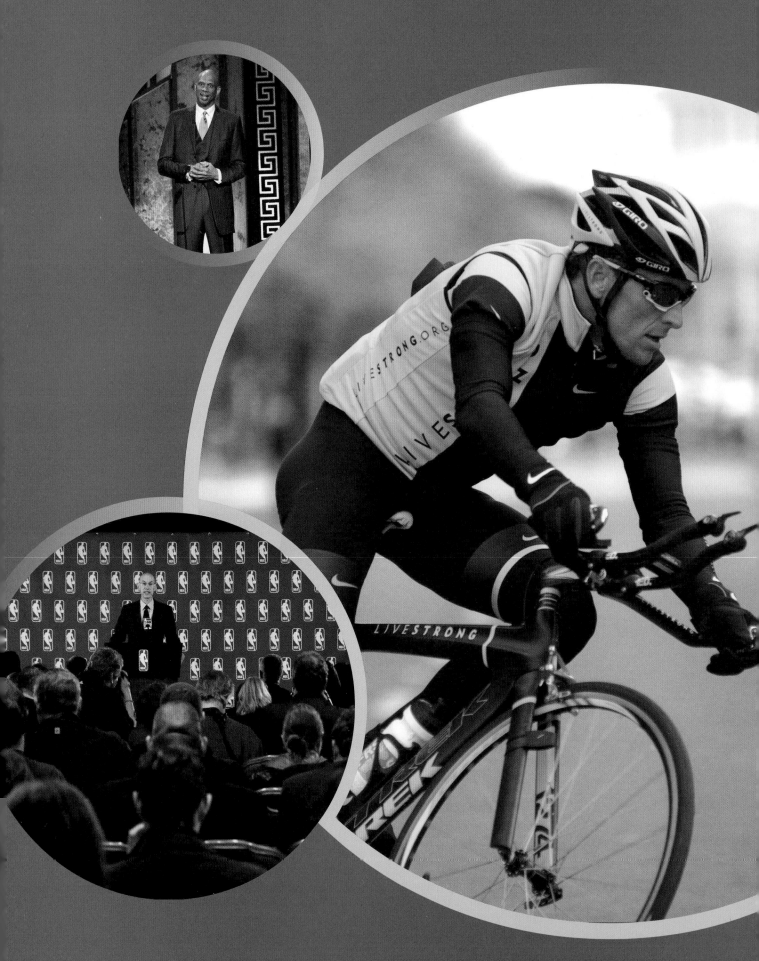

# Ethics and Evidence-Based Decisions: Using Best Practices to Lead the Profession into the Future

*How do ethics impact your ability to be a "good" leader? What are the common ethical principles that drive people to make "good" decisions, and how do you reconcile your ethical principles with evidence-based practice standards when making decisions?*

**LESSON 1** INTEGRATING ETHICS AND KINESIOLOGY

**LESSON 2** EXAMPLES OF APPLYING ETHICS TO THE KINESIOLOGY SUBDISCIPLINES

## Learning Objectives

*After completing this chapter, you will be able to:*

**Explain** the common terms associated with ethics and ethical practices within the field of kinesiology.

**Justify** the importance of ethics and values in kinesiology.

**Explain** how ethics and values are related to participation in physical activity within the various subdisciplines of kinesiology.

**Describe** the historical importance of ethical best practices within the field of kinesiology.

**Integrate** the historical understanding of ethical behavior in terms of physical activity principles across the physical activity continuum and the various subdisciplines of kinesiology.

**Explain** the common ethical practices that encompass all of kinesiology and its subdisciplines.

**Give** examples of situational ethical decisions within the practice of kinesiology.

**Critically** review the positive and negative consequences associated with situational ethical decisions.

**Develop** a personal code of ethics based upon the rules and guidelines of the kinesiology subdiscipline that you wish to practice.

# INTEGRATING ETHICS AND KINESIOLOGY

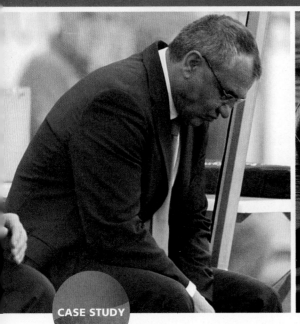

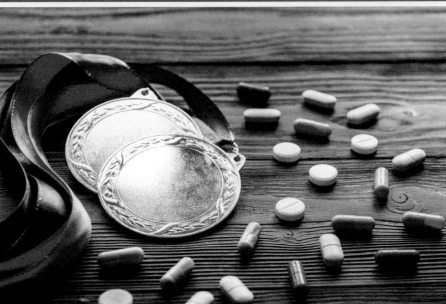

**CASE STUDY**

## In the real world . . .

Coach Glenn, as you might recall from Chapter 8, coaches cross-country at Cara and Amy's high school. You may also remember that prior to coaching at the high school he was an assistant college coach. Recently, a rumor that Coach Glenn was fired from his previous college position due to inappropriate behavior with a student began to circulate among the school board members. To determine if this rumor is true, the school board decides to hold a closed meeting with Coach Glenn so that he can answer some of the lingering questions about his departure from the college. At the meeting, Coach Glenn is asked to explain why he left his college coaching position. Coach Glenn responds, "I was asked to resign my position after making an ethical decision to report what I believed to be unethical behavior of the cross-country program to the NCAA. The behaviors were in direct conflict with my values and interpretation of the rules." The president of the school board asks Coach Glenn to clarify his statement by explaining the circumstances of the ethical decision. Coach Glenn explains that he found out that the strength and conditioning coaches at the college were offering athletes a new ergogenic aid that improved the speed of runners. The ergogenic aid had just become available on the market and had effects similar to those of an amphetamine-based drug, but was not detectable by

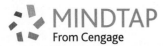
**From Cengage**

Go to your MindTap course now to answer some questions and discover what you already know about ethics and evidence-based decisions in kinesiology.

## INTERACTIVE ACTIVITIES

### Research Focus

Go to your MindTap course to complete an activity researching your school's code of ethics and policies in place for plagiarism and cheating in academics.

### Career Focus

Go to your MindTap course to complete an activity using the ethical decision making model introduced in Table 14.2. You will use this model to determine if your neighborhood is ethically supporting public health.

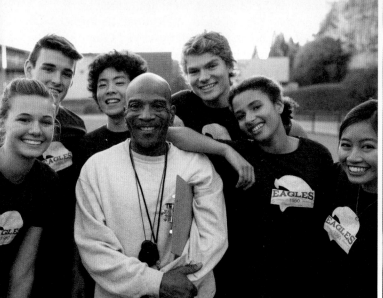

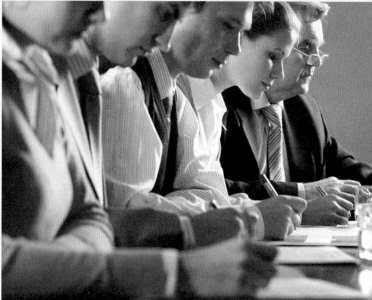

current drug tests and was not yet named specifically on the banned substances list of the NCAA. Upon learning about the program's promotion of this ergogenic aid, Coach Glenn went to the head coach to explain his concerns. The head coach told Coach Glenn that, in his opinion, if an ergogenic aid is not specifically on the banned substance list and is not detectable with current drug tests, then it is all right for the athletes to take it. The head coach also reminded Coach Glenn that their teams were competing for the national title and most of the other schools were most likely using the ergogenic aid. So, what do you think about the decision Coach Glenn made? Do you think it was the correct decision? What values do you think Coach Glenn addressed when he made the decision? Is it unethical to do something

that seems wrong even if no laws or guidelines specific to the situation are in place? Does Coach Glenn's decision make him a better or worse coach for his athletes? We will revisit this later.

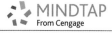

### What Do You Think about Coach Glenn's Decision?

**Go to your MindTap course** and use the "Take Action" folder to record your responses to the questions raised above about Coach Glenn's decision.

# Introduction: Ethics in Kinesiology

This chapter will shift direction from a focus on the integration of the field of kinesiology and its subdisciplines to applying this knowledge to real-world experiences in an effort to improve decision-making skills. Evidence-based decision-making is very important in kinesiology; however, it must be recognized that many decisions are not clear-cut, black-and-white decisions.[1] Furthermore, when making a decision, unintended consequences that may result from the decision should also be considered.

Any decision an individual makes will, to some extent, be subjective, based upon that individual's values and current cultural or societal norms. For example, in professional sports, many athletes use accentuated movements or actions, such as a fake injury, in hopes to slow the game or force the referee to call a foul or penalty on the other team. Many coaches would view these actions as a strategy to improve the chance of winning; conversely, some coaches may view these actions as deceitful and therefore equate them with cheating. Whether faking an injury is defined as a strategy or as cheating is dependent on the **values** to which the coach adheres.[2] Values are defined as the ideals, customs, and institutions that a society or a group uses as guidelines for living. Many times the values of an individual may affect his or her interpretation of evidence and therefore affect the decision-making process. So how are values developed within a group? Values are developed through the acceptance of specific moral principles—in other words, the group defines certain actions as right or wrong. In the United States, as in many other countries, lying, cheating, and stealing are considered wrong; therefore, U.S. citizens' moral principles identify lying, cheating, and stealing as "bad" behaviors whereas truthfulness, fairness, and honesty are accepted as "good" behaviors. The moral principles that a group or society recognizes are adopted as rules of acceptable conduct ("good" behavior).[3,4] These moral principles or rules of acceptable conduct that a group recognizes are called **ethics**.

Ethics guide behavior and the decision-making process by providing a moral framework within which to behave, as well as a means to interpret and use the evidence-based outcomes deemed acceptable within the prevailing societal and cultural norms. Some may equate the laws of a country or state with ethical guidelines; however, this is not always accurate. Most federal and state laws are intended to curb socially defined bad behavior as defined by the majority within a democracy, but some laws may directly violate the ethics of smaller groups within society.

An example of a conflict between a federal law and a group's ethics emerged during the Vietnam War. The federal government invoked the military draft to enlist males over the age of 18 into military service. In 1967, a boxer by the name of Cassius Clay (better known now as Muhammad Ali) refused to be inducted at the Houston, Texas, induction center. He told the induction board that he was a conscientious objector because of his religious faith, Islam. War, he explained, went against the teachings of its primary religious text, the Qur'an. He further stated, "I ain't got no quarrel with those Viet Cong." He was arrested, tried, and found guilty of draft dodging. Because he was now a felon, Clay's boxing license was suspended and he lost his heavyweight title. It wasn't until the Supreme Court overturned the conviction in 1971 (*Clay* v. *United States*) that he was able to continue his boxing career. In this example, you see that a federal law that was accepted by many came into direct conflict with the values or ethics guiding a few.

Your professional and personal ethics will help determine your own integrity. **Integrity** is the quality of being honest and standing up for truthfulness. Integrity is based on value systems and on consistency and accuracy. Your professional integrity in kinesiology should be primarily based on evidence-based decision making and ethics.

Because ethics are rules of acceptable behavior, many professional organizations have published ethical standards that guide individuals on how they should behave when practicing their profession. Also, many groups that offer specific certifications and licensures have published ethical standards and require that these be followed to maintain the certification or license. In the field of kinesiology, the American Kinesiology Association (AKA) has yet to adopt an inclusive set of ethical standards; however, many of the subdisciplines in the field have their own ethical standards of practice.

## Groups with Ethical Standards That Affect the Kinesiology Profession

The following groups have published ethical standards that impact the subdisciplines within kinesiology:

> • American Medical Association
> • American Psychological Association
> • National Association of Sport and Physical Education
> • American College of Sports Medicine (Certification Standards)
> • National Strength and Conditioning Association
> • Association for Applied Sport Psychology
> • North American Society for the Psychology of Sport and Physical Activity
> • American Council on Exercise

Table 14.1 provides you with one example of a code of ethics for kinesiology professionals.

**Table 14.1** | Code of Ethics for ACSM Certified and Registered Professionals

### F.1 PURPOSE

This Code of Ethics is intended to aid all certified and registered American College of Sports Medicine Credentialed Professionals (ACSMCP) to establish and maintain a high level of ethical conduct, as defined by standards by which an ACSMCP may determine the appropriateness of his or her conduct. Any existing professional, licensure, or certification affiliations that ACSMCPs have with governmental, local, state, or national agencies or organizations will take precedence relative to any disciplinary matters that pertain to practice or professional conduct.

This Code applies to all ACSMCPs, regardless of ACSM membership status (to include members and non-members). Any cases in violation of this Code will be referred to the ACSM CCRB Executive Council and the CCRB Ethics subcommittee, and if appropriate the ACSM Committee on Ethics and Professional Conduct as well.

### F.2 PRINCIPLES AND STANDARDS

**Responsibility to the Public**

ACSMCPs shall be dedicated to providing competent and legally permissible services within the scope of the Knowledge and Skills (KSs) of their respective credential. These services shall be provided with integrity, competence, diligence, and compassion.

ACSMCPs provide exercise information in a manner that is consistent with evidence-based science and medicine.

ACSMCPs respect the rights of clients, colleagues, and health professionals, and shall safeguard client confidences within the boundaries of the law.

Information relating to the ACSMCP/client relationship is confidential and may not be communicated to a third party not involved in that client's care without the prior written consent of the client or as required by law.

ACSMCPs are truthful about their qualifications and the limitations of their expertise and provide services consistent with their competencies.

**Responsibility to the Profession**

ACSMCPs maintain high professional standards. As such, an ACSMCP should never represent him/herself, either directly or indirectly, as anything other than an ACSMCP unless he/she holds other license/certification that allows him/her to do so.

ACSMCPs practice within the scope of their knowledge, skills, and abilities. ACSMCPs will not provide services that are limited by state law to provision by another health care professional only.

An ACSMCP must remain in good standing relative to governmental requirements as a condition of continued Credentialing.

ACSMCPs take credit, including authorship, only for work they have actually performed and give credit to the contributions of others as warranted.

Consistent with the requirements of their certification or registration, ACSMCPs must complete approved, additional educational course work aimed at maintaining and advancing their knowledge and skills.

### F.3 PRINCIPLES AND STANDARDS FOR CANDIDATES OF THE CERTIFICATION EXAM

Candidates applying for a credentialing examination must comply with all eligibility requirements and to the best of their abilities, accurately complete the application process. In addition, the candidate must refrain from any and all behavior that could be interpreted as "irregular" (please refer to the policy on irregular behavior).

### F.4 DISCIPLINE

Any ACSMCP may be disciplined or lose their certification or registry status for conduct which, in the opinion of the Executive Committee of the ACSM Committee on Certification and Registry Boards, goes against the principles set forth in this Code. Such cases will be reviewed by the ACSM CCRB Ethics subcommittee, which may include a liaison from the ACSM Committee on Ethics and Professional Conduct, as needed, based on the ACSM membership status of the ACSMCP. The ACSM Ethics subcommittee will make an action recommendation to the ACSM Committee on Certification and Registry Boards Executive Council for final review and approval.

*Note:* Code of Ethics approved by the CCRB Executive Council, May 2005 and approved by the ACSM Board of Trustees, June, 2005.

*Source:* American College of Sports Medicine, available at certification.acsm.org/faq-new/faq28-codeofethics

Ethics and evidence-based decisions also need to be made with considerations related to the concepts associated with the physical activity continuum. As you recall, the physical activity continuum is based on the principles of overload, specificity, and adaptation along with many other training principles that can impact successful and on-going positive outcomes along the continuum. 🏃

## Understanding Ethics: Development, Practice, and Use

The practice of and adherence to professional ethics in kinesiology is paramount to maintaining integrity and the reliability of practice within the profession. The development and practice of ethical guidelines, however, are not as simplistic as it at first may seem. Ethical guidelines development and compliance can in fact be very complicated. The cause for this complexity lies in the nature of the many different value systems that may exist within a society.

Furthermore, ethical guidelines can be interpreted through either of two differing theories: deontological theory and teleological theory.[5] The deontological theory of ethics and subscribers to **deontological ethics** believe that the moral principles expressed by the group are universally accepted, concrete guidelines that prescribe acceptable behavior and elicit fair decisions and practice for the whole of the society. Universities, for example, rely on the practice of deontological ethics when enforcing their honor codes. Most university ethics or honor codes define cheating as a punishable infraction and require students to report any known cheating incidences immediately. Furthermore, knowingly allowing cheating and not reporting it is also deemed as an infraction of the code. Notice that both cheating and not reporting cheating incidences are considered bad behavior regardless of any extraneous circumstances, and therefore are ethical violations. Another example may be lying or being deceitful. In the United States, being deceitful is considered bad behavior. Specific ethical guidelines prevent physicians from deceiving their patients, or lawyers from deceiving the court system. In kinesiology, however, specifically in sports, deceit is part of the strategy to win. What would football be like if players were unable to misdirect the other team by using fake passes or fake punts? Notice that although deceit is unacceptable behavior in daily life among the general population, in sports like football it is acceptable behavior within the context of the game.

This conundrum brings us to the second theory in the study of ethics. **Teleological ethics** suggests that moral ambiguity exists within society and no behavior is inherently wrong but rather the amount of good the behavior produces determines whether it is morally right; in other words, the ends justify the means. An example of a teleological ethical decision is the one Harry S. Truman made near the end of World War II when he decided to use the atomic bomb on Japan. President Truman had to weigh the great loss of life among the Japanese people that would result from dropping such a devastating weapon against the deaths of hundreds of thousands of Americans that would result from trying to invade Japan. As history tells us, Truman decided it was morally right to save American lives and therefore would be ethical to sacrifice Japanese lives to accomplish those ends.

Now, you might at this point suppose that most rules and decisions made in kinesiology are teleologically derived. For the most part, the field of kinesiology subscribes to the deontological theory of ethics, but most kinesiology professionals would agree that the interpretation of the rules and guidelines may be structured based on the situation.[6,7] **Situational ethics** recognizes the deontological ethics of the group but accepts that certain situations might require interpretation based upon the virtue of the consequences specific to the situation. As described before, although being deceitful is deemed bad behavior and interpreted as unethical within society as a whole, within the rules of football, some deceit, such as play misdirection, is acceptable as a strategy and therefore is considered ethical behavior. Getting a competitive advantage by "bending" rules in a sport is common practice. For example, players do not always incur a penalty for tripping an opponent in hockey, but is this behavior ethical?

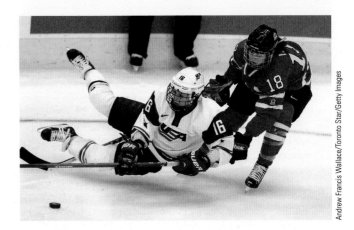

## Historical Context of Modern Ethics in Kinesiology

Many of the modern ethical guidelines developed for the profession of kinesiology research and practice can trace their roots back to the 1947 Nuremberg Code.[8] The Nuremberg Code was developed in the aftermath of the court decisions from the post–World War II Nuremberg Trials, where Nazi scientists were convicted of crimes against humanity for their infamous research with human subjects. Based upon the court decision, 10 moral, ethical, and legal concepts were codified to give future researchers a framework within which to develop their human research. Although the code was meant for the protection of human research subjects, the tenets of the code have been adopted by most groups that work and interact with humans. The 10 tenets of the Nuremberg Code are:

1. Consent of the human subject is absolutely essential and all participation is voluntary.

2. The outcomes of the experiment should benefit society, and human subjects should only be used when other methods or means of study are impossible, and not at random or when unnecessary.

3. The experiment should be designed based on the results of animal experimentation and knowledge of natural history of the disease or other problems under study so that the anticipated results will justify the performance of the experiment.

4. All unnecessary physical and mental suffering and injury should be avoided.

5. Human subjects should not be used when it is previously known or believed that death or disabling injury will occur.

6. The amount of risk taken should never exceed that determined to be justified by the humanitarian importance of the problem to be solved.

7. Proper preparations should be made and adequate facilities provided to protect the subjects against even remote possibilities of injury, disabilities, or death.

8. Studies should be conducted only by qualified persons. The highest degree of skill and care should be required through all stages of the study for those who conduct or engage in the study.

9. During the course of the study, human subjects should be able to quit the study at any time.

10. The person in charge of the study must be prepared to terminate the study at any stage if he/she has probable cause to believe that a continuation of the study may result in injury, disability, or death to the subject.

In reviewing these tenets, which represent an ethical foundation for interacting with humans, notice how they may apply to the profession of kinesiology. The first tenet indicates that individuals must give consent to participate in a physical activity and have the autonomy to determine whether or not to participate. **Autonomy** refers to the freedom and independence an individual has to make her or his own decisions; therefore, when interacting with another person, the kinesiology professional must recognize that it is unethical to coerce the individual into participating.[9] The role of an exercise psychologist is to use the evidence from behavior modeling research to determine the best way to entice individuals to voluntarily participate in physical activity. Notice, also, that based on the tenth tenet of the Nuremberg Code, the kinesiology professional, who is a leader, has the duty and authority to stop any participation in physical activity that may pose a risk of severe injury or death. **Authority**, in the case of the kinesiology professional, refers to the ability to control, determine, and settle issues. Kinesiology professionals need to recognize that they not only have the authority to allow individuals to participate in physical activity but also have the duty to protect these individuals from severe injury or bodily harm. Coaches, for example, must remember that their ethical obligation to protect their players from injury should supersede their desire to win.

Following World War II and the implementation of the 1947 Nuremberg Code, the United States, along with most of Europe, saw unprecedented economic expansion. The economic expansion in the United States was accompanied by numerous medical and technological advances. The advances in medicine included mass production of antibiotics, improved diagnosis and treatment of heart disease, and a better understanding of and newer treatments for mental disorders. Many of the post–World War II advances[10] were a direct result of a boom in research that included the use of human subjects. Some of these human research trials, such as the Tuskegee syphilis study—in which researchers intentionally withheld the positive diagnosis and treatment of syphilis from some African-American people with syphilis—and the thalidomide drug trials—in which researchers found that pregnant women who were given thalidomide to treat nausea would give birth to children with birth defects but did not inform them of this risk—brought about a new discussion of medical ethics around the globe. As a direct result of these studies and several others, a new document known as the **Helsinki Declaration** was developed in 1964 by the World Medical Association (link to WMA: www.wma.net/policies-post/wma-declaration-of-helsinki-ethical-principles-for-medical-research-involving-human-subjects/). The Helsinki Declaration further explained and expanded upon the tenets of the 1947 Nuremberg Code. The Helsinki declaration also emphasized the need and duty of researchers to receive informed consent from research subjects, including consent from proxies or guardians of individuals who lack the cognitive ability to understand the potential risks of the experimentation.

In 1974, the National Research Act (Public Law 93–348) was enacted in the United States and codified in the regulations of the Department of Health and Human Services as the Protection of Human Subjects of Biomedical Research (Title 45 Code of Federal Regulations [CFR] 46, Subpart A). Title 45 CFR 46 established the guidelines for **Institutional Review Boards (IRBs)**, which require independent peer review of research proposals as a means for the ethical protection of human subjects. IRBs are panels of professionals that review research protocols prior to allowing the researcher to collect data. These boards verify that all necessary steps have been taken by the researcher to prevent any unnecessary harm and discomfort to the subjects and that the researcher will receive **informed consent** from the participants. Informed consent is the permission granted by the subject for the researcher to conduct the research only after a full description of the research; possible consequences associated with the research including but not limited to dangers to the subject, side effects, and/or issues of discomfort and stress must be explained in detail to the subject.

The previously described codes, declarations, and acts are an important part of the rules that guide research in kinesiology. These rules provide a framework for some of the most important ethical standards in the kinesiology profession: those that ensure the protection of the human subjects who participate in physical activity research.

## Academic/Professional Honesty and Integrity

**Academic/professional honesty and integrity** refers to ethical standards that support truth and the accurate dissemination of one's acquired professional knowledge, skills, and abilities. For example, you have probably already heard that as a student at your college or university you are supposed to follow an honor code of ethics regarding your own academic work. Penalties are common and often harsh for those who plagiarize (take the work of others and pass on as their own) individual and group works or for those who cheat (e.g., exams, assignments). **Plagiarism** and cheating are highly unethical and are unacceptable behaviors and practices for kinesiology professionals in their academic training or career fields. Obviously, we have all seen or heard of individuals or groups who have plagiarized or cheated and they have not been caught in the act. However, when cases are exposed, the individuals or groups involved can face career ending or limiting effects (e.g., expelled from school, fired at work, public scorn and scrutiny). The International Center for Academic Integrity reports that 39% of undergraduate and 17% of graduate students have reported cheating on at least one exam. The number of students who reported cheating on at least one assignment increased to 62% of undergraduate and 40% of graduate students. The total percentages of cheating incidences reported were 68% of undergraduate and 43% graduate students cheated either on a written assignment and/or an exam.[11] In fact, academic dishonesty and lack of proper disclosures (see the next paragraph) can potentially create legal problems for those who ignore ethical professional standards (see Chapter 16 for more about legal issues).

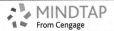

**Plagiarism and Cheating in Academics**

**Go to your MindTap course** to complete an activity researching your school's code of ethics and policies in place for plagiarism and cheating in academics.

Other ethical considerations that apply to kinesiology professionals and that you should become aware of include disclosure, disclaimers, and conflicts of interest. **Disclosure** generally refers to admitting or revealing, for example, that if you are providing professional advice, promoting a technique, or endorsing a product you may or may not have personal interests that benefit yourself monetarily or professionally. A specific example of disclosure might be a situation where you have a full-time job with a governmental or corporate organization and want to make additional money part time (e.g., consulting) pursing other interests. It is very common for governmental or corporate organizations to require you to disclose, as part of company policy, your time and work efforts involving the part-time work so as to limit any negative effects on your full-time job performance.

**Disclaimers** are oral and/or written statements that provide disclosures about your (or an associated group's) legal links to things like providing professional advice, specific technique promotion, or product endorsement. Another example of providing a disclaimer might be where you as personal trainer or a group you work for inform individuals who use your fitness facility that they do so at their own risk and assume their own liability for injury. We often see such statements of disclosure, but it is important for you to realize that just providing a disclaimer may not release you or others from legal liability (see Chapter 16 for more on legal issues).

**Conflict of interest** refers to situations where kinesiology professionals provide no disclosure or hide personal interests that potentially benefit them monetarily and/or professionally. For example, we have all seen media testimonials in which fitness experts promote fitness techniques or products that they make money from and use to expand their professional reputations. Ethically, such conflicts of interest should all be disclosed and disclaimers provided ahead of any promotion regarding professional kinesiology advice and technique using product endorsements.

## The Ethical Decision-Making Process

As previously discussed in this chapter, the kinesiology professional generally subscribes to the deontological theory of ethical decision making while understanding that in certain situations, a decision may need to be made without a rule for guidance, or by interpreting rules for the situation that are ambiguous or unclear. In these cases, the kinesiology professional needs to base his or her decision on a logical construct that will best improve the situation while minimizing the harm the decision will have on the profession.[12] To arrive at a sound, defensible, and ethical decision, the individual must develop and weigh four possible alternatives based upon the accepted rules that best fit the situation, the situation itself, the means by which the decision will be morally judged, and the ends or benefits to all of those affected by the decision. One way of making a sound ethical decision is to weigh the best four possible outcomes as demonstrated in Table 14.2.

Table 14.2 outlines four possible arguments to use when considering an ethical decision.[13,14] When interpreting this decision rubric, rules describe specific, written guidelines that regulate the actions to take in a given situation, while situation expressly recognizes that the situation is beyond the scope of the current rules, or unique and current rules do not apply to the situation. Means and ends in the rubric describe the group that the decision will impact. Means refers to the community at large, while ends refer specifically to those individuals who are directly affected by the situation or are involved in the specific situation. When developing an argument for a **rules-means decision**, one must weigh the rules

**Table 14.2 | Ethical Decision Making Scenarios**

|  | RULES | SITUATION |
|---|---|---|
| **MEANS** | Rules-means argument | Means-situation argument |
| **ENDS** | Rules-end argument | Ends-situation argument |

that apply to the decision against what is morally acceptable to the community (means). When developing a **rules-end argument**, one must weigh the rules that apply to the decision against how the decision will affect the majority of the people in the situation (ends). When developing a **means-situation argument**, one must take the perspective that the situation is unique, so that no accepted rule applies, and therefore the facts of the situation (situation) must be weighed against what is morally acceptable (means) to the community. Finally, when developing an **ends-situation argument**, one must take the perspective that the situation is unique, so that no accepted rule applies, and that therefore the facts of the situation (situation) must be weighed against what is best for the majority of those impacted by the decision (end). Once all four arguments have been developed, they must be carefully considered to determine which argument will lead to the best decision based upon its impact to the individual, the majority, the profession, the community, and society.

An example that can be used to better explain this process is the NBA's decision to force LA Clippers owner Donald Sterling to sell the team in 2014. Mr. Sterling made racially charged statements in a private setting that were recorded and later released to the public by his significant other. When the recordings made national news, the NBA had to decide how to sanction Mr. Sterling. The final decision by the NBA was to force Mr. Sterling to sell the Clippers franchise. How might they have come to that decision based upon the four arguments previously discussed?

## Rules-Means Argument

NBA owners sign agreements that include clauses protecting the NBA brand from undue harm (rule). Since Mr. Sterling brought negative publicity on the franchise as well as the NBA by making racist comments unacceptable to the community (means) he violated the ownership rule and therefore negated his contract with the NBA. Since the owner's contract was negated by his actions, he could no longer own the team and therefore he had to sell it.

An alternative decision in this example might have been that the NBA determined the comments did not bring undue harm to the NBA brand (rule) but rather Mr. Sterling violated the morality clause (rule) in the contract, which is adjudicated by fines. Although Mr. Sterling's racist comments were unacceptable to the community (means), the rule that fits the situation is adjudicated by a fine and therefore Mr. Sterling could retain ownership of the team.

## Rules-Ends Argument

As already stated in the rules-means argument, Mr. Sterling brought negative publicity on the franchise by

making racist comments that might have harmed the reputation of the African-American athletes on his team as well as those playing for other teams. The NBA ownership is a business, and the selling of the team would have minimal impact on Mr. Sterling's income since the team could be sold for more than he paid to purchase it (ends). Moreover, the impact on the players would be positive because they would gain a new franchise owner who was not labeled as a bigot (ends). Thus, Mr. Sterling should sell the team.

Alternatively, the NBA could have determined that the impact of selling the team might be far more detrimental to Mr. Sterling's financial well-being (end) than to the impact on the players (end) and therefore Mr. Sterling should be fined rather than forced to sell.

## Means-Situation

Using this argument, Mr. Sterling used speech that was unacceptable to the community (means). Although his remarks are constitutionally protected, they were deemed morally unacceptable within the community of players, coaches, fans, and other owners. The remarks were made in private, but once they were released into the public venue they negatively impacted Mr. Sterling's integrity as an owner of an NBA team. Furthermore, the comments would have a negative impact on the players' trust in him and would possibly create a hostile work environment for the players and coaches (situation). Since the sanction with least impact on the players and coaches would be a change in ownership, Mr. Sterling should sell the team.

Alternative to this decision, the NBA could have determined that although the remarks were unacceptable to the community (means), there were no previous reports from players or coaches of his bigotry, therefore the work environment (situation) would not change and was separate from Mr. Sterling's private activities. In this argument, the NBA could dismiss the accusations with a warning or fine and Mr. Sterling could have maintained ownership of the team.

## Ends-Situation

Using this argument, current and future players would be negatively impacted by continued ownership of the team by a person who has been publicly labeled a bigot (ends), and the team could be sold for more than its purchase price (ends). Since it will permit the NBA to maintain a high moral code that supports diversity and deplores racism (situation), then Mr. Sterling should sell the team.

Alternatively, Mr. Sterling had owned the Clippers for 33 years without negatively impacting the players (ends), and the sale of the team might cause a financial hardship for Mr. Sterling (ends). Also, Mr. Sterling had an ethnically diverse team that included African-American head coaches such as Alvin Gentry, Dennis Johnson, and Doc

Rivers during the 33 years of ownership. Furthermore, the racially charged comments were made in a private setting while he was going through a contentious divorce (situation) and therefore his actions might be attributed to extreme stress and a lapse in judgement (situation). With these extenuating factors, the NBA could have decided to fine Mr. Sterling and require him to go to cultural sensitivity training rather than ban him from professional basketball and force the sale of the team.

Upon reviewing the four ethical arguments, the best supportable ethical arguments for the decision were (1) Mr. Sterling violated the NBA contract by bringing undue harm to the brand (rule), (2) the speech was unacceptable to the community (means), (3) the comments had a negative impact on the players' trust in him and would create a hostile work environment for the players and coaches (situation), (4) the NBA needs to maintain a high moral code that supports diversity and deplores racism (situation), and (5) the sale of the team would not have a negative impact on Mr. Sterling's financial well-being since the team could be sold for more than he paid to purchase it (ends). Using these arguments, the NBA decided that Mr. Sterling would sell the team and be banned from investing in any future NBA teams. By forcing the sale of the team, the NBA was able to ethically sanction Mr. Sterling for his actions without causing a loss of revenue and helped maintain a work environment for the players and coaches that is supportive of diversity and fairness. NBA Commissioner Adam Silver is shown in the picture on page 306, explaining the NBA's decision to the national media. What type of decision do you think you would have made?

## Summary

Ethical decision making is steeped in history, philosophy, and societal acceptance. Ethical decision making will help the kinesiology professional maintain her or his integrity while achieving an outcome that is fair. For the most part, kinesiology professionals use the deontological theory of ethical decision making while understanding that sometimes the rules may not apply directly to the situation. In these cases, decision making must be accomplished by comparing arguments based upon the rules, situation, means, and end. The final decision must meet societal norms as well as professional expectations to maintain a high level of integrity.

# EXAMPLES OF APPLYING ETHICS TO THE KINESIOLOGY SUBDISCIPLINES

*Requiring high ethical standards in kinesiology is paramount in order to maintain the integrity of the profession. Most subdisciplines in kinesiology have some uniform code of standards to which the kinesiology professional must adhere. In those situations without clear standards, the ethical decision-making task can be performed by developing four arguments based upon the rules, situation, means, and ends. This lesson will help the student understand how to* *use ethical decision making in the context of several of the subdisciplines within the kinesiology profession.*

- Exercise Physiology
- Biomechanics
- Public Health
- Sport/Exercise Psychology
- The Practice of Kinesiology

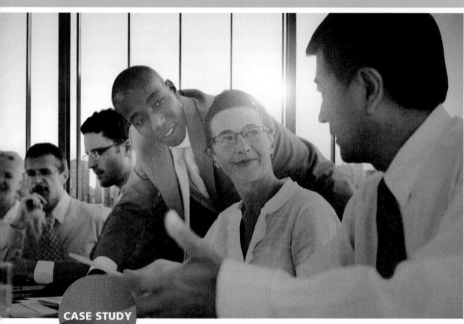

**CASE STUDY**

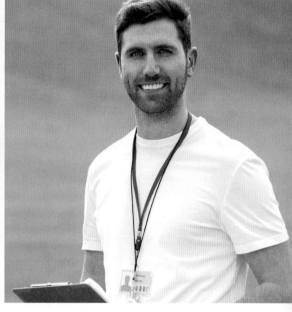

## In the real world . . .

As stated previously, Coach Glenn told the school board that he resigned his college coaching position because of an ethical decision he made when his values came in direct conflict with the head coach's beliefs. Coach Glenn had found out that the strength and conditioning coach at the college was offering the athletes a new ergogenic aid that improved the runners' speed—a product that had just become available on the market and had effects similar to an amphetamine-based drug but was not detectable by current drug tests and was not yet specifically named on the NCAA's banned substances list. Develop four arguments

using the rules, situation, means, and end process to determine whether or not Coach Glenn made a proper ethical decision to report the use of the ergogenic aid to the NCAA review board. Remember when assessing the means and ends of this portion of the assignment that the community associated with the means portion of the rubric of argument does not just encompass the sports program, but also the university and its students

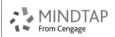
**MINDTAP**
From Cengage

Go to your MindTap course to complete the Case Study activity for this chapter.

# Exercise Physiology

Obtaining informed consent is part of the process of standardized clinical graded exercise testing (GXT) as recommended by the American College of Sports Medicine.[15] Informed consent, as you have learned, is an ethical process in which kinesiology professionals disclose appropriate information to individuals or groups who then can make a voluntary choice to undergo treatment or participate in a procedure or a project (like a research study). A typical informed consent for GXT (which takes the form of a document) includes the following sections: purpose of and explanation for the test; attendant risks and discomforts; responsibilities; benefits to be expected; inquiries; freedom of consent; and signatures of the individual, a witness, and sometimes a parent (if required for testing minors).

Often, as part of the attendant risks and discomforts section of the informed consent, individuals or groups are informed that during maximal GXTs there is some risk for atypical physiological responses such as abnormal blood pressure, fainting, irregular heart rhythms, and, in rare circumstances, heart attack, stroke, or death. Of course, when most people read that there is a chance of dying during the test they become very concerned, as anyone should. While the risk of dying during GXTs varies largely based on an individual's health risks and clinical status, it is estimated that there are 0 to 5 deaths per 10,000 tests.[16] Because the risk of death is very low during GXTs, do you think it would be ethical to not tell individuals about the risk so as to prevent them from worrying about the testing procedures? If you answered "yes," you would be violating the Code of Ethics for ACSM Certified and Registered Professionals, which requires certified professionals to disclose complete and reasonable information that would maximize the odds that the GXT provides far more benefits to the individual or group than discomforts. A signed standardized informed consent provides kinesiology professionals with legal documentation that they have followed ethical procedures as part of their standards of care and can be most valuable in cases of litigation due to implied negligence (see Chapter 16 for more).

# Biomechanics

Technological advancements in biomechanical devices in the past 20 years have improved the quality of life for many disabled athletes. Current trends in biomechanics include the introduction of new nanomaterials in clothing that reduce friction and improve muscular contractile velocity, "blade" prosthetics for individuals who have lower limb amputations, and exoskeletons that can help the paraplegic walk through human-computer interfaces. Although each of these new inventions has improved the quality of life for many of the disabled, they have also sparked a new debate regarding their ethical use in competitive sports. Several ethical questions arise as technological advances improve the capabilities of the disabled who participate in competitive physical activities.

One of the major ethical questions that has arisen recently in competitive running is whether lower limb amputees should be allowed to compete against non-amputees in competitive running events. The argument for allowing the use of blade prosthetics in competitive events is that it gives the lower limb amputee acceptance into "normal" societal activities that they were barred from only a few years earlier. At the same time, as materials and biomechanical devices are continually improved through research, at what point does the blade prosthetic give an undue advantage to the lower limb amputee as compared with a non-amputee? Furthermore, at what point do scientific advancements

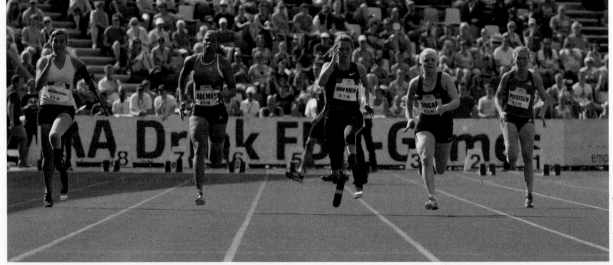

Helene Wiesenhaan/Getty Images

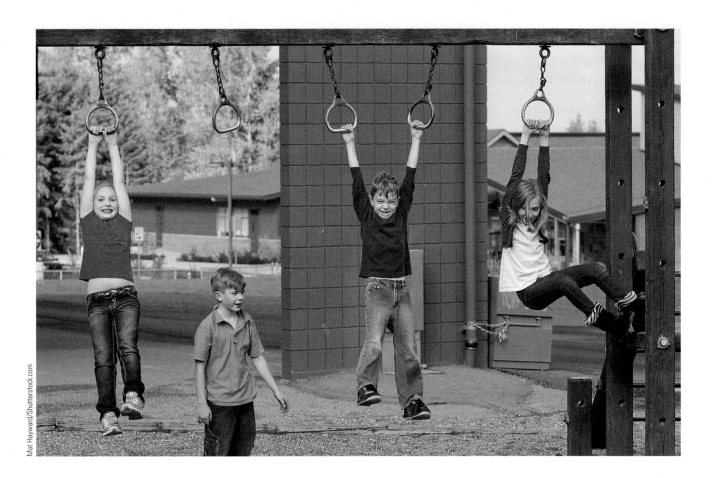

Mat Hayward/Shutterstock.com

remove the "human" from human performance? Develop four arguments based upon the rules, situation, means, and ends that will support and refute the use of blade prosthetics in competitive running events. Which is the best ethical decision?

## Public Health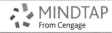

Public health practice, like medicine, is guided by a series of ethical principles. One of these key principles is that public health programs and policies should be implemented in a manner that most likely will benefit the physical and social environment. How does this relate to physical activity and kinesiology? In Chapter 13, we learned about the profound role that the built environment can have on physical activity, particularly transport-related physical activity. Neighborhoods that are connected with sidewalks and bicycle paths, that provide destinations such as shops and cafes to which people can actively travel, and that have easy access to places where people can be active such as parks and green spaces promote health more than neighborhoods without such characteristics. Where we live affects our health, and physical inactivity is no different than other health concerns in this regard.

A fundamental ethical principle in public health is to focus on the physical and social environment: the situation.

We know that the physical environment is strongly associated with physical activity participation (rules), and because physical activity participation is needed for optimal health, development, and maturation (ends), it follows that all neighborhoods should be designed to support healthy physical activity. Do you agree? Look around the neighborhood where you live now, the route you travel to school, or the neighborhoods where you grew up. Are they supportive of physical activity? Are you concerned about speeding or out-of-control traffic if you ride your bicycle? Are these neighborhoods safe, clean, and free of crime? Are sidewalks well lit and continuous? Are there cut-away curbs?

---

### ⁎ MINDTAP
From Cengage

**Ethical Decision Making Scenarios**

Go to your MindTap course to complete an activity using the ethical decision making scenarios model introduced in Table 14.2. You will use this model to help determine if your neighborhood is ethically supporting public health.

---

## Sport/Exercise Psychology

Interest in the fields of sport and exercise psychology has grown significantly in the last 20 years. Sport and exercise psychologists are concerned about behaviors, mental health strategies, and the health and well-being of individuals, teams, and organizations involved in pursuing high levels of physical activity performance. Sport and exercise psychologists often work with star athletes and championship teams, which is exciting and glamorous, but can create ethical challenges such as the maintenance of confidentiality.

For sport and exercise psychologists, **confidentiality** refers to duties (moral and legal obligations or responsibilities) they must perform when working with individuals or groups to maintain privacy and secrecy. The need for confidentiality can influence many areas of communication such as disclosing individual injuries, reporting on team mood or confidence issues, or discussing individual or team health test results. Confidentiality of individuals and groups is protected by several forms of national and state legislation and regulations in the United States, including the Health Information Portability and Accountability Act of 1997 (HIPAA), which requires professionals such as sport and exercise psychologists to protect the privacy of individual health-related information including electronic data.

What ethical concerns would you have to consider if you were the sport/exercise psychologist for the next Super Bowl championship team? Or for the next Master's professional golf champion? What level of education and certifications prepares and improves your likelihood in being a successful sport psychologist in these situations? What strategies would you need to acquire to develop and maintain ethical standards during your personal and professional relationships? Is it ethical to consider yourself a sport psychology professional with a bachelor's degree in kinesiology?

## The Practice of Kinesiology 🧍

Have you had to make professional ethical decisions yourself yet? If so, did you find that your decisions were difficult? Did you learn anything about your own integrity when trying to make your choices? Were you disappointed in yourself or others based on your decisions? What skills do you think might help you in the future to make ethical and informed decisions?

Let's imagine that you are the head men's basketball coach at a university that is eligible to advance to post-season NCAA-Division I play if you qualify. You have one excellent player who most likely will be an NBA top five draft pick and sign a large professional contract. During his annual team physical exam in October of his senior year, he is diagnosed with hypertrophic cardiomyopathy (HCM), which is an abnormally enlarged heart that can cause sudden death, particularly during exercise. He is given a high-dose beta blocker, a medication that lowers heart rate and blood pressure at rest and during exercise and helps control abnormal heart rhythms.

What ethical challenges would you face as his coach once you are informed that he has HCM? What concerns do you think the team physician might have? What about the player? Will he take his medicine regularly since the side effects may cause him to feel tired and listless? Will the team doctor let him play? Will you play him if the doctor doesn't want him to play? Why or why not? What ethical obligations do you have to the player? To the team? To the player's family? To the university? To the community? What ethical obligations does the player have to the team? To his family? To the university? To the community? To himself?

The answers to all of these questions and the many more that will arise later are complex and are not easy to determine without considering your own integrity and the ethical standards that involve medical, university, and personal ethics. One suggestion for optimizing ethical decision making related to this case might be to organize a diverse athletic committee review group (physician, coach, team parent representative, athletic trainer, school attorney, etc.) that can provide advisement and develop a consensus regarding the best course of action for all involved.

## The Teaching of Physical Education

School physical education has been promoted very strongly as a way to increase physical activity levels of children and adolescents (see Chapter 11). Despite the efforts of groups like NASPE and SHAPE America, in many situations physical education remains a setting where humiliation, intimidation, ridicule, physical inactivity, and other poor behaviors are dominant. Physical education should be health-oriented physical education that:[17]

- Focuses on health-related activities and fitness
- Keeps students physically active (50% of class time)
- Engages all students
- Ultimately, provides students with knowledge, skills, abilities, and confidence to be physically active for life

Ethically, schools have a duty to all students who take physical education classes to help them develop physical activity skills and behaviors that they can use for a lifetime. Unfortunately, many school administrators and leaders (knowingly or unknowingly) stack physical education classes with too many students (often 40 to

# People Matter  Jeremy Knous, Professor of Kinesiology*

**Q:** **Why and how did you get into the field of kinesiology?**

**A:** *My journey in kinesiology began very early on, being drawn to sports and having an active childhood. It developed into a passion as I got older and I became a competitive athlete always looking to improve my performance. As I entered college with great interest and aptitude for the sciences, I was mentored by a professor who opened my eyes to the career opportunities and knowledge in the field of kinesiology. Through unique opportunities, research, and scholarly presentation at the undergraduate level, I found my passion in kinesiology.*

**Q:** **What was the major influence on you to work in the field?**

**A:** *I was fortunate enough to have professors who mentored me throughout my entire educational experience as a student. Each of these mentors were willing to involve me in various research projects and trust enough in my abilities to place me in leadership roles. These experiences made me grow as an individual and influenced me to work in the field of kinesiology.*

**Q:** **What are your current research interests, and how do you translate your research results to practitioners?**

**A:** *My research interest lies in athlete performance. Currently, I work with numerous athletic teams and the strength and conditioning staff at a university to conduct research that provides data that essentially will dictate their training. From basic athlete movement screening to sport-specific testing, myself and a team of undergraduate students work to fine-tune each athlete to prevent injury and improve performance. This research is reported directly to the coaching staff of each sport as well as the strength and*

*conditioning staff to improve the individual athlete or team. Additionally, the data gathered is disseminated through peer-review presentations and publications.*

**Q:** **How do you stay physically active yourself and promote good health to others directly around you?**

**A:** *For me, exercising daily, whether lifting weights, running, or just being physically active by doing yard work, all are a means to improving my body physically while providing stress relief. I am passionate about hiking, backpacking, and climbing, thus maintaining a physically activity lifestyle allows for me to maintain the required fitness level to participate in my various adventures. I am avid in sharing the benefits of a physically active lifestyle to those all around me. I will be the first person to invite you to join me for a run or for a weekend hiking trip.*

**Q:** **How have you had to integrate the subdisciplines of kinesiology in your professional practice?**

**A:** *One of the easiest ways I integrate a subdiscipline of kinesiology is through my teaching. Every semester I teach a couple sections of the exercise physiology course. In addition, through my scholarship I implement aspects of exercise physiology, biomechanics, motor development, strength and conditioning, and sport psychology in the research conducted with sports teams. Finally, some aspects of sport management as well as other subdisciplines are utilized in my service to the university, for example, when I serve on committees.*

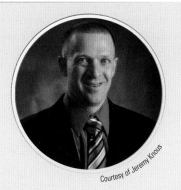
Courtesy of Jeremy Knous

*Jeremy Knous, an associate professor in the department of Kinesiology at Saginaw Valley State University, obtained his Ph.D. in Kinesiology from Michigan State University. He has taught a number of courses across the exercise science curriculum, with his main focus being exercise physiology. Dr. Knous's current research interests are related to athlete performance to prevent injury and enhance physiologic performance.

50 or more per one certified physical education teacher), hindering the teacher's ability to effectively get or keep students moving. Physical education classes are often perceived as not being academically credible; some perceive a good year for a school's physical education program as a year "when no one breaks a leg or has a serious injury." Physical educators themselves fall into unethical behaviors—such as becoming or remaining physically

inactive, just rolling out the ball, or minimally teaching appropriate skills and activities—when asked to teach such large numbers of students for many years, especially when their performances are not perceived by their teaching/administrative peers to be of importance.

Many national organizations and states are now trying to implement accountability measures into physical education teaching settings in order to improve teaching standards and increase the integrity of physical education as a profession. The implementation of standards such as those from the Institute of Medicine Report that you learned about in Chapter 11 will help provide professional ethical teaching pathways for future physical educators.[18]

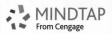 **MINDTAP** From Cengage | Now that you have completed this chapter, go to your MindTap course to complete all assigned activities. Check out the additional resources developed to help you apply the material in this chapter to your course and career goals.

## Chapter Summary

‣ Values are defined as the ideals, customs, and institutions that a society or a group uses as guidelines for living. Many times the values of an individual may affect that individual's interpretation of evidence and therefore affect the decision-making process.

‣ Ethics guide behavior and the decision-making process by providing a moral framework for behavior, as well as interpretation and use of the evidence-based outcomes deemed acceptable within the prevailing societal and cultural norms.

‣ Since ethics are rules of acceptable behavior, many professional organizations have published ethical standards that guide individuals on how they should behave when practicing their profession. Also, many groups that offer specific certifications and licensures have published ethical standards that are required to be followed to maintain the certifications or license.

‣ Institutional review boards are panels of professionals that review research protocols prior to allowing the researcher to collect data. These boards verify that all necessary steps have been taken by the researcher to prevent any unnecessary harm and discomfort to the subjects and that the researcher will receive informed consent from the subjects.

‣ To make a sound, defensible, and ethical decision, the individual must develop and weigh four possible alternatives based upon the accepted rules that best fit the situation, the situation itself, the means by which the decision will be morally judged, and the ends or benefits to all of those affected by the decision.

‣ Ethical decision making is steeped in history, philosophy, and societal acceptance. In the kinesiology profession, ethical decision making will help the professional maintain his or her integrity while achieving an outcome that is fair.

‣ For sports and exercise psychologists, confidentiality refers to duties (moral and legal obligations or responsibilities) they must perform when working with individuals or groups to maintain privacy and secrecy. The need for confidentiality can influence many areas of communication such as disclosing individual injuries, reporting on team mood or confidence issues, or discussing individual or team health test results.

## Remember This

| | | | |
|---|---|---|---|
| Academic/professional honesty and integrity | deontological ethics | informed consent | plagiarism |
| authority | disclaimer | Institutional Review Board (IRB) | rules-end argument |
| autonomy | disclosure | integrity | rules-means decision |
| confidentiality | ends-situation argument | means-situation argument | situational ethics |
| conflict of interest | ethics | | teleological ethics |
| | Helsinki Declaration | | values |

# For More Information

Access these websites for further study of topics covered in the chapter:

- Search for further information about ethical decision making from the University of California at San Diego at http://blink.ucsd.edu/finance/accountability/ethics/path.html.

- Search for information about and resources for the American College of Sports Medicine (ACSM) Code of Ethics at www.acsm.org/join-acsm/membership-resources/code-of-ethics.

- Search for information about the Nuremberg Code in the *New England Journal of Medicine* at www.nejm.org/doi/full/10.1056/NEJM199711133372006.

- Search for more information about the Helsinki Declaration by the World Medical Association at www.wma.net/en/30publications/10policies/b3/17c.pdf.

- Search for more information about IRBs and human subjects at www.hhs.gov/ohrp/assurances/irb/.

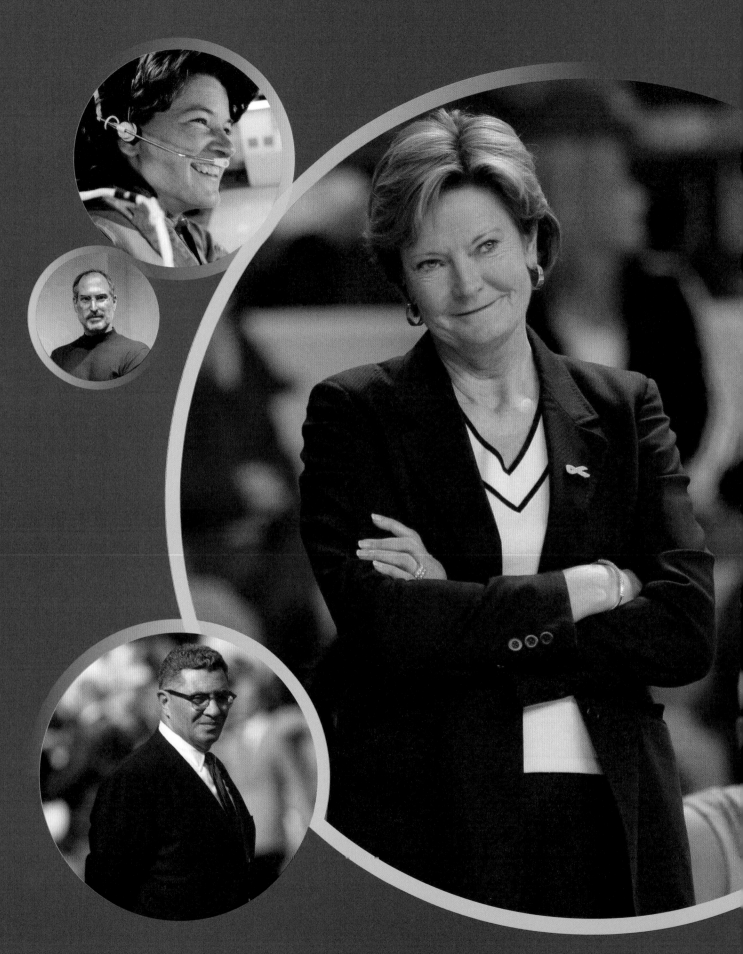

324

# Best Practices for Leadership in the Kinesiology Profession

*What are the different types of leadership styles? What are the common attributes that make a "good" leader? In what situations should a specific leadership style be used?*

**LESSON 1** LEADERSHIP IN KINESIOLOGY

**LESSON 2** EXAMPLES OF APPLYING LEADERSHIP TO THE KINESIOLOGY SUBDISCIPLINES

## Learning Objectives

*After completing this chapter, you will be able to:*

**Explain** common leadership styles and how they can be applied to the field of kinesiology.

**Justify** the importance of leadership with regard to participation in physical activity and the various subdisciplines of kinesiology.

**Explain** the leadership styles that work best in various situations across the various subdisciplines of kinesiology.

**Explain** the common goals and objectives for leaders in the kinesiology profession.

**Describe** the behavioral characteristics of a good leader.

**Explain** the model for leadership and supervision in the field of kinesiology.

**Give** examples of situations of good and poor leadership within the profession of kinesiology.

**Critically** evaluate the positive and negative consequences associated with the examples of good and poor leadership within the profession of kinesiology.

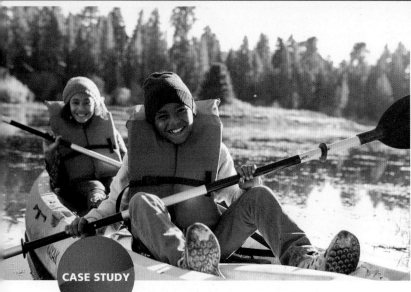

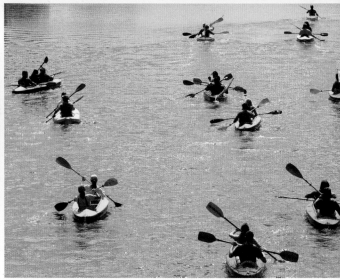

**CASE STUDY**

# In the real world . . .

Remember Dan, the kayaker from Chapter 5? The Buffalo Kayaking Club has asked Dan to lead the outreach committee in the development of a program that will promote and market kayaking to inner city youth. The committee consists of five members from the club, of which one is a founding member, three have extensive knowledge of competitive kayaking, and one is a new junior member who is a senior in high school and has just learned to kayak. In the first meeting, Dan realizes that the founding member is concerned with the ecological impact more kayakers will have on the river, two of the three competitive kayakers want to hold open races in which the inner-city children can participate, and the junior member is concerned that the older members do not know how to relate to high school students. Dan and his committee have three months to bring a proposal to the kayak club members to determine if they will go forward with the promotional campaign. What are some of the things Dan needs to do as a leader to lead the committee to complete a great proposal? How can Dan include the concerns and ideas of the committee, while

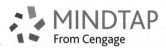

**From Cengage**

Go to your MindTap course now to answer some questions and discover what you already know about best practices for leadership in the kinesiology profession

## INTERACTIVE ACTIVITIES

### Research Focus

Go to your MindTap course to complete an activity based on the six leadership styles and the Badgett-Kritsonis Supervision Leadership Model (BK-SLM) discussed later in this chapter.

### Career Focus

Go to your MindTap course so see a list of leadership opportunities for the undergraduate kinesiology major. You can also complete an activity based on specific leadership opportunities offered by organizations such as the American Physical Therapy Association, the National Strength and Conditioning Association, the Association for Applied Sport Psychology, the American College of Sports Medicine (ACSM), and the American Kinesiology Association (AKA).

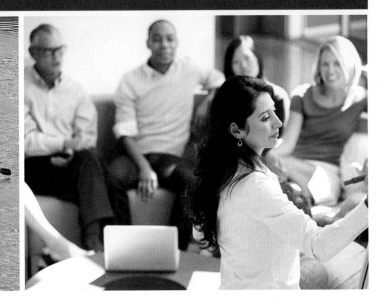

at the same time not allowing these ideas to distract from accomplishing the development of the promotion proposal? We will revisit this challenge later in the chapter.

# Introduction: Leadership and Kinesiology

**Leadership** is the process used to influence a group to reach a common goal or outcome. The success of a leader depends on his or her leadership style, communication skills, and recognition of the individual differences among the group members. Good leaders should strive to use evidence-based decision-making practices accompanied by a set of ethical guidelines when making decisions and guiding the group (see Chapter 2 about evidence-based skills and Chapter 14 on ethical decision making). Furthermore, good leaders should be able to accept responsibility for their decisions and be aware of and minimize any biases that may negatively impact the outcome of the group.[1,2]

A degree in kinesiology will likely ensure that at some time in your professional career you will be asked to be a leader. Kinesiology leadership comes in many forms, whether it is as a coach of a sports team, a teacher in the classroom, a researcher, a fitness trainer, a public health official, or a corporate employee. In all of these areas, and many more, you may be asked to work with a small group, a large group, a professional organization, or a government body to see a project to fruition. How a leader interacts with these groups will determine the success or failure of every project attempted. This chapter will focus on the tools that an individual will need to be a successful leader in the field of kinesiology and its subdisciplines.

---

### Leadership Opportunities for the Undergraduate Kinesiology Major

The following are a list of groups that have leadership opportunities:

▸ American Physical Therapy Association
▸ National Strength and Conditioning Association
▸ Association for Applied Sport Psychology
▸ American College of Sports Medicine (ACSM)
▸ American Kinesiology Association (AKA)
▸ Society of Health and Physical Educators (SHAPE)

---

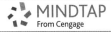
MINDTAP
From Cengage

### Take Action: Leadership Opportunities

**Go to your MindTap course** to see an expanded list of leadership opportunities and read profiles of leaders in the field of kinesiology. You will also be able to link to some of the organizations mentioned above and complete an activity based on leadership opportunities offered.

## Leadership Styles: Development, Practice, and Use

Numerous researchers have tried to describe the types of leadership styles used to guide groups to common goals and outcomes.[3] Some suggest that the leadership style is based on the style of interaction between the leader and the group, while others have suggested that it is based on the emotional characteristics of the leader. For the purpose of this chapter, three leadership styles will be discussed, with further discussion of how the emotional style of the leader may enhance or detract from the positive outcomes elicited by each.

Three styles of leadership commonly recognized are: authoritarian style, democratic style, and laissez-faire style (Table 15.1). Each of these styles has both positive and negative effects on project completion, depending on the group with which the leader is interacting. As these styles are discussed, think about the leadership styles used by coaches, teachers, or others in your life, and recall how you reacted to them.

The **authoritarian** or autocratic leadership style places all decision-making, goal-setting, and policy-making power with the leader. Most authoritarian leaders control all aspects of a project, from project vision and goal setting to implementation. The authoritarian leader has a top-down approach to directing the group, giving each member specific tasks and expectations without regard to members' input. Many times authoritarian leaders view the members of the group as subordinates with less knowledge and understanding of the project. The authoritarian leader follows a specific hierarchy, which limits autonomy of the rest of the group, allowing for full control of the project direction as the sole priority and accomplishment of the leader. One major drawback to this style of leadership is that it minimizes input from group members while maximizing the bias of the leader, which may affect project decisions, direction, and completion. Minimization and disregard of group members' input can cause low morale, create animosity, and reduce work productivity and efficiency of the members. Although it might seem as if the authoritarian leadership should never be used, in fact, it sometimes is

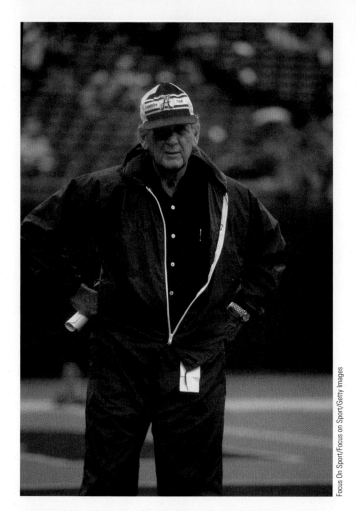

Legendary Alabama football coach, Paul William "Bear" Bryant.

necessary for project completion. The authoritarian leadership style is best used when project completion is time sensitive and tasks required of the members are not complex. To reduce some of the negative effects of the authoritarian leadership style, the leader should have good communications skills, be consistent when explaining and enforcing rules, be respectful of group members, give credit to group members for positive accomplishments, and listen to group members' ideas although they may not be prudent to use.

**Table 15.1** | Leadership Styles and Characteristics

| LEADERSHIP STYLE | | |
|---|---|---|
| **AUTHORITARIAN** | **DEMOCRATIC** | **LAISSEZ-FAIRE** |
| ▸ Controlling of all aspects of decisions | ▸ Group equality in decision-making process | ▸ Delegative leader |
| ▸ Top-down approach to communication | ▸ Encourages group participation in all decision making | ▸ Uses hands-off approach |
| ▸ Minimal input from team members | | ▸ Relinquishes control of decision making to the members |
| ▸ Members are treated as subordinates | ▸ Members are treated as colleagues | ▸ Maximizes the autonomy of the members |
| ▸ Limits autonomy of the members | ▸ Recognizes expertise of members and makes decisions based upon consensus | |

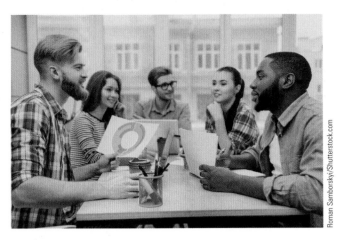
Group members sharing in decision making.

The **democratic** or participatory leadership style allows the group members to participate in the decision-making process, give input into the direction of the project, and voice their expertise to solve problems that arise. Although the democratic leader still has final say on project direction and veto power over ideas, this type of leader encourages participation in every aspect of the project's development, goals, and implementation. The democratic leader will distribute control of activities for the project to specific members of the group based upon their expertise or willingness to commit to the activities. A good democratic leader must be well organized and able to communicate effectively for this type of leadership style to work. Democratic leaders interact with other group members as colleagues rather than subordinates and therefore need better-developed interpersonal skills compared to the authoritarian leader. Leaders who use the democratic style of leadership make decisions through consensus with the group members, emphasize teamwork, and have two-way communications with group members. Democratic leadership emphasizes problem solving within the group and reduces the risk of individual confrontations through open communications and direct, open management of the problem. Democratic leaders will recognize differences among individuals in the group and use individual expertise to minimize friction between the group members. Democratic leaders will also be more likely to publicly recognize individual accomplishments and minimize any punishments for mistakes. One pitfall when using the democratic leadership style is the likelihood of loss of focus on the problem to be solved by the group when consensus building, which will minimize the effectiveness of the group. To reduce this risk, the democratic leader must be able to manage discussions and return conversations back to the problem being discussed.

Finally, the **laissez-faire** or delegative leader uses a hands-off approach when interacting with the group. Unlike the authoritarian leader, who holds strict control of the decision-making process, or the democratic leader, who works with the group for consensus in the decision-making process, the laissez-faire leader relinquishes control of the decision-making process to the group members. Laissez-faire leaders will supply the group with a broad overview of the project to be completed along with the tools and resources necessary to complete the project, but will allow and expect the group members to complete the problem solving for the project among themselves. Externally, laissez-faire leaders are viewed as detached and uninvolved with the daily management of the group or team. Internally, the group may perceive the laissez-faire leader as noncommittal and unconcerned with the project, which will detract from productivity. The laissez-faire leadership style works well with a group that is highly motivated, knowledgeable, self-directed, and independent. If any group member lacks these traits, however, the cohesiveness of the group deteriorates and members become resentful toward each other. In this case, the laissez-faire leader will generally shift the blame for failure toward group members and attempt to minimize the impact of failure toward them. Failure of this style of leadership usually occurs when the leader avoids making decisions, refuses to interact with group members, or refuses to be decisive or becomes reactionary when the problem solving exceeds the expertise of the group members. The positive side of this type of leadership style is that it allows independence and free thinking of group members, which in turn may lead to new problem-solving strategies and innovative ideas.

Each of the three styles of leadership discussed here has its place in the kinesiology profession. Although the democratic style of leadership is generally most preferred by professionals, the authoritarian and laissez-faire leadership styles may be better suited for certain situations, projects, or group dynamics. It is the job of the kinesiology professional to determine which style is best suited for these and to use the style to maximize the productivity and performance of the group.

## Behavioral Characteristics of a Good Leader

Although leadership styles are a major part of the equation for successful completion of a complex task or group project in the kinesiology profession, the personality and behaviors of the leader will impact each of the leadership styles either positively or negatively. The personality or behavioral characteristics that are most often observed among leaders are shown in Table 15.2 and can be described as commanding, charismatic (democratic), visionary, affiliative, pacesetting, and coaching. Each of these behaviors has their place among leadership styles; while most leadership styles will incorporate to some extent a combination of these behaviors depending on specific

**Table 15.2** | The Six Leadership Styles (Goleman)

| | COMMANDING | VISIONARY | AFFILIATIVE | DEMOCRATIC | PACESETTING | COACHING |
|---|---|---|---|---|---|---|
| The leader's modus operandi | Demands immediate compliance | Mobilizes people toward a vision | Creates harmony and builds emotional bonds | Forges consensus through participation | Sets high standards for performance | Develops people for the future |
| The style in a phrase | "Do what I tell you." | "Come with me." | "People come first." | "What do you think?" | "Do as I do now" | "Try this." |
| Underlying emotional intelligence competencies | Drive to achieve, initiative, self-control | Self-confidence, empathy, change catalyst | Empathy, building relationships, communication | Collaboration, team leadership, communication | Conscientious-ness, drive to achieve, initiative | Developing others, empathy, self-awareness |
| When the style works best | In a crisis, to lick start a turnaround, or with problem employees | When changes require a new vision, or when a clear direction is needed | To heal rifts in a team or to motivate people during stressful circumstances | To build buy-in or consensus, or to get input from valuable employees | To get quick results from a highly motivated and competent team | To help an employee improve performance or develop long-term strengths |
| Overall impact on climate | Negative | Most strongly positive | Positive | Positive | Negative | Positive |

Goleman, Daniel, "Leadership that Gets Results," *Harvard Business Review.* March–April 2000 p. 82–83.

situations, it is paramount that the kinesiology professional understand these behaviors and recognize which ones will produce the best results.[4]

**Commanding behavior** is considered the classic military behavior of giving orders and expecting group members to follow them without question. While commanding behavior is most often used by leaders, it may create the most problems and least productivity of the group, especially among groups whose members have high levels of expertise in specific areas being addressed. The commanding behavior is best used during a crisis, when time is of the essence, or when there is an impasse among individuals in the group. Commanding behavior is the predominant behavior of the authoritarian leader and when overused can cause animosity, a decline in new idea generation, and declines in morale among the group. These changes in the group dynamic will reduce productivity and maximize inefficiency.

**Charismatic (democratic) behavior** is the energetic and powerful behavior that influences and motivates group members simply through the charm and personality of the leader. The charismatic approach assumes that the leader's personality and charm will motivate the group members, whether or not the leader has any external power or authority. Charismatic behavior requires the leader to relate to individuals within a group at a personal level, making each individual feel that she or he is the most important person in the group. To effectively use this type of behavior, the leader must be sensitive to the group dynamics and the individual needs of the members of the group. Furthermore, this type

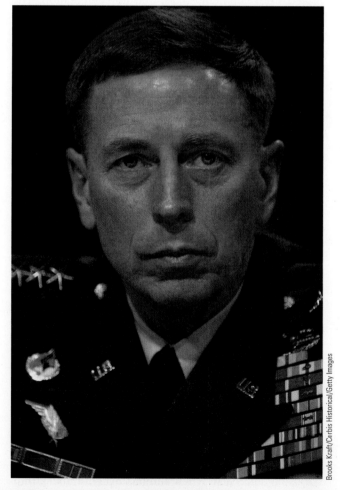

Brooks Kraft/Corbis Historical/Getty Images

| Retired U.S. Army General David Petraeus.

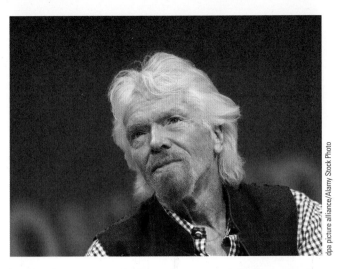

Richard Branson is a business magnate. His business empire grew from a small chain of record stores and the successful launch of the recording label, Virgin Records.

of behavior requires clear vision and articulation of the goals desired to produce the best outcomes of the project. Charismatic behavior works well to motivate individuals and should be used in developing group cohesion among the members at the start of the project; when used properly, it will create a highly motivated group of individuals with a single vision for success. One of the downsides of using charismatic behavior is that it tends to create an attitude of supported risk taking among group members. Although some risk taking is supported and acceptable, too much risk taking by members can negatively impact project success.

**Visionary behavior** directs the group through clear articulation of the innovation involved and vision of what the specific project will produce. This type of leadership behavior works well with the democratic and laissez-faire styles of leadership when group members are internally motivated and have high levels of expertise in specific areas of the project. A leader will use visionary behavior to broadly describe a vision of the results expected upon project completion but will allow the group members to determine the best way to get to those results. This allows the members to be creative in problem solving, relying on their expertise to innovatively approach a problem. With a clear vision of the expectations of the resultant project, the group members can many times improve problem solving in project tasks and increase morale. Leaders using this type of behavior alone may fail if they themselves do not have a clear vision of what is to be expected or when members of the group lack motivation or the expertise to complete the project.

**Affiliative (or team-building) behavior** builds upon the cohesiveness of the team by creating harmony among members through emphasizing emotional bonds among them. A leader using affiliative behaviors will emphasize the "we" and the "team" while deemphasizing the

"I" and the needs of the individual. This type of behavior relies heavily upon member communication, supportive relationships among group members, and the empathy and understanding of the leader. Affiliative behavior is best used during times of high stress and when group cohesion dissolves. Good leaders of all three leadership styles will use this type of behavior when addressing rifts among team members or when trying to eliminate factions within the group. Affiliative behavior can improve morale during stressful situations by letting each individual know that failure is not individualized and that success is dependent on the team as a whole. Although affiliative behavior has mostly positive effects, sometimes the emphasis on the team can detract from recognizing individual poor performance, which may negatively affect project outcomes.[5]

**Pacesetting behavior** allows the leader to set the standards of performance for the group. When using pacesetting, the leader will set high standards for the whole group and act as a role model by maintaining those high standards. Pacesetting emphasizes achievement, initiative, and conscientiousness among all members of the group, including the leader. Generally, this behavior works well with highly motivated members and, when used properly, can increase efficiency and productivity. When used improperly (e.g., when standards are set so high that they are unachievable), this type of behavior can have catastrophic results and decrease member morale and productivity, ensuring complete failure of the project. Although pacesetting behavior can be used within all three leadership styles with both success and failure, it is predominantly observed in the authoritarian style of leadership.

**Coaching behavior** allows the leader to act as a teacher for individual group members. Leaders use coaching behavior to improve upon an individual's skills and performance. When using this behavior, the leader is assuming that she or he is developing the individual for future accomplishments and not for immediate results. This type of behavior is effective when the long-term goals of the leader are more important than the current task or project. Leaders using the coaching behavior need to have empathy and understanding for each individual, recognizing their strengths and weaknesses. Leaders using coaching behavior will deemphasize the negative qualities of the weaknesses and will communicate clear ideas for improvement. When used correctly, coaching behavior can enhance professional development and initiative of the individual. Coaching behavior can negatively affect team cohesiveness when the individual being coached has an exaggerated view of self-importance and self-esteem. In this case, the leader can be perceived as a micromanager and lose the respect of team members.

All six leadership behaviors have specific positive effects when used at the appropriate time by the kinesiology leader. Each behavior will impact how group members respond to specific leadership styles. It is the job of the kinesiology professional to determine which behavior to use with which leadership style in a specific situation to improve the productivity, performance, and results of the group.[6,7]

# A Model for Leadership and Supervision in Kinesiology

Up to this point, the chapter has focused on the styles and behaviors leaders in the kinesiology profession use to interact with the group being led. The discussion will now shift from styles and behaviors of the kinesiology professional to how the kinesiology leader should supervise a group or team. As with the many different leadership behaviors and styles discussed previously, there are also many different leadership models that can be used to direct the supervision of group members. One such model that seems to work with most of the "good" leadership behaviors and that best fits the profession of kinesiology is the Badgett-Kritsonis Supervision Leadership Model (BK-SLM).[8] The BK-SLM relies on clarity of communications and feedback as they relate to expectations and results of the group and its individuals (see Figure 15.1). Good communication is essential for

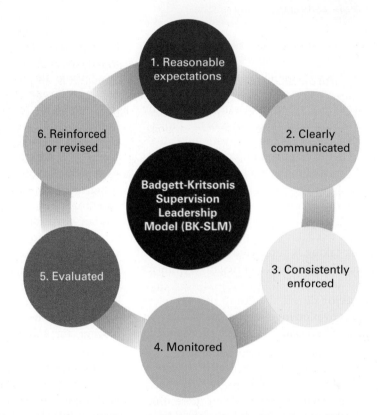

The *Badgett-Kritsonis Supervision Leadership Model (BK-SLM)* focuses on six fundamental principles of effective supervision. *Step One*: Expectations must be reasonable. *Step Two*: Expectations clearly communicated. *Step Three*: Expectations consistently enforced. Once these foundational steps are established, the supervisor advances to the fourth, fifth, and sixth steps. *Step Four*: Results monitored. *Step Five*: Results evaluated for effectiveness. *Step Six*: Expectations reinforced or revised in a systematic, measured, and safe manner. This model is grounded on effective decision making.

| FOUNDATION LEVELS | ADVANCED LEVELS |
|---|---|
| Step One: Expectations must be reasonable | Step Four: Results monitored |
| Step Two: Expectations clearly communicated | Step Five: Results evaluated for effectiveness |
| Step Three: Expectations consistently enforced | Step Six: Expectations reinforced |

**Figure 15.1** | Badgett-Kritsonis Supervision Leadership Model (BK-SLM)

any leadership model to succeed. The BK-SLM model is divided into a foundation level and an advanced level of supervision. Each level has an important role in the success of a project, and the model can be used with any of the three leadership styles and any of the six leadership behaviors.

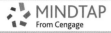
MINDTAP
From Cengage

**More on Leadership Styles**

**Go to your MindTap course** to complete an activity based on the six leadership styles and the Badgett-Kritsonis Supervision Leadership Model (BK-SLM) discussed in this section.

The foundation level of the BK-SLM requires the leader to develop reasonable expectations, clearly communicate these expectations to the group and its individual members, and then consistently enforce these expectations among the group and its members. To develop reasonable expectations for the group and its individuals, the kinesiology leader must know the strengths and weaknesses of each of the group members and the size and scope of the project to be completed. The kinesiology leader should rely on evidence-based and ethical decision-making strategies to develop the expectations for the group. This may require the kinesiology professional to review the related literature for the specific project, talk with other professionals who have previously worked on a similar project, put together a focus group to aid in the development of the expectations, and finally rely on his or her own expertise. Once the expectations have been defined, these expectations must be clearly communicated to the members of the group. Clear communication is necessary to ensure success of the project. Time must be allowed to answer all questions that may arise when presenting the expectations to the members. Once all questions have been answered, it is important that the kinesiology leader enforces the expectations consistently across all members of the group. Consistent enforcement of expectations is paramount to reduce friction among group members and to maintain group cohesion.[9]

Once the foundation stage is completed, the kinesiology leader can begin the advanced stage of supervision. The advanced stage of supervision requires the kinesiology leader to monitor the work of the group and evaluate the performance of the group and its members in the context of the defined expectations. During the monitoring phase, the kinesiology leader can improve productivity by providing specific formative feedback that will help improve the productivity of the group. Once the evaluation phase is completed, summative feedback (evaluation) describing both positive accomplishments that met the expectations and negative results that fell short of the expectations should be given to the group. When the evaluation process is completed, the kinesiology leader should review the negative results of the evaluation to determine whether reinforcement or further clarification of the expectations is needed, or if the expectations should be revised. Whether reinforcement or revision of the expectations is required, the kinesiology leader needs to communicate the results and changes to the group. When either reinforcement or revision of the expectations occurs, the leader will begin at the foundation phase for another cycle of monitoring and evaluation. Although the BK-SLM is independent of leadership style and behavior, specific leadership styles or behaviors may affect the amount and type of feedback given in the foundation stage. For instance, commanding leaders who use an authoritarian style assume that their direction, instructions, and feedback are clear and understandable. With this type of leader, it is imperative that the members of the group ask questions when feedback is unclear, or the project will fail. Conversely, charismatic leaders who use the laissez-faire leadership style may be good at motivating the members of the group, but feedback will be infrequent, and necessary corrections to the project may be overlooked. In this instance, members of the group may need to seek feedback from other group members to ensure project success. Ensuring success of any project when using the BK-SLM model requires good communication skills of the leader. Leaders should also have a self-awareness of their dominant leadership style and leadership behavior and determine if the use of another leadership behavior or style that is not dominant to their personality would work better with an individual member when presenting instruction and feedback. Self-awareness of the leadership styles and behaviors will improve the kinesiology leader's success. It is necessary for the kinesiology leader to keep in mind that regardless of leadership style or behavior, clarity in expectations and feedback will enhance the overall outcome and results of the project.

## Summary

In the kinesiology profession, leadership skills are necessary in every subdiscipline. Kinesiology professionals should recognize and evaluate which leadership style best fits the situation and group they are asked to lead. For the most part, kinesiology professionals have had the most experience with the authoritarian style of leadership. Although kinesiology professionals have historically used this style, it is the least likely to produce consistent results, especially when working with highly trained experts within a group. The democratic style of leadership accompanied by charismatic, affiliative, and coaching behaviors can produce better results in more situations while maintaining high levels of group cohesiveness. Finally, though the laissez-faire leadership style may be ineffective in most situations, kinesiology leaders should recognize that in certain situations where the group is highly motivated and has advanced expertise, this style may improve innovation when accompanied by visionary leadership behavior.[10]

Regardless of the leadership style and behavior, to supervise the group, the kinesiology leader should rely on a supervision model that emphasizes clearly defined expectations and communications. The BK-SLM stresses clearly defined and reasonable expectations and communication of these expectations to the group. The model further stresses consistent enforcement of the expectations accompanied by monitoring, feedback, and evaluation of the process. By keeping all of this information in mind, kinesiology professionals can excel in leadership.

# EXAMPLES OF APPLYING LEADERSHIP TO THE KINESIOLOGY SUBDISCIPLINES

*In all subdisciplines of kinesiology, at some point the kinesiology professional will be asked to lead a project to conclusion. When this situation arises, a determination of which leadership style and leadership behaviors will increase the chance for successful completion must be made. Once the kinesiology professional has determined which type of leadership style will enhance performance of the group and which behaviors will have the greatest impact on success, she or he should develop the expectations for the group, clearly communicate them to the group, and consistently enforce them. Monitoring and feedback during the supervision process will enhance the evaluation of the productivity of the group while helping the*

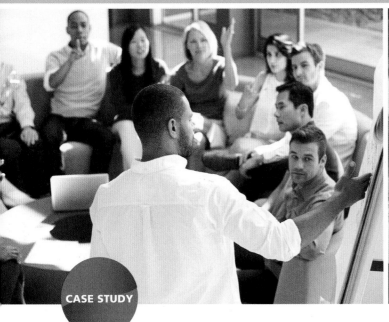

**CASE STUDY**

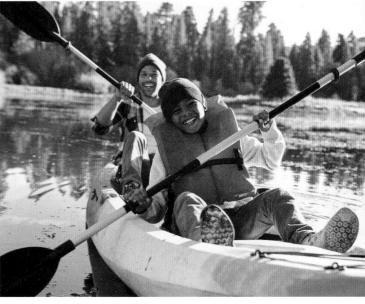

## In the real world . . .

As stated previously, Dan the kayaker has been asked to lead the outreach committee in the development of a program that will promote and market kayaking to inner city youth. The five committee members have divergent views on what type of promotion campaign should be accomplished and what impact the promotion and subsequent increase in activities will have on the bayou and on the club. Dan realizes that with such divergent viewpoints of the members, the authoritarian style of leadership may cause undue strife among members and negatively impact friendships and camaraderie among the members—perhaps well beyond the committee. There is enough time for discussion that authoritarian leadership may be inefficient at this juncture. Dan also realizes that with such divergent viewpoints, a laissez-faire style of leadership would likewise be inefficient because each member would develop her or his own promotional plan and there would not be enough time to address all of the plans. Therefore, Dan decides

to use the democratic style of leadership with the group. Using a visionary type of behavior in the first meeting, Dan speaks to the committee about the plight of the inner-city youth and their need to become involved in safe physical activities that promote opportunities for involvement in society with nurturing communities. Once Dan has shared his vision with the committee, he shifts his behavior to an affiliative style, explaining to the members that most of these children have never had access to kayaks and so are novices. If the committee desires to develop them into competitive kayakers, the kayaking club must first peak their interest in the activity. Dan also states that if the demand for learning kayaking expands—such that the added number of people on the bayou may have a short-term impact on the bayou's environment—the potential positive long-term impact of having greater numbers to participate in bayou habitat protection would ultimately benefit the group and the bayou's ecology. Notice how Dan uses the affiliative type of behavior to foster cohesiveness among the group by turning their concerns into positive situations for the club and

*kinesiology leader to revise expectations when necessary. Lesson 2 will help you understand how to use leadership styles and behaviors in the context of several of the subdisciplines within the kinesiology profession.*

‣ Exercise Physiology
‣ Biomechanics
‣ Public Health
‣ Sport/Exercise Psychology
‣ Practice of Kinesiology

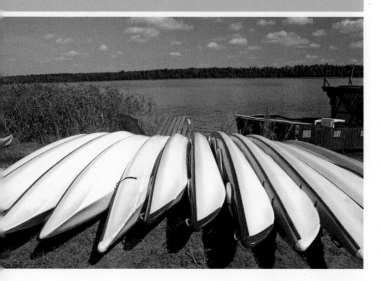

the river's sustainability. After hearing Dan's explanation of the vision and benefits for this opportunity to include inner-city youth in a new activity that will improve their physical activity levels as well as be beneficial to the kayaking club and the bayou, all members are ready to promote kayaking.

Now that Dan's committee is ready to develop a kayaking promotional campaign targeted to inner-city youth, what types of leadership skills will he need to sway inner-city youth to participate in kayaking? What issues do you think Dan and his committee should address to make the promotion a success? Imagine that you are the leader and identify two barriers that may impede the inner-city youth from participating in kayaking; then develop solutions to overcome the barriers. Develop a leadership strategy describing the type of leadership style you would use along with the behaviors that would positively affect the outcome of your solutions.

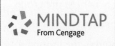
Go to your MindTap course to complete the Case Study activity for this chapter.

# Exercise Physiology

Assume you have been hired by a cardiac rehabilitation clinic to improve the efficiency of a post-rehabilitation evaluation of the patients. The evaluation unit consists of two supervising physicians, a physical therapist, and five technicians who set up and run standardized clinical graded exercise tests (GXT). Remember that a GXT of a post-rehabilitation cardiac patient entails risks for atypical physiological responses such as abnormal blood pressure, fainting, irregular heart rhythms, and, in rare circumstances, heart attack, stroke, or death. What leadership style would you suggest the physician use to supervise these individuals to maximize efficiency? What dynamics of the group may affect the capacity to lead it? How might you minimize friction among members of the team while maximizing safety of the patient?

# Biomechanics

Technology continues to influence the design and production of running shoes. Current trends in biomechanics include the introduction of new nanomaterials in shoe soles that improve the rebound effect of the shoe when it strikes the ground. This rebound effect is thought to reduce the energy needed in muscular contraction of the legs while enhancing contractile velocity.

Imagine that a large, international sporting goods company has asked you to lead a team to test varying amounts of the nanotech in the soles to determine which would meet performance requirements while producing the most cost-effective shoe model. Generally, you consider yourself a laissez-faire style of leader who uses affiliative behaviors to lead. To evaluate the shoe soles, you will need a team of three technicians, an accountant, and a marketing expert. What types of characteristics and knowledge would you desire in each of these individuals? What would be your expectations for the group and each of its members? What possible situations might arise that could cause your project to fail?

# Public Health

How would a public health leader whose agency has a physical activity focus promote advocacy in a leadership model that would motivate his team to become successful at developing and implementing programs, policy, and built environmental changes? One method might be to introduce a model for global advocacy for physical activity as described by Shilton.[11]

Shilton suggests that there are five imperatives for advancing physical activity globally. They are:

1. Urgency: Translate and articulate the physical activity evidence (science) as urgent—promote national physical activity guidelines and plans.

2. Present physical activity as policy relevant—demonstrate how physical activity intersects with health, environment sustainability, the economy, and social policy.

3. Present solutions and outline an agenda for action.

4. Mobilize an action strategy that includes political action, media resources, professional mobilization, community mobilization, and advocacy from within organizations.

5. Provide persuasive communication by releasing physical activity promotion success stories to various media sources.

Once the team has learned about the model and had the opportunity to ask questions, the public health leader can encourage them to become active participants and subscribe to the newsletter of the Global Physical Activity Network (www.globalpanet.com). The GlobalPANet rapidly communicates the latest research from around the globe via its unique e-newsletter and website. GlobalPANet users are informed about recent physical activity developments, careers, and events, as well as being linked to a global network of individuals with professional and personal interests in physical activity. By providing and articulating clear vision about the global importance and relevance of physical activity, the public health leader can motivate his team and help them more clearly understand their collective professional importance.

## Sport/Exercise Psychology 🧩

The female athlete triad, a syndrome comprised of eating disorders, amenorrhea, and osteoporosis, has been observed among female high school athletes. One of the primary factors that may drive this disorder is negative comments coaches make about their female athletes' bodies. As the athletic director for Cypress Normal High School, you have been made aware that one of the high school track coaches has been telling his female runners that they are "too fat" and need to weigh less than 100 pounds to compete. You understand how these statements might negatively affect the athletes' body image. Using the BK-SLM as a guide, develop a supervision plan for the coach to remedy this situation. Be sure to include specific expectations and describe how you will monitor and evaluate the coach's remediation progress.

## The Practice of Kinesiology 🧍

Now that you have had the chance to consider different types of leadership styles based upon specific subdisciplines and situations, it is time for a self-evaluation and reflection on your inherent leadership style and leadership behaviors. Have you had a chance to be a leader in some form or fashion prior to taking this course? Do you aspire to become a leader at some time in your career? Do you think you will have leadership thrust upon you at any time during your career? If you answered "yes" to any of these questions, then you should start evaluating the type of leadership style you previously used and compare it with the information in this chapter.

In previous chapters, this section was used to introduce a specific scenario that might arise during your career. For this chapter, rather than giving you a scenario to evaluate, we want you to evaluate yourself and reflect upon the type of leadership styles you use currently and how you might change your style to improve your leadership capabilities. Truthfully answer the following questions and then reflect on how your answers might change now that you have reviewed this chapter's content.

What type of leadership style do you use most often when working with a group? What leadership behaviors are your "go to" behaviors when placed into a leadership situation? Which leadership behaviors make you feel the most uncomfortable when you are a member of the group and not a leader? Which leadership behaviors do you need to practice to become a more proficient leader?

After answering all of the questions, reflect back upon what makes a good leader and determine how you might improve upon your leadership skills. One suggestion for preparing for a leadership role is to become involved with a local chapter of one of the many public health associations, such as the American Heart Association, the American Cancer Society, or the American Diabetes Association. You might also actively participate in your school's student government or seek a leadership role in your local kinesiology club.

### The Teaching of Physical Education

The HEALTHY Study was funded by the National Institutes of Health. This project was designed to reduce the risk of developing type 2 diabetes among middle school students (primarily minorities) in 42 schools over three years at multiple sites in the United States. One of the interventions of the study included a physical education (PE) component that was designed to increase the amount of moderate to vigorous physical activity (MVPA) in PE classes.[12]

In order to evaluate whether the HEALTHY Study was effective at increasing MVPA, a feasibility pilot study was conducted to determine if PE teachers taught classes that were composed of the following: instant class start-up activity, a health-related physical activity (HRPA), and a skill-related physical activity. The pilot study showed that teachers did a fairly good job at complying with the daily lesson components with a 10 to 15% drop-off in delivering the start-up activity and the HPRA at

## People Matter Tomas Green, Corporate and Business Development Director*

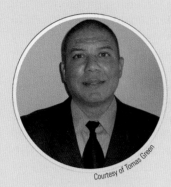

*Courtesy of Tomas Green*

**Q:** **Why and how did you get into the field of kinesiology?**

**A:** *As a first-generation college student and not knowing much about college career tracks, my first instinct was to select what was most natural and something I could relate to the best. For me, this was something related to sports and in my case, specifically coaching. I overheard someone in college say one day that he had considered coaching and I thought, wow if I could go to college, I think I would coach.*

**Q:** **What was the major influence on you to work in the field?**

**A:** *I had a few great coaches who hung in there for me. Even when I was 85 pounds as a freshman, and ran a 70-second 400-meter dash, they encouraged me not to drop out of athletics and treated me with respect. Thus, I saw vast improvement in physique and performance. I felt like I owed it to them to pay it forward by helping others see the magic of kinesiology.*

**Q:** **What are your current research interests, and how do you translate your research results to practitioners?**

**A:** *My current research interest is on community preventive wellness screenings; this includes identifying unknown health risks to individuals and providing them with resources available to treat conditions. The fear of the unknown pales in comparison to the benefit of knowing your health status. In a medical center, our practitioners consist of our medical providers who are able to act upon screening results.*

**Q:** **How do you stay physically active yourself and promote good health to others directly around you?**

**A:** *I incorporate a daily routine of physical activity into my day. This includes going to the fitness center five to six times per week. In addition, I actively engage family members and colleagues through self-awareness of current fitness levels and opportunities for wellness.*

**Q:** **How have you had to integrate the subdiscipline of kinesiology in your professional practice?**

**A:** *The field of kinesiology is a hand with subdisciplines, its fingers that work together to accomplish various tasks of wellness. Tasks may include fitness, health, performance, social/emotional, and aesthetic. Synergistically, the subdisciplines such as exercise physiology, pedagogy, sport psychology, motor learning/development, biomechanics, and sports medicine/management are necessary to fulfill these tasks. Depending on the specific task on hand, a different subdiscipline may come to the forefront, but undoubtedly integration occurs for each case.*

*Tomas Green is the director of Corporate and Business Development at UT Physicians, the medical group practice of McGovern Medical School in Houston, Texas USA. He currently leads health promotion teams in the greater Houston area in providing corporate and community wellness biometric screenings.

---

the beginning of the last year of the study. Based on the results, a PE coordinator/leader at each study site was asked to coach her or his fellow teachers on how to improve compliance.

Each PE coordinator/leader used a coaching model of leadership to encourage three to four PE teachers under their leadership to practice strategies to increase lesson compliance. They asked teachers to volunteer individual strategies that they found helpful and to demonstrate techniques to their peers. In addition, the PE coordinator/leader recruited teacher volunteers to be evaluated in their classes and to serve as evaluators and coaches to others at their school. As a result of the feasibility study follow-up and coaching leadership style follow-up, the HEALTHY Study group was able to successfully meet their PE objectives.

---

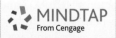

**MINDTAP** From Cengage

Now that you have completed this chapter, go to your MindTap course to complete all assigned activities. Check out the additional resources developed to help you apply the material in this chapter to your course and career goals.

---

# Chapter Summary

- Leadership is a process used to influence a group to reach a common goal or outcome. The success of a leader depends on the leadership style used in a given situation, the communication skills of the leader, and recognition of the individual differences among the group members.

- Authoritarian or autocratic leaders make all decisions, set all goals, and make all policy decisions. Most authoritarian leaders control all aspects of a project, from project vision and goal setting to implementation. Authoritarian leadership requires the leader to also accept all ramifications from decisions.

- Democratic leaders encourage participation of the group members in every aspect of the project's development, goals, and implementation. The democratic leader distributes control of activities for the project to specific members of the group based upon their expertise or willingness to commit to the activities.

- Laissez-faire leaders use a hands-off approach to leading the group. This type of leader relinquishes control of the decision-making process to the group members. Although this action gives the group autonomy, it many times creates a lack of direction that can have catastrophic consequences.

- While leadership styles are a major part of the equation for successful completion of a complex task or group project in the kinesiology profession, the personality and behaviors of the leader will impact each of the leadership styles either positively or negatively. The personality or behavioral characteristics that are most often observed among leaders can be described as commanding, charismatic, visionary, affiliative, pacesetting, and coaching.

- The commanding and pacesetting leadership behaviors should be used with caution because of their negative effects on group cohesion. Charismatic, visionary, affiliative, and coaching behaviors have greater positive responses among group members; however, certain situations may limit their effect upon group dynamics.

- The Badgett-Kritsonis Supervision Leadership Model (BK-SLM) is one of the better models that fits into the profession of kinesiology. The BK-SLM relies on clarity of communications and feedback as they relate to expectations and results of the group and its individual members. The model is divided into a foundation level and an advanced level of supervision.

# Remember This

| | | | |
|---|---|---|---|
| affiliative (or team building) behavior | charismatic (democratic) behavior | commanding behavior | leadership |
| authoritarian leader | coaching behavior | democratic leader | pacesetting behavior |
| | | laissez-faire leader | visionary behavior |

# For More Information

Access these websites or twitter sites for further study of topics covered in the chapter:

- Find updates and quick links to these and other evidence-base practice-related sites in MindTap.

- American Medical Association: www.ama-assn.org /life-career/residency-career-planning

- American Physical Therapy Association: www.apta .org/Advocacy/Involvement/

- American College of Sports Medicine Interest Groups: www.acsm.org/join-acsm/interest-groups

- National Strength and Conditioning Association: www .nsca.com/foundation/

- Association for Applied Sport Psychology: www .appliedsportpsych.org/students-center/

- American Kinesiology Association: www.americanki nesiology.org/

- Society of Health and Physical Educators: www .shapeamerica.org/_

- Institute for Social Change: http://sisgigroup.org/isc /intro-leadership/

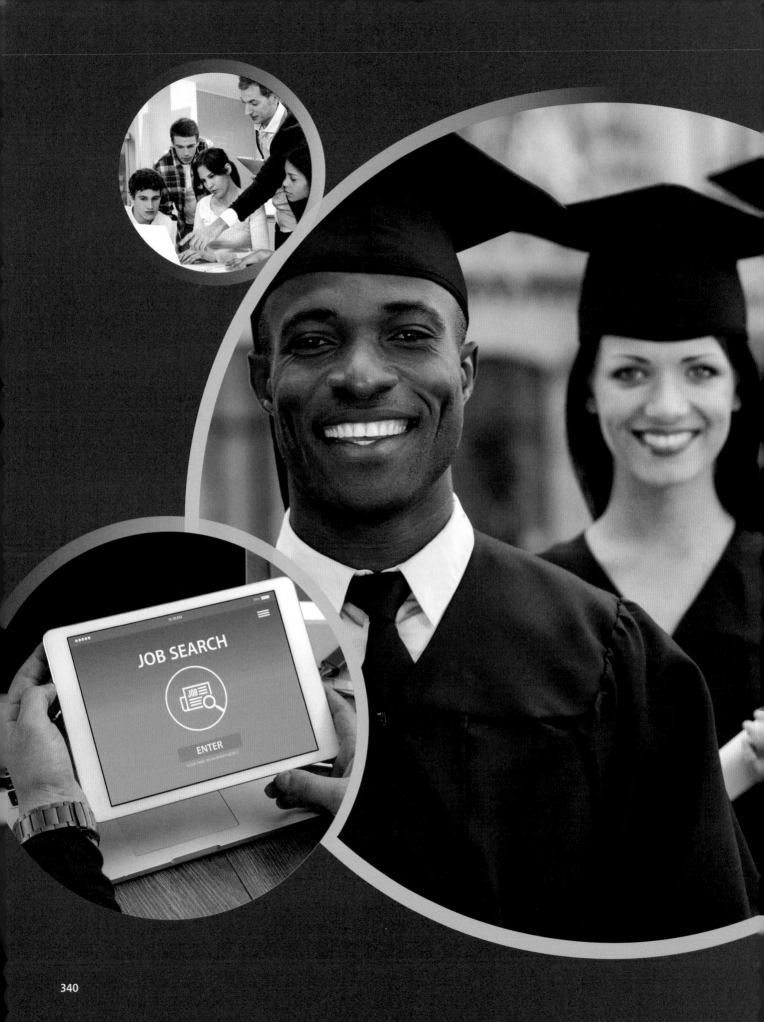

# Summary of Key Concepts and Your Future in the Kinesiology Profession

**16**

*What are the foundations of kinesiology? How are the subdisciplines integrated? How will you use this course going forward?*

**LESSON 1** UNIFYING THEMES IN KINESIOLOGY

**LESSON 2** THE FUTURE AND FINAL THOUGHTS

## Learning Objectives

*After completing this chapter, you will be able to:*

**Explain** the common unifying themes associated with the field of kinesiology.

**Justify** the importance of the physical activity continuum, dose/response, and the unifying principles (overload, specificity, and adaptation) in the various subdisciplines of kinesiology.

**Explain** how to use evidence-based approaches to problem solving in kinesiology.

**Give** examples of ways in which you can find your career niche in kinesiology.

**Explain** how you can adapt and move on to new careers as necessary within and outside the field of kinesiology.

**Describe** the personal future KSAs (knowledge, skills, and abilities) that you should strive to achieve in your lifetime of learning as a kinesiology professional.

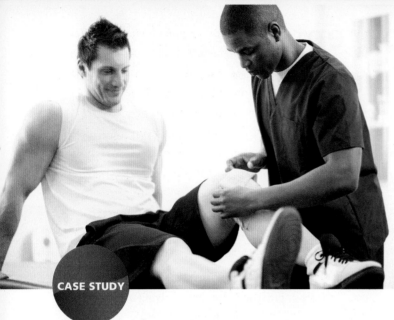

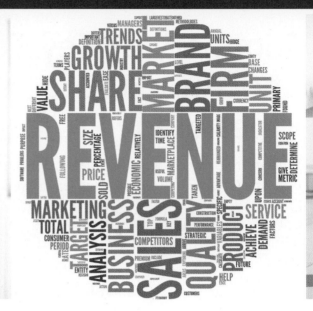

**CASE STUDY**

# In the real world . . .

Recall Martijn from Chapter 2. He was an undergraduate kinesiology major who could not get into physical therapy (PT) school but was successful at gaining admission to a master's graduate program in health administration. Martijn's undergraduate degree in kinesiology served him well as he ultimately completed his master's degree in two years and wrote a thesis that focused on alternate revenue resources for PT programs/clinics.[1] He gained employment as a junior executive in a health promotion company and works with preventive/rehabilitative professionals with undergraduate kinesiology backgrounds similar to his.

Martijn's thesis work focused on the changing economic landscape for the PT profession with regard to the Affordable Care Act of 2010. He was able to turn his passion for PT into a study to help PT practices/clinics explore new revenue options to replace traditional sources of revenue (such as third-party insurance company reimbursement and Medicare) that were projected to decrease in the near future.

Martijn used financial modeling to evaluate additional revenue streams for PT programs/clinics such as workers' compensation testing, post-offer employment testing (POET), drug testing, and fitness management programming. He determined break-even analyses for each revenue stream; for example, his projections for

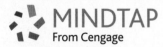

# MINDTAP
### From Cengage

Go to your MindTap course now to answer some questions about the key concepts in kinesiology and your future in the profession.

## INTERACTIVE ACTIVITIES

### Research Focus

Go to your MindTap course to learn more about policy statements to promote physical activity from international, national, state, and local organizations.

### Career Focus

Go to your MindTap course to complete an activity based on 22 career strategies and tips presented at the end of this chapter as a final summary of items to consider as you prepare to enter the kinesiology profession or to move on after obtaining your undergraduate degree in kinesiology.

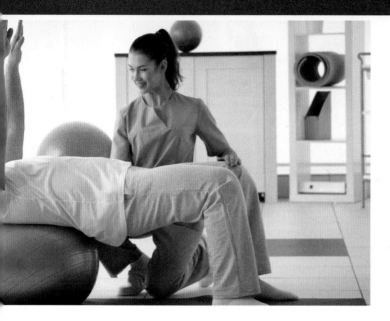

break-even point for profit development with post-offer employment testing implementation indicates that once the PT program/clinic has completed more than 45 tests, they will be making a profit by adding this new selected revenue stream. By integrating his educational experiences from kinesiology and health management, Martijn was able to provide practical future economic options that will allow PT programs/clinics to maintain or increase profits as they adjust to the changing health care landscape. Martijn was successful at earning his undergraduate degree in kinesiology and then used his integrated knowledge, skills, and abilities (KSAs) to earn his master's degree and a career in a field that matched his evolving professional goals. His case example is consistent with the overall goal of this text, to help you learn to integrate the subdisciplines of kinesiology to prepare for all your future career opportunities.

post-offer employment testing are shown in Figure 16.1. The three lines graphed in Figure 16.1 illustrate how costs, revenue, and profit shift as the number of new service line POET unit tests, represented by the x-axis, increases. The

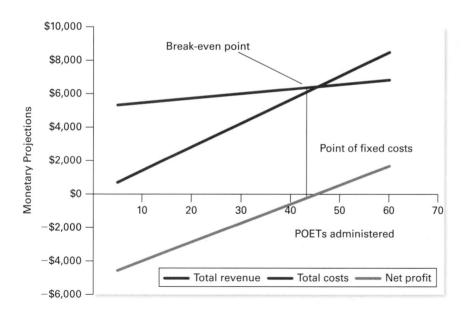

**Figure 16.1** Financial Modeling and Projections for Post-Offer Employment Testing (POET). Total revenue, total costs, and the net profits are shown. Once 45 tests have been administered in the PT clinic, the break-even point is achieved and additional tests will generate profits.

*Source:* M. Van Oort, "The Use of Additional Revenue Streams to Expand Case-Mix in Outpatient Physical Therapy Management," Master's Thesis, Texas State University, 2011, accessed January 11, 2016, https://digital.library.txstate.edu/bitstream/handle/10877/2414/VAN-OORT-THESIS.pdf?sequence=1.

# Introduction

In the previous 15 chapters, you learned about how kinesiology is an integrated field with many subdisciplines. In this chapter, we will summarize key take-away points that will reinforce why you should learn to integrate the variety of academic discipline exposures (like coursework and internships) you will experience as an undergraduate kinesiology major. We will also use our crystal ball to highlight additional KSAs you should acquire to find future opportunities as a professional in the field of kinesiology.

Several professional kinesiology leaders and organizations have emphasized the need for all kinesiology practitioners to study current and future trends related to our rapidly changing field.[2,3,4] Although the future is difficult to predict, the information in this text will help prepare you to look forward in the field of kinesiology. To understand emerging and future trends, you should be able to integrate the following principles and experiences:

▸ Physical activity in health, wellness, and quality of life

▸ Scientific foundations of physical activity

▸ Cultural, historical, and philosophical dimensions of physical activity

▸ The practice of physical activity

Lawson suggests that understanding the following additional integrated concepts can help you prepare for your future career in kinesiology and promote the field as a whole:[5]

▸ The need to produce public goods or tangible products that contribute to solving societal problems. Examples of public goods in kinesiology are developing physical activity plans at the community level for specific populations or helping implement physical activity policies at the national, regional, or state levels. Examples of tangible kinesiology products are the development of wearable technology or programs like pop-up yoga classes conducted in park settings.

▸ The need to show that the kinesiology field and your role in the profession will continue to be valuable to society and that there are professional agendas that integrate kinesiology into national policy decisions and legislative actions such as public health-oriented goals.

▸ The need to focus on the future by being willing to change rapidly to meet emerging societal needs and able to evaluate the effectiveness of interventions, monitor them, and adjust them as needed.

By mastering the knowledge base of kinesiology, translating that knowledge, and communicating it by developing effective ways to enhance human movement, you can become better prepared to help solve societal challenges.

**"Do what you can, with what you have, where you are" —Theodore Roosevelt, 1913**

In 2014, The **Canadian Council of University Physical Education and Kinesiology Administrators (CCUPEKA)** developed a position statement entitled "The Role of Kinesiologists and the Promotion of Physical Activity and Exercise in the Canadian Health Care System."[6] The CCUPEKA statement is the first formal scientific document encouraging government leaders to integrate kinesiology as an emerging health care profession that should be incorporated into a health care system. The CCUPEKA approach is consistent with the promotion of kinesiology and integrated concepts that you have learned about in the previous 15 chapters.

CCUPEKA defines *kinesiology* as "an evolving term to describe a multi-disciplinary academic discipline that spans the biophysical, socio-cultural, psychological, and neuromotor control aspects of human movement and performance. The discipline includes knowledge generation through research and translation of that knowledge into practice by professionals who work with a broad spectrum of populations—from those who are physically inactive due to choice or injury or disease, through to those who are performance athletes or who have physically demanding occupations." The CCUPEKA and **American Kinesiology Association (AKA)** definitions of kinesiology are very similar to what you learned in Chapter 1: "Kinesiology is the study of movement and how physical activity and physical fitness affect health, behavior, community, and quality of life." Although the field has its roots in physical education, it includes many subdisciplines today.

## Kinesiology: A View of the Discipline

The American Kinesiology Association definition of kinesiology is "the academic discipline which involves the study of physical activity and its impact on health, society, and quality of life." As a discipline, kinesiology draws on several sources of knowledge including knowledge gained from personal and corporate physical activity experiences, professional practices centered in physical activity, and knowledge gained through scholarly study and research into physical activity itself. Although the discipline is most often associated with the last of these, the AKA recognizes that the body of knowledge of kinesiology is informed by and defined by the other two sources as well. Ultimately, the uniqueness of kinesiology as a discipline is its embrace and integration of a multi-dimensional study and application of physical activity—biological, medical, and health-related aspects, but also psychological, social-humanistic, and a variety of professional perspectives. Although individual departments may choose to shape their curricula and research agendas around select aspects of the discipline, such institutional preferences should not be interpreted as a complete and comprehensive definition of the discipline.[7]

The CCUPEKA position paper summary emphasizes several issues central to physical activity:

- Health management should focus more on the prevention of negative health consequences due to a lack of physical activity and exercise. Exercise aimed at preventing or managing disease and injury has the potential to reduce health care costs by billions of dollars annually.
- The kinesiologist is an exercise expert trained to prescribe exercise as a preventive and rehabilitative intervention against disease and injury.
- The kinesiologist plays an integral role with the interprofessional health care/promotion team.
- Provinces should recognize kinesiologists in legislation as regulated health professionals, and by doing so acknowledge that the specialized nature of their education and training is integral to the interprofessional health care/promotion team.
- Relevant metrics should be developed to demonstrate the long-term health and economic benefits of integrating kinesiologists within the health care system.

Table 16.1 contains the scope of practice statements for kinesiologists and exercise physiologists within

**Table 16.1** | Scope of Practice Statements for the Kinesiologist and Exercise Physiologist

| PROVINCE | ORGANIZATION | PRACTICE STATEMENT |
| --- | --- | --- |
| Alberta | Alberta Kinesiology Association | *"Kinesiologists provide services through the application of the science of human movement and deliver quality solutions through prevention, objective assessment, and evidence-based intervention."* |
| British Columbia | British Columbia Kinesiology Association | *"Kinesiologists conduct fitness and human movement tests and assessments. They design and implement programs to maintain, rehabilitate, or enhance movement and performance in the areas of sports, recreation, work, and exercise."* |
| Manitoba | Transitional Council of the College of Kinesiologists of Manitoba | *"Kinesiologists promote and provide best practices in prevention, assessment, and intervention to enhance and maintain fitness, health and wellness, performance, and function, in the areas of sport, recreation, work, exercise, and activities of daily living."* |
| Newfoundland and Labrador | Newfoundland and Labrador Kinesiology Association | *"The practice of Kinesiology is the assessment of movement, performance, and function and the rehabilitation, prevention, and management of disorders to maintain, rehabilitate, and enhance movement, performance, and function, in the areas of sport, recreation, work, and exercise."* |
| Ontario | College of Kinesiologists of Ontario | *"The assessment of human movement and performance and its rehabilitation and management to maintain, rehabilitate, or enhance movement and performance."* |
| Ontario | Ontario Kinesiology Association | *"Kinesiologists are committed to enhancing quality of life through the promotion of physical activity and workplace health and safety, the prevention and management of injury and chronic disease, and the overall improvement of health and performance."* |
| Québec | Fédération des kinésiologues du Québec | *"Le kinésiologue évalue la dynamique du mouvement humain, et ses déterminants, d'une personne présentant ou non des facteurs personnels perturbés s'étalant de la dimension fonctionnelle à la haute performance selon des fondements biopsychosociaux. Il établit un plan d'intervention et en assure sa réalisation afin d'obtenir un rendement fonctionnel optimal incluant ses capacités d'adaptation/réadaptation dans une perspective de santé globale et l'acquisition de saines habitudes de vie durable."* |
| **The following provinces currently have Chapters of the CKA:** | | |
| Saskatchewan, Manitoba, Prince Edward Island, Nova Scotia, Yukon, Northwest Territories, Nunavut | Canadian Kinesiology Alliance | *Organization advocates for the profession of kinesiology in the areas of health promotion, clinical rehabilitation, ergonomics, health and safety, disability, and case management.* |
| All provinces | Canadian Society for Exercise Physiology | *"A CSEP-CEP\* performs assessments, prescribes conditioning exercise, as well as exercise supervision, counseling, and healthy lifestyle education in apparently healthy individuals and/or populations with medical conditions, functional limitations, or disabilities associated with musculoskeletal, cardiopulmonary, metabolic, neuromuscular, and aging conditions.*<br><br>*\*Certified Exercise Physiologist* |
| Kinesiology Act 2007 | Government of Ontario Ontario Regulation 401/12 | *"The assessment of human movement and performance and its rehabilitation and management to maintain, rehabilitate, or enhance movement and performance."* |

G. Bergeron et al., Council of University Physical Education and Kinesiology Administrators Position Statement: The Role of Kinesiologist and the Promotion of Physical Activity and Exercise in the Canadian Health Care System, 2014, www.ccupeka.ca/en/images/Position_Statement_-_Role_of_Kin_in_Health.pdf.

Canada, which are relevant to any country. The common kinesiology scope of practice definitions (from the various Canadian provinces) are much like the themes you have learned about throughout the topics covered in this text and the course and include the following:

*What?*—Study of human movement

*How?*—Physical activity and exercise prescription

*Why?*—Prevent, rehabilitate, and improve/enhance performance, health, and function

*With What?*—Biomechanics, anatomy, physiology, exercise psychology, or neuroscience

The CCUPEKA position paper represents a significant step forward in moving the field of kinesiology toward branding the scope of practice for practitioners and the importance of the integration of the subdisciplines.

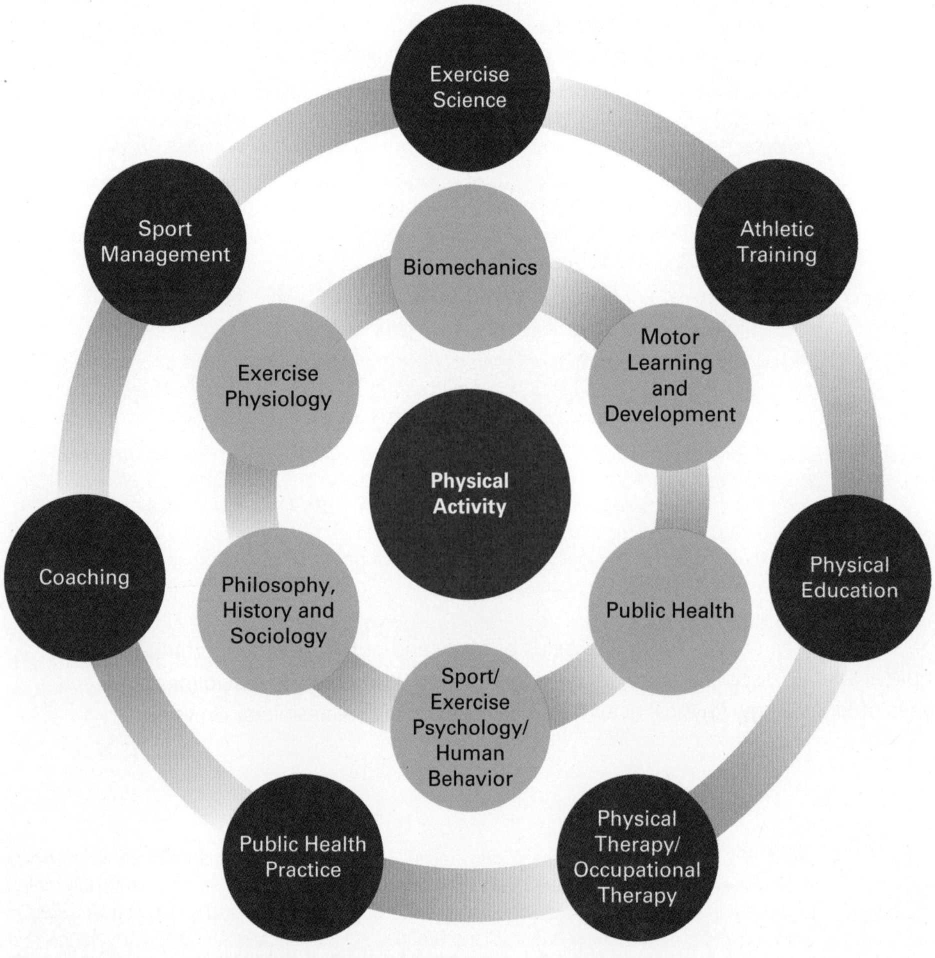

## Physical Activity Integration and Kinesiology

As you learned in Chapter 1, physical activity is everywhere, and kinesiology and its subdisciplines are unified and should help promote the science of physical activity and produce problem-solving products for society. The following section focuses on key messages from the textbook chapters regarding the importance of being able to integrate your kinesiology undergraduate KSAs into professional practice.

From Figures 1.1 and 1.4 (pages 6 and 11) you learned that all human movement involves physical activity. Physical activity can then be conceptualized as the center of kinesiology. In our model, the ring directly surrounding physical activity consists of six academic subdisciplines, or areas of specialization, all of which focus on some aspect of physical activity. The six areas of specialization—biomechanics; motor learning and development; public health; human behavior; philosophy, history, and sociology; and exercise physiology—provide the research and training core of kinesiology. These selected specialization areas link directly to the American Kinesiology Association's common core or knowledge base you learned about in Chapter 2, while the outer rings (or satellites) include "the practice" of kinesiology or selected career options. (See Figures 16.2 and 16.3.)

In Chapter 2, you learned that the AKA and other professional organizations and societies recommend that kinesiology majors be able to integrate KSAs acquired through undergraduate courswork. Your future career success is dependent on recognizing that physical activity and exercise are for everyone and that the field of kinesiology is continuing to expand regarding career opportunities to serve traditionally underserved populations.

Chapter 3 focused on evidence-based practice, which refers to a model in which

**Figure 16.2** | An Integrated Vision of Careers and Fields of Study in Kinesiology.
Fields of study (green spheres) are united around physical activity as the center of kinesiology. Red spheres (outer ring) indicate possible careers toward which various fields of study in kinesiology can lead.

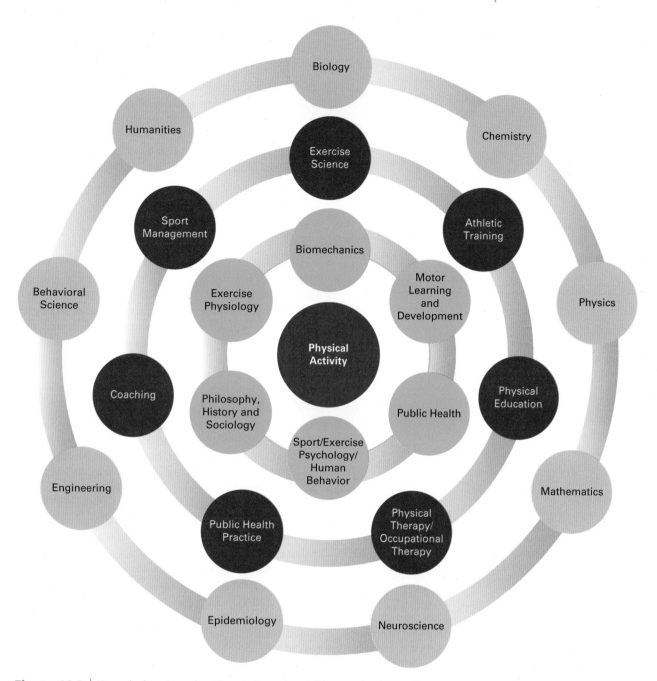

**Figure 16.3** | **Knowledge Base for Kinesiology.** In addition to the fields of study and potential careers, the kinesiology universe is highly influenced by multiple academic disciplines. The yellow spheres show the academic disciplines that inform the practice-based subdisciplines of kinesiology. Physical activity is the center of the "Kinesiology Universe."

clinical decisions are based on the best research knowledge or evidence available.[8] Evidence-based practice is essentially professional practice in which decisions are based on, or are informed by, the best available science. Your professional decisions in exercise and physical activity kinesiology practice should rely on the body of evidence, the big picture, rather than on random facts. You should strive to integrate evidence-based practices

into kinesiology. Use the scientific method to solve professional questions that you regularly encounter.

In Chapter 4 you learned to integrate physical activity as a continuum—from sedentary behavior (sleeping and sitting) to the intense exercise needed to train for marathon competition. The continuum includes the difficulty (intensity) of physical activity and the frequency with which the physical activity is performed (e.g., times per week), as well as the duration of an individual physical activity bout. Together the frequency, intensity, and duration of training represent the total volume of training. The dose of physical activity or exercise helps one determine the threshold for expected or desired health, physical fitness, and peak performance benefits. When training the body's systems with physical activity, you should also integrate three unifying training principles—overload, specificity, and adaptation—across the physical activity continuum.

In Chapters 5–8, you learned to integrate common health, physical fitness, and peak performance principles of physical activity and exercise within the following areas of the kinesiology knowledge base: aerobic physical activity, strength and conditioning, energy balance and body composition, and mental and psychological challenges. For each of these areas you learned the following:

» How to define and explain common terms and how they relate to health and human performance.

» How to justify the importance of understanding numerous physical activity principles in relationship to the various subdisciplines of kinesiology.

» How to describe and explain the specific health and performance benefits of participating in physical activities across the physical activity continuum and how the acquisition of the health benefits can influence the prevention and management of chronic diseases and affect longevity.

In Chapters 9–13, you learned to integrate common and current professional and occupational settings that are dependent upon acquired kinesiology-related discipline KSAs. Several of the sectors highlighted in the U.S. National Physical Activity Plan were summarized in relationship to the subdisciplines of kinesiology; these include the workplace (business and industry); leisure time, recreation, and personal training (community, recreation, and parks); schools (education); sports; transportation; and home environments (transportation, land use, and community design). For each of these areas, the following concepts were emphasized:

» How to define and explain the common terms associated with physical activity principles that promote health, physical fitness, and optimal human performance.

» How to justify the importance of understanding several occupational and professional settings with participation in physical activities integrating the various subdisciplines of kinesiology

» How to think about and implement effective strategies to describe and explain the specific health and human performance benefits for those who participate in physical activity programs in various occupational and professional settings in relationship to the physical activity continuum.

In the final Chapters 14–15, you learned how to integrate ethical decision making and the importance of developing a strong ethical base from which to operate. You also learned about leadership styles and the qualities associated with effective and ethical leadership. Specifically, you learned:

» How to define and explain the common terms associated with ethics and ethical leadership practices within the field of kinesiology.

» How to justify the importance of ethics, values, and leadership and explain their relationships with physical activity participation within the various subdisciplines of kinesiology.

» How to think about and implement effective strategies common to ethical practices and leadership that encompass all of kinesiology and its subdisciplines.

## Public Health and Kinesiology

Throughout this text, public health has been emphasized as a key subdiscipline in the field of kinesiology. This is a somewhat new development, but one that is fundamentally important to the future kinesiologist as well as to the field in general. Historically, kinesiology has focused on the study of human movement for performance—from elite athletic performance to rehabilitation services for people with a fundamental need to move more, such as cardiac or musculoskeletal rehabilitation. The historical vision of kinesiology is that it is a clinical specialty that focuses on responses, effects, and consequences of physical activity in individuals.

Public health involves the study of communities and populations. And a major part of public health involves prevention—doing what is necessary to stop a disease or disability from occurring in the first place rather than treating it once it develops. Physical activity is a key component of disease prevention across the life span, across populations, and across the world. It transcends gender, race, and ethnicity and even such important determinants of health as poverty and education. People who are more physically active are healthier and are more likely to live longer, fuller lives than their inactive peers.[9,10]

What images come to mind when you read the words "public health"? Screening children for nutritional deficiencies? Quarantine practices that isolate a tuberculosis patient to prevent the transmission of the bacteria to others? Disaster responses to prevent disease transmission during and after a hurricane or earthquake?

Immunizations for prevention of influenza? If you answered yes to any of these questions, then you are correct. Public health is all this and more. **Public health** seeks to promote and protect health and prevent disease and disability in defined populations and communities. An important future trend in kinesiology is the application of the principles covered in this text beyond the individual to populations.

Clearly, then, public health should be focused on problems that affect, or could affect, a substantial portion of the population of concern. Physical inactivity is very much a part of this picture. Worldwide, fewer than 30% of adults and approximately 80% of adolescents are physically active enough to enjoy the health benefits that come from the behavior.[11] This is why the problem of physical inactivity has been framed as a pandemic affecting the entire world.[12] Trends in urbanization (people moving from rural life to city life) and motorized transportation, particularly in developing countries, strongly suggest that physical activity associated with active transportation and jobs that require physical activity will continue to decline. How will this activity be replaced?

Moreover, from a population standpoint, physical inactivity has been identified as being every bit as important for health and disease development as cigarette smoking.[13] As seen in Figure 16.4, physical inactivity was responsible for more deaths in the world in 2008 than cigarette smoking or obesity. Annually, approximately 5.3 million deaths due to any cause can be attributed specifically to physical inactivity. Because tobacco use and (more recently) obesity have been framed as public health problems, it only makes sense that physical inactivity, given its prevalence throughout the world as well as its importance in determining the health of populations, should be an urgent public health issue. The well-prepared kinesiologist will understand this and, along with the clinical or individual view, understand the importance of work in populations as well.

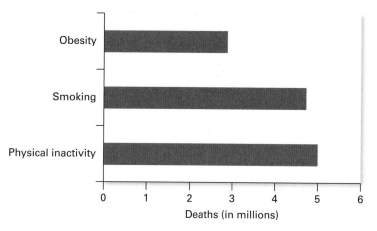

**Figure 16.4** | Global Mortality Burden of Physical Inactivity in 2008. Physical inactivity was responsible for more deaths in the world in 2008 than cigarette smoking or obesity.

*Source:* I. M. Lee et al., "Effect of Physical Inactivity on Major Non-Communicable Disease Worldwide: An Analysis of Burden of Disease and Life Expectancy," *The Lancet* 380, no. 9838 (2012): 219–229.

# THE FUTURE AND FINAL THOUGHTS

*In this final section of the text, we will use our crystal ball to focus on a few general topics that may help you frame your professional preparation for a career in kinesiology. This* *section provides tips for enhancing your resume/curriculum vitae, management of professional legal issues, continuing education, and lifelong learning.*

## Your Resume and Curriculum Vitae

In Chapter 2, you learned to search for items like resume development, writing cover letters, and interviewing tips at your university career services office or website. By now, you should have a basic resume, which many conceive to be a one-page document listing your academic credentials, work experience, collegiate experiences, volunteer activities, and awards/honors. References are often listed on a separate page or noted to be available upon request.

As you accomplish more professionally, you may find that your originally one-page resume will grow because you are adding new skills and accomplishments that require more categories. An expanded resume or **curriculum vitae** (several pages) reflects more of your life's work than a brief, standard resume and usually includes many additional categories such as grants, presentations, workshops, and publications.

To improve future professional opportunities, you should consider the following recommendations for making additions to your standard resume or for developing a curriculum vitae as you gain more experience and desire to acquire higher professional and leadership status:

1. Make sure you update your resume quarterly—think in terms of pushing yourself to professionally achieve new skills and accomplishments every three months (or, as stated in the business world, quarterly). Focus on acting scholarly by adding skills as a *teacher* (good leaders are good teachers), performing professional and/or community *service* (like serving on a professional or community organization board/staff), and *speaking* and/or *writing* (like presenting at a workshop or writing for a group newsletter).

2. Make sure you have a strong reference list of at least three professionals and three friends/colleagues with complete contact information (addresses, mobile numbers, email addresses). These individuals should know you well and be aware you are using them as references. Use your references to help you find your dream kinesiology job, as knowing key people always helps your chances even if you already have great experience. As you gain professional experience,

update your reference list regularly with top-credentialed professionals you work with to optimize your chance for advancement.

## Legal Issues

As a kinesiology professional, you will undoubtedly encounter some situations that increase your legal liability (such as working as a gymnastics instructor, conducting exercise tests on individuals with chronic disease, or organizing a mass participation event like a city 5K). It is important that you recognize your legal vulnerabilities and understand how you can protect yourself professionally by minimizing your legal risks. Most likely you will have an additional course or two in your undergraduate training that addresses legal issues related to kinesiology, but if you do not, you should seek professional advice to develop your own legal risk management plan. We have provided the following tips as a starting point:

1. Get to know the basics of kinesiology-related lawsuits in which there have been violations of contracts, failure to obtain informed consent (see Chapter 14; violation of sharing personal information), civil wrongs (torts) through acts of negligence or malpractice, and violations of national and international standards of care (policies, protocols, forms, and equipment).

2. Secure liability insurance to protect yourself from financial losses in the event of a lawsuit. Contact the leadership in your workplace to find out just what legal support you already have, and then discuss with your organization's counsel how you can minimize your professional liability.

## Continuing Education/Lifelong Learning

As a kinesiology professional, you should recognize that continuing education is often required (and at least preferred) to maintain or improve your professional employment status. You learned in Chapter 2 that there are many kinesiology certifications offered by professional organizations to enhance your academic training and professional development they can help you stay abreast of new changes in the field.

Another professional trend promoted by educational experts is **lifelong learning**, which is the acquisition of new KSAs related to personal, civic, social, and/or employment-related desires. By becoming a lifelong learner, you can challenge yourself to not only improve professionally but also become a better person and more globally informed.

Here are a few suggestions on how you can more effectively participate in continuing education/professional development experiences and lifelong learning:

1. Join a professional organization or society and attend local, regional, state, or national meetings. Joining will enable you to network with colleagues and learn new techniques and strategies. Remember, many organizations have discounted membership rates for students and encourage student involvement through incentives like scholarships. These experiences provide lifelong professional development, long-time personal friendships, and personal and professional fulfillment.

2. Volunteer to work with a professional organization or society so that you learn more about how professional groups function and how policies related to kinesiology are developed and implemented.

3. Challenge yourself to learn more about what interests you professionally as well as your personal hobbies or sidelines. By challenging yourself to continue to learn new things, you can expand your formal and informal learning experiences in a fun way and at your own pace.

## Local to Global Awareness

Kinesiology policies in the United States are influenced by international, national, state, regional, and local informal and formal rules and legislation. As you gain more professional experience, it will be important for you to further understand what determines various policies related to your professional role in kinesiology and how you can advocate for or against current and future polices. By having a local to global awareness spectrum, kinesiology professionals can more effectively influence policy changes that improve the delivery of their products and make their jobs more enjoyable. For example, the following groups have advocated policy statements to promote physical activity at various hierarchical levels:

▸ International level: The Toronto Charter
▸ National Level: The U.S. National Physical Activity Plan
▸ State level: The West Virginia Physical Activity Plan
▸ Local level: The Mayor's Fitness Council of San Antonio

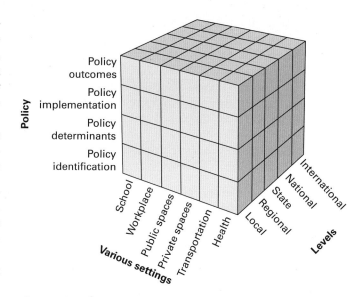

**Figure 16.5** | **Physical Activity Matrix.** Physical activity policies may impact the effective promotion or inhibition of physical activity in various settings (schools, workplace, and so on) and at various levels (local, regional, and so on).

*Source:* H. W. Kohl III and T. D. Murray, *Foundations of Physical Activity and Public Health* (Champaign, IL: Human Kinetics, 2012), 236.

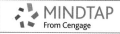

### Physical Activity Policy Statements: From International to Local

**Go to your MindTap course** to learn more about policy statements to promote physical activity at various hierarchical levels.

Physical activity policies that may impact the effective promotion or inhibition of physical activity in various settings (schools, the workplace, public spaces, private spaces, transportation, or health) at the local, regional, state, national, and international levels are shown in Figure 16.5. At the bottom-left corner of the cube, policies are initially identified (what they are and how they work); then they are evaluated to determine what they require and whether they are effective. Third, the effectiveness of the policy and the consequences of its implementation are determined. Finally, the outcomes of the policy—how it affects physical activity participation, either positively or negatively—are evaluated, and avenues for improving these outcomes are explored.

## Career Strategies and Tips

As with any professional or career choice, it is important to learn from those who preceded you and who have been successful. We have included the following 22 career strategies and tips as a final summary of items to consider as you prepare to enter the kinesiology profession or to move on after obtaining your undergraduate degree in kinesiology. Gene Del Vecchio, who is affiliated with University of Southern California's Marshall School of Business, is a widely known expert in marketing and entertainment who developed the list.[14] He is also a widely known author and draws from his more than 30 years of experiences to share this sound professional advice for your future:

1. **Discover the Career Trifecta:** Most never know what they are looking for in a career, and so they can't find it. The career you select should be one that you love, in which your skills will help you excel, that provides an income large enough to support the life you want to live. Sadly, many people achieve none of these. Some attain just one or two. When you attain all three, it is magic!

2. **Find a Rocket:** When searching for your career trifecta, pay close attention to industries that are growing, to premier growth companies within those industries, and to smart bosses who can teach you a lot and are destined to move upward. If you find a position that has all three, it greatly increases the odds that your career will blast off into the stratosphere.

3. **Own a Unique Expertise:** As your career advances, find an important niche within your industry where knowledge, products, and/or services are sorely lacking, and then deliver them well. Keep learning and advancing knowledge. You will become indispensable.

4. **Learn the Surrounding Disciplines:** If you are the marketing specialist, learn about finance. If you are the artist, learn the business side. This reveals the big picture, makes you more valuable, and helps you become management material.

5. **Be a Leader Before Anyone Expects It:** Early in your career, focus on the big stuff like company vision, objectives, and strategies. The more that your work helps your organization achieve the important things, the faster you will rise. Take the initiative, take ownership of projects, take responsibility, and have an optimistic can-do attitude. Others will follow.

6. **Exceed Expectations:** If your boss needs results by Friday, deliver them Thursday. If she asks for two good solutions for some challenge, give her four great ones. Over-delivering is key.

7. **Use Both Hemispheres of Your Brain:** Some use a rational approach to decision making. Others use more of an emotional/creative approach. Those who use both stand out.

8. **Make Your Contributions Known on the Inside:** If your boss does not know of your efforts, the work will not count. Sorry. You must find a way to make your contributions known. It could be as easy as issuing a weekly status report.

9. **Communicate Your Ideas to the World:** You must develop a reputation outside of your company's walls. Without that, you are invisible to the world. Speak at conferences, write for journals and blogs. The greater you expand your reach, the greater your opportunities.

10. **Take Measured Risks:** Fear is ever-present. It prevents you from many things like voicing your ideas or asking for a promotion. Defeat it. At worst, you will fail. That's no big deal. Babe Ruth is remembered for his 714 home runs and not for his 1,330 strike-outs.

11. **Network Before You Need It:** Success is 33% of what you know and 67% of who you know. Cultivate contacts early.

12. **Know Your Worth:** Search salaries online for jobs that are reflective of your experience. When a potential employer asks for your salary requirements, use the data. If you are currently underpaid in your current position, use the data to ask for more. The worst they can say is "no."

13. **Never Let Your Ego Outweigh Your Talent:** If your ego gets larger than your talent, you will eventually be fired. If your talent stays well above your ego, you will be cherished.

14. **Avoid Company Politics:** Don't disparage other employees. Ever! Because they will find out. Don't pick sides when others battle. Just be considerate of others, do good work for all, and make your contributions known.

15. **Keep Your Ears Open:** Companies are always making changes. It's advantageous to know what's ahead. Make friends with your CFO (central financial officer) and head of human resources. They know everything.

16. **Don't Suffer Demon Bosses:** If you cannot resolve problems through your own mediation, go to human resources or use outside means. When all else fails, quit. Life is too short. But always have an exit strategy. Interview even when you're happy because environments change.

17. **Hire People Better Than You:** Don't be intimidated by potential new hires who are better. Good underlings make you look good and free you up to do higher-level work. So hire those with skills you

# People Matter  Lynn Zhang, Assistant Director of Performance Nutrition*

**Q:** **Why and how did you get into the field of kinesiology?**

**A:** *The human body is an amazing machine. From the innate functions and mechanisms that fundamentally dictate how the body operates, to the capability of the body to learn and adapt, learning about how the body works is fascinating to me. I am a dietitian by trade and have become more involved in the kinesiology and exercise realm through working in athletics.*

**Q:** **What was the major influence on you to work in the field?**

**A:** *I currently work in a university athletic department. I had a bicultural upbringing that presented me with differences and challenges growing up; however, a topic commonly shared and understood among everyone was sports. Sport is universal and has the power to bring humankind together, despite all the differences and conflicts that exist across the globe. The power of sports has greatly impacted me and left me with a huge passion for what it can represent.*

**Q:** **What are your current research interests, and how do you translate your research results to practitioners?**

**A:** *I am currently a practitioner and do not work in research. However, part of my job does involve keeping up with the latest science, whether that be through reading journal articles or collaborating with our athletic*

*performance lab. Research regarding optimizing performance through nutrition (quantity, timing, ergogenic aids, etc.) are of primary interest.*

**Q:** **How do you stay physically active yourself and promote good health to others directly around you?**

**A:** *I stay physically active primarily by jogging a few times a week. I also do occasional workout videos at home. I promote good health through leading by example, as well as by working with individuals and discussing how healthy habits can support their personal goals.*

**Q:** **How have you had to integrate the subdisciplines of kinesiology in your professional practice?**

**A:** *As a performance dietitian, my job entails integrating nutrition and exercise. The relationship between the two go hand-in-hand, as both play fundamental, integrated roles in health and performance. Understanding the physiology and physical demands of each sport allows me to appropriately tailor nutrition regiments to best support health and activity levels.*

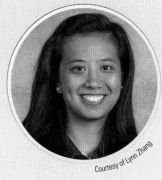
Courtesy of Lynn Zhang

*Lynn Zhang is an assistant director of performance nutrition for the University of Nebraska Athletic Department. She holds one-on-one nutrition meetings with student-athletes, provides her teams with nutrition education, and assists with menu selections. She also provides body composition analysis, hydration assessments, and supplement evaluation. The nutrition staff collaborates with strength and conditioning staff, athletic medicine staff, and team coaches to help student-athletes reach their goals.

---

lack. Good employees know that one of their tasks is to get you promoted.

18. **Remember What Mama Said:** Don't lie, cheat, steal, break promises, or engage in illegal activities. Your behavior is not invisible, nor is it forgotten when you are socializing with co-workers after work. Your reputation is never "off the clock."

19. **Mark the Moments You Enjoy:** All jobs are shiny when new. Then they get older and more dull. If 80% of your career tasks becomes mundane, focus on the 20% that still excite you. Mentally mark the moments.

20. **Manage Your Expectations:** In generations past, the primary objective of a job was to pay the bills. Many of today's students expect jobs to satisfy a grand lifestyle. Wake up, kids. You need to work your butt off to pay for that lifestyle. You still must pay your dues.

21. **Don't Be Afraid to Change Careers:** Most people do. What you thought was the trifecta in your twenties may not be the trifecta in your thirties. In later years, many people such as myself found great rewards not by finding new jobs but by creating them. It's immensely rewarding.

22. **Remember What Really Matters:** When in the trenches, it is easy for employees to succumb to mass hysteria because sales are down 1%, or because Baltimore didn't get its product shipment, or because the numbers sent to the CFO included errors. Just fix what you can and move on. My wife is a nurse and has worked primarily in labor and delivery. Any problems I have had on the job cannot compare to any one of the lives she has saved. When corporate panic strikes, put it into perspective.[15]

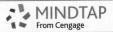

**Career Lesson for Grads**

**Go to your MindTap course** to complete an activity based on the list of career tips and strategies discussed here. You will find this activity in the "Take "Action" folder in MindTap.

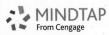

Now that you have completed this chapter, go to your MindTap course to complete all assigned activities. Check out the additional resources developed to help you apply the material in this chapter to your course and career goals.

# Chapter Summary

▸ You should be able to integrate the concepts of (1) physical activity in health, wellness, and quality of life; (2) scientific foundations of physical activity; (3) cultural, historical, and philosophical dimensions of physical activity; and (4) the practice of physical activity.

▸ "Kinesiology is the study of movement and how physical activity and physical fitness affect health, behavior, community, and quality of life." Although the field has its roots in physical education, today it includes many subdisciplines.

▸ The clinical practice of kinesiology includes the *What?* (study of human movement), the *How?* (physical activity and exercise prescription), the *Why?* (prevent, rehabilitate, and improve/enhance performance, health, and function), and the *With What?* (biome-chanics, anatomy, physiology, exercise psychology, or neuroscience).

▸ Physical activity is everywhere, and kinesiology and its subdisciplines are unified. They should help promote the science of physical activity and produce problem-solving products for society.

▸ Develop a concise but thorough resume or curriculum vitae and keep it updated quarterly with key references that continue to evolve during your career.

▸ Prepare yourself professionally to effectively reduce your legal liability risk as a practitioner and engage regularly in continuing education activities as well as lifelong learning activities.

▸ Develop a local to global awareness of how kinesiology policies influence physical activity opportunities for all populations.

# Remember This

American Kinesiology Association (AKA)

The Canadian Council of University Physical Education and Kinesiology

Administrators (CCUPEKA)
curriculum vitae

lifelong learning
public health

# For More Information

Access these websites for further study of topics covered in the chapter:

- Find updates and quick links to these and other evidence-based practice related sites in MindTap.

- Search for information about international physical activity policy recommendations at www.interamericanheart.org/images/PHYSICALACTIVITY/TorontoCharterPhysicalActivityENG.pdf

- Search for more information about the U.S. National Physical Activity Plan at www.physicalactivityplan.org.

- To learn more about state physical activity plans, see West Virginia's at www.wvphysicalactivity.org.

- To learn more about local city physical activity plans, see the Mayor's Fitness Council of San Antonio, TX, at www.fitcitysa.com.

- To learn more about legal liability protection, perform an Internet search using your favorite web search engine.

- To find career options in kinesiology, review the American Kinesiology Association website at www.americankinesiology.org.

# American Heart Association (AHA) and American Association of Cardiovascular and Pulmonary Rehabilitation (AACVPR)/ Guidelines for Physical Activity and Exercise Science Counseling

## Physical Activity Counseling

### Evaluation

▶ Assess current physical activity level (e.g., self-report or wearable device) and determine domestic, occupational, and recreational needs.

▶ Evaluate activities relevant to age, gender, and daily life, such as driving, sexual activity, sports, gardening, and household tasks.

▶ Assess readiness to change behavior, self-confidence, barriers to increased physical activity, and social support in making positive changes.

### Interventions

▶ Provide advice, support, and counseling about physical activity needs on initial evaluation and in follow-up. Target exercise program to meet individual needs (see Exercise Training section). Provide educational materials as part of counseling efforts. Consider exercise tolerance or simulated work testing for patients with heavy labor jobs.

▶ Consistently encourage patients to accumulate 30 to 60 minutes per day (150 minutes/week minimum) of moderate-intensity physical activity on five (preferably all) days of the week. Explore daily schedules to suggest how to incorporate increased physical activity into usual routine (e.g., parking farther away from building entrances, walking two flights of stairs, and walking during lunch break).

▶ Advise low-impact aerobic physical activity to minimize risk of musculoskeletal injury. Recommend gradual increases in the volume of physical activity over time.

▶ Caution patients to avoid performing unaccustomed vigorous physical activity (e.g., racquet sports and manual snow removal).

▶ Reassess the patient's ability to perform such activities as exercise training program progresses.

### Expected Outcomes

▶ Patient shows increased participation in leisure-time, occupational, transportation-related, and household physical activities.

▶ Patient shows improved psychosocial well-being, reduction in stress, facilitation of functional independence, prevention of disability, and enhancement of opportunities for independent self-care to achieve recommended goals.

▶ Patient shows improved aerobic fitness and body composition and reduced coronary risk factors (particularly for the sedentary patient who has adopted a lifestyle approach to regular physical activity).

## Exercise Training

### Evaluation

▶ Symptom-limited exercise testing (treadmill or bicycle) prior to participation in an exercise-based cardiac rehabilitation program is strongly recommended.

▶ The evaluation may be repeated as changes in clinical condition warrant. Test parameters should include heart function, perceived exertion, and exercise capacity.

▶ On the basis of patient assessment and the exercise test if performed, risk stratify the patient to determine the level of supervision and monitoring required during exercise training. Use risk stratification schema as recommended by the AHA and the AACVPR.

## Interventions

▸ Develop an individualized exercise prescription for aerobic and resistance training that is based on evaluation findings, risk factors for heart disease, comorbidities (e.g., peripheral arterial disease and musculoskeletal conditions), and patient and program goals.

▸ The exercise regimen should be reviewed by the program medical director or referring physician, modified if necessary, and approved. Exercise prescription should specify frequency, intensity, duration, type, and progression.

▸ For aerobic exercise: frequency of three to five days per week; intensity of 50% to 80% of exercise capacity; duration of 20 to 60 minutes; and type such as walking, treadmill, cycling, rowing, stair climbing, arm/leg ergometry, and others using continuous or interval training as appropriate.

▸ For resistance exercise: frequency of two to three days per week; intensity of 10 to 15 repetitions per set to moderate fatigue; duration of one to three sets of 8 to 10 different upper and lower body exercises; and type such as calisthenics, elastic bands, cuff/hand weights, dumbbells, free weights, wall pulleys, or weight machines.

▸ Include warm-up, cool-down, and flexibility exercises in each exercise session.

▸ Provide progressive updates to the exercise prescription and modify further if clinical status changes.

▸ Supplement the formal exercise regimen with activity guidelines as outlined in the Physical Activity Counseling section.

## Expected Outcomes

▸ Patient understands safety issues during exercise, including warning signs/symptoms.

▸ Patient achieves increased cardiorespiratory fitness and enhanced flexibility, muscular endurance, and strength.

▸ Patient achieves reduced symptoms, attenuated physiologic responses to physical challenges, and improved psychosocial well-being.

▸ Patient achieves reduced global cardiovascular risk resulting from an overall program of cardiac rehabilitation/secondary prevention that includes exercise training.

# Glossary

**1 RM**  One-repetition maximum is the maximum amount of weight one can lift or move one time. Sometimes used as an overall indicator of strength.

**Absenteeism**  Missing work, school, or other regular commitments due to illness or minor ailments which may be associated with unhealthy behaviors such as low levels of physical activity.

**Academic/professional honesty and integrity**  Ethical standards that support truth and the accurate dissemination of one's acquired professional knowledge, skills, and abilities.

**Acceleration**  Change in velocity over time.

**Accessibility**  Availability of resources for positive health promotion education and experiences.

**Action**  A Stage of Motivational Readiness in which an individual or population has become physically active at a minimum threshold (such as 150 minutes per week).

**Active transport**  Walking, cycling, or other human-powered methods (e.g., skate boarding) of transportation.

**Active travel**  Physical activity that helps a person to reach a destination.

**Adaptation principle**  How the body (muscles, tissues, organ systems) reacts over time to overload and specificity related to physical activity.

**Adjunct therapy**  A physical activity treatment modality that provides health benefits other than treating the disorder.

**Adverse events**  Undesired health events, such as musculoskeletal injures or heat-related illness.

**Aerobic**  Activities that depend on good heart/lung (cardiorespiratory) function and heavily on metabolic reactions in muscle cells that require large amounts of oxygen (hence the word "aerobic") and that allow an individual to reach steady state.

**Aerobic capacity**  A broad measure of a human's ability to work for several minutes and an indicator of how well the body is able to deliver oxygen and fuel to, and clear metabolic products from, working muscles.

**Affiliative (or team-building) behavior**  Behavior that builds upon the cohesiveness of the team by creating harmony among members through emphasizing emotional bonds among them.

**Affordable Care Act of 2010**  Federal legislation that prioritized the quality and efficiency of health care for all Americans, while improving attention to preventing chronic diseases and improving public health. Currently being reviewed by national legislators for repeal or modification.

**Age-related decline in cognitive function**  Gradual decreases in the ability to process, select, manipulate, or store information over time.

**Aging workforce**  Current trend in which U.S. employees are working longer than ever prior to retirement, thus increasing the average age of the workforce. An older employee population is at higher risk for work-related injuries (e.g., falls) and chronic diseases.

**American Kinesiology Association (AKA)**  A professional organization in the United States for which the purpose is to promote and enhance kinesiology as a unified field of study and advance its many professional applications.

**Anaerobic**  Activities that depend heavily on metabolic reactions (or bioenergetics) in muscle cells that do not require high levels of oxygen to provide chemical energy for movement.

**Anorexia nervosa**  Disordered eating characterized by limiting food intake and becoming excessively lean.

**Anxiety**  A condition of nervousness, uneasiness, or apprehension about a future event or events.

**Arousal**  The mental, emotional, and physiological state that prepares your body to engage in physical activity or exercise at peak levels (competition), related to the trait and state anxiety of competitors.

**Arterial-Venous Oxygen Difference (A-VO$_2$ diff)**  The amount of oxygen tissues (such as skeletal muscles) can extract or use from arterial blood and return to venous blood.

**Associate**  The action of an athlete focusing on their body's feedback (e.g., breathing, heart rate, muscle pain) during exercise and adjust their movements accordingly.

**Atrophy**  Loss of muscle strength and muscular endurance or other wasting due to disuse, disease, or both.

**Augmentation**  A physical activity treatment modality that uses other methods in addition to therapies, such as medication.

**Authoritarian leadership style**  A leadership style that places all decision-making, goal-setting, and policy-making power with the leader.

**Authority**  The ability to control, determine, and settle issues.

**Autonomy**  The freedom and independence an individual has to make her or his own decisions.

**Basal metabolic rate (BMR)**  A person's absolute minimal metabolic rate, measured at rest and under rigid, standardized conditions.

**Biomechanics**  The study of the relationship between physics and physical movement during sports and other physical activities.

**Biometric tests/health screenings**  Opportunities to assess clinical measures in large groups of people such as blood pressure, body composition, blood cholesterol, blood glucose, skin cancer risk, and others evaluated away from a traditional medical setting. Screening examinations are not intended to be diagnostic.

**Biostatistics**  The statistical methods applied to biomedical and public health research.

**Body composition**  A general term that refers to the body's content of fat, lean tissue, water, and minerals, usually presented as percentages.

**Body of evidence**  An accumulation of all the facts, usually developed with the scientific method, in a particular area.

**Built environment**  Human-constructed surroundings that are thought to positively or negatively affect physical activity opportunities.

**Bulimia nervosa** Disordered eating characterized by bingeing and purging.

**Business and industry or corporate culture** Norms or "how things get done" within a company. A particular set of attitudes or behaviors that define a company and how its employees work together.

**Business and industry or corporate image** The external or public perception of a company.

**Business sector** A part of the economy comprised of organizations designed to provide goods and/or services to consumers, governments, or other businesses.

**Canadian Council of University Physical Education and Kinesiology Administrators (CCUPEKA)** A professional organization developed to represent the administration of physical education and kinesiology programs at universities in Canada.

**Capital** Resources related to health and well-being.

**Cardiac output** The volume of blood being pumped by the heart in one minute. Calculated as heart rate (HR) × stroke volume (SV), and measured in liters/minute.

**Charismatic behavior** The energetic and powerful behavior that influences and motivates group members simply through the charm and personality of the leader.

**Classroom-based physical activity breaks** All activity, regardless of intensity, performed in the classroom during normal classroom time.

**Coaching** According to Cote and Gilbert[1]: "The consistent application of integrated professional, interpersonal, and intrapersonal knowledge to improve athletes' competence, confidence, connection, and character in specific coaching contexts".

**Coaching behavior** Behavior that allows the leader to act as a teacher for individual group members.

**Commanding behavior** The classic military behavior of giving orders and expecting group members to follow them without question.

**Comprehensive worksite health promotion program** Includes health-related programming, implementation of health-related policies, health benefits package (insurance plus other services or discounts regarding health), and environmental supports that promote health and physical activity.

**Concussion** A type of traumatic brain injury (TBI) caused by a bump, blow, or jolt to the head, with or without loss of consciousness, that can change the way the brain normally works.

**Conditioning** The persistent physiological changes or adjustments resulting from training or training adaptation.

**Confidentiality** Duties (moral and legal obligations or responsibilities) that kinesiology professionals must perform when working with individuals or groups to maintain patient and/or client privacy.

**Conflict of interest** A situation where multiple interests (financial, professional, social, etc.) might overlap to bias decision-making.

**Contemplation** A Stage of Motivational Readiness in which an individual or population is starting to think about being physically active but has not started the process.

**Cost-benefit ratios** Ratios that represent the dollars saved—or "earned"—for each dollar spent.

**Cost-effectiveness evaluation** Evaluation that involves determining if the program costs and potential income (if applicable) are appropriate or might be improved with alternative approaches.

**Culture of health and physical activity** Norms regarding how an organization promotes health and physical activity to its employees or members and recognizes the benefits of a healthy environment.

**Curriculum vitae** An expanded résumé that reflects more of one's life's work than a brief, standard resume and usually includes many additional categories such as grants, presentations, workshops, and publications.

**Decisional balance** A person's ability to weigh the pros and cons of being physically active and to take action based on that balance.

**Delayed onset muscle soreness (DOMS)** Muscular soreness and/or stiffness that arises 24 to 48 hours after participation in physical activity unusual (in intensity, duration, mode) than one is unaccustomed to.

**Democratic leadership style** A leadership style that allows the group members to participate in the decision-making process, give input into the direction of the project, and voice their expertise to solve problems as they arise.

**Deontological ethics** Belief that the moral principles expressed by the group are universally accepted, concrete guidelines that prescribe acceptable behavior and elicit fair decisions and practice for the whole of the society.

**Depression** A mental state that can cause difficulty concentrating and making decisions, loss of interest in hobbies and activities, feelings of hopelessness and helplessness, insomnia, and even thoughts of suicide.

**Detraining** The negative physiological, psychological, and biomechanical effects of extended periods without physical activity.

**Disassociate** When athletes ignore or suppress their body's feedback during exhaustive exercise.

**Disclaimers** Oral and/or written statements that provide disclosures about legal or other links to professional advice, specific technique promotion, or product endorsement.

**Disclosure** The act of admission or revelation that if you are providing professional advice, promoting a technique, or endorsing a product you may or may not have personal interests that benefit yourself monetarily or professionally.

**Dose** Amount or volume of physical activity or exercise including frequency, intensity, and duration.

**Drive theory** A theory that suggests that the more a coach or kinesiology practitioner motivates a competitor, the higher that competitor's arousal and, therefore, the better her or his performance will be.

**Duration** The length in time of a specific physical activity or exercise event.

**Dynamic exercise** Activities that depend on both aerobic and anaerobic pathways and involve concentric (shortening) and eccentric (lengthening) through a large range of motion around major skeletal joints.

**Economy** The quantification of energy utilization during exercise. It is usually measured as oxygen cost (used) at given speed or workload.

**Emotional capital** The mental health and psychological benefits of regular participation in physical activity and exercise.

**Employee health insurance** Employer-subsidized health insurance.

**Employee recruitment** The process of searching, recruiting, screening, and hiring of new employees.

**Employee retention** Retention of current employees in the workforce.

**Ends-situation argument** An ethical argument that an individual makes when no accepted rule applies to a situation, and therefore the facts of the situation must be weighed against the outcome of the decision for what is best for the majority of those impacted by the final decision.

**Energy balance**   The relationships among energy intake (the calories provided by the foods and beverages you eat and drink each day), energy expenditure (the calories you burn each day), and energy storage associated with the maintenance of body weight.

**Environmental health**   The field of study that is used to assess the role that the physical environment and environmental characteristics play in health and health indicators.

**Epidemiology**   The study of the distribution and determinants of disease, disability, and health characteristics in a population. Epidemiology is the basic science of public health.

**Ergonomics**   Scientific study of how humans interact with design features of systems, products, and processes.

**Essential fat**   The amount of fat necessary for normal body function and good health.

**Ethics**   The moral principles that a group or society recognizes and adopts as rules of acceptable conduct.

**Eustress**   Normal, everyday stress.

**Evidence-based practice (EBP)**   A model in which clinical decisions are based on the integration of the best research knowledge or evidence available.

**Exercise**   A specific type of physical activity that is planned, repetitive, and done for a specific purpose.

**Exercise order**   Varying the sequence of exercises for a specific training outcome, such as starting with smaller muscle mass recruitment followed by recruitment of larger muscle mass groups to reduce the rate of muscular fatigue, especially for beginners.

**Exercise physiology**   The study of the physiological/biological responses to physical activity and the effects of these responses on biological adaptations that occur with acute and chronic exercise.

**Exercise type**   The type or mode of exercise such as aerobic, anaerobic, static, or dynamic. Exercise type selection determines the amount of muscle mass required to perform physical activities.

**Extrinsic motivation**   External input, such as encouragement from a coach or kinesiology practitioner or incentives such as a trophy or cash to improve performance.

**Fads**   Activities that produce high levels of individual and group enthusiasm for brief periods of time.

**Fast twitch**   Muscle fibers that are primarily anaerobic and highly related to speed and strength performance.

**Feedback**   Knowledge about the results of an individual's performance including suggestions for improvement.

**FICK equation**   A method used to calculate maximal oxygen uptake. Maximal Oxygen Uptake ($VO_2$ max) = (Maximal Heart Rate × Stroke Volume) × Arterial-Venous Oxygen Difference

**Financial capital**   Job success and productivity and lower health care costs associated with regular participation in physical activity and exercise.

**Fitness test**   Usually a field-based method to estimate cardiorespiratory or musculoskeletal fitness. Sometimes included with biometric testing, fitness test assessments may be offered to employees or students and can vary based on the physical activity continuum and the population.

**Flexibility**   The amount of movement (range of motion) around a joint that a person can achieve and involves muscles and connective tissue such as tendons and ligaments.

**Formative evaluation**   An evaluation process where feedback is given at every step. Determining the needs, utility, and design features of a physical activity program.

**Frequency**   The number of occasions (or bouts) of physical activity that occur within a unit of time.

**Functional abilities**   Abilities such as physical movement for self-care, transportation, walking, and preventing avoidable falls.

**Functional health**   The ability to maintain health and wellness by reducing or controlling your health problems and maintaining your physical independence through functional abilities.

**Games**   According to Woods[2]: Forms of play "that have greater structure and are competitive. Games have clear participation goals … [and] are governed by informal or formal rules".

**General adaptation syndrome (GAS)**   Stress (psychological, physiological, or environmental) causes numerous physiological reactions beyond rest or homeostasis.

**Graded exercise testing (GXT)**   Clinical testing for cardiorespiratory fitness and heart disease risk screening.

**Health**   According to the Wolrd Health Organization[3]: "A state of complete physical, mental and social well-being, and not merely the absence of disease".

**Health-related fitness**   Fitness attributes that are related to improved health. Health-related fitness includes cardiorespiratory endurance, muscular strength, muscular endurance, and flexibility.

**Health risk appraisals (HRAs)**   Screening tools used to help identify health risks in individuals. HRAs can be used for baseline data and reviewed over time to track changes in health risks.

**Healthy weight**   For adults, a BMI of 18.5 to 24.9.

**Helsinki Declaration**   A set of ethical principles used to guide scientific study of humans. Developed in 1964 by the World Medical Association, it further explained and expanded upon the tenets of the 1947 Nuremberg Code.

**Homeostasis**   A condition of constancy in a biologic system. Often refers to equilibrium while sitting at rest.

**Human behavior**   A study area that incorporates the traditional kinesiology study areas of sport/exercise psychology as well as behavioral science for changes in physical activity.

**Human Capital Model (HCM)**   Participation in and socialization through physical activity contribute holistically to the development of positive individual and population attributes; these attributes, in turn, can yield successful societal investments such as well-being, economic worth, academic achievement, and so on.

**Hyperplasia**   Increase in the number of cells (such as fibers in a muscle) in an organ.

**Hypertrophy**   Increase in the overall size of the muscle fiber and mass of a muscle.

**Imagery**   The ability of a person to create or recreate in his or her mind a physical activity, exercise or sport performance experience.

**Individual capital**   The positive character developmental factors associated with regular participation in physical activity and exercise.

**Individual point theory**   A theory that suggests that a coach or kinesiology practitioner needs to tailor motivation and feedback to the needs of each individual he or she works with to optimize arousal levels for peak performance.

**Industry**   According to Pronk[4]: "A separate economic subdivision, is involved in activities related to the creation of finished products as the result of the manufacturing of raw materials into goods and products".

**Informed consent**   The permission granted by a participant in a research study for the researcher to conduct the research only after a full description of the research.

**Institutional Review Board (IRB)**   An independent committee that is designed to oversee all aspects of human and/or animal research.

**Integrity**   The quality of being honest and truthful. Integrity is based on value systems and on consistency and accuracy.

**Intellectual capital**   The cognitive developmental, academic, and educational gains associated with regular participation in physical activity and exercise.

**Intensity**   The amount of work that a single session of physical activity or exercise requires.

**Intervals**   Activities that require participation in a high-intensity (more anaerobic than aerobic) bout of activity followed by participation in a lower-intensity (more aerobic than anaerobic) bout of activity, or vice versa.

**Intrinsic motivation**   Internal input that provides feelings of pleasure and success.

**Inverted U theory**   A theory that suggests that individuals reach an optimal level of arousal, beyond which their arousal levels drop off and their peak performance decreases.

**Isokinetic**   Muscle contractions that are dynamic, work-producing movements that include concentric and eccentric components at a constant speed and are performed through a large range of motion.

**Isolated facts**   Ideas and concepts that tend to generalize simple solutions to complex problems.

**Kilocalories (kcal) (Calories)**   A common unit of measure of energy.

**Kinesiology**   The scientific study of movement.

**Knowledge base of kinesiology**
According to Lawson[5]: (Integration) "of information gained through experiencing physical activity, through professional application, and through multidimensional scholarly approaches to the study of physical activity—biological, medical, and health-related aspects, psychological and social-humanistic".

**Knowledge of performance (KP)**   How a movement felt or what observers said about it.

**Knowledge of results (KR)**   Personal interpretation or official ruling.

**Laissez-faire leader**   A leader who uses a hands-off approach when interacting with a group and allows the group to make all decisions.

**Leadership**   The process used to lead, direct, and influence a group to reach a common goal or outcome.

**Leisure time physical activity**
Participation during discretionary time in exercise, recreation, or hobbies that are not part of essential activities such as one's occupation, school or household work, or transportation.

**Licensure**   Granting of a license to practice.

**Lifelong learning**   The acquisition of new KSAs (Knowledge, Skills, Abilities) related to personal, civic, social, and/or employment-related desires.

**Load (intensity)**   The amount of weight one lifts or resistance one moves against, the number of repetitions of the exercise performed, and the number of sets of the strength and conditioning activity performed.

**Logic models**   Frameworks that provide an integrated approach with which to plan, implement, evaluate, and report interventions requiring accountability.

**Maintaining weight**   A weight change in a given unit of time of less than 3% (gain or loss).

**Maintenance**   A Stage of Motivational Readiness in which an individual or population has remained physically active for at least six months.

**Maximal heart rate (MHR)**   The highest heart rate that an individual can attain during vigorous physical activity. Rarely measured, maximal heart rate (HR) in beats per minute can be estimated by subtracting your age (in years) from 220.

**Maximal oxygen uptake or VO₂ max**
One's maximum capacity for using oxygen at peak or maximal intensities of physical activity.

**Means-situation argument**   An ethical argument that an individual makes when the situation is unique and no accepted rule applies; therefore, the facts of the situation must be weighed against what is morally acceptable to all within the community and not just with the majority.

**Mental health**   A state of well-being in which every individual realizes his or her own potential, can cope with the normal stress of life, can work productively and fruitfully, and is able to make a contribution to her or his community.

**Metabolic equivalent of task (MET)**
The typically used unit of measure for energy expenditure. 1 MET is equivalent to energy expenditure sitting quietly at rest.

**Metabolic syndrome**   A syndrome that includes combinations or clustering of factors such as hypertension, abnormal blood lipids–fats, abnormal glucose or insulin levels, and increased waist girth that are associated with chronic diseases such as coronary heart disease and diabetes.

**Moderate-intensity physical activity**
Physical movements that require 3 to 5.9 METs of energy expenditure.

**Monotherapy**   A physical activity treatment modality that includes only treatment.

**Motor behavior**   The learning and performance of coordinated movement resulting from the combination of motor learning, motor control, and motor development.

**Motor control**   Process of the brain and one's cognition to activate and coordinate muscles performing various movement skills.

**Motor development**   The study of changes in motor behavior over time or the lifespan.

**Motor learning**   The study of the relationship between neural sciences and biology as it applies to physical movement during sports and physical activity, and methods to produce permanent changes that will enhance these movements.

**Motor unit**   The basic unit of skeletal muscle contraction and includes a motor nerve and all the fibers that it controls.

**Muscle dysmorphia**   A preoccupation with muscularity.

**Muscular strength**   The maximum force that a person can generate one time at a given speed.

**Obesity**   The accumulation of excess fat mass that can be detrimental to health. For adults, obesity is classified as a BMI > 30.0 kg/m².

**Osteoarthritis**   A form of arthritis characterized by breakdown of cartilage and bone, and associated with lasting stiffness and swelling of joints.

**Osteoporosis**   Low bone density associated with loss of bone minerals.

**Outcome evaluation**   Evaluation that involves determining the direct impact of the programming on physical activity.

**Overload principle**   Increasing the dose of physical activity and exercise to stress the body's physiologic systems beyond normal homeostasis (rest) in order to improve function.

**Overtraining**   When stress of physical activity or exercise persists long enough or with a great enough intensity that the individual begins to experience a decline in performance.

**Overweight**   For adults, a BMI of 25 to 29.9 kg/m².

**Pacesetting behavior**   Behavior that allows the leader to set the standards of performance for the group.

**Pedagogy**   The art and science of teaching.

**Personal training**   An occupation in which fitness professionals, usually with an academic training background in kinesiology and national professional certification, teach and coach individuals and groups how to achieve functional health, improved levels of physical fitness, high levels of performance fitness, wellness, and adopt other healthy behaviors.

**Physical activity**   Any bodily movement that results in energy expenditure.

**Physical activity continuum**   A possible progression (and regression) of movement of individuals or populations from sedentary behaviors (physical inactivity) toward functional health, then goal-specific physical fitness outcomes (such as weight loss, improved cardiorespiratory fitness, or others), and ultimately, if desired, toward peak performance.

**Physical capital**   The direct benefits of participating regularly in physical activity and exercise and the prevention/treatment effects of physical activity on disease processes.

**Physical culture**   A social movement with its origins in the 1800s designed to promote wellness with physical activity as a cornerstone.

**Physical activity energy expenditure (PAEE)**   Energy expenditure resulting from physical activity, as opposed to metabolism. Includes daily activities such as exercising and bathing, as well as additional physical work one may do.

**Physical education**   A formal, standards-based content area of study in schools that encompasses assessment according to standards and benchmarks.

**Physical fitness**   A set of measurable physiological parameters related to health and/or increased levels of physical activity and peak performance.

**Plagiarism**   Taking the work of others and passing it on as one's own.

**Play**   According to Woods[6]: A "free activity that involves exploration, self-expression, dreaming, and pretending".

**Point-of-decision prompting**   A scientifically proven strategy for physical activity promotion designed to help a person select the more active choice at the point when an active choice can be made.

**Power**   Work per unit of time.

**Precontemplation**   A Stage of Motivational Readiness in which an individual or population is not even thinking about being physically active.

**Preparation**   A Stage of Motivational Readiness in which an individual or population has started making small changes in behavior toward becoming physically active.

**Prepartication physical exam**   A brief physical exam that a student must take before participating in school-based sports, often required by state law and administered, at least in part, by a physician.

**Presenteeism**   Nonproductivity due to working while sick or covering job related tasks of others who are unable to be present due to illness or other employee leave considerations.

**Prevention of weight re-gain**   Less than 5% of weight loss is regained over a period of time.

**Primary prevention**   Efforts to prevent a condition or disease outcome from emerging by affecting its precursors (like normalizing or lowering blood pressure with regular participation in physical activity).

**Primordial prevention**   Efforts to prevent disease precursors from manifesting, and therefore preventing disease from occurring. The most basic level of disease prevention.

**Process evaluation**   Evaluation that focuses on the quality of the program and delivery options.

**Productivity**   Effective employee performance associated with a healthy and motivated individual.

**Professional certification**   Documentation that you possess the essential knowledge, skills, and abilities—KSAs (Knowledge, Skills, Abilities)—to perform a specific job.

**Profile of Mood States (POMS)**   A tool in human behavior studies used to measure transient mood states.

**Proprioceptors**   Body position receptors in the nervous system.

**Psychological distress**   Mental stressors that are not congruous with good health or well-being.

**Public health**   The science and practice of protecting, promoting, and improving the health of populations and communities.

**Recess**   The time of day set aside for students to take a break from their class work, engage in play with their peers, and take part in independent, unstructured activities.

**Recreation**   That part of the time spent in leisure and is associated with fun, enjoyment, and pleasure.

**Rehabilitation**   The fifth area where kinesiology is related to treatment of conditions designed to promote recovery from disease or disability.

**Relapse**   A Stage of Motivational Readiness where an individual or population has stopped participating in physical activity after starting, which is commonly due to factors such as illness, injury, or vacations, but may also be due to other, preventable barriers.

**Resting metabolic rate (RMR)**   Metabolism occurring at rest. For a 70-kg person, approximately 1 kcal/minute while sitting or about 1,440 kcal per 24 hours.

**Restoration**   The process (including strategies) recovering from participation in physical activities.

**Rules-end argument**   An ethical argument or decision that an individual makes when a specific rule applies to the situation and how that rule will impact the majority of the people affected by the decision.

**Rules-means decision**   An ethical argument that an individual makes when a specific rule applies to the situation and how that rule affects the outcome of what is morally acceptable to all in the community.

**Sarcopenia**   Loss of mainly fast twitch muscle fibers and reduced size of muscle fibers.

**Scientific method**   A systematic process for testing hypotheses and acquiring new knowledge.

**Secondary prevention**   A focus on individuals rather than populations and acts to prevent progression of a disease condition after it has been detected.

**Self-confidence**   One's self-assurance regarding one's personal judgments.

**Self-efficacy**   One's confidence in performing specific skills.

**Self-esteem**   One's response to others and what one hears from those in one's social network; feelings of self-worth and value that can positively influence mental health.

**Self-talk cues**   Mental skills that allow athletes both to associate and to disassociate.

**Situational ethics**   Recognizes the deontological ethics or rules of the group but accepts that certain situations might require interpretation based upon the virtue of the consequences or outcomes specific to the situation.

**Skill-related fitness**   Attributes that are the most important for successful movement and sports participation (like speed, strength, muscular endurance, agility, balance, and others).

**SLOTH model**   Sleep, leisure-time, occupation, transportation, and home-based activities.

**Slow twitch**   Muscle fibers that are primarily aerobic and fatigue resistant. Slow twitch muscle fibers are mainly recruited for endurance physical activities.

**Social capital**   The effects related to interactions with people and groups during regular participation in physical activity and exercise experiences.

**Social support**   Perception and/or reality that one is cared for and is receiving assistance to overcome health challenges.

**Special populations**   Those individuals who have either acute or chronic conditions that limit or require modifications to standard physical activity practices.

**Specificity principle**   Training adaptations are very specific and directly related to the imposed demands on the body.

**Sport and exercise psychology**   The study of psychology in relation to sports performance and physical activity.

**Sport management**   The organization of educational and business aspects of sports and sports-related physical activities.

**Sports**   A specialized or higher order of play or games with special characteristics.

**State anxiety**   A person's existing or current emotional state, which can be situational and can change quickly.

**Static exercise (isometric exercise)**   Physical activities that rely primarily on the anaerobic metabolic pathways. Muscles contract and increase force, with little range of motion.

**Steady state**   Working at a level at which your heart and lungs can deliver adequate oxygen through the blood stream to meet the demands for oxygen by the working muscles.

**Stroke volume (SV)**   The amount of blood pumped per beat of your heart in milliliters/minute.

**Subcutaneous fat**   The layer of fat cells just under the skin.

**Surveillance**   The ongoing, systematic collection, analysis, and interpretation (e.g., regarding physical activity, risk factors, or health events) essential to planning, implementation, and evaluation of public health.

**Systems approach**   In kinesiology, the realization and tactics to understand that physical activity behavior in individuals is part of an open "system" that includes environment, policy, and unknown barriers.

**Teleological ethics**   Moral ambiguity exists within society and no behavior is inherently wrong but rather the amount of good the behavior produces determines whether it is morally right.

**Termination/adoption**   An individual or population is successful at adopting regular physical activity or terminates the behavior.

**Tertiary prevention**   Improving or maintaining quality of life for people with diseases, their complications, and disabilities.

**Thermic effect of food (TEF)**   Energy required to absorb, digest, and metabolize food.

**Total energy expenditure (TEE)**   (1) Your resting metabolic rate (RMR; for a 70-kg person, approximately 1 kcal/minute while sitting or about 1,440 kcal per 24 hours), (2) the thermic effect of food (TEF; energy required to absorb, digest, and metabolize food) for your diet, and (3) your physical activity energy expenditure (PAEE) that includes daily activities like bathing, as well as additional physical work you may do.

**Training**   A consistent or chronic progression of exercise sessions designed to improve physiologic function for better health or sports performance.

**Training principles**   Fundamental guidelines that form the basis for training the body's systems with physical activity.

**Trait anxiety**   A broad pattern of anxiety that reflects a person's personality, which is more long term and usually more stable.

**Transtheoretical model (Stages of Change model)**   A behavior change theory is used to assess a person's initial readiness to make a change and then is used to help deliver a "stage" appropriate intervention.

**Traumatic brain injury (TBI)**   For this text, an externally oriented injury to the brain associated with participation in physical activity (like a concussion).

**Trends**   Physical activity developments or changes that appear to be sustained over several years.

**Understudied populations**   Groups who have not been scientifically studied as extensively as others.

**Underweight**   For adults, those with a BMI < 18.5.

**Values**   The ideals, customs, and institutions that a society or a group uses as guidelines for living.

**Vigorous-intensity physical activity**   Physical movements that require more than 6 METs of energy expenditure.

**Visceral fat**   Fat that surrounds vital organs, such as the stomach in the abdominal area.

**Visionary behavior**   Leadership behavior that directs the group through clear articulation of the innovation involved and vision of what the specific project will produce.

**Volume of physical activity**   The total calories burned; V (volume) = F (frequency) $\times$ I (intensity) $\times$ D (duration).

**Walkability**   The extent to which an area of the built or physical environment is conducive to walking. In relation to school transportation, a term that encompasses specific features such as directness of the route to school, sidewalk infrastructure, and greater intersection and residential density.

**Walking school bus**   A form of active transport that often entails one or two adult volunteers escorting a group of children from pick-up points (walking school bus stops) or their homes to school along a fixed route, starting with the pick-up point or home that is farthest from the school and stopping at other pick-up points or homes along the way.

**Wearables**   Consumer devices useful to begin to increase and monitor physical activity. Wearables are useful for tracking steps per day in order to monitor physical activity over time and are often used as incentives for challenges among different subgroups of workers.

**Weight loss**   A loss of at least 5% of initial body weight over a defined period of time.

**Wellness**   A concept redesigned in the 1980s to describe the constant and deliberate efforts to stay healthy in the following domains: physical, emotional, mental, social, environmental, occupational, and spiritual.

**Worker's compensation costs (WCC)**   Costs of work-related injuries or incidences that are preventable (not all are) and due to unhealthy behaviors.

**Worksite health care costs**   Health care costs for the workplace associated with modifiable unhealthy behaviors such as low levels of physical activity, tobacco use, and obesity.

**Worksite health promotion or wellness program**   Various education and participation activities that a worksite implements to promote healthy lifestyles for employees and their families and produce a healthier workforce.

# References

## Preface

1. P. Freedson, "Back to the Future: Reflecting on the Past and Envisioning the Future for Kinesiology Research," *Kinesiology Review*, 3 (2014): 1–3.

2. H. Lawson, "The American Kinesiology Association and the Future of Kinesiology—American Kinesiology Association White Papers," accessed January 11, 2016, www.americankinesiology.org/white-papers/white-papers/.

## Chapter 1

1. C. J. Caspersen and K. E. Powell, "Physical Activity, Exercise, and Physical Fitness: Definitions and Distinctions for Health-Related Research," *Public Health Reports* 100 (1985): 126–131.

2. J. N. Morris et al., "Coronary Heart Disease and Physical Activity of Work," *The Lancet* 265 (1953): 1053–1057, 1111–1120.

3. I. M. Lee et al., "Effect of Physical Inactivity on Major Non-Communicable Diseases Worldwide: An Analysis of Burden of Disease and Life Expectancy," *The Lancet* 380, no. 9838 (2012): 219–229.

4. H. W. Kohl III et al., "The Pandemic of Physical Activity: Global Action for Public Health," *The Lancet* 380, no. 9838 (2012): 295–305.

5. P. Freedson, "Back to the Future: Reflecting on the Past and Envisioning the Future for Kinesiology Research," *Kinesiology Review* 3 no. 1 (2014): 1–105.

6. J. Mausner and A. K. Bahn, *Epidemiology: An Introductory Text* (Philadelphia, PA: W. B. Saunders, 1974).

7. World Health Organization, "A Comprehensive Global Monitoring Framework and Voluntary Global Targets for the Prevention and Control of NCDs," December, 2011, accessed April 4, 2016, www.who.int.

8. J. F. Sallis et al., "Co-Benefits of Designing Communities for Active Living: An Exploration of Literature," *The International Journal of Behavioral Nutrition and Physical Activity* 12 (2015): 30, doi:10.1186/s12966-015-0188-2.

9. N. Palmateer et al., "Evidence for the Effectiveness of Sterile Injecting Equipment Provision in Preventing Hepatitis C and Human Immunodeficiency Virus Transmission among Injecting Drug Users: A Review of Reviews," *Addiction* 105 (2010): 844–859.

10. D. L. Gill, "Integration: The Key to Sustaining Kinesiology in Higher Education," *Quest* 59 (2007): 270–286.

11. J. F. Sallis et al., "Physical Education's Role in Public Health: Step Forward and Backward over 20 Years and HOPE for the Future," *Research Quarterly for Exercise and Sport* 83, no. 2 (2012): 125–135.

## Chapter 2

1. H. A. Lawson, "Renewing the Core Curriculum," *Quest* 59 (2007): 219–243.

2. T. G. Reeve, "Core Knowledge Competencies, Learning Outcomes and Assessment." Paper presented at the meeting of the American Kinesiology Association, Orlando FL, February 2009.

3. P. R. Cavanagh and R. Kram, "The Efficiency of Human Movement: A Statement of the Problem," *Medicine and Science in Sports and Exercise* 17 (1985): 304–308.

4. P. B. Raven et al., *Exercise Physiology: An Integrated Approach* (Cengage Learning, 2013).

5. W. E. Amonette, K. L. English, and K. J. Ottenbacher, "Nullius in Verba: A Call for the Incorporation of Evidence-Based Practice into the Discipline of Exercise Science," *Sports Medicine* 40 (2010): 449–457.

6. A. Bauman, N. Murphy, and V. Matsudo, "Is a Population-Level Physical Activity Legacy of the London 2012 Olympics Likely?" *Journal of Physical Activity and Health* 10 (2012): 1–4.

7. J. Berryman, "The Tradition of the 'Six Things Non-Natural': Exercise and Medicine from Hippocrates through Ante-Bellum America," *Exercise & Sports Science Reviews* 17 (1989): 515–559.

8. SHAPE America, Society of Health and Physical Educators, "National Standards for K-12 Physical Education," accessed April 9, 2016, www.shapeamerica.org/standards/pe.

9. J. Ivy, "Exercise Physiology: A Brief History and Recommendations Regarding Content Requirements for the Kinesiology Major," *Quest* 59 (2007): 34–41.

10. J. Hamill, "Biomechanics Curriculum: Its Content and Relevance to Movement Sciences," *Quest* 59 (2007): 25–33.

11. B. D. Ulrich and T. G. Reeve, "Studies of Motor Behavior: 75 Years of Research in Motor Development, Learning, and Control," *Research Quarterly for Exercise and Sports* 76, Suppl. 2 (2005): S62–70.

12. H. W. Kohl and T. D. Murray, *Foundations of Physical Activity and Public Health* (Champaign, IL: Human Kinetics, 2012).

13. T. L. McKenzie, "The Preparation of Physical Educators: A Public Health Perspective, *Quest* 59 (2007): 346–357.

14. P. McCullough and G. Wilson, "Psychology of Physical Activity: What Should Students Know?" *Quest* 59 (2007): 42–54.

15. D. L. Gill, "Integration: The Key to Sustaining Kinesiology in Higher Education," *Quest* 59 (2007): 270–286.

16. D. H. Perrin, "Athletic Training: From Physical Education to Allied Health, *Quest* 59 (2007): 111–123

17. S. A. Herring, W. B. Kibler, and M. Putukian, "The Team Physician and Return-to-Play Decision: A Consensus Statement—2012 Update," *Medicine and Science in Sports and Exercise* 44 no. 12: 2446–2448.

18. Active Texas 2020, accessed April 9, 2016, sph.uth.edu/content/uploads/2012/06/Active-Texas-2020-full.pdf.

19. E. Elliott et al., "Experiences in Developing State Physical Activity Plans," in *Implementing Physical Activity Strategies*, ed. R. R. Pate and D. Buchner (Champaign, IL: Human Kinetics Publishers, 2013), Chapter 29.

20. The Community Guide, accessed April 9, 2016, www.thecommunityguide.org/pa/index.html.

21. J. McCubbin, "Adapted Physical Activity: Influential Impacts to Establish a Field of Study," *Kinesiology Reviews* 3 (2014): 53–58.

## Chapter 3

1. W. E. Amonette, K. L. English, and K. J. Ottenbacher, "Nullius in Vebra: A Call for the Introduction of Evidence-Based Practice into the Discipline of Exercise Science," *Sports Medicine* 40, no. 6 (2010): 449–457.

2. D. Knudson, "Evidence-Based Practice in Kinesiology: The Theory to Practice Gap Revisited," *Physical Educator* 62, no. 4 (2005): 212–221.

3. G. H. Guyatt, D. L. Scakett, and D. J. Cook, "Users' Guides to Medical Literature. I. How to Get Started. Evidence-Based Medicine Working Group," *Journal of the American Medical Association* 270, no. 17 (1993): 2093–2095.

4. Amonette et al., 451–452.

5. Ibid.

6. F. S. Sizer and E. Whitney, *Nutrition: Concepts and Controversies*, 12th ed. (Cengage Learning, 2011).

7 S. R. Colberg et al., "Exercise and Type 2 Diabetes: The American College of Sports Medicine and American Diabetes Association, Joint Statement," *Diabetes Care* 33, no. 12 (2010): e147–e167.

8 Colberg et al., e155–e156.

9. J. T. Daniels, *Daniel's Running Formula,* 2nd ed. (Human Kinetics, 2005).

10. T. Grund and V. Senner, "Traction Behavior of Soccer Shoe Stud Designs under Different Game-Relevant Loading Conditions," *Procedia Engineering* 2, no. 2 (June 2010): 2783–2788.

11. J. P. Farthing et al., "Neuro-Physiological Adaptations Associated with Cross-Education of Strength," *Brain Topogr* 20, no. 2 (Winter 2007): 77–88.

12. T. J. Carroll et al., "Contralateral Effects of Unilateral Strength Training: Evidence and Possible Mechanisms," *J Appl Physiol* 101, no. 5 (2006): 1514–1522.

13. C. B. Corbin, "C. H. McCloy Lecture: Fifty Years of Advancements in Fitness and Activity Research," *Research Quarterly for Exercise & Sport* 83, no. 1 (2012): 1–11.

14. C. C. Giza et al., "Summary of Evidence-Based Guidelines Updates: Evaluation and Management of Concussion in Sports: Report of the Guideline Development Subcommittee of the American Academy of Neurology," *Neurology* 80 (2013): 2250–2257.

15. Giza et al., 2250–2257.

## Chapter 4

1. C. J. Caspersen and K. E. Powell, "Physical Activity, Exercise, and Physical Fitness: Definitions and Distinctions for Health-Related Research," *Public Health Rep.* 100, no. 2 (1985): 126–131.

2. M. J. Karvonen, E. Kentala, and O. Mustala, "The Effects of Training on Heart Rate: A Longitudinal Study," *Ann. Med. Exp. Biol. Fenn.* 35 (1957): 307–315.

3. Nike, Inc., "Designed to Move: A Physical Activity Action Agenda," 2012, www.designedtomove.org.

4. H. W. Kohl III, H. D. Cook, and the Institute of Medicine, *Educating the Student Body: Taking Physical Activity and Physical Education to School* (Washington, DC: The National Academies Press, 2013).

5. J. Berryman, "History of 'Six Things Non-Natural:' Exercise Is Medicine from Hippocrates (BC) to Ante-Bellum America (1850's)," *Exercise & Sports Science Reviews* 17 (1989): 515–553.

6. Physical Activity Guidelines Advisory Committee, *Physical Activity Guidelines Advisory Committee Report, 2008* (Washington, DC: U.S. Department of Health and Human Services, 2008).

7. U.S. Department of Health and Human Services, *2008 Physical Activity Guidelines for Americans* (Washington, DC: U.S. Department of Health and Human Services, 2008).

8. *National Physical Activity Plan*, accessed April 20, 2016, www.physicalactivityplan.org.

9. Department of Health and Human Services, *2008 Physical Activity Guidelines for Americans*.

10. R. Bailey et al., "Physical Activity as an Investment in Personal and Social Change: The Human Capital Model," *Journal of Physical Activity and Health* 9 (2012): 1053–1055.

11. Bailey et al., 1055.

12. M. Pratt et al., "Economic Interventions to Promote Physical Activity: Applications of the SLOTH Model," *American Journal of Preventive Medicine* 27, supple 3 (2004): 136–145.

13. H. Selye, "Stress and the General Adaptation Syndrome," *British Medical Journal* 1, no. 4667 (June 17, 1950): 1383–1392.

14. D. K. McQuire et al., "A 30-Year Follow-Up of the Dallas Bedrest and Training Study: I. Effect of Age on the Cardiovascular Response to Exercise," *Circulation* 104, no. 12 (2001): 1380–1387.

15. H. W. Kohl III and T. D. Murray, *Foundations of Physical Activity and Public Health* (Champaign, IL: Human Kinetics, 2012).

16. Bailey et al., 1053–1055.

17. H. W. Kohl III et al., "The Pandemic of Physical Activity: Global Action for Public Health," *Lancet* 380 (2012): 295–305.

18. G. J. Balady et al., "Core Components of Cardiac Rehabilitation/Secondary Prevention Programs: 2007 Update," *Circulation* 115 (2007): 2675–2682.

19. H. W. Kohl III, H. D. Cook, and the Institute of Medicine, *Educating the Student Body: Taking Physical Activity and Physical Education to School* (Washington, DC: The National Academies Press, 2013).

20. J. O. Prochaska, J. C. Norcross, and C. C. DiClemete, *Changing for Good* (New York: William Morrow, 1994).

21. A. E. Price, "Heart Disease and Work," *Heart* 90, no. 9 (2004): 1077–1084.

## Chapter 5

1. K. H. Cooper, *Aerobics* (New York: Bantam Books, 1968).

2. U.S. Department of Health and Human Services, *Physical Activity and Health: A Report of the Surgeon General* (Atlanta, GA: U.S. Department of Health and Human Services, Centers for Disease Control and Prevention, National Center for Chronic Disease Prevention and Health Promotion, 1996).

3. Physical Activity Guidelines Advisory Committee, *Physical Activity Guidelines Advisory Committee Report* (Washington, DC: Department of Health and Human Services, 2008), www.health.gov/paguidelines.

4. M. J. Karvonen, E. Kentala, and O. Mustala, "The Effects of Training on Heart Rate: A Longitudinal Study," *Ann Med Exp Biol Fenn.* 35: 307–315.

5. Physical Activity Guidelines Advisory Committee, *Physical Activity Guidelines Advisory Committee Report.*

6. Ibid.

7. American College of Sports Medicine, *ACSM's Guidelines for Exercise Testing and Prescription,* 9th ed. (Riverwoods, IL: Wolters Kluwer /Lippincott Williams and Wilkins, 2014).

8. Physical Activity Guidelines Advisory Committee, *Physical Activity Guidelines Advisory Committee Report.*

9. H. W. Kohl III, H. D. Cook, and the Institute of Medicine, *Educating the Student Body: Taking Physical Activity and Physical Education to School* (Washington, DC: The National Academic Press, 2013).

10. A. S. Jackson et al., "Role of Lifestyle and Aging on the Longitudinal Change in Cardiorespiratory Fitness," *Arch. Int. Med.* 169, no. 19: 1781–1787.

11. U.S. Department of Health and Human Services, *Physical Activity and Health: A Report of the Surgeon General* (Atlanta, GA: U.S. Department of Health and Human Services, Centers for Disease Control and Prevention, National Center for Chronic Disease Prevention and Health Promotion, 1996).

12. C. J. Caspersen, K. E. Powell, and G. M. Christenson, "Physical Activity, Exercise, and Physical Fitness: Definitions and Distinctions for Health-Related Research," *Public Health Rep* 100 (1985): 126–131.

13. K. R. Barnes et al., "Effects of Resistance Training on Running Economy and Cross-Country Performance," *Med Sci. Sports Exerc.* 45 (2013):12, 2322–2331.

14. S. N. Blair et al., "Physical Fitness and All-Cause Mortality: A Prospective Study of Healthy Men and Women," *JAMA* 262 (1989): 2395–2401.

15. S. N. Blair et al., "Changes in Physical Fitness and All-Cause Mortality: A Prospective Study in Healthy and Unhealthy Men," *JAMA* 273 (1995): 1093–1098.

## Chapter 6

1. S. M. Phillips and R. A. Winett, "Uncomplicated Resistance: Training and Health-Related Outcomes: Evidence for a Public Health Mandate," *Current Sports Medicine Reports* 9, no. 4 (2010): 208–213.

2. Ibid.

3. M. A. Fiatarone et al., "Exercise Training and Nutritional Supplementation for Physical Frailty in Very Elderly People," *New England Journal of Medicine* 330 (1994):1769–1765.

4. N. A. Ratamess et al., "Progression Models in Resistance Training for Healthy Adults, American College of Sports Medicine (ACSM) Position Statement," *Medicine & Science in Sports & Exercise* 41, no. 3(2009): 687–708.

5. N. T. Triplett et al., "Strength and Conditioning Professional Standards and Guidelines," 2014, www.nsca-lift.org.

6. M. Brzycki, "Strength Testing: Predicting a One-Rep Max from Reps-to-Fatigue," *JOPERD* 68 (1993): 88–90.

7. A. D. Faigenbaum et al., "Youth Resistance Training: Updated Position Statement Paper from The National Strength and Conditioning Association," *Journal of Strength and Conditioning Research* 23, no. 5 (2009): S60–S79.

8. V. G. Payne et al., "Resistance Training in Children and Youth: A Meta-Analysis," *Research Quarterly for Exercise and Sports* 68 (1997): 80–88.

9. T. Moritani and H. Devries, "Neural Factors vs. Hypertrophy in the Time Course of Muscle Strength Gain," *American Journal of Physical Medicine* 58 (1979): 115–130.

10. M. W. Thompson and A. H. Mokhtar "Enhanced Performance with Elastic Resistance During the Eccentric Phase of a Countermovement Jump," *Int J Sports Physiol Perform.* 8, no. 2 (2013):181–187, PMID:23428490.

11. M. S. Silbernagel, S. E. Short, and L. C. Ross-Stewart, "Athletes' Use of Exercise Imagery during Weight Training," *J Strength Cond Res* 21, no. 4 (2007): 1077–1081, PMID:18076239.

12. S. Di Stasi, G. D. Myer, and T. E. Hewett, "Neuromuscular Training to Target Deficits Associated with Second Anterior Cruciate Ligament Injury," *J Orthop Sports Phys Ther.* 43, no. 11 (2013): 777–792, A1–A11, doi: 10.2519/jospt.2013.4693, Epub October 11, 2013, PMID: 24175599.

13. B. Lauber et al., "Cross-Limb Interference During Motor Learning," *PLoS One* 8 no. 12 (2013): e81038, doi: 10.1371/journal.pone.0081038.

14. B. Saltin, G. Blomquist, and J. H. Mitchell, "Response to Exercise After Bed Rest and After Training: A Longitudinal Study of Adaptive Changes in Oxygen Transport and Body Composition," *Circulation* 37/38, Suppl. VH (1968): VII-1–VII-78.

15. D. K. McGuire et al., "A 30-Year Follow-Up of the Dallas Bed Rest and Training Study: I. Effects of Age on Cardiovascular Response to Exercise," *Circulation* 104 (2001): 1350–1357.

## Chapter 7

1. R. P. Shook et al., "What Is Causing the Worldwide Rise in Body Weight?" *U.S. Epidemiology* 10, no. 1 (2014): 44–52.

2. U.S. Department of Health and Human Services, *2008 Physical Activity Guidelines for Americans*, www.health.gov/paguidelines

3. Centers for Disease Control and Prevention, Division of Nutrition, *Physical Activity, and Obesity*, accessed July 27, 2015, www.cdc.gov/healthyweight/assessing/bmi/adult_bmi/index.html

4. H. W. Kohl III and T. D. Murray, *Foundations of Physical Activity and Health* (Champaign, IL: Human Kinetics, 2012).

5. C. L. Ogden et al., "Prevalence of Obesity in the United States, 2009–2010," *NCHS Data Brief, no. 82* (Hyattsville, MD: National Center for Health Statistics, 2012).

6. Y. Wang et al., "Will Americans Become Overweight or Obese? Estimating the Progression and Cost of the U.S. Obesity Epidemic," *Obesity* 16 (2008): 2323–2330.

7. J. O. Hill, H. R. Wyatt, and J. C. Peters, "Energy Balance and Obesity," *Circulation*, 126 (2012): 126–132.

8. J. O. Hill, H. R. Wyatt, and J. C. Peters, "The Importance of Energy Balance," *U.S. Endocrinology* 9, no. 1 (2013): 27–31.

9. U.S. Health and Human Services, *Physical Activity Guidelines Advisory Committee Report, 2008*, www.health.gov/paguidleines/report

10. C. A. Slentz et al., "Inactivity, Exercise, and Visceral Fat. STRIDE: A Randomized, Controlled Study of Exercise Intensity and Amount," *Journal of Applied Physiology* 99, no. 4 (2005): 1613–1618.

11. J. A. Harris and F. G. Benedict, "A Biometric Study of Basal Metabolism in Man," *Proceedings of the National Academy of Sciences* 4, no. 12 (1918): 370–373.

12. H. C. Del Porto et al., "Biomechanical Effects of Obesity on Balance," *International Journal of Exercise Science* 5, no. 4 (2012): 301–320.

13. N. K. Janz, V. L. Champion, and V. J. Streche, "The Health Belief Model." In *Health Behavior and Health Education*, edited by K. Glanz, F. M. Lewis, B. K. Rimer (San Francisco: Jossey-Bass, 2002), 45–66.

14. I. Ajzen, "The Theory of Planned Behavior," *Organizational Behavior and Human Decision Processes* 50 (1991): 179–211.

15. A. Bandura, 1986. *Social Foundations of Thought and Action* (Englewood Cliffs, NJ: Prentice Hall, 1986).

16. R. M. Ryan, and E. L. Deci, "Self-Determination Theory and the Facilitation of Intrinsic Motivation, Social Development, and Well-Being," *American Psychology* 55 (2000): 68–78.

17. J. O. Prochaska and C. C. DiClemente, "Stages and Processes of Self-Change of Smoking: Toward an Integrative Model of Change," *Journal of Consulting Clinical Psychology* 51 (1983): 390–395.

18. S. V. Gill and M. K. Walsh, "Use of Motor Learning Principles to Improve Motor Adaptation in Adult Obesity," *Health* 4, no. 12A (2012): 1428–1433, doi: dx.doi.org/10.4236/health.2012.412A206.

## Chapter 8

1. D. M. McNair, M. Lorr, and L. F. Droppleman, *Profile of Mood States Manual* (San Diego, CA: Educational and Industrial Service, 1971).

2. W. P. Morgan and M. L. Pollock, "Psychological Characterization of the Elite Distance Runner," *Annals of the New York Academy of Science* 301 (1977): 382–403.

3. B. J. Cardinal, "Physical Activity Psychology Research: Where Have We Been? Where Are We Going?" *Kinesiology Reviews* 3 (2014): 42–52.

4. World Health Organization Constitution, International Health Conference, New York, 1946, accessed August 6, 2015, www.who.int/about/en/index.html

5. World Health Organization, accessed August 6, 2015, www.who.int/features/facilities/mental_health/en/.

6. World Health Organization, accessed August 6, 2015, www.who.int/topics/mental_health/en/.

7. H. W. Kohl III and T. D. Murray, *Foundations of Physical Activity and Public Health* (Champaign, IL: Human Kinetics, 2012).

8. American Psychiatric Association, *Diagnostic and Statistical Manual of Mental Disorders*, 5th ed. (Arlington, VA: Author, 2013).

9. Physical Activity Guidelines Advisory Committee, *Physical Activity Guidelines Committee Report, 2008* (Washington, DC: U.S. Department of Health and Human Services, 2008).

10. Physical Activity Guidelines Advisory Committee, *Physical Activity Guidelines Committee Report, 2008*.

11. American Psychiatric Association, *Diagnostic and Statistical Manual of Mental Disorders*, 5th ed.

12. U.S. National Institute of Mental Health, accessed August 6, 2015, www.numh.nih.gov/.

13. Physical Activity Guidelines Advisory Committee, *Physical Activity Guidelines Committee Report, 2008*.

14. U.S. Department of Health and Human Services, National Guideline Clearinghouse, *Adult Primary Care Depression Guidelines 2006*, accessed August 6, 2015, www.guideline.gov/summary.aspx?doc_id=6007.

15. Physical Activity Guidelines Advisory Committee, *Physical Activity Guidelines Committee Report, 2008*.

16. Centers for Disease Control and Prevention, *Sleep and Sleep Disorders*, accessed August 6, 2016, www.cdc.gov/sleep/index.htm.

17. G. Corbari, "Goal Setting and Record Keeping," presentation at the Texas High School Coaches Association Annual Meeting, Ft. Worth, TX, 2009.

18. The Community Guide, *Physical Activity: Stand Alone Mass Media Campaigns* (Atlanta, GA: Centers for Disease Control and Prevention, 2010), accessed August 9, 2015, www.thecommunityguide.org.

19. P. Ekkekakis et al., "The Pleasure and Displeasure People Feel When They Exercise at Different Intensities," *Sports Medicine* 41, no. 8 (2011): 641–671.

20. Centers for Disease Control and Prevention, "Insufficient Sleep Is a Public Health Epidemic," accessed August 9, 2015, www.cdc.gov/sleep/.

21. Physical Activity Guidelines Advisory Committee, *Physical Activity Guidelines Committee Report, 2008* (Washington, DC: U.S. Department of Health and Human Services, 2008).

22. M. Barrera, "Distinctions between Social Support Concepts, Measures, and Models," *American Journal of Community Psychology* 14 (1986): 413–445.

23. Morgan and Pollock, pp. 382–403.

24. W. P. Morgan, "Negative Addiction in Runners," The Physician and Sports *Medicine* 7, no. 2 (1979): 56–63; 67–69.

25. Physical Activity Guidelines Advisory Committee. *Physical Activity Guidelines Committee Report, 2008.*

26. See www.healthypeople.gov/2020 /topicsobjectives2020/nationaldata. aspx?topicId=33.

27. J. Daniels, *Daniels' Running Formula*, 3rd ed. (Champaign, IL: Human Kinetics, 2013).

28. Kohl and Murray.

## Chapter 9

1. K. R. McLeroy et al., "An Ecological Perspective on Health Promotion Programs," *Health Educ Behav* 15 (1988): 351.

2. D. H. Chenoweth, *Worksite Health Promotion*, 2nd ed. (Champaign, IL: Human Kinetics, 2007).

3. N. P. Pronk, "Physical Activity Promotion in Business and Industry: Exercise, Context, and Recommendations for a National Plan," *Journal of Physical Activity and Health* 6, Suppl. 2 (2009): S220–S235.

4. S. Marshall and D. Gyi, "Evidence of Health Risks from Occupational Sitting: Where Do We Stand?" *Am J Prev Med.* 39, no. 4 (2010): 389–391.

5. Pronk, 2009.

6. K. Proper and W. van Mechelen, "Effectiveness and Economic Impact of Worksite Interventions to Promote Physical Activity and Healthy Diet," World Health Organization, 2012 accessed May 19, 2016, www.who.int.

7. Pronk, 2009

8. Pronk, 2009.

9. Chenoweth, 2007.

10. Chenoweth, 2007.

11. L. Linnan, M. Bowling, and P. Royall, "Results of the 2004 National Worksite Health Promotion Survey," *American Journal of Public Health* 98, no. 8 (2008): 1503–1509.

12. Centers for Disease Control and Prevention, *Steps to Wellness: A Guide to Implementing the 2008 Physical Activity Guidelines for Americans in the Workplace* (Atlanta: U.S. Department of Health and Human Services, 2012), www.cdc .gov/nccdphp/dnpao.

13. Worksite Health Promotion, www .thecommunityguide.org/worksite/index.html.

14. Centers for Disease Control and Prevention, "Workplace Health Model," updated October 23, 2013, www.cdc.gov/workplacehealthpromotion /model/index.html.

15. Pronk, 2009.

16. Grossmeier et al., "2010 Best Practices in Evaluating Worksite Health Promotion Programs," *The Art of Health Promotion* (Jan/Feb 2010).

17. S. B. Thacker and R. L. Berkelman, "Public Health Surveillance in the United States," *Epidemiology Review*s 10 (1988): 164–190.

18. U.S. Army Over 40 Cardiovascular Screening Program, "Chapter 14: Army Physical Fitness Test," accessed September 9, 2015, www.apft-standards.com/files/14ch.pdf.

19. N. Pronk et al., "Reducing Occupational Sitting Time and Improving Worker Health: The Take-a-Stand Project, 2011," *Preventing Chronic Disease* 9 (2012): 110323, www.cdc .gov/pcd/issues/2012/11_0323.htm.

20. Pronk et al., 2012.

21. C. Fowler, "Addressing the Work Performance of Individuals with Mild Stroke," *Work and Industry Special Interest Section Quarterly* 27, no. 1 (2013): 1–4.

22. Fowler, 2013.

23. D. Roberts, "Fit to Drive: Integrated Injury Prevention, Health, and Wellness for Truck Drivers," in *Implementing Physical Activity Strategies*, ed. D. Roberts, R. R. Pate, and D. M. Bucher (Champaign, IL: Human Kinetics, 2013), Chapter 23.

24. Roberts, 2013.

## Chapter 10

1. A. J. Mowen and B. L. Baker, "Park, Recreation, Fitness, and Sport Sector Recommendations for a More Physically Active America: A White Paper for the United States Physical Activity Plan, *Journal of Physical Activity and Health* 6, Suppl 2 (2009): S236–S244.

2. Mowen and Baker, 2009.

3. W. R. Thompson, "Worldwide Survey of Fitness Trends for 2016," *ACSM's Fitness Journal* 19, no. 6 (2015): 8–17.

4. Physical Activity Guidelines Advisory Committee, *Physical Activity Guidelines Advisory Committee Report, 2008* (Washington, DC: U.S. Department of Health and Human Services, 2008), www.health.gov /paguidelines.

5. Bureau of Labor Statistics, *American Time Use Survey* (Washington, DC: U.S. Department of Labor, 2013).

6. Centers for Disease Control and Prevention, *Behavioral Risk Factor Surveillance System* (Washington, DC: U.S. Department of Health and Human Services, 2011), www .cdc.gov/brfss/.

7. Centers for Disease Control and Prevention, *National Health and Nutrition Examination Survey* (Washington, DC: U.S. Department of Health and Human Services, 2011), https://www.cdc.gov/nchs/nhanes /index.htm.

8. Moore et al., "Trends in No Leisure-Time Physical Activity—United States, 1988–2010," *Research Quarterly for Exercise and Sport* 83, no. 4 (2012): 587–591.

9. Centers for Disease Control and Prevention *National Health Interview Survey* (Washington, DC: U.S. Department of Health and Human Services, March 11, 2011), www.cdc.gov /nchs/data/nhis/earlyrelease/201103_07.pdf

10. Centers for Disease Control and Prevention, *Youth Risk Factor Surveillance System* (Washington, DC: U.S. Department of Health and Human Services, 2013), www .cdc.gov/brfss.

11. CDC, YRBSS, 2013.

12. C. A. Schoenborn, S. Carlson, J. Fulton, and F. Loustalot, *Monitoring Leisure-Time Physical Activity among U.S. Adults* (Washington, DC: Division of Health Statistics, CDC, 2010), www.cdc.gov/nchs/ppt/nchs2010/06 _schoenborn.pdf.

13. R. C. Brownson and T. K. Boehmer, "Declining Rates of Physical Activity in the United States: What Are the Contributors?" *Annual Review of Public Health* 26 (2005): 421–443.

14. C. A. Schoenborn and P. E. Adams, "Health Behaviors of Adults: United States, 2005–2007," *Vital Health Stat Mar* 245 (2010): 1–132.

15. Moore et al., 2012; CDC, *National Health Interview Survey*; Brownson and Boehmer, 2005.

16. A. R. Hurd and D. M. Anderson, *The Park and Recreational Professional's Handbook* (Champaign, IL: Human Kinetics, 2011).

17. A. Mowen, A. Kaczynski, and D. Cohen, "The Potential of Parks and Recreation in Addressing Physical Activity and Fitness," *President's Council on Physical Fitness and Sports Research Digest* 9 (March 2008): 1.

18. Mowen et al., 2008.

19. G. Godbey and A. Mowen, "The Benefits of Physical Activity Provided by Park and Recreation Services: The Scientific Evidence," *National Parks and Recreation Research Series* (2010), www.NRPA.org.

20. Godbey and Mowen, 2010.

21. R. J. Brustad, "The Role of the Family in Promoting Physical Activity," *President's Council on Physical Fitness and Sports Research Digest*, 10 (March 2010): 3.

22. Mowen et al., 2008.

23. H. A. Starnes et al., "Trails and Physical Activity: A Review," *Journal of Physical Activity and Health* 8 (2011): 1160–1174.

24. Starnes et al., 2011.

25. Starnes et al., 2011.

26. Godbey and Mowen 2010.

27. Godbey and Mowen, 2010.

28. Bureau of Labor Statistics, U.S. Department of Labor, *Occupational Outlook Handbook, 2016–2017, Fitness Trainers and Instructors.*

29. J. D. Massengale, *Trends Toward the Future in Physical Education* (Champaign, IL: Human Kinetics, 1987).

30. W. R. Thompson, "Worldwide Survey of Fitness Trends for 2016," 10th Anniversary Edition, *ACSM's Health and Fitness Journal* 19, no. 6 (2016): 9–18.

31. H. W. Kohl III and T. D. Murray, *Foundations of Physical Activity and Public Health* (Champaign, IL: Human Kinetics, 2012).

32. D. Bassett et al., "Policies to Increase Youth Physical Activity in School and Community Settings," *Research Digest* 14, no. 1 (March 2013).

33. Kohl and Murray, 2012.

## Chapter 11

1. P. C. Hallal et al., for the Lancet Physical Activity Series Working Group, "Global Physical Activity Levels: Surveillance Progress, Pitfalls, and Prospects," *The Lancet* 380, no. 9838 (2012): 247–257.

2. H. W. Kohl III, H. D. Cook, and the Institute of Medicine, *Educating the Student Body: Taking Physical Activity and Physical Education to School* (Washington, DC: The National Academies Press, 2013).

3. Ibid.

4. National Association for Sport and Physical Education & American Heart Association, *Shape of the Nation Report: Status of Physical Education in the USA* (Reston, VA: American Alliance for Health, Physical Education, Recreation, and Dance, 2012).

5. A. Weston, *The Making of American Physical Education* (New York, NY: Appleton-Century-Crofts, 1962).

6. National Association for Sport and Physical Education, *National Physical Education Standards* (Reston, VA: American Alliance for Health, Physical Education, Recreation, and Dance, 2012).

7. M. T. Mahar et al., "Effects of a Classroom-Based Program on Physical Activity and On-Task Behavior," *Medicine and Science in Sports and Exercise* 38, no. 12 (2006): 2086–2094.

8. J. E. Donnelly et al., "Physical Activity Across the Curriculum (PAAC): A Randomized Controlled Trial to Promote Physical Activity and Diminish Overweight and Obesity in Elementary School Children," *Preventive Medicine* 49, no. 4 (2009): 336–341.

9. N. D. Ridgers et al., "Day-to-Day and Seasonal Variability of Physical Activity During Recess," *Preventive Medicine* 42, no. 5 (2006): 372–374.

10. R. Woods, *Social Issues in Sport*, 3rd ed. (Champaign, IL: Human Kinetics, 2011).

11. S. Kretchmar, *Understanding and the Delights of Human Activity: Examining a Teaching Games for Understanding Model* (Champaign, IL: Human Kinetics, 2004).

12. Centers for Disease Control and Prevention/ (CDC)/National Center for Health Statistics, National Survey of Children's Health, 2007 Accessed at: https://www.cdc.gov/nchs/slaits/nsch.htm on 04/05/17.

13. Centers for Disease Control and Prevention, *Trends in the Prevalence of Physical Activity; YRBS 1991–2009* (Washington, DC: Author, 2012).

14. Ibid.

15. N. Colabianchi, L. Johnston, and P. M. O'Malley, *Sports Participation in Secondary Schools: Resources Available and Inequalities in Participation – A BTG Research Brief* (Ann Arbor, Bridging the Gap Program, Survey Research Center, Institute for Social Research, University of Michigan, 2012).

16. U.S. Government Accountability Office, "Students with Disabilities: More Information and Guidance Could Improve Opportunities in Physical Education and Athletics" (2010), www.gao.gov/products /GAO-10-519

17. S. A. Ham, S. Martin, and H. W. Kohl III, "Changes in the Percentage of Students Who Walk or Bike to School – United States, 1969 and 2001," *J Phys Act Health* 5 (2008): 205–215.

18. Ibid.

19. D. R. Bassett et al., "Walking, Cycling, and Obesity Rates in Europe, North America, and Australia," *J Phys Act Health* 5 (2008): 795–814.

20. H. W. Kohl III, H. D. Cook, and the Institute of Medicine.

21. M. G. Boarnet et al., "Evaluation of the California Safe Routes to School Legislation: Urban Form Changes and Children's Active Transportation to School," *American Journal of Preventive Medicine* 28, no. 2, Suppl. 2 (2005): 134–140.

22. D. C. A. Collins and R. A. Kearns, "The Safe Journeys of an Enterprising School: Negotiating Landscapes of Opportunity and Risk," *Health and Place* 7, no. 4 (2001): 293–306.

23. L. Turner, J. Chriqui, and F. Chaloupka, "Walking School Bus Programs in U.S. Public Elementary Schools," *Journal of Physical Activity & Health* (2012).

24. Ibid.

25. H. W. Kohl III, H. D. Cook, and the Institute of Medicine.

26. J. Eldridge et al., "Comparison of Academic and Behavioral Performance between Athletes and Non-athletes," *International Journal of Exercise Science,* 7, no. 1 (2014): 3–13.

27. R. Jago, et al., "Modifying Middle School Physical Education: Piloting Strategies to Increase Physical Activity," *Pediatric Exercise Science* 21 (2009): 171–185.

28. Ibid.

29. J. Daniels et al., "Differences and Changes in VO2 among Young Runners 10 to 18 Years of Age, *Medicine and Science in Sports* 10 (1978): 200–203.

30. R. M. Malina, "Fitness and Performance: Adult Health and the Culture of Youth," in *New Possibilities, New Paradigms?*, ed. R. J. Park and H. M. Eckert (Champaign, IL: Human Kinetics), 30–38.

31. J. McNamee et al., "High Activity Skills Progression: A Method for the Madness," *JOPHERD* 78, no. 7 (2007): 17–21.

## Chapter 12

1. B. Van der Smissen, "Sport Management: Its Potential and Some Developmental Concerns," in J. D. Massengale (Ed.), *Trends Toward the Future in Physical Education* (Champaign, IL: Human Kinetics, 1987), Chapter 8.

2. Ibid.

3. Ibid.

4. Ibid.

5. Physical Activity Council, "The 2016 Physical Activity Council Participation Report," accessed March 1, 2017, www .physicalactivitycouncil.com.

6. J. Cote and W. Gilbert, "An Integrated Definition of Coaching Effectiveness and Expertise," *International Journal of Sports Science and Coaching* 4, no. 3 (2013) 307–323.

7. R. R. Pate, B. McClenaghan, and R. Rotella (Eds.), *Scientific Foundations of Coaching* (New York, NY: Saunders College Publishing, 1984).

8. Ibid.

9. National Collegiate Athletic Association, "Probability of Competing in Sports Beyond High School," accessed December 7, 2015, www.ncaa.org.

10. E. B. Power and T. D. Murray, *101 Healthy Lifestyle Tips for Coaches* (Monterey, CA: Coaches Choice Publisher, 2013).

11. National Association for Sport and Physical Education, *Quality Coaches, Quality Sports: National Standards for Sport Coaches,* 2nd ed. (Reston, VA: Author, 2006).

12. Physical Activity Guidelines Advisory Committee, *Physical Activity Guidelines Advisory Committee Report, 2008* (Washington, DC: U.S. Department of Health and Human Services, 2008).

13. Ibid.

14. M. A. Mittleman et al., "Triggering of Acute Myocardial Infarction by Heavy Physical Exertion: Protection Against Triggering by Regular Exertion: Determinants of Myocardial Infarction Onset Study Investigators," *New England Journal of Medicine* 329 (1993):1677–1683.

15. S. N. Blair, H. W. Kohl, and N. N. Goodyear, "Rates and Risks for Running and Exercise Injuries: Studies in Three Populations," *Research Quarterly for Exercise and Sport* 58, no. 3 (1987): 221–228.

16. Ibid.

17. B. H. Jones et al., "Epidemiology of Injuries Associated with Physical Training among Young Men in the Army," *Medicine and Science in Sports and Exercise* 25 (1993): 197–203.

18. Ibid.

19. CDC, "Injury Prevention and Control: Traumatic Brain Injury and Concussion," 2014, www.cdc.gov/traumaticbraininjury /get_the_facts.html.

20. P. McCrory et al., "Consensus Statement on Concussion in Sport—the 4th International Conference on Concussion in Sport held in Zurich, November 2008," *British Journal of Sports Medicine* 47 (2012): 250–258.

21. M. Marar, N. M. McIlvain, S. K. Fields, et al., "Epidemiology of Concussions among United States High School Athletes in 20

Sports," *The American Journal of Sports Medicine*, 40: 747–755, 2012.

22. T. D. Murray, M. Sardo, and G. Keeton, *101 Cheerleading Facts, Tips, and Drills* (Monterey, CA: Coaches Choice Publishers, 2007).

23. G. Keeton et al., *101 Tips and Activities for Dance/Drill Team Directors* (Monterey, CA: Coaches Choice Publishers, 2012).

24. J. D. MacDougall and H. A. Wenger, *Physiological Testing of the High-Performance Athlete*, 2nd ed. (Champaign, IL: Human Kinetics Publishers, 1991).

25. W. E. Prentice, *Principles of Athletic Training: A Competency Based Approach*, 15th ed. (New York, NY: McGraw-Hill, 2014).

26. Ibid.

27. National Research Council et al., *Sports-Related Concussions in Youth: Improving the Science, Changing the Culture* (Washington, DC: National Academies Press, 2014).

28. A. Ripley, "The Case against High School Sports," *The Atlantic* (October 2013).

29. L. Mooney, "Five Key Trends That Are Driving the Business of Sports," Stanford Graduate School of Business (2014), www.gsb.stanford.edu/news/headlines/five-key-trends-are-driving-business-sports.

30. Masters in Sport Management, "30 Unique Career Paths with a Sports Management Degree" (2011), accessed December 10, 2015, www.mastersinsportsmanagement.org/2011/30-unique-career-paths-with-a-sports-management-degree/.

## Chapter 13

1. Centers for Disease Control and Prevention. Guide for Community Preventive Services. https://www.thecommunityguide.org/findings/physical-activity-built-environment-approaches. Accessed 18 July 2017.

2. S. A. Ham, S. Martin, and H. W. Kohl III, "Changes in the Percentage of Students Who Walk or Bike to School—United States, 1969 and 2001," *J Phys Act Health* 5 (2008): 205–215.

3. A. Goodman, "Walking, Cycling and Driving to Work in the English and Welsh 2011 Census: Trends, Socio-economic Patterning and Relevance to Travel Behaviour in General," *PLoS ONE* 8, no. 8 (2013): e71790.

4. L. M. Besser and A. L. Dannenberg, "Walking to Public Transit: Steps to Help Meet Physical Activity Recommendations," *American Journal of Preventive Medicine* 29, no. 4 (2005): 273–280.

5. K. K. Davison, J. L. Werder, and C. T. Lawson, "Children's Active Commuting to School: Current Knowledge and Future Directions," *Preventing Chronic Disease* 5, no. 3 (2008): A100.

6. B. Giles-Corti et al., "Increasing Walking: How Important Is Distance to, Attractiveness, and Size of Public Open Space?," *American Journal of Preventive Medicine* 28, no. 2S2 (2005): 169–176.

7. G. Beirao and J. A. Sarsfield Cabral, "Understanding Attitudes Towards Public Transport and Private Car: A Qualitative Study," *Transportation Policy* 14, no. 6 (2007): 478–489.

8. L. Østergaard et al., "Cross Sectional Analysis of the Association between Mode of School Transportation and Physical Fitness in Children and Adolescents," *International Journal Behavioral Nutrition Physical Activity* 10, no. 91 (2014).

9. F. G. O'Connor et al., "Functional Movement Screening: Predicting Injuries in Officer Candidates," *Medicine and Science in Sports and Exercise* 43, no. 12 (2011): 2224–2230.

10. G. Cook, L. Burton, and B. Hoogenboom, "Pre-Participation Screening: The Use of Fundamental Movements as an Assessment of Function – Part 1," *North American Journal of Sports Physical Therapy* 1, no. 2 (2006): 62–72.

11. Ibid.

12. E. Hansson et al., "Relationship Between Commuting and Health Outcomes in a Cross-Sectional Population Survey in Southern Sweden," *BioMed Central Public Health* 11, no. 834 (2011): 1–14.

13. D. Merom et al., "Predictors of Initiating and Maintaining Active Commuting to Work Using Transport and Public Health Perspectives in Australia," *Preventive Medicine* 47 (2008): 342–346.

14. S. A. Eckel, "Good Excuse to Stay Home from the Gym, Fashion and Style," *The New York Times* (March 24, 2010).

15. J. Smith, "How to Build the Perfect Home Gym" (December 22, 2015), www.shape.com.

## Chapter 14

1. G. S. Fain, "Ethics in Health, Physical Education, Recreation, and Dance," *Eric Digest* (1992).

2. E. F. Zeigler, "Application of a Scientific Ethics Approach to Sport Decisions," *Quest* 32, no. 1 (1980): 8–21.

3. Ibid.

4. J. H. Conn and D. A. Gerdes, "Ethical Decision-Making: Issues and Applications to American Sport," *Physical Educator* 55, no. 3 (1998): 121–126.

5. R. S. Kretchmar, "Philosophy of Ethics," *Quest* 45 (1993): 3–12.

6. E. J. Shea, *Ethical Decisions in Physical Education and Sport* (Springfield, IL: Charles C. Thomas, 1978), 228.

7. Conn and Gerdes, 121–126.

8. W. Kroll, "Ethical Issues in Human Research," *Quest* 45 (1993): 32–44.

9. L. L. Bain, "Ethical Issues in Teaching," *Quest* 45 (1993): 69–77.

10. Office of History, NIH, "Selected Research Advances of NIH," accessed June 7, 2016, https://history.nih.gov/about/timelines_research_advances.html.

11. International Center for Academic Integrity, "Statistics," www.academicintegrity.org/icai/integrity-3.php.

12. E. Howe, "Ethical Considerations When Making Exceptions to 'Rules' in Psychiatry," *Innovations in Clinical Neuroscience* 11, no. 32 (2014).

13. Kretchmar, 3–12.

14. R. Martens, "Business, Ethics, and the Physical Activity Field," *Quest* 45 (1993): 120–132.

15. American College of Sports Medicine, *ACSM's Guidelines for Exercise Testing and Prescription*, 9th ed. (Baltimore, MD: Wolters Kluwer/Lippincott Williams & Wilkins, 2014).

16. Ibid.

17. J. F. Sallis and T. L. McKenzie, "Physical Education's Role in Public Health," *Research Quarterly for Exercise and Sport* 62 (1991): 124–137.

18. H. W. Kohl and H. D. Cook (Eds.), *Institute of Medicine Report: Educating the Student Body* (Washington, DC: National Academies Press, 2013).

## Chapter 15

1. O. J. Odetunde, "Influence of Transformational and Transactional Leaderships, and Leaders' Sex on Organisational Conflict Management Behaviour," *Gender & Behaviour* 11, no. 1 (June 2013).

2. Y. Inandi, B. Tunc, and F. Gilic, "School Administrator's Leadership Styles and Resistance to Change," *International Journal of Academic Research* 5, no. 5 (September 2013).

3. D. D. Warrick, "Leadership Styles and Their Consequence," *Journal of Experiential Learning and Simulation* 3–4 (1981): 155–172.

4. D. Goleman, "Leadership That Gets Results" *Harvard Business Review* (March–April 2000): 82–83.

5. M. Watts and S. Corrie, "Growing the 'I' and the 'We' in Transformational Leadership: The Lead, Learn & Grow Model," *The Coaching Psychologist* 9, no. 2 (December 2013).

6. Warrick, 155–172.

7. Goleman, 82–83.

8. K. Badgett and W. Kritsonis, "Badgett-Kritsonis Supervision Leadership Model (BK-SLM)," *International Journal of Organizational Behavior in Education* 2, no. 1 (2014).

9. Ibid.

10. R. J. Sternberg, "Perspectives: Leadership Styles for Academic Administrators: What Works When?," *Change* 45, issue 5 (2013): 24–27.

11. T. Shilton, "Creating and Making the Case: Global Advocacy for Physical Activity," *Journal of Physical Activity and Health* 5 (2008):765–776.

12. R. McMurray et al. (Writing Group on Behalf of HEALTHY Study Group), "Rationale, Design and Methods of the HEALTHY Study Physical Education Intervention Component," *International Journal of Obesity* 33 (2009): S37–S43.

## Chapter 16

1. M. Van Oort, "The Use of Additional Revenue Streams to Expand Case-Mix in Outpatient Physical Therapy Management," Master's Thesis, Texas State University, 2011, accessed January 11, 2016, https://digital .library.txstate.edu/bitstream/handle /10877/2414/VAN-OORT-THESIS. pdf?sequence=1.

2. J. D. Massengale (Ed.), *Trends Toward the Future in Physical Education* (Champaign, IL: Human Kinetics, 1986).

3. J. M. Dunn, "Honoring the Past—Embracing the Future," *Quest* 53, no. 4 (2001): 495–506.

4. P. Freedson (Ed.), "The Academy Papers: Back to the Future: Reflecting on the Past and Envisioning the Future for Kinesiology Research," *Kinesiology Review* 3, no. 1 (2014):1–106.

5. Lawson, H. The American Kinesiology Association and the Future of Kinesiology — American Kinesiology Association White Papers, accessed January 11, 2016, www .americankinesiology.org/white-papers /white-papers/.

6. G. Bergeron et al., Council of University Physical Education and Kinesiology Administrators Position Statement: The Role of Kinesiologist and the Promotion of Physical Activity and Exercise in the Canadian Health Care System, 2014, www.ccupeka.ca/en /images/Position_Statement_-_Role_of _Kin_in_Health.pdf.

7. American Kinesiology Association White Papers, accessed January 11, 2016, www .americankinesiology.org/white-papers /white-papers/.

8. G. H. Guyatt, D. L. Scakett, and D. J. Cook, "Users' Guides to Medical Literature. I. How to Get Started. Evidence-Based Medicine Working Group," *Journal of the American Medical Association* 270, no. 17 (1993): 2093–2095.

9. Physical Activity Guidelines Advisory Committee, *Physical Activity Guidelines Advisory Committee Report, 2008* (Washington, DC: U.S. Department of Human Services, 2008), accessed January 11, 2016, health.gov /paguidelines/report/pdf/CommitteeReport .pdf

10. F. Booth, "Is Health One Future for Kinesiology?," *Kinesiology Review* 3 (2014): 13–18.

11. P. Hallal et al., "Global Physical Activity Levels: Surveillance Progress, Pitfalls, and Prospects," *The Lancet* 380, no. 9838 (2012): 247–257.

12. H. W. Kohl III et al., "The Pandemic of Physical Inactivity: Global Action for Public Health," *The Lancet* 380, no. 9838 (2012): 294–305.

13. I. M. Lee et al., "Effect of Physical Inactivity on Major Non-Communicable Disease Worldwide: An Analysis of Burden of Disease and Life Expectancy," *The Lancet* 380, no. 9838 (2012): 219–229.

14. G. Del Vecchio, "A Final Lesson for Grads: Learn 22 Keys to Career Success," *The Huffington Post*, April 29, 2014, accessed January 11, 2016, www.huffingtonpost .com/gene-del-vecchio/a-final-lesson-for -grads-_b_5233343.html.

15. Ibid.

## Glossary

1. J. Cote and W. Gilbert, "An Integrated Definition of Coaching Effectiveness and Expertise," *International Journal of Sports Science and Coaching* 4, no, 3 (2013): 307–323.

2. R. Woods, *Social Issues in Sports*, 3rd ed. (Champaign, IL: Human Kinetics, 2011).

3. World Health Organization, Preamble to the Constitution of WHO as adopted by the International Health Conference, New York, 19 June–22 July 1946; signed on 22 July 1946 by the representatives of 61 States (Official Records of WHO, no. 2, p. 100) and entered into force on 7 April 1948.

4. N. P. Pronk, "Physical Activity Promotion in Business and Industry: exercise, Context, and Recommendations for a National Plan," *Journal of Physical Activity and Health* 6, Suppl 2 (2009): S220–S235.

5. H. A. Lawson, "Renewing the Core Curriculum," *Quest* 59, no. 2 (2007): 219–243.

6. R. Woods, *Social Issues in Sports*, 3rd ed. (Champaign, IL: Human Kinetics, 2011).

# Photo Credits

**Chapter 1**
**Opener Images:** © TunedIn by Westend61/Shutterstock.com; © ARCHITECTE/Shutterstock.com; © Bikeriderlondon/Shutterstock.com; © DayOwl/Shutterstock.com.
**Lesson 1 Case Study Images:** © Sean Locke Photography/Shutterstock.com; © Tracy Whiteside/Shutterstock.com; © Rob Marmion/Shutterstock.com; © bikeriderlondon/Shutterstock.com.

**Chapter 2**
**Opener Images:** © Cyrus McCrimmon/Denver Post/Getty Images; © BSIP/Getty Images; © DGLimages/Getty Images; © kali9/E+/Getty Images.
**Lesson 1 Case Study Images:** © Sean Locke Photography/Shutterstock.com; © Tyler Olson/Shutterstock.com; © Rob Marmion/Shutterstock.com.
**Lesson 2 Case Study Images:** © docstockmedia/Shutterstock.com; © Africa Studio/Shutterstock.com; © lightwavemedia/Shutterstock.com.

**Chapter 3**
**Opener Images:** © Puwadol Jaturawutthichai/Shutterstock.com; © Yellow Dog Productions/Iconica/Getty Images; © Hero Images/Getty Images.
**Lesson 1 Case Study Images:** © Rob Marmion/Shutterstock.com; © Umpaporn/Shutterstock.com; © Dariush M/Shutterstock.com.
**Lesson 2 Case Study Images:** © Keith Bell/Shutterstock.com; © Monkey Business Images/Shutterstock.com; © Andrey_Popov/Shutterstock.com.

**Chapter 4**
**Opener Images:** © bikeriderlondon/Shutterstock.com; © kali9/E+/Getty Images; © Hero Images/Getty Images; © Buena Vista Images/DigitalVision/Getty Images.
**Lesson 1 Case Study Images:** © pixelheadphoto digitalskillet/Shutterstock.com; © Tewan Banditrukkanka/Shutterstock.com; © GagliardiImages/Shutterstock.com.
**Lesson 2 Case Study Images:** © digitalskillet/Shutterstock.com; © Thinglass/Shutterstock.com; © Pavel L Photo and Video/Shutterstock.com; © funnyangel/Shutterstock.com.

**Chapter 5**
**Opener Images:** © Monkey Business Images/Shutterstock.com; © Jaren Jai Wicklund/Shutterstock.com; © lightpoet/Shutterstock.com; © Monkey Business Images/Shutterstock.com.
**Lesson 1 Case Study Images:** © goodluz/Shutterstock.com; © CroMary/Shutterstock.com; © Tom Wang/Shutterstock.com.
**Lesson 2 Case Study Images:** © Kzenon/Shutterstock.com; © sportpoint/Shutterstock.com; © Dean Drobot/Shutterstock.com.

**Chapter 6**
**Opener Images:** © belushi/Shutterstock.com; © Ververidis Vasilis/Shutterstock.com; © Nestor Rizhniak/Shutterstock.com.
**Lesson 1 Case Study Images:** © Ruslan Shugushev/Shutterstock.com; © Iakov Filimonov/Shutterstock.com; © Sean Locke Photography/Shutterstock.com.
**Lesson 2 Case Study Images:** © digitalskillet/Shutterstock.com; © Ruslan Shugushev/Shutterstock.com; © kwanchai.c/Shutterstock.com.

**Chapter 7**
**Opener Images:** © kali9/iStock/Getty Images; © Maxisport/Shutterstock.com; © wavebreakmedia/Shutterstock.com.
**Lesson 1 Case Study Images:** © Ruslan Shugushev/Shutterstock.com; © Mat Hayward/Shutterstock.com; © Zerbor/Shutterstock.com.
**Lesson 2 Case Study Images:** © wavebreakmedia/Shutterstock.com; © wavebreakmedia/Shutterstock.com; © oliveromg/Shutterstock.com; © Light And Dark Studio/Shutterstock.com.

## Chapter 8

**Opener Images:** © REUTERS/Alamy Stock Photo; © dotshock/Shutterstock.com; © LatinContent/STR/LatinContent WO/Getty Images.

**Lesson 1 Case Study Images:** © Shawn Pecor/Shutterstock.com; © DonLand/Shutterstock.com; © littleny/Shutterstock.com; © antoniodiaz/Shutterstock.com.

**Lesson 2 Case Study Images:** © Joseph Sohm/Shutterstock.com; © holbox/Shutterstock.com; © Air Images/Shutterstock.com; © Mark Herreid/Shutterstock.com.

## Chapter 9

**Opener Images:** © istock.com/xavierarnau; © Tyler Olson/Shutterstock.com; © Rawpixel.com/Shutterstock.com; © Monkey Business Images/Shutterstock.com.

**Lesson 1 Case Study Images:** © Monkey Business Images/shutterstock.com; © Ghislain & Marie David de Lossy/Getty Images; © Ruslan Kudrin/Shutterstock.com; © Sean Locke Photography/shutterstock.com.

**Lesson 2 Case Study Images:** © Monkey Business Images/Shutterstock.com; © michaeljung/Shutterstock.com; © one photo/shutterstock.com.

## Chapter 10

**Opener Images:** © Dreaming Poet/Shutterstock.com; © Alextype/Shutterstock.com; © dotshock/Shutterstock.com.

**Lesson 1 Case Study Images:** © Bikeriderlondon/Shutterstock.com; © sirtravelalot/Shutterstock.com; © Spotmatik Ltd/Shutterstock.com; © maxpro/Shutterstock.com; © Giuseppe Elio Cammarata/Shutterstock.com.

**Lesson 2 Case Study Images:** © ImageFlow/Shutterstock.com; © Visionsi/Shutterstock.com; © Colin Underhill / Alamy Stock Photo.

## Chapter 11

**Opener Images:** © Robert Kneschke/Shutterstock.com; © Dasha Rosato/Shutterstock.com; © Pat Canova/Alamy Stock photo.

**Lesson 1 Case Study Images:** © wizdata/Shutterstock.com; © Monkey Business Images/Shutterstock.com; © Southern Stock/Stockbyte/Getty Images; © Monkey Business Images/Shutterstock.com.

**Lesson 2 Case Study Images:** © kentoh/Shutterstock.com; © Lisa F. Young/Shutterstock.com; © Sergey Novikov/Shutterstock.com; © Sergey Novikov/Shutterstock.com.

## Chapter 12

**Opener Images:** © Christian Bertrand/Shutterstock.com; © Blend Images/Alamy Stock Photo; © Otto Greule Jr/Getty Images.

**Lesson 1 Case Study Images:** © View Apart/Shutterstock.com; © Yellow Dog Productions/Iconica/Getty Images; © Shawn Pecor/Shutterstock.com.

**Lesson 2 Case Study Images:** © Rawpixel.com/Shutterstock.com; © Rawpixel.com/Shutterstock.com; © View Apart/Shutterstock.com.

## Chapter 13

**Opener Images:** © Artens/Shutterstock.com; © LarsZ/Shutterstock.com; © stockphoto mania/Shutterstock.com.

**Lesson 1 Case Study Images:** © Marjorie Kamys Cotera/Bob Daemmrich Photography/Alamy Stock Photo; © CAN BALCIOGLU/Shutterstock.com; © Roman Tiraspolsky/Shutterstock.com; © Sean Locke Photography/Shutterstock.com.

**Lesson 2 Case Study Images:** © Burlingham/Shutterstock.com; © Dragon Images/Shutterstock.com; © goofyfoottaka/Shutterstock.com.

## Chapter 14

**Opener Images:** © Randy Miramontez/Shutterstock.com; © REUTERS/Alamy Stock Photo; © Trish Tokar/Getty Images.

**Lesson 1 Case Study Images:** © dpa picture alliance archive/Alamy Stock Photo; © 279photo Studio/Shutterstock.com; © Hero Images Inc./Alamy Stock Photo; © Pressmaster/Shutterstock.com.

**Lesson 2 Case Study Images:** © Rawpixel.com/Shutterstock.com; © DGLimages/Shutterstock.com.

## Chapter 15

**Opener Images:** Courtesy of NASA; © Anton_Ivanov/Shutterstock.com; © Tony Tomsic/Getty Images Sport/Getty Images; © ZUMA Press Inc./Alamy Stock Photo.

**Lesson 1 Case Study Images:** © Monkey Business Images/Shutterstock.com; © Andrii Zhezhera/Shutterstock.com; © Monkey Business Images/Shutterstock.com.

**Lesson 2 Case Study Images:** © Monkey Business Images/Shutterstock.com; © Monkey Business Images/Shutterstock.com; © Dj7/Shutterstock.com.

## Chapter 16

**Opener Images:** © goodluz/Shutterstock.com; © garagestock/Shutterstock.com; © g-stockstudio/Shutterstock.com.

**Lesson 1 Case Study Images:** © FatCamera/E+/Getty Images; © Rafal Olechowski/Shutterstock.com; © Africa Studio/Shutterstock.com.

# Index

Body composition (*Continued*)
    standards for evaluating body composition of
        adults, 160T
    subcutaneous fat, as type of, 151
    typical body composition of an adult man and
        woman, 150F
    visceral fat, as type of, 151
    waist circumference, and disease risk, 157T
    waist circumference values for European
        American children and adolescents, 157F
Body Mass Index (BMI)
    and body composition, 153
    calculation of, 145
    for children, 143F
    for females ages 14–18, 156F
    in evaluation of evidence, 62
    and health, 167
    *vs*. mortality rate, 151F
    and obesity, 162
    of overweight children, 161–162
    weight classifications using BMI, 62T

C
Caloric intake and expenditure
    adult gradual weight gain due to caloric
        imbalance (intake vs. expenditure), 148F
    caloric balance equation, 144T
    caloric balance, role in, 144
    caloric expenditure of children and
        adolescents, 238T
    caloric imbalance and weight, 148F
    caloric imbalance in weight gain, 148
    caloric intake and caloric strategies for weight
        management, 153T
    calories expended per hour for common home
        maintenance activities, 298T
    caloric strategies for weight management, 153R
    differences between self-reported and actual
        daily caloric intake in obese individuals
        attempting to lose weight, 150F
    and moderate-intensity physical activity,
        vigorous-intensity physical activity, 143
    and obesity, 144
    in weight loss, 149
Canadian Council of University Physical Education
    and Kinesiology Administrators, 344–346
Cardiac rehabilitation
    in exercise science, 32
    after heart attack, 72
    in kinesiology, 87
    leadership for maximum efficiency of, 336
    mental health, role of, 191
    and physical activity continuum, 91
    returning to work after heart attack, 91–92
Cardiovascular disease
    and graded exercise testing (GXT), 213
    in kinesiology, 104
    and physical inactivity, 104
    screening of for health promotion in
        workplace, 211
Careers in kinesiology; *see also* Kinesiology
    practitioners
    and continuing education/lifelong learning,
        350–351
    examples of 91; *see also* Kinesiology practitioners
        and individual subdiscipines
    financial modeling and projections for post-offer
        employment testing (POET), 343F
    future predictions for, 341–355
    integrated vision of careers and fields of study in
        kinesiology, 346F
    key concepts for success, 341–355
    strategies for, 351–353

Career preparation
    for careers in kinesiology, 37–38
    for coaching, 273–274
    for physical therapists, 39
    sources for, 40
    for sports management, 273–274, 277–278
Children and adolescents; *see also* Physical activity
    in school settings
    changes in physical activity needs with
        increasing age of children and adolescents,
        259F
    health of, 48, 143
    motor skills of, 259
    obesity of, 118, 145
Classroom-based activity breaks, 248
Clinical exercise physiology, 91
Coaching
    adverse events in, 277–282
    behavioral guidelines for youth sport and
        coaching, 277T
    and creating positive environment, 284
    coachability in, 275T
    and concussions, 35
    ethics of, 308–309
    exercise physiology in, 285
    and goal setting, record keeping, 179
    inappropriate behavior in, 308
    incompetence in, 266–267
    and mental health of athletes, 173
    and mental state of runners, 186
    motivation in, 180
    national standards for sports coaching, 276T
    and performance-enhancing drugs,
        308–309
    physiological testing programs in, 285
    professional training in, 17
    safety guidelines for, 283–284
    strategies for providing an autonomy-supportive
        coaching environment, 277T
College admissions
    for physical therapy programs, 38–39, 342
Concussions
    in coaching, 35
    concussion modifiers, 282T
    in kinesiology, 66
    in public heath, 286
    in sports, 281–282
Cooper Institute, 113
Curriculum vitae development, 350

D
Dallas Bed Rest Study, 137F
Diabetes
    logic model for the HEALTHY Middle School
        Diabetes Intervention and Prevention
        Study, 166F
    resistance training in treatment for, 46
Disabilities
    mental health disorders, role in, 184–1855
    physical activity of individuals with physical
        disabilities, 185T
    prevention of with physical activity, 24
    of understudied populations, 185
Disease prevention and control
    epidemiology, role of, 14
    physical activity, role in, 9
    stages of disease prevention and how they relate
        to high blood pressure, 8F
Disease prevention types
    primary prevention, 8
    primordial prevention, 8
    secondary prevention, 8
    tertiary prevention, 8

Dose
    definition of, 78
    physical activity and exercise dose response
        curves that influence health outcomes, 78F

E
Economy
    definition of, 24
Energy balance
    achievement of, 147, 153–154
    in achieving peak performance, 152
    chart of, 144F
    definition of, 143
    energy expenditure for three different levels of
        physical activity, 147F
    energy requirements for individuals at varying
        amounts of exercise, 147T
    illustration of the hypothesis that energy
        balance may be easier to achieve at high
        energy expenditure, which represents the
        regulated zone, 149F
    and kinesiology practitioners, use by, 145
    measurement of energy expenditure at rest
        (RMR), 154–155
    model of energy balance that includes a
        focus on factors related to physical activity
        expenditure, 148F
    in physical activity, 147F
    physiologic responses to participation in
        physical activities affecting energy
        balance, 152
    physical activity energy expenditure (PAEE),
        definition of, 146
    resting metabolic rate (RMR), definition of, 146
    in sport/exercise psychology, 164
    thermic effect of food (TEF), definition of, 146
    total energy expenditure (TEE), composition
        of, 146F
    and weight loss, 143
Environmental health
    description of, 14
Epidemiology
    definition of, 15
Ethics
    academic/professional honesty and integrity, as
        type of, 313
    conflict of interest in, 313
    in coaching, 308–309
    deontological ethics, definition of, 311
    disclaimers, role of, 314
    disclosure in, 313
    ethical decision making, arguments for, 314–316
    ethical decision-making scenarios, 314
    in evidence-based decision making, 310
    in kinesiology, 310
    in sports medicine, 311T
    situational ethics, definition of, 312
    teleological ethics, definition of, 312
Evidence-based practice
    in athletic training, 65
    in biomechanics, 63
    Body Mass Index, application of, 62
    ethics in, 310
    evaluation of, 51, 63
    examples of, 56, 60
    in exercise physiology, 61
    in human behavior studies, 60
    history, philosophy, and sociology, integration
        of, 64
    in kinesiology, 47
    and incorporation of evidence, 57, 60
    vs. isolated facts, 48
    and motor learning, 63